BASIC MEDICAL HISTOLOGY

Basic

The Biology of Cells, Tissues, and Organs

New York   Oxford

Medical Histology

RICHARD G. KESSEL

OXFORD UNIVERSITY PRESS   1998

Oxford University Press

Oxford   New York
Athens   Auckland   Bangkok   Bogota
Bombay   Buenos Aires   Calcutta   Cape Town
Dar es Salaam   Delhi   Florence   Hong Kong   Istanbul
Karachi   Kuala Lumpur   Madras   Madrid
Melbourne   Mexico City   Nairobi   Paris
Singapore   Taipei   Tokyo   Toronto   Warsaw

and associated companies in
Berlin   Ibadan

Published by Oxford University Press, Inc.
198 Madison Avenue, New York, New York 10016

Oxford is a registered trademark of Oxford University Press

Library of Congress Cataloging-in-Publication Data
Kessel, Richard G., 1931-
Basic medical histology: the biology of cells, tissues, and organs/
by Richard G. Kessel.
p. cm.
Includes bibliographical references and index.
ISBN 0-19-509528-6
1. Histology.   I. Title.
QM551.K47   1998   611'.0189—dc21   97-6576

9 8 7 6 5 4 3 2 1

Printed in the United States of America
on acid free paper

Acknowledgments

This book is the culmination of teaching histology (cell, tissue, and organ biology) at the University of Iowa for nearly 35 years. Histology is a basic and diverse course that complements information presented in anatomy, physiology, cell biology, biochemistry, endocrinology, and immunology courses. The course content has changed markedly over the decades, and this has contributed greatly to the excitement in both teaching and learning this subject matter. However, the explosion of new information and the time constraints on teaching have challenged us to make critical judgments about the selection of course content. Thus, it is necessary to package information as efficiently as possible to facilitate maximum learning and retention. The extensive summary tables and line drawings inserted throughout this text, as well as the many transmission and scanning electron micrographs should facilitate learning by the students who read this book. The use of selected color plates in the book is intended to serve this purpose further. I welcome suggestions from students, professors, and other readers who may want to provide suggestions for improving the book.

It is a pleasure to acknowledge the skilled work of John Birkbeck, who made most of the line drawings that appear in the book. A number of colleagues have made useful contributions by reading parts or all of the chapters for accuracy and have provided suggestions for shortening the book and improving its overall organization. Their suggestions have all been extremely useful. Special thanks are extended to Dr. Nina Zanetti, Biology Department, Siena College, for her remarkably thorough review of the entire manuscript and for her numerous very helpful suggestions for improving and shortening the text and illustrations. Her contributions were invaluable. I also extend my sincere thanks and appreciation to Dr. Amy Aulthouse, Department of Anatomy, University of Oklahoma Health Science Center; Dr. Douglas Paulsen, Department of Anatomy, Morehouse School of Medicine; Dr. Daniel Neufeld, Department of Anatomy, University of South Dakota School of Medicine; Dr. Robert Ogilivie, Department of Cell Biology and Anatomy, Medical University of South Carolina; and Dr. Gene Spaziani, Department of Biological Sciences, The University of Iowa. The contributions of these individuals are all greatly appreciated. I would also like to acknowledge with appreciation two students, Doug Squire and Randy Lovstuen, who read selected portions of the book and provided useful input.

I am indebted to Jenny Ritchie and Marge Zalesky of the Department of Biological Sciences, The University of Iowa, for their conscientious and tireless efforts to process the manuscript and make the extensive revisions necessary to reduce its length to an acceptable level. Thank you for your contributions.

Finally, I convey my appreciation to individuals at Oxford University Press for their work to make this book a reality: Kirk Jensen, Nancy Wolitzer, and Donna Miller.

Iowa City, Iowa   R. G. K.
October 1996

Contents

Techniques for the Study of Cells, Tissues, and Organs

Historically, studies of cells, tissues, and organs have relied on a variety of microscopes and related procedures. The first compound microscope was constructed by Hans and Zacharias Janssen in 1590 in Holland. Antioni Van Leeuwenhoek is credited with using a magnifying glass and a specimen holder as early as 1673 to observe microorganisms in pond water at a magnification of about 275×. The microscope has been an important tool for those who have worked to improve our understanding of cells and their internal organization.

BRIGHT-FIELD MICROSCOPE (BFM)

The most widely used microscope has been the BFM because it is inexpensive, relatively movable, and capable of providing a great deal of information about cell, tissue, and organ structure. Living cells and small portions of tissues or organs can be studied with the BFM, but the information generated is limited by a number of factors, including specimen size, resolution, magnification, and contrast. The BFM consists of three ground glass lenses (a condenser, an objective, and an ocular or projector lens), a stage on which the specimen is placed, and coarse and fine focus controls for focusing the image, as well as controls for adjusting the size of the lens aperture and for centering the lenses and light source (Fig. 1.1). Parallel rays of light, usually from an electric bulb, are focused on the specimen by the condenser lens. The light then passes through the specimen, if it is sufficiently thin, where the light is modified. This modified beam of light then enters the objective lens system, where an image is formed in the focal plane of the objective lens. The ocular or eyepiece then magnifies the image formed by the objective lens and presents it to the eye.

Magnification is the ratio of image size to object size. The upper effective limit of magnification is 1000 to 1200 diameters. The approximate magnification and field diameter for a representative BFM are given in the accompanying table. As the magnification increases, the field diameter decreases, as does the ability to judge overall shapes of larger objects. The resolution of the BFM is about 0.25 μm (250 nm). Objects cannot be resolved or distinguished as separate if they lie closer than approximately one-half the wavelength of the illumination being used. Therefore, *resolution* refers to the ability to distinguish objects located close together.

Eyepiece	Objective	Magnification	Field Diameter
10×	10× (low power)	100×	1500 μm
10×	40× (high dry)	400×	375 μm
10×	100× (oil immersion)	1000×	150 μm

The units of measure presently used in cell biology and histology are listed in the accompanying table.

Unit of Measure	Symbol	Value
Micrometer (formerly called *micron*)	μm	0.001 mm or 10^{-6} m or 10^{-4} cm or 10^{-3} nm
Nanometer (formerly called *millimicron*)	nm	0.001 μm (1/1000 μm): 10^{-9} m or 10^{-7} cm

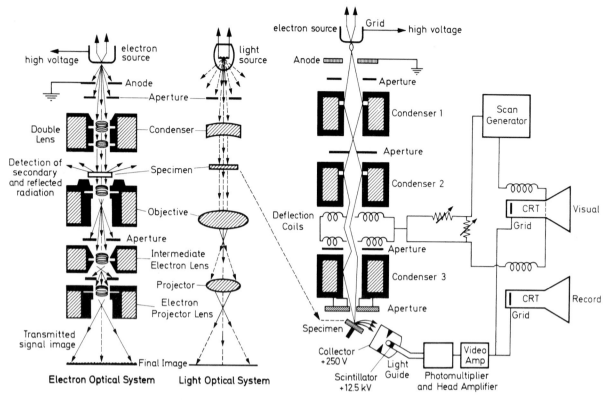

Figure 1.1. Figures illustrate the basic organization of a TEM (left), LM or BFM (middle), and SEM (right). (From

P.E. Mee. Microscopy and its contribution to computer technology. *Microstructures*, Oct./Nov. 1972, with permission)

HISTOLOGIC TECHNIQUES FOR LIGHT MICROSCOPY (LM)

While cells in culture and individual cells such as protozoa or spermatozoa can be observed in the living organism by either bright field or phase contrast microscopy, many specimens (e.g., kidney, liver) are too large or thick to be studied in such a manner. Therefore, it is necessary to preserve these tissues and to prepare sections (~5–10 μm) that can be stained before observation. The preservation of tissues or organs is called *fixation*, and many different combinations of chemicals were used in the past to preserve or immobilize different macromolecules in the cell. Many proteins (nucleoproteins, lipoproteins, glycoproteins) are retained in cells after fixation because proteins are denatured and new cross-linkages are formed, making the proteins insoluble. Small molecules such as sugars, amino acids, and electrolytes are easily washed out of tissues during processing. Triglycerides and lipids are usually dissolved from tissue sections if solvents such as acetone, chloroform, and xylol are used. Glycogen is soluble in water but insoluble in alcohol, so this feature must be recognized if it is desirable to retain glycogen in tissue sections. Many enzymes are inacti-

vated by fixation. The staining of tissues with contrasting colors brings out additional structural details when such sections are examined with the BFM. The steps for preparing stained slides will now be briefly outlined.

FIXATION

The primary objective of fixation is to preserve cells with minimal alteration; thus the fixative should rapidly penetrate the tissue block so as to cross-link and immobilize the molecules present. The fixative should also harden the tissue for sectioning and increase its affinity for staining. Many fixatives have been used for light microscopy, including *Champy's* (*potassium bichromate, chromic acid,* and *osmium tetroxide*), 10% neutral buffered formalin, *Bouin's* (*picric acid, formalin, glacial acetic acid*), and *Carnoy's* (*acetic acid, alcohol, chloroform*), among others. A fixative regimen currently in use for LM is one developed for electron microscopy and involves a primary fixation with buffered paraformaldehyde/glutaraldehyde followed by secondary exposure to buffered osmium tetroxide. Both paraformaldehyde and glutaraldehyde are good cross-linkers of proteins, while osmium tetroxide immobilizes lipids.

DEHYDRATION

Following fixation, all water must be removed from the tissue prior to encasement in a paraffin block. The water is removed by passing the tissue specimen through graded ascending concentrations of ethanol (or acetone) to absolute (100%) ethanol (Fig. 1.2).

CLEARING

Since alcohol and paraffin do not mix, it is necessary to use a transition fluid (clearing agent) that will mix with both alcohol and paraffin. During clearing, the tissue samples are passed through several changes to remove all traces of alcohol.

INFILTRATION

In order for melted paraffin to permeate throughout the tissue block, the block is transferred from the clearing agent into several changes of melted paraffin (52°–60°C) over a period of several hours.

EMBEDDING

The tissue block is then placed in a small container of fresh, melted paraffin and removed from the warming oven (Fig. 1.2). The paraffin will solidify, encasing the tissue block.

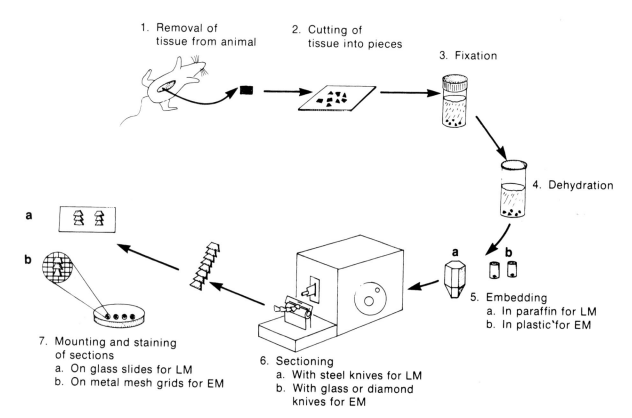

Figure 1.2. Major steps in the preparation of sections for study in the LM and transmission electron microscope (EM); major differences are in the embedding and sectioning procedures. During dehydration, water is removed by passing tissue blocks through graded, ascending concentrations of ethanol (or acetone) to absolute (100%) ethanol. For clearing, samples are passed through several changes of xylol to remove alcohol and provide a chemical (xylol) that is miscible with paraffin. During infiltration and embedding, the tissue blocks are transferred through several changes of melted paraffin (52°C to 60°C) over a period of several hours. The tissue and melthed paraffin are removed from the oven, and the paraffin solidifies. The paraffin and tissue can then be trimmed and section cut (usually 5–10 μm thick) with a steel blade or razor blade using a microtome. The paraffin sections are transferred to a glass microscope slide, dried, and are ready for staining. (From C.J. Flickinger, *Medical Cell Biology*, W.B. Saunders Co., Philadelphia, 1979, with permission)

SECTIONING

When the paraffin solidifies, the paraffin block containing the tissue is trimmed and sections are cut with a microtome (Fig. 1.2). The knife used can be a steel blade or a razor blade, and the sections obtained are typically 5–10 μm thick.

MOUNTING

The tissue sections are fixed to a glass slide and stained. Staining requires several steps. The slides with the tissue sections are deparaffinized using xylol. These sections must be gradually hydrated by being passed through different descending concentrations of ethanol and finally into distilled water. Most stains are prepared as aqueous solutions.

STAINING AND SLIDE MOUNTING

The hydrated sections can then be stained with one of a large number of possible stains. Once the tissue section is stained, a permanent slide is made. In this process, the section is once again dehydrated by passing the stained slide through ascending series of ethanols to absolute ethanol. The slide is then placed in xylene (a transition fluid for alcohol and mounting medium). When it is removed, a mounting medium (Permount, Balsam) that will harden is placed over the sections and a coverglass applied. After drying, the slide can be viewed with the LM.

STAINING TECHNIQUES FOR LM

Unfortunately, methods for staining cells while maintaining cell viability are severely limited. *Vital* stains that do not kill living cells usually exist as colloidal particles rather than as true solutions; examples include *trypan blue*, *India ink*, and *thorotrast*. *Supravital stains* eventually kill cells exposed to them but not immediately. These stains obviously have limited usefulness. In the past, *Janus green B* was useful for staining mitochondria in cells. *Neutral red* has been used for staining lysosomes in cells. *Procein yellow* can be injected into nerve cells to delineate their axons and dendrites.

Staining sections for LM is an extremely broad and diverse field. Stains can be distinguished by whether their coloring radicals are positively or negatively charged. If the color is due to the acid radical (which in ionic form is negatively charged), then the stain is referred to as an *anionic stain* or *acid stain*. If, however, the coloring is due to the basic radical of the stain (which in ionic form is positively charged), then the stain is called a *cationic stain* or *basic stain*. In fact, basic and acid stains are neutral salts but have either an acid

or a basic radical. Basophilic substances in cells are negatively charged and therefore have an affinity for basic stains. Acidophilic substances are positively charged and have an affinity for acid stains. *Hematoxylin* is both a basic stain and a cationic stain; similarly, *eosin* is both an acid stain and an anionic stain. Other basic dyes include *basic fuchsin*, *toluidine blue*, and *methylene blue*. Among the structures in cells displaying a relative basophilia are chromatin, nucleoli, and rough-surfaced endoplasmic reticulum because they contain nucleic acids which are rich in PO_4^{3-} groups. Examples of other *acid dyes* include *orange G*, *phloxine*, *aniline blue*, and *light green*.

Histologic slides are commonly stained both with hematoxylin (blue) a nuclear stain, and eosin (red); the latter is a cytoplasmic stain. Two triple stains are commonly used for histologic staining, and in each, three stains are employed to provide three different colors to the components in the section. *Mallory's* triple stain contains acid fuchsin, aniline blue, and orange G. *Masson's* triple stain contains iron hematoxylin, acid fuchsin, and light green.

HISTOCHEMISTRY/CYTOCHEMISTRY

The use of chemistry on cell, tissue, and organ sections to precisely localize specific macromolecules is useful because morphologic relationships can be maintained, a situation that is impossible in many procedures used in biochemistry and molecular biology. Cytochemical analysis can be carried out on fixed tissue and on frozen or freeze-dried sections. It is necessary for a cytochemical test to be based on a specific chemical identifying reaction that produces an insoluble, colored product. For the reaction product to be visible in the LM, it must be colored. Specificity of the reaction must also be determined by the use of appropriate controls. In addition, it is important to prevent nonspecific binding, and the sensitivity must be established. For enzyme cytochemistry, the enzyme may not be directly localized, but rather the reaction product that indicates the catalytic activity of the enzyme. More precise localization of the reaction product, often to cisternae of specific membranous organelles, can be achieved by applying histochemistry to the transmission electron microscope.

FEULGEN REACTION

The Feulgen reaction is one of the oldest cytochemical reactions and is used for demonstrating DNA in cells. The procedure is described in Figure 1.3.

PERIODIC ACID–SCHIFF (PAS)

The PAS technique for the localization of carbohydrates or polysaccharides is described in Figure 1.4. While this

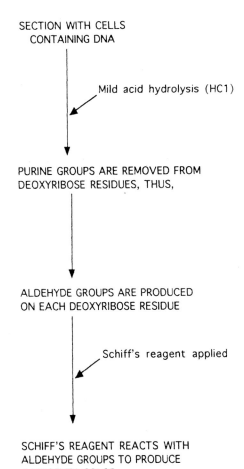

Figure 1.3. Steps involved in Feulgen cytochemical reaction.

procedure identifies glycoproteins and glycogen, it is usually possible to distinguish between these substances. For example, if some of the sections are treated with saliva (amylase), the glycogen is digested and removed from the section. Comparison of untreated and treated sections can, therefore, identify the glycogen.

PHOSPHATASES

Phosphatases are enzymes that split the phosphate group from specific substrates. Phosphatases thus hydrolyze the ester linkages of natural organic phosphates (examples are adenosine triphosphate, glucose-6-phosphate, and glycerophosphate) and release the phosphate ions, which can be trapped by the lead in a lead salt. Lead phosphate is insoluble and precipitates, thus appearing opaque in the transmission electron microscope (Figs. 1.6, 1.7). Calcium ions can be used to form an insoluble reaction product visible in the LM. The procedure for demonstrating acid phosphatase, an enzyme commonly found in lysosomes, is illustrated in Figure 1.5

TRANSMISSION ELECTRON MICROSCOPE (TEM)

The first TEM was built by Ruska and colleagues in 1931, and the first commercial TEM was built by Siemens in 1939. Porter, Claude, and Fullam used an electron microscope in 1945 to view whole cells grown in tissue culture after exposure to osmium tetroxide. By 1948, Pease and Baker were able to obtain thin sections of biologic material that were about 0.1 to 0.2 μm thick. In the early 1950s, Palade, Porter, Sjostrand, and Blum made improvements in fixation and thin sectioning of biologic

Figure 1.4. Steps in the histochemical demonstration of carbohydrates by the PAS reaction.

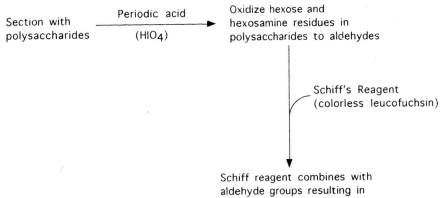

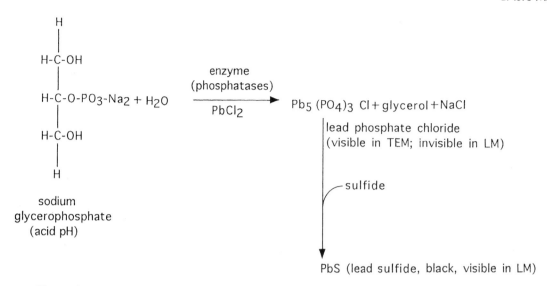

$$
\begin{array}{c}
H \\
| \\
H\text{-}C\text{-}OH \\
| \\
H\text{-}C\text{-}O\text{-}PO_3\text{-}Na_2 + H_2O \\
| \\
H\text{-}C\text{-}OH \\
| \\
H
\end{array}
\quad
\xrightarrow[\text{PbCl}_2]{\substack{\text{enzyme}\\ \text{(phosphatases)}}}
\quad
Pb_5(PO_4)_3\ Cl + glycerol + NaCl
$$

sodium
glycerophosphate
(acid pH)

lead phosphate chloride
(visible in TEM; invisible in LM)

sulfide

PbS (lead sulfide, black, visible in LM)

Figure 1.5. Steps in the localization of acid phosphatase.

materials. Initially, osmium tetroxide fixation and embedding in methacrylate (*n*-butyl and methyl methacrylate mixtures) were employed. Methacrylate polymerization, however, caused polymerization damage (shrinkage) and created substantial amounts of heat. Glauert and colleagues first used the epoxy resin Araldite for embedding in 1956, and Luft introduced Epon 812 resin embedding in 1961.

INSTRUMENT, THEORY, OPERATION

Electrons are used as the illuminating source because they have a very short wavelength. The TEM is some-

what similar to an inverted LM, with the electrons derived by electrically heating a V-shaped tungsten filament called a *cathode* (Fig. 1.1). The electrons are accelerated toward an anode by a potential difference that is variable (usually 50,000–100,000 volts). The electrons pass through an opening in the anode and are focused by a *condenser electromagnetic lens* onto an extremely thin specimen. The electrons that pass through the sample are focused by the *objective electromagnetic lens* to produce an *image* that is further *enlarged* by the *intermediate* electromagnetic lens. The *projector* electromagnetic *lens projects* the image onto a *fluorescent* screen, where the image can be viewed with a binocular microscope just outside of the specimen viewing area. Immediately below the fluorescent screen is a camera or photographic

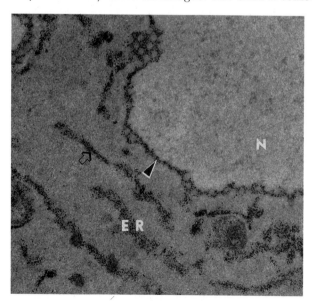

Figure 1.6. Ultrastructural localization of acid phosphatase reaction product in perinuclear cisterna (arrowhead) and ER (arrow). ×23,600.

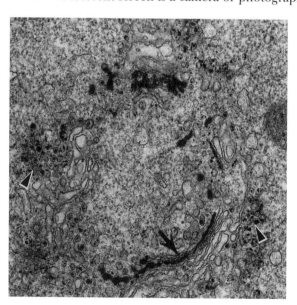

Figure 1.7. Ultrastructural localization of reaction product for inosine 5'-diphosphatase (IDPase) in Golgi saccules (arrow) and Golgi vesicles (arrowheads). ×32,400.

film plates for recording images. The image, once photographed, can be enlarged further if required. Electrons cannot be visualized by the human eye; therefore the fluorescent screen is required to produce an image. The resolution of the TEM for most biologic samples is approximately 0.10 nm.

SPECIMEN PREPARATIONS FOR TEM

Because of the utility of using dialdehydes for cross-linking proteins and osmium tetroxide for reacting with fatty acids, tissues are now routinely subjected to a dual fixation schedule. The primary fixative consists of *buffered glutaraldehyde* (*3%, phosphate* or *cacodylate buffer*) or a combination of *paraformaldehyde* (*2–3%*) and *glutaraldehyde* (*1–3%*), using either phosphate or cacodylate as buffers. After primary fixation in the cold for several hours followed by several buffer rinses, the tissues are postfixed in ice-cold 1% osmium tetroxide, using similar buffer and pH, for 2–4 hours. The tissues are then rinsed with buffer, dehydrated through an ascending series of cold ethanols, and then passed through three or four changes of absolute ethanol at room temperature. The tissues are then treated with propylene oxide (a transition fluid between ethanol and epoxy resins) and infiltrated in a mixture of propylene oxide and resin before being placed in fresh resin mixture in small capsules. The capsules are placed in an oven (~60°C) for 1–3 days so that the resin hardens.

The tissue blocks are trimmed and placed in a chuck of an ultramicrotome for sectioning with either glass or diamond knives. The sections, usually 50–100 nm thick, come off in ribbons onto a fluid in a knife trough. The sections are then picked up onto a circular grid that contains many openings but still supports the delicate sections (Fig. 1.2). Sometimes a thin membrane (e.g., formvar) is placed on the grid for additional support. After drying, the sections are stained, usually in *aqueous uranyl acetate*, washed, and stained again in lead salts (such as *lead citrate*). After drying, the grid containing the ribbon of sections is placed in the specimen holder and inserted into a TEM to be studied and photographed.

EXPERIMENTAL PROCEDURES FOR TEM

Negative staining

Negative staining is particularly useful for illustrating details of small, isolated structures such as bacteriophage, fibers, mitochondria, and ribosomes and for monitoring the composition of various cell fractions that are obtained by cell fractionation and differential centrifugation. The isolated sample of cell constituents is placed on a formvar-coated grid, then negatively stained with salts of phosphotungstate or molybdate, examined, and photographed.

Cytochemistry

This technique involves reacting a cell or tissue slice in appropriate biochemical solutions to localize a specific macromolecule or enzyme or its reaction product in sections (Figs. 1.6, 1.7).

Autoradiography

This technique is used for visualizing a newly synthesized cell product after the cells are exposed to radioactive precursor molecules for varying lengths of time either under in vitro or in vivo conditions (Figs. 1.8, 1.9).

Freeze fracture (etch)

This technique involves splitting membranes down the lipid bilayer; a thin platinum-carbon replica of the new membrane faces is made and examined (Fig. 1.10). Fresh tissue or tissue briefly prefixed is transferred through glycerol, which serves as a cryoprotectant and prevents ice crystal damage. The samples are frozen in freon that is, in turn, cooled by liquid nitrogen. After freezing, the specimens are quickly transferred to the evacuated chamber of a freeze etch machine that is also cooled with liquid nitrogen. The specimens are then fractured with a cold knife. This tends to split the cells such that the fracture plane passes through the lipid bilayers, but the fracture jumps from one membrane to another. The fractured specimen is then coated with a thin layer of platinum at an angle to give a shadowed effect that brings out fine surface features. Etching, if desired, is accomplished by "warming" the specimen to sublimate the ice (etch) for a short distance into the specimen. This reveals membrane surfaces in addition to the membrane faces exposed by the fracture. A thin layer of carbon is evaporated onto the specimens from another electrode in the specimen chamber to complete the replica and to provide stability. Following this procedure, the specimens with overlying replicas are removed to room temperature, and the replicas are floated off the adhering tissue in spot depression plates. The replicas are then placed on a grid for TEM observation, study, and photography (Fig. 1.11).

Immunogold labeling

Specific proteins in cells can be localized by immunogold labeling. An antibody is labeled with colloidal gold particles of different sizes. After the antibody-gold is reacted with a cell or tissue, interaction of the antibody-gold complex with the antigen occurs. The complex can be viewed in either the TEM or the BFM (Figs. 1.12, 1.13). Colloidal gold is useful for immunoelectron microscopy because it appears as electron-dense particles. The colloidal gold can be prepared with different diameters (e.g., 10 or 20 nm), and double labeling can be performed.

Figure 1.8. Diagrams show major steps in preparation of an autoradiograph for LM or TEM. After exposure to isotope, specimen is fixed, dehydrated, infiltrated, and embedded in paraffin (for LM) or epoxy resins (for TEM). Sections are placed on slides (LM) or grids (TEM) and coated with liquid photographic emulsion in the darkroom, covering the specimen with a monolayer of silver bromide particles. After exposure, the slides are developed similarly to a photograph in the darkroom. Thus, a silver halide crystal that has been struck by a beta particle from the isotope is converted into metallic silver, which can be seen in the LM or TEM.

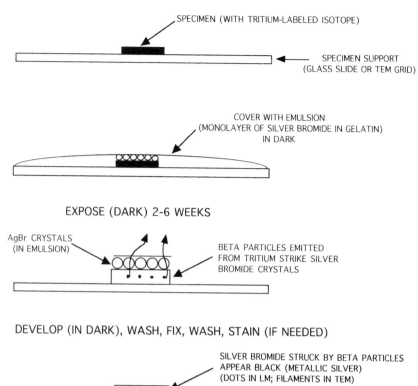

SPECIMEN (WITH TRITIUM-LABELED ISOTOPE)

SPECIMEN SUPPORT
(GLASS SLIDE OR TEM GRID)

COVER WITH EMULSION
(MONOLAYER OF SILVER BROMIDE IN GELATIN)
IN DARK

EXPOSE (DARK) 2-6 WEEKS

AgBr CRYSTALS
(IN EMULSION)

BETA PARTICLES EMITTED
FROM TRITIUM STRIKE SILVER
BROMIDE CRYSTALS

DEVELOP (IN DARK), WASH, FIX, WASH, STAIN (IF NEEDED)

SILVER BROMIDE STRUCK BY BETA PARTICLES
APPEAR BLACK (METALLIC SILVER)
(DOTS IN LM; FILAMENTS IN TEM)

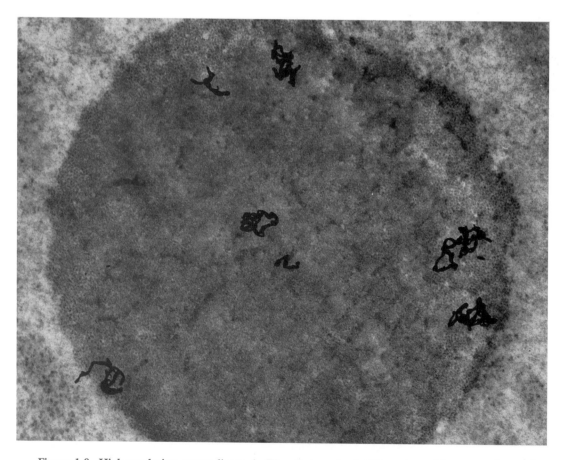

Figure 1.9. High-resolution autoradiograph. The silver grains indicate sites of incorporation of ^{3}H-uridine into the nucleolus. ×32,800.

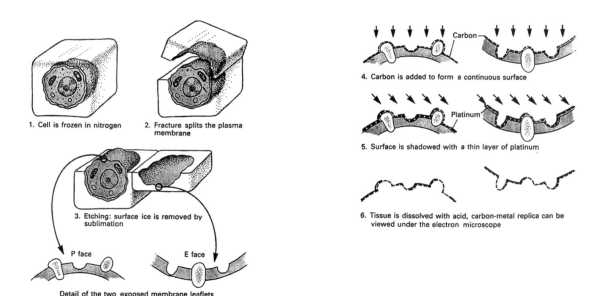

1. Cell is frozen in nitrogen

2. Fracture splits the plasma membrane

3. Etching: surface ice is removed by sublimation

P face

E face

Detail of the two exposed membrane leaflets

4. Carbon is added to form a continuous surface

Carbon

5. Surface is shadowed with a thin layer of platinum

Platinum

6. Tissue is dissolved with acid, carbon-metal replica can be viewed under the electron microscope

Figure 1.10. Diagram depicts major steps in the preparation of a freeze fracture replica for study in the TEM. (From J. Darnell, H. Lodish, and D. Baltimore, *Molecular Cell Biology*. Scientific American Books, Inc., New York, 1986, with permission)

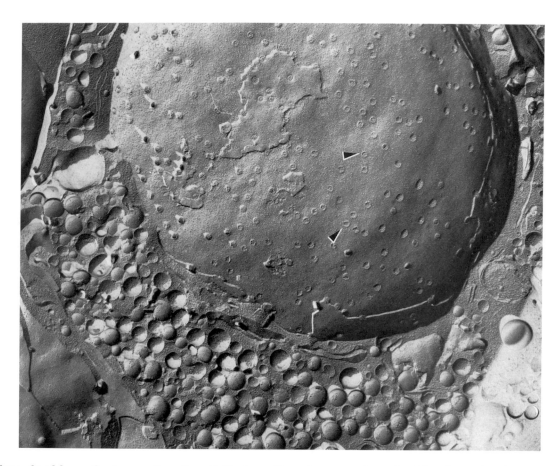

Figure 1.11. Example of freeze fracture replica of a cell. Nucleus with nuclear pores (arrowheads) and cytoplasmic granules are illustrated. ×8250.

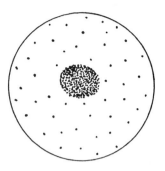

PEROXISOME LABELED WITH
CATALASE - PROTEIN A - COLLOIDAL GOLD

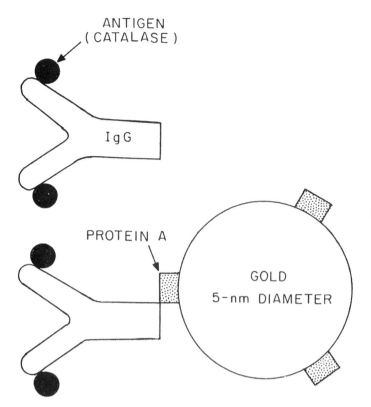

Figure 1.12. Diagram illustrates the use of protein A-colloidal gold labeling and TEM. In this example, the antigen catalase, a protein present in peroxisomes, is coupled to the antibody IgG and to 5-nm diameter gold particles.

The catalase-gold localization appears in the peroxisome. (Reproduced by permission from G. E. Karp, *Cell and Molecular Biology*, John Wiley & Sons, Inc., New York, 1996)

SCANNING ELECTRON MICROSCOPE (SEM)

INSTRUMENT, THEORY, OPERATION

The SEM became commercially available in 1965 and was widely used in biological research in the late 1960s. In the SEM, in the normal mode of operation, the primary electron beam does not pass through the specimen, as in the TEM; instead, the electron beam is "scanned" back and forth across the surface of a specimen that is located in a large chamber at the bottom of the SEM column (Fig. 1.1). The electron beam is produced by an electron gun that is basically similar to that of a TEM. Several condenser electromagnetic lenses then focus the electron probe into a fine point onto the specimen surface. The electron beam is scanned across the specimen by scan coils or deflection coils. One result of this scanning of a fine probe of electrons over the specimen is that low-energy *secondary electrons* are emitted from the specimen's surface. Specimens are typically coated with *gold-palladium* to increase the output of secondary electron emission when the specimen is scanned by the primary electron beam.

For the conventional mode of SEM operation, the secondary electrons are drawn or attracted to a collector and then strike a scintillator, where each electron produces many *photons* (a flash of light). The photons are then guided through a quartz rod to a photomultiplier, where many *photoelectrons* are excited. The photoelectrons comprising the signal are delivered to two *cathode ray tubes* (*CRTs*). One CRT is used to view the image, while the other CRT, with greater resolution (more lines per inch), is used to photograph the image.

The magnification in an SEM ranges from about $10\times$ to $100,000\times$ or more, with a resolution of 0.10–0.20 nm, depending upon how the instrument is used. A unique and useful feature of the SEM is the fact that the *depth of field* is some 300–500 times that of the LM at equivalent magnification (Fig. 1.14). The SEM can provide images of three-dimensional object surfaces because, in its conventional mode of operation, it records not the electrons passing through the specimen, but rather the secondary electrons that are released from the specimen by the impinging electron beam. As the magnification increases in the SEM, the relative depth of field does not decrease but remains constant. In addition, very large samples can be viewed in the specimen chamber of an SEM. Like the TEM, the SEM is under vacuum to permit control of the electron beam. Therefore, in most cases, preserved biologic materials must be viewed in the instrument. The SEM can be used

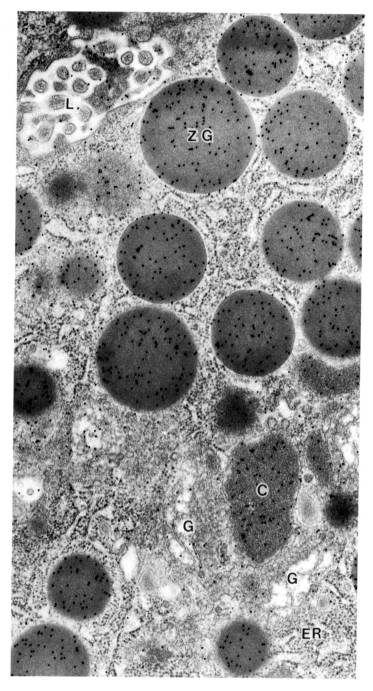

Figure 1.13. Rat pancreatic acinar cell stained with gold-protein A after incubation in antiamylase antibody. The 15-nm-diameter gold particles appear as small black dots and denote the location of amylase over the acinar lumen (L), secretory (zymogen) granules (ZG), and those forming as condensing vacuoles (C) in the Golgi complex (G). ER, rough endoplasmic reticulum. (Illustration courtesy of Dr. M. Bendayan, University of Montreal)

in other modes of operation because photons and x-rays are generated in an SEM.

SEM SPECIMEN PREPARATION

For optimum preservation of large organs such as the liver or kidney, for example, in a mammal such as a rat or guinea pig, the fixative (2.5% or 3% glutaraldehyde or a mixture of 2% paraformaldehyde and 2% glutaraldehyde in $0.1M$ phosphate or cacodylate buffer, pH 7.2) is usually infused through the heart into the cir-

culatory vessels of the organism. After several hours of exposure to the primary fixative, organs are sectioned into smaller slices in the fixative. After several buffer rinses, the samples are placed in a secondary fixative consisting of a buffered osmium tetroxide (for 1–2 hours at 4°C). The tissue samples are rinsed in buffer and dehydrated through a graded series of ethanols (or acetone) of increasing strength, and the specimens are cut, teased, or sheared in 70% or 100% ethanol. In other cases, the tissue samples are transferred from 100% ethanol into liquid nitrogen and fractured with a cold knife. This results in the formation of additional frac-

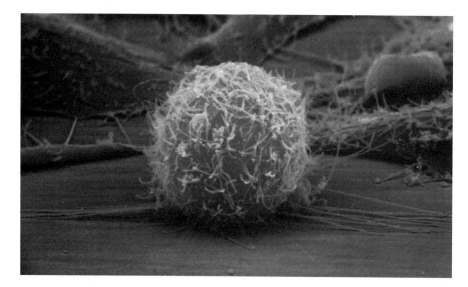

Figure 1.14. SEM of a rounded (mitotic) HeLa cell in culture. Note the many surface microvilli and long filopodia that anchor the cell to the substratum. ×3250.

tured surfaces that may be useful for study. After dehydration in absolute (100%) ethanol, specimens are dried by the critical point method using liquid carbon dioxide. Drying by this method prevents destructive surface tension forces that could affect the fine morphology of the cells or tissues. Once dried, the sample is attached to a specimen holder by copper conducting tape and coated with a layer of heavy metal such as gold and palladium, as well as carbon, to prevent buildup of electric charge during observation in the SEM.

HIGH-VOLTAGE ELECTRON MICROSCOPY (HVEM)

Because of the low energy of electrons, it is necessary to use extremely thin sections so that the electron beam can penetrate. With a conventional 100-kV TEM, specimens are limited in thickness to about 10 times the desired resolution—about 40–70 nm for plastic-embedded biologic samples. Thus, for one cell 15 μm in diameter, it would be necessary to examine over 200 sections. A 1-MeV (1 million volt) HVEM developed in the 1960s demonstrated that whole mounts of entire cells or thick sections of fixed biologic materials could be usefully studied. Because of their high cost, the instruments (1000 to 3000 kV) are limited to several central facilities. Entire cells ~3 μm thick can be observed in an HVEM with a resolution of ~0.2 nm. In addition, it is possible to take stereopairs of photographs that provide three-dimensional information. If thick sections are examined, the preparative techniques used are similar to those for TEM except for some modifications in staining. The use of stereoimages with the HVEM permits one to sort out relationships of overlapping images within the cytoplasm of a cell.

OTHER MICROSCOPES

PHASE CONTRAST MICROSCOPE

The components of an unstained cell observed by BFM have very similar optical density and thus reduce the amplitude of light rays rather equally. Therefore, staining is required to provide additional detail with the LM. The constituents of cells, however, do alter the phase of the light waves. The eye cannot observe these phase alterations by various cellular components, but this can be achieved by the phase contrast microscope, which converts invisible phase differences into amplitude differences that can be observed. This microscope can reveal considerable detail in living cells. The thickness of the specimen is a limiting factor; thus the microscope is used for studying living cells in tissue culture, protozoa, spermatozoa, and other rather small, dispersed cells.

NORMARSKI DIFFERENTIAL INTERFERENCE MICROSCOPE

The Nomarski (or differential, interference) microscope is also useful for studying unstained living cells. In this microscope, a prism splits the incident light beam so that one portion of the beam passes through one region of a specimen, while the other portion of the beam passes through a nearby region of the specimen. Very small differences in thickness or refractive index in the adjacent sample parts are converted into a bright image or a dark image, depending upon whether the two beams are in phase or out of phase after recombination.

FLUORESCENCE MICROSCOPE (FM) (IMMUNOFLUORESCENCE MICROSCOPY)

The FM can be used to detect and localize intracellular proteins that have been tagged with fluorescent antibodies for the specific protein. A chemical is defined as fluorescent if it absorbs light at one wavelength and emits light at another, longer wavelength within the visible spectrum. In the FM, the exciting wavelength that induces the fluorescence is absorbed by filters, so that only fluorescent light emitted by the sample is used to form an image. A number of fluorescent dyes are available, such as fluorescein (emits a green light) and rhodamine (emits a red light). These and other dyes can be chemically coupled to purified antibodies so that the dye-antibody complex, when applied to a tissue section or permeabilized cell, can then be illuminated by the exciting wavelength and observed (Fig. 1.15). It is also possible to localize specific proteins in cells using an an-

tibody that is labeled with colloidal gold particles and observed in TEM (Fig. 1.13).

CONFOCAL SCANNING MICROSCOPE (CSM)

The CSM can provide markedly improved fluorescent images. In FM, fluorescent images are generated from many molecules at different depths in a specimen, which often results in confusion about actual three-dimensional molecular arrangements. In contrast, the CSM permits fluorescent molecules in a single plane of focus to be observed. As a consequence, a much sharper image is obtained because only a small part of the sample is illuminated with exciting light from a focused laser beam. However, many different spots in the sample can be sequentially illuminated, and the images from these spots can be recorded with a video camera and stored on a computer screen. Numerous individual images can

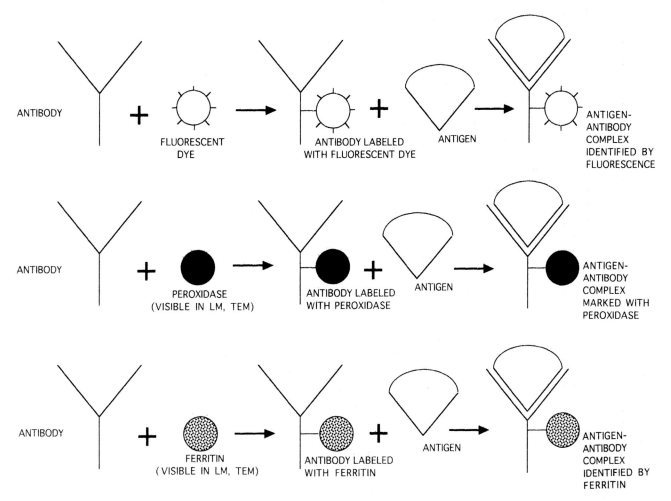

Figure 1.15. Diagram illustrates ways in which antigen-antibody complexes can be visualized. Antibodies can be tagged with fluorescent dye, peroxidase, or ferritin and then coupled to the specific antigen to visualize the antigen-antibody complex by fluorescence microscopy, LM, or TEM.

then be incorporated or stacked into a three-dimensional image that markedly improves image clarity.

ANTIGEN-ANTIBODY COMPLEXES: IMMUNOCYTOCHEMISTRY

Antibodies are unique proteins of many different forms, each of which has a different binding site that specifically recognizes molecules, called *antigens*, that caused the antibody to be formed. To produce antibodies, a protein is injected two or three times into an animal. To produce antibodies to myosin in mouse tissues, purified myosin from mouse muscle is prepared and injected several times into a rabbit. After several weeks, the rabbit blood serum will contain antibodies that the rabbit has produced against the antigenic mouse myosin. The antibodies are then purified from the serum of the immunized rabbit. The purified antibodies are combined with a fluorescent dye, without loss of immunologic specificity. The fluorescent antibody can be used to localize the antigen in tissue sections. This staining procedure is called *direct immunofluorescence,* since the fluorescent antibody binds directly to the antigen in cell or tissue slices. Antibodies can also be labeled with electron-dense particles such as ferritin or colloidal gold and used to locate specific molecules with the high resolution of the TEM (Fig. 1.15). In *indirect immunofluorescence*, a tissue section is exposed to unlabeled specific antibody generated in a certain species of mammal. The section is then washed, and the unlabeled antibody that has bound to areas in the section is visualized in the FM after application of a fluorescent-labeled antibody that was produced using a different species of mammal and that is directed against the immunoglobulin of the first mammalian species used. Because each antibody molecule can bind five molecules of fluorescent anti-antibody, the indirect immunofluorescence procedure is more sensitive than direct immunofluorescence.

Antibodies can also be used to detect and quantify molecules in cell extracts and to identify specific proteins that have been fractionated by electrophoresis in polyacrylamide gels. An alternative system uses the high binding affinity of *biotin*, a small, water-soluble vitamin, for *streptavidin* (a bacterial protein). If the primary antibody is covalently coupled to biotin, streptavidin can be directly labeled with a marker and used in place of a secondary antibody. Another very sensitive method uses an enzyme, alkaline phosphatase, as the marker molecule. The enzyme-linked immunosorbent assay (ELISA) permits small amounts of antigen to be detected.

The specificity of an antiserum for a particular antigen is sharpened by the *monoclonal antibody technique,* which involves propagating a clone of cells from a single antibody-secreting B lymphocyte, thereby obtaining a homogeneous preparation of antibodies in large quantity. Since B lymphocytes have a limited life span in culture, individual antibody-producing B lymphocytes from an immunized mouse are fused with cells derived from an "immortal" B-lymphocyte tumor. From the heterogeneous mixture of hybrid cells, those hybrids that have both the ability to make a particular antibody and the ability to proliferate in culture are screened and selected. The resulting *hybridomas* are propagated as individual clones, each of which provides a permanent source of specific *monoclonal antibodies.* An important feature of the hybridoma technique is that monoclonal antibodies can be made against molecules that comprise only a minor component of a complex mixture.

AUTORADIOGRAPHY

Autoradiography utilizes a radioactive precursor molecule introduced to an animal (cell) by injection (in vivo) or added to cells in culture (in vitro). After a period of exposure to the radioactive precursor, the specimen is processed so that the isotope or its site of incorporation can be localized in the cell. The procedure is summarized in Figure 1.8. The radioisotope is detected using a photographic emulsion that is developed in a manner similar to that of a photograph. This technique requires some knowledge of biochemistry and biochemical pathways. Amino acids and nucleotides usually labeled with β-emitters such as carbon-14 or tritium-(^{3}H) are commercially available, in addition to hundreds of labeled metabolic intermediates. The most widely used isotope for LM and TEM is tritium (radioactive form of hydrogen, ^{3}H), and some common ^{3}H-labeled precursors used to study specific synthetic events in cells are listed in the accompanying table. The basic procedure for autoradiography is outlined in Figure 1.8.

Cellular Event to Be Studied	*Common Isotope Used*
DNA synthesis	^{3}H-thymidine
RNA synthesis	^{3}H-uridine
Protein synthesis	^{3}H-amino acid (e.g., leucine)
Polysaccharide synthesis	^{3}H-sugar (e.g., fucose)
Lipid synthesis	^{3}H-fatty acid

Cells are exposed to isotopes for several minutes in *pulse labeling* experiments in which *sites* of *synthesis* are to be investigated. If, however, it is desirable to obtain information about intracellular transport, a *pulse chase* experiment is necessary. For example, after pancreatic cells are exposed to ^{3}H-leucine for 5 minutes and processed for autoradiographic study, the grains that indicate the site of incorporation will be associated with the endoplasmic reticulum in the cell base. If, however, the cells are exposed to isotope for 5 minutes and then placed in medium without isotope (or cold isotope) for 2 hours, most of the label in the subsequent autoradiograms will be located over the secretory (zymogen) granules at the apical end of the cells or just outside the cell. This indicates that once the amino acids are synthesized into proteins in the endoplasmic reticulum, they are packaged into secretory granules that are discharged.

CELL AND ORGAN CULTURE (TISSUE CULTURE)

Refined and sterile media are now commercially available for culturing many different cell lines that are available for research. It is possible to study cell growth, division, and differentiation, as well as cellular responses to various drugs and hormones. Cell culture procedures require considerable attention to the constituents of the nutritive media, as well as optimum temperature and sterile conditions. Living cells in culture can be observed and studied by various kinds of microscopes, such as phase contrast, confocal, Nomarski optics (interference), and fluorescence microscopes. Cultured cells can be preserved for examination by SEM or by TEM. Microsurgical procedures, the use of laser and ultraviolet microbeams, and microcinematography (motion pictures) are only some of the experimental manipulations that have been made on living cells in culture under observation with phase contrast microscopy.

CELL FRACTIONATION AND DIFFERENTIAL CENTRIFUGATION

Cells can be homogenized and their constituents separated by differential centrifugation. This technique was first used by Bensely and Hoerr in 1934 to isolate mitochondria from liver cells. Cells are disrupted mechanically by grinding them in glass homogenizers so that their components are mixed in an isolation medium. When the solution containing the cell constituents is centrifuged at certain speeds, the cell parts sediment according to their density. Thus, the more dense parts settle out or sediment at lower centrifugal speeds, while the less dense parts require higher speeds. To separate smaller components relatively close to each other in density, a sucrose gradient is used. With the use of a gradient pump and 15% and 30% sucrose stock solutions, a tube of sucrose can be prepared in which 30% sucrose is located at the bot-

tom of the tube and 15% sucrose is located at the top; gradients ranging from 15% to 30% are located in the remainder of the tube from top to bottom. When a mixed suspension of small organelles or other substances is placed on top of the sucrose gradient and centrifuged at high speeds for a specified time period, the constituents settle to the point at which the *organelle density matches* that of the particular *concentration of sucrose.* The various fractions obtained at different sucrose concentrations can be monitored for content and purity by negative staining or by processing and sectioning for TEM examination. The constituents of the pellet can also be determined by fixation, embedding, sectioning, staining, and study in the TEM. An example of how organelles are isolated from a liver cell is illustrated in Figure 1.16.

SOME CURRENT TECHNIQUES IN CELL AND MOLECULAR BIOLOGY

Proteins have either a positive or a negative charge, depending upon the net charges of the amino acids they contain. When an electric field is applied to a solution containing protein molecules, the dissolved proteins migrate at a rate depending on their net charge, size, and shape. *Sodium dodecyl sulfate polyacrylamide gel electrophoresis* (SDS-PAGE) uses a gel as an inert matrix through which proteins migrate. The gel is made by polymerization (cross-linking) of polyacrylamide monomers, and the pore size of the gel can be varied to retard the migration of specific proteins of interest. The proteins are not in simple solution, but in a strong negatively charged detergent called *sodium dodecyl sulfate (SDS).* The detergent binds to hydrophobic regions of protein molecules, so that they unfold into extended polypeptide chains and the individual protein molecules become freely soluble in the detergent solution. A reducing agent (e.g., mercaptoethanol) is added to break S-S (disulfide) bonds that might be present.

When a mixture of SDS-solubilized proteins is electrophoresed through a slab of polyacrylamide gel, each protein molecule binds large numbers of the negatively charged detergent molecules. This causes the protein to migrate toward the positive electrode when a voltage is applied. Proteins of the same size respond similarly. In the meshes of the polyacrylamide gel, which actually acts as a molecular sieve, large proteins are retarded more than small ones, such that a complex mixture of proteins is fractionated into a series of discrete protein bands arranged in order of their molecular weight. Since polypeptides are separated according to size, information is obtained about the molecular weight and subunit composition of the protein complexes. The proteins are detected by staining the gel with a dye such as Coomassie blue or with silver stain, and as little as 10 ng of protein can be detected. Two-dimensional gel

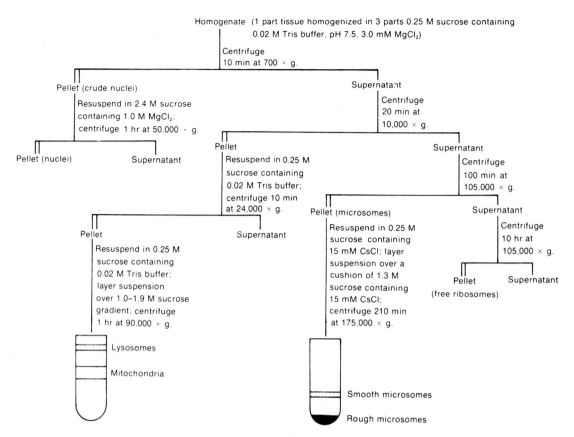

Figure 1.16. Stages in the separation of cellular constituents using the techniques of cell fractionation and differential centrifugation. (From C.J. Flickinger, *Medical Cell Biology*, W.B. Saunders Co., Philadelphia, 1979, with permission) 1. Pieces of liver are homogenized in sucrose solution with a homogenizer. 2. The homogenate is centrifuged at low speed (~1000 × *g*) for 10 minutes. 3. The resulting pellet at the bottom of the tube contains chiefly unbroken cells, large plasma membrane fragments, and nuclei. The supernatant contains remaining cellular constituents. 4. The supernatant is transferred to a new centrifuge tube and centrifuged at higher speed (~10,000 × *g*) for 20 minutes. 5. The pellet formed at the bottom of this tube contains mitochondria, lysosomes, and peroxisomes, for example. 6. The pellet can then be layered over a tube containing a sucrose gradient and centrifuged at still higher speed for a longer period. This will separate the mitochondria from the peroxisomes and lysosomes. With the use of another sucrose gradient and additional centrifugation, the lysosomes can be separated from the peroxisomes. 7. If the supernatant from the second centrifugation step in No. 5 is centrifuged at about 100,000 × *g* for 1–2 hours, a pellet will result that contains microsomes (including fragments of ER and plasma membrane), while the supernatant contains ribosomes (polyribosomes) that are not bound to membranes, as well as various soluble molecules.

electrophoresis can be used, if required, to resolve many closely positioned protein bands.

In *Western blotting* or immunoblotting, the proteins that have been separated by gel electrophoresis are transferred using an electric field to a sheet of nitrocellulose paper. The nitrocellulose paper is soaked in a solution containing the antibody specific for the protein of interest. The antibody can be coupled to an enzyme, a radioactive isotope, or a fluorescent dye. Then the membrane is developed with an enzyme-linked antibody that identifies the band containing the protein.

SELECTED BIBLIOGRAPHY

Bradbury, S. (1984). *An Introduction to the Optical Microscope.* Oxford University Press, Oxford.

Celis, J., and Bravo, R., eds. (1983). *Two-Dimensional Gel Electrophoresis of Proteins.* Academic Press, New York.

deDuve, C. (1975). Exploring cells with a centrifuge. *Science* **189**, 186–194.

Everhart, T., and Hayes, T. (1972). The scanning electron microscope. *Sci. Am.* **226**, 54–69.

Freshney, R. (1987). *Culture of Animal Cells: A Manual of Basic Technique.* Alan R. Liss, New York.

Glauert, A. Ed. (1980). Freeze-fracturing and freeze-etching. In *Practical Methods in Electron Microscopy*, Vol. 8, North-Holland, Amsterdam.

Lesko, L., Donlon, M., Marinetti, G., and Hare, J. (1973). A rapid method for the isolation of rat liver plasma membranes using an aqueous two-phase polymer system. *Biochim. Biophys. Acta* **311**, 173–179.

Pease, D.C., and Porter, K.R. (1981). Electron microscopy and ultramicrotomy. *J. Cell Biol.* **91**, 287s–292s.

Ploem, J., and Tanke, H. (1987). *Introduction to Fluorescence*

Microscopy. Royal Microscopy Handbook No. 10, Oxford Scientific Press, Oxford.

Polak, J., and Priestley, J. (eds). (1992). *Electron Microscopic Immunocytochemistry. Principles and Practice.* Oxford University Press, Oxford.

Pool, R. (1992). Optics' new focus: beams of atoms. *Science* **255**, 1513–1515.

Rogers, A.W. (1979). *Techniques of Autoradiography.* Elsevier/North Holland, New York.

Smith, R.F. (1990). *Microscopy and Photomicrography: A Working Manual.* CRC Press, Boca Raton, FL.

Spencer, M. (1982). *Fundamentals of Light Microscopy.* Cambridge University Press, Cambridge.

Taylor, D., Nederlof, M., Lanni, F., and Waggoner, A. (1992). The new vision of light microscopy. *Am. Sci.* **80**, 322–335.

Yatchmenoff, B. (1988). A new confocal scanning optical microscope. *Am. Lab.* **20**, 58–66.

Yelton, D.E., and Scharff, M. (1981). Monoclonal antibodies; a powerful new tool in biology and medicine. *Annu. Rev. Biochem.* **50**, 657–680.

CHAPTER 2

The Eukaryotic Cell: The Plasma Membrane and Cytoplasmic Organelles

A multitude of activities can be performed by eukaryotic cells (for examples, see the accompanying table). Cells differ, however, in the number and extent of basic activities that they can perform (for example, see table)

Some Basic Activities of Eukaryotic Cells

DNA replication, cell division	Locomotion
RNA synthesis	Shape changes
Protein synthesis	Nuclear pore translocation
Carbohydrate synthesis	Nuclear import
Lipid synthesis	Intracellular organelle movements
Intracellular digestion	Intracellular membrane trafficking
Transport, translocation of molecules across membranes	

Examples of Structural and Functional Cell Diversity

Cell Type	Principal Function
Polymorphonuclear leukocyte	Phagocytosis, intracellular digestion of bacteria
Osteoclast	Erode bone
Chondroblast	Synthesize cartilage matrix

Cell Type	Principal Function
Muscle cell	Contractility
Neuron	Nerve impulse transmission
Epithelial cells	Secretion, absorption, transport
Gland cell	Synthesis, packaging, discharge of secretory products

THE PLASMA (CELL) MEMBRANE

INTRODUCTION

That a barrier separates the cell from its surrounding environment was evident from the time of early micromanipulation with fine needles. Information generated by x-ray diffraction provided evidence that the plasma membrane consists of two lipid layers, each a single molecule thick, that is, a *bimolecular layer of lipid*. In addition, protein was found to be associated with the plasma membrane, indicating that it is a lipoprotein complex. Covalently attached carbohydrate is associated with the plasma membrane's external surface as the cell coat or *glycocalyx*. Plasma membrane molecules play important roles in cell recognition, signal transduction, cell adhesion, and coupling of the cytoskeleton to the cell surface. The cell membrane is a semipermeable barrier; the forces of diffusion, osmosis, and active transport are important functional events involving the plasma membrane.

18

MEMBRANE STRUCTURE (TEM)

The plasma membrane of eukaryotes contains lipid, protein, and carbohydrate molecules. The *lipids* constitute a *permeability barrier* to the cellular exterior and serve to compartmentalize the cellular interior. The *membrane proteins* are responsible for most *dynamic functions* performed by the membranes. The *carbohydrates* contribute to cellular *recognition* and *specific binding* phenomena.

High-resolution TEM studies on the plasma membrane have demonstrated two narrow, electron-dense lines separated by an electron-lucent region. This trilaminar appearance has been called the *unit membrane model* since it is so widely observed in sections of membranes examined by TEM. The two electron-dense lines are each ~2.5–3 nm wide and are the plasma membrane's *outer leaflet* and *inner leaflet* (Figs. 2.1–2.2). The outer leaflet faces the extracellular space, and the inner leaflet faces the cytoplasmic matrix. The electron-lucent interior is also about 2.5–3 nm wide; therefore, the entire plasma membrane is approximately 7.5–9 nm across. The electron-lucent interior appears to correspond to the hydrophobic lipid tails of the bilayer. The electron-dense inner and outer leaflets appear to correspond to the polar, hydrophilic lipid heads and some peripheral proteins. As shown by freeze fracture techniques (Fig. 2.3), *integral membrane proteins* are embedded in the lipid bilayer, while *peripheral proteins* are bound to the surface. A fine, filamentous network also radiates from the plasma membrane's external leaflet and represents the cell coat or glycocalyx. It is not surprising that the plasma membrane, which covers the en-

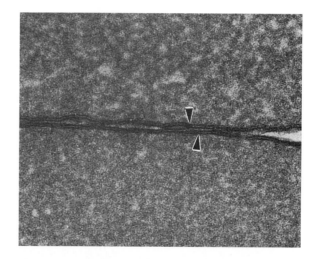

Figure 2.2. TEM illustrates the trilaminar unit membrane (arrowheads) in two erythrocytes. ×210,000.

tire cell, exhibits both structural and biochemical heterogeneity, thus facilitating division of labor in cellular activities. Different structural specializations of the plasma membrane of cultured cells are illustrated by the SEM (Figs. 2.4–2.7).

MEMBRANE LIPIDS

Membrane lipids are small molecules with both *hydrophilic* (water-loving or water-soluble) and *hydrophobic*

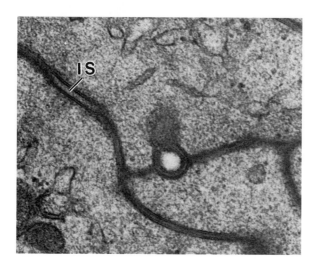

Figure 2.1. TEM image of the folded plasma membranes of two adjacent cells. In places where the section is perpendicular to the plasma membrane, a narrow intercellular space of about 25 nm (IS) is evident; in these regions, it is possible to visualize the trilaminar unit membrane structure (two electron-dense lines and an intermediate electron-lucent layer) of each cell membrane, as denoted by the arrowheads. ×60,000.

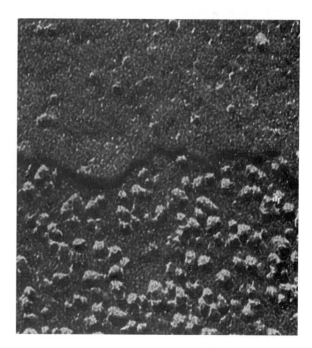

Figure 2.3. Freeze fracture replica of a small part of an erythrocyte plasma membrane. The P fracture face contains many intramembranous particles that represent integral membrane proteins. ×300,000.

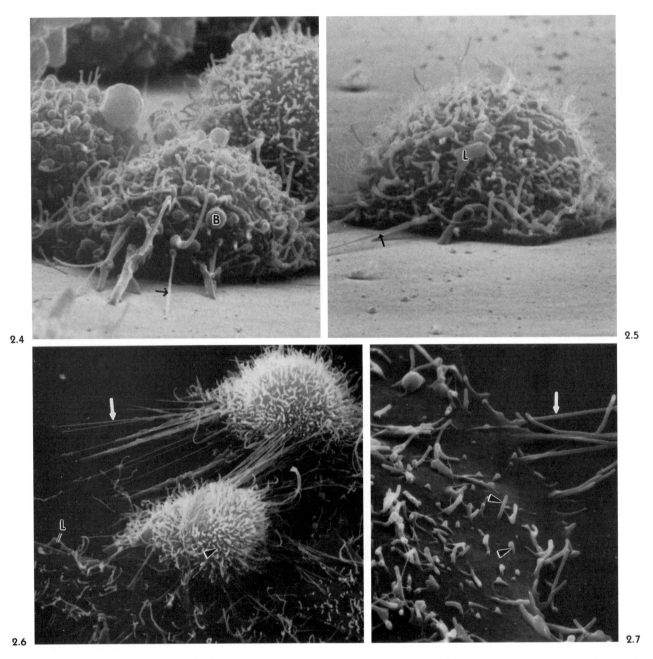

Figures 2.4–2.7. SEM images of mitotic and interphase HeLa and KB cells in culture display a variety of surface specializations. Long filopodia (arrows) attach the cells to substratum; many finger-like processes called *microvilli* extend from both (arrowheads) rounded and flattened cells, and they are of different lengths. Other plasma membrane specializations shown include zeiotic blebs (B) and flap-like lamellipodia (L). Figure 2.4, ×4940; Figure 2.5, ×6175; Figure 2.6, ×2860; Figure 2.7, ×6825.

(water-insoluble) constituents (Fig. 2.8). For this reason, they are called *amphipathic* molecules. In the membrane bilayer, the *polar head groups* are external and the *hydrocarbon tails* (hydrophobic portion) are oriented toward the interior bilayer. Lipid bilayers tend to close upon themselves, so there are no exposed hydrocarbon chains.

In 1925, when the plasma membrane of erythrocytes was extracted with acetone and floated onto a water surface, a monomolecular film formed that covered twice the surface area of the original erythrocytes. This finding suggested that a bimolecular layer of lipid constituted the plasma membrane, a finding supported by x-ray diffraction data a few years later. In general, about 50% of the cell membrane mass is protein. In a typical animal cell, there are approximately 10^9 lipid molecules.

There are three main types of membrane lipids. *Phospholipids* are the most abundant, and diffuse laterally in the plane of the membrane but do not flip-flop (Fig. 2.8). There are four major types: *phosphatidyl-*

Figure 2.8. Diagram illustrates the parts of a phospholipid molecule in the plasma membrane.

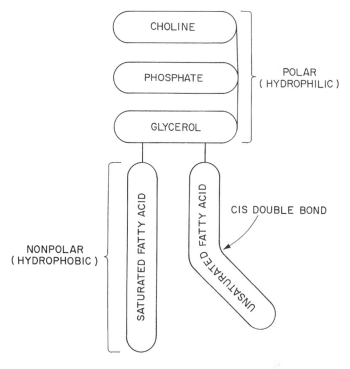

choline, phosphatidylserine, phosphatidylethanolamine, and spingomyelin. A phospholipid molecule is illustrated in Figure 2.8. *Cholesterol* reduces membrane fluidity at higher temperatures and increases fluidity at lower temperatures. Cholesterol can flip-flop in the membrane. While cholesterol occurs in eukaryotic cell membranes, it is not present in bacterial membranes. *Glycolipids* are sugar-containing lipids; the simplest glycolipid is cerebroside, which has only one sugar residue (either glucose or galactose). Gangliosides are more complex glycolipids that have branched chains and several sugar residues including sialic acid. Glycolipids comprise only about 5% of the membrane lipids.

Fatty acid chains in phospholipids and glycolipids typically contain an even number of carbon atoms, usually between 14 and 24, with 16- and 18-carbon fatty acids being most common. Fatty acids can be saturated or unsaturated, and the degree of unsaturation affects membrane fluidity. Fluidity is greater when a high percentage of the membrane phospholipids is polyunsaturated. Membrane fluidity also depends upon temperature and lipid composition. Fluidity increases at higher temperatures and decreases as temperature declines.

Hydrophobic properties of lipids provide a major force for bilayer self-assembly. In addition, *van der Waals attractive forces* between the hydrocarbon tails of the lipid molecules cause close packing. *Electrostatic forces* and *hydrogen bonding* between polar groups of lipid molecules stabilize molecular interactions in membranes. Lipid molecules diffuse in the plane of the membrane. Lipid bilayers have low permeability to ions and polar molecules because the hydrophobic membrane interior

makes it energetically unfavorable for charged molecules and ions to cross.

MEMBRANE PROTEINS

Integral membrane proteins tend to extend partially or completely through the lipid bilayer and interact with the hydrocarbon chains of membrane lipids, so they are more difficult to dissociate (Fig. 2.9). *Peripheral proteins* are associated either with the periphery of the lipid membrane bilayer or with the external surface of some integral proteins. Both lipid molecules and membrane proteins diffuse in the plane of the membrane, but the diffusion of protein molecules is slower than that of lipids, partly due to the protein's larger size. Some membrane proteins do not move in the plane of the membrane since they are anchored to cytoskeletal elements. One way to study membrane proteins involves SDS-PAGE, which was briefly described in Chapter 1.

Functionally different proteins are present in the plasma membrane. *Pumps*, such as the sodium pump, actively transport sodium ions. *Channel proteins*, such as sodium, potassium, calcium, and chloride channels permit passage of these small ions down a concentration or voltage gradient. *Receptor proteins* include immunoglobulin molecules and others that permit recognition and binding of substances to the plasma membrane, as in receptor-mediated endocytosis or hormonal response. *Transducers* couple receptors to enzymes following ligand binding. A *ligand* is any molecule that binds to a receptor. An enzyme can act through a transducer to activate a second messenger such as cyclic

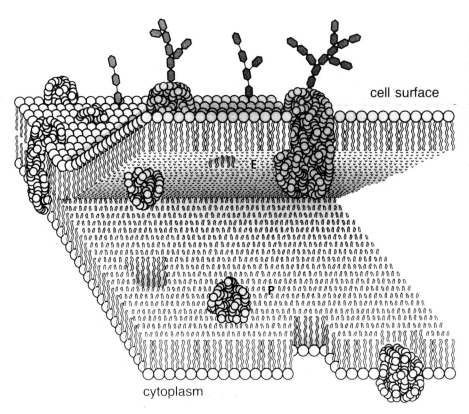

cell surface

cytoplasm

Figure 2.9. Model of a plasma membrane illustrates lipids, cholesterol, peripheral and integral membrane proteins, and the oligosaccharide chains that extend from the external leaflet of the bimolecular layer of lipid that comprises the extracellular coat or glycocalyx. (From S.L. Wolfe, *Molecular and Cellular Biology*, reprinted by permission of Wadsworth Publishing Co., Belmont, CA, © 1993)

adenosine monophosphate (cAMP). *Enzymes* such as adenosine triphosphatase (ATPase) are also bound to the plasma membrane. *Structural proteins*, like those in tight junctions, represent this type of molecular differentiation. *Integrins* include a group of plasma membrane receptors for extracellular matrix proteins.

SIGNAL TRANSDUCTION

When an appropriate ligand binds to and activates a plasma membrane receptor-G protein complex, a plasma membrane-bound enzyme, called *adenylyl cyclase* is activated, which causes the synthesis of *cAMP* from *ATP* (Fig. 2.10). Cyclic AMP is hydrolyzed by cAMP phosphodiesterase. Trimeric G proteins consist of three polypeptide chains that are closely associated with cell surface receptors. Cycling of the guanosine nucleotides associated with the G protein between inactive and active states is coupled to activation and inactivation of adenylyl cyclase. Cyclic AMP acts by activating the enzyme *cAMP-dependent protein kinase*, which catalyzes the transfer of phosphate from ATP to certain serines or threonines of selected proteins. The *phosphorylation* of the appropriate *amino acids* serves to regulate the activity of the target protein (Fig. 2.10).

In another pathway, the binding of a signaling molecule to a G-protein-linked receptor in the plasma membrane can activate the enzyme *phospholipase C*, which cleaves *phosphatidylinositol biphosphate* (*PIP₂*), which is lo-

cated in the inner leaflet of the plasma membrane, into two substances: *inositol triphosphate* (*IP₃*) and *diacylglycerol* (*DAG*) (Fig. 2.11). IP₃ diffuses to and binds IP₃-gated calcium-release channels in the endoplasmic reticulum, resulting in the *release* of *calcium* from this storage site. IP₃ is rapidly dephosphorylated, and the calcium is pumped from the cytoplasm to limit the response. DAG, together with calcium and phosphatidylserine, activate *protein kinase C* (*PKC*), which is calcium dependent. PKC *phosphorylates* various *proteins* in target cells (Fig. 2.11).

The extracellular space and cytosol (cytoplasm) are both aqueous, but the plasma membrane allows cells to maintain large concentration gradients. Certain membrane proteins transport charged and polar molecules into and out of cells; this *protein-mediated transport* includes *facilitated* and *active transport*. In facilitated transport (facilitated diffusion), proteins allow molecules to cross the membrane down their concentration gradient; energy is not required. Active-transport systems move uncharged molecules against a concentration gradient and ions against an electrochemical gradient. Active transport requires energy. Most cells maintain ion gradients across their plasma membrane. For example, extracellular Na^+ and Cl^- concentrations are much higher than intracellular concentrations. Conversely, the cytoplasmic K^+ concentration is much higher than the extracellular K^+ concentration. Many cells use the potential energy of the Na^+ electrochemical gradient in cotransport systems. Cotransport systems drive molecules and ions into the cell against a concentration gradient using energy provided

Figure 2.10. Glucagon acts on liver cells by binding to plasma membrane receptors (#1); this activates the receptor, which triggers the synthesis of cAMP (#2–4) from adenylate cyclase via a G protein (#2); cAMP activates a series of protein kinases. Protein kinase A has two regulatory (R) and two catalytic (C) subunits in inactive form. Cyclic AMP combines with R subunits (#5), producing a conformational change that releases and activates the C subunits. When active, protein kinase A phosphorylates two enzymes, phosphorylase kinase and glycogen synthase. Phosphorylase kinase is activated by phosphate groups added to the protein kinase A (#6). The activated phosphorylase kinase adds a phosphate group to glycogen phosphorylase (#7) an enzyme that catalyzes the breakdown of glycogen to glucose (#8). Glycogen synthase is inactivated by phosphorylation catalyzed by protein kinase A (#9). (From S.L. Wolfe, *Molecular and Cellular Biology*, reprinted by permission of Wadsworth Publishing Co., Belmont, CA, © 1993)

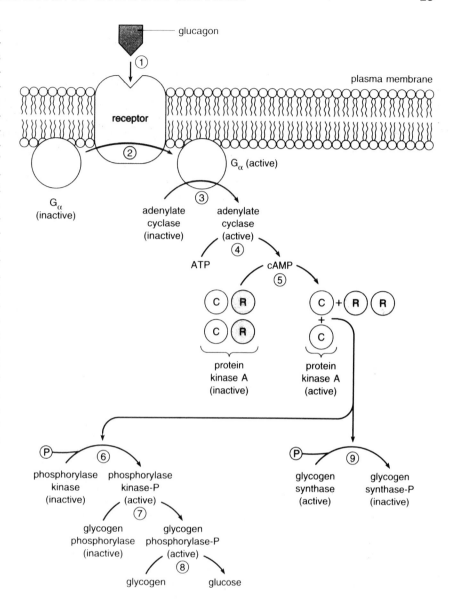

by Na^+ moving into the cell down its concentration gradient. The Na^+ gradient results from the activity of Na^+,K^+-*ATPase*, a membrane protein that transports *three* Na^+ ions out of the cell and *two* K^+ ions into the cell, with the energy released by the hydrolysis of *one ATP* molecule (described in Chapter 10).

MEMBRANE CARBOHYDRATES

Sugar residues or oligosaccharides are attached to either integral membrane proteins to form a *glycoprotein* or to the polar heads of lipid molecules to form *glycolipids* (Fig. 2.9). Sugar residues are attached only to the outer or external surface of the plasma membrane. This arrangement confers asymmetry to the membrane (Fig. 2.12). Oligosaccharide side chains possess a *net negative charge* owing to the abundant *sialic acid* (an amino sugar)

termini. The carbohydrates on the membrane's external surface play an important role in cell recognition and adhesion.

Membrane mobility

Lipids and many proteins are in constant lateral motion in the plasma membrane. To demonstrate this, membrane receptors of a mouse cell are labeled with a green fluorescent dye. In contrast, the membrane receptors of a human cell can be labeled with a red fluorescent dye. The mouse cell and human cell then can be fused into one cell (called a *heterokaryon*) in the presence of Sendai virus. Initially, the red and green fluorescent receptors are separate. However, within 1 hour at 37°C, the red and green fluorescent colors become intermixed, demonstrating that membrane receptor proteins can diffuse in the plane of the membrane.

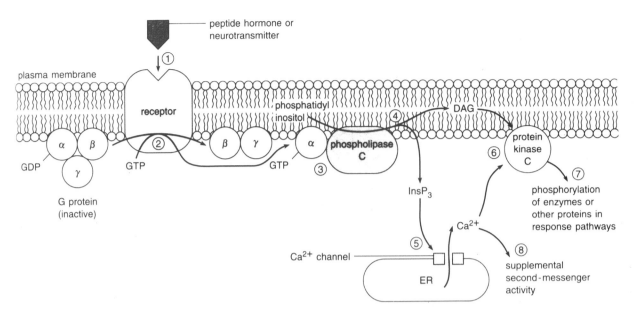

Figure 2.11. Diagram illustrates important signaling pathway involving phospholipase C, inositol triphosphate (InsP$_3$), and diacylglycerol (DAG). (From S.L. Wolfe, *Mole-* *cular and Cellular Biology*, **reprinted by permission of Wadsworth Publishing Co., Belmont, CA, © 1993)**

Membrane specializations

Lateral interdigitations. Epithelial cells are closely packed sheets of cells that possess a variety of specializations. The narrow intracellular space between cells in a sheet is about *25 nm wide* (Fig. 2.2). When the membranes become twisted with respect to

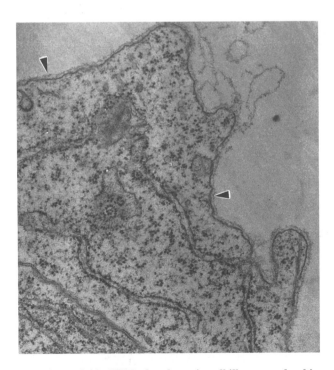

Figure 2.12. TEM of embryonic cell illustrates the thin glycocalyx (arrowheads) or extracellular coat that is located just outside of the plasma membrane. ×23,600.

the section plane, the clarity of the unit membrane structure is reduced. The plasma membranes of epithelial cells commonly interdigitate along their lateral borders, a device that could anchor the cells and stabilize their organization.

Microvilli and glycocalyx. The apical surfaces of some epithelial types contain numerous finger-like plasma membrane evaginations called *microvilli* (Fig. 2.13), which increase the surface area of cells possessing them. A single intestinal epithelial cell may contain 2000 or 3000 apical microvilli. The organization of microvilli is described in Chapter 4.

Basal lamina and basement membrane. The basal lamina is an external amorphous layer about 50–80 nm thick associated with the base of epithelial cells (Fig. 2.14). In this particular region, the basal lamina is closely associated with fine connective tissue fibers (collagen or reticular fibers) to collectively form a basement membrane. The basement membrane is described in more detail in the Chapter 4.

Basal plasma membrane infoldings. The plasma membrane at the base of epithelial cells may be infolded into the basal cytoplasm (Fig. 2.14). This structural specialization is common to cells involved in active transport of ions and water (e.g., kidney tubule cells, duct cells of glands). Mitochondria are located between the basal plasma membrane folds and are favorably situated to provide a ready supply of energy to sustain active transport in this region. The membrane infoldings serve to locally amplify this cell region and its associated function.

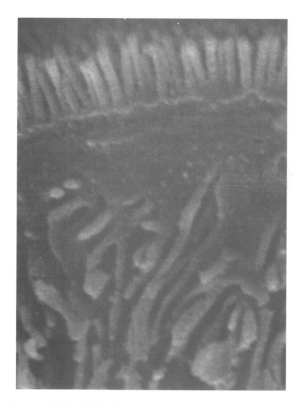

Figure 2.13. SEM shows short microvilli extending from apical plasma membrane of epithelial cell. ×21,875.

Endocytosis, exocytosis, micropinocytotic vesicles. Eukaryotic cells take up materials from the surrounding medium by endocytosis. There are three distinct but related pathways. *Bulk-phase endocytosis* refers to the uptake of fluid from the surrounding medium and does not involve surface receptors. A second endocytotic pathway, called *phagocytosis*, involves the uptake of large, insoluble aggregates or cell parts or entire cells. A third pathway, *receptor-mediated endocytosis*, involves incorporation of material (ligand) into the cell after being bound to specific cell surface receptors. Nonselective uptake of fluid into cells occurs in *smooth-surfaced vesicles*. Material becomes located in depressions (*caveolae*) that then detach from the plasma membrane to internalize material within the cell. This type of endocytosis is referred to as *micropinocytosis* ("cellular drinking on a small scale"). Non-clathrin-coated caveolae of plasma membranes contain a transmembrane protein called *caveolin*. Endothelial cells commonly illustrate extensive micropinocytotic activity (Figs. 2.15, 2.16) in the transport of materials from the blood to the extracellular space surrounding the capillaries (transcytosis). Micropinocytotic pits pinch off from the plasma membrane of the capillary endothelium on the blood side and become micropinocytotic vesicles that fuse with the

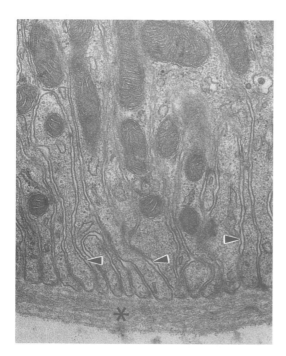

Figure 2.14. TEM of basal portion of kidney cell. Note the extracellular basement membrane (*), the infolded basal plasma membrane (arrowheads), and the many mitochondria. ×32,800.

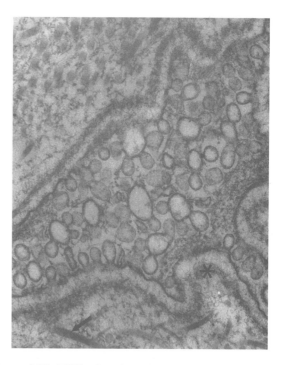

Figure 2.15. TEM of endothelial cell illustrates basal lamina (*) and many micropinocytotic vesicles, a number of which are attached to the plasma membrane. Fusion of vesicles inside the endothelial cell cytoplasm is also evident. Microvesiculation of the plasma membrane is a method for the transendothelial movement of fluid materials from the capillary lumen to the pericapillary space. Connective tissue fibers (arrow) are also associated with the basal lamina. ×48,000.

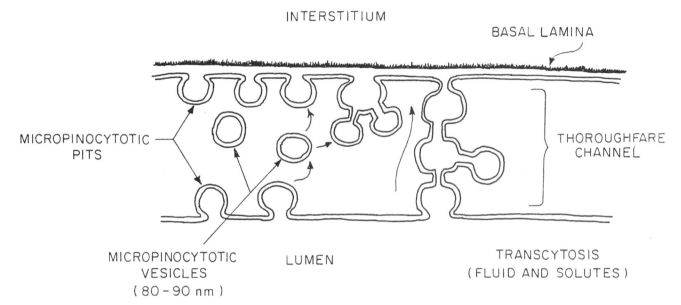

INTERSTITIUM

BASAL LAMINA

MICROPINOCYTOTIC
PITS

THOROUGHFARE
CHANNEL

MICROPINOCYTOTIC
VESICLES
(80 - 90 nm)

LUMEN

TRANSCYTOSIS
(FLUID AND SOLUTES)

Figure 2.16. Diagram depicts the fusion and fission of micropinocytotic pits and vesicles in the process of transcytosis in endothelial cells. The diagram considers that thor- oughfare channels may be formed under some conditions to provide more rapid transcapillary transport.

plasma membrane on the tissue side of the capillary so as to release their content. Receptor-mediated endocytosis by cells occurs in *clathrin-coated vesicles* (Fig. 2.17). Clathrin consists of three large polypeptides and three small polypeptides that form a three-legged structure called a *triskelion*. The formation of a *clathrin* coat on clathrin-coated pits and vesicles appears to provide a mechanical force that causes bud and vesicle formation, and it participates with adaptins to capture specific receptors and the bound cargo molecules. *Adaptin* is another coat protein that binds to both clathrin and cargo receptors. The peptide signal for endocytosis involves an amino acid sequence of the cargo receptor that is recognized by the adaptin. The invagination of a coated pit in the plasma membrane is believed to be driven by forces generated by the assembly of clathrin and other coated proteins. Clathrin and adaptin are stripped off the coated vesicle, once formed, and return to the plasma membrane. After entry into the cell, the receptor and ligand are separated or sorted by a proton pump that acidifies the membrane-bound endosome (Fig. 2.17). Receptors return to the plasma membrane, while the endosome with ligand fuses with a lysosome. The coated pits and vesicles comprise a major pathway for the uptake of extracellular fluid and membrane-bound ligands. Coated pits and vesicles can form from the plasma membrane, the endoplasmic reticulum membrane, and the trans-Golgi network to endolysosomes. Not all coated vesicles, however, have clathrin. *Coatomer-coated vesicles* are involved in transport from the endoplasmic reticulum to the Golgi complex, from one Golgi cisterna to another, and from the trans-Golgi network to the plasma membrane.

Substances can enter the cell by diffusion, by the use of pumps, by the use of channel proteins, or by *endocytosis*. In contrast to endocytosis, *exocytosis* is the fusion of membrane-bound vesicles with the plasma membrane and the consequent release of the material to the exterior. There are two main pathways for exocytosis. The *constitutive pathway* is a continual process of release and is not induced; an example is the release of humoral antibody by a plasma cell. The *regulated pathway* for exocytosis refers to the fact that the release must be activated. An example of a regulated pathway is the release or exocytosis of secretory granules (zymogen granules) from the pancreatic exocrine cell in response to hormone.

Receptor-mediated endocytosis. A general pathway for receptor-mediated internalization of peptide ligands has been established based on studies of the low-density lipoprotein receptor system (Fig. 2.17). Cholesterol is needed to make new membrane. It circulates in the blood and is bound to protein in the form of complexes called *low-density lipoprotein* (*LDL*). A cell that needs cholesterol to make new membrane synthesizes LDL receptor molecules and inserts them into its plasma membrane. After a peptide ligand binds to a receptor, clustering of the ligand-receptor complexes occurs over clathrin-coated regions of the plasma membrane called *clathrin pits*. These coated pits invaginate and pinch off from the plasma membrane. The receptor-ligand complex is thereby sequestered in membrane-bound, clathrin-coated vesicle. The clathrin coat is then lost. The vesicle is acidified by an *ATP-dependent proton pump*, releasing the ligand from the receptor. The

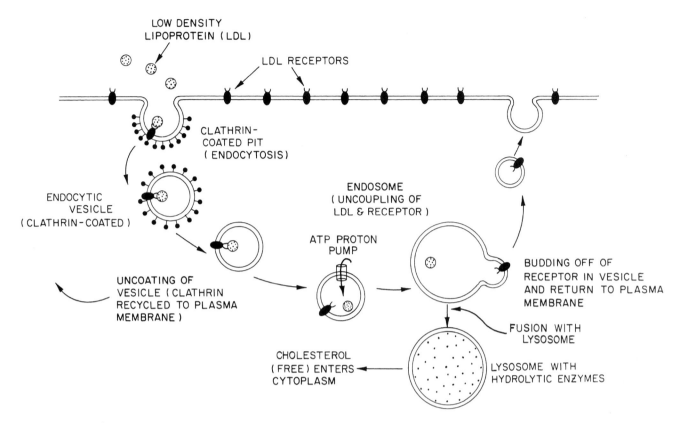

Figure 2.17. Diagram illustrates pathway for LDL uptake and conversion to cholesterol (see text for details). (Redrawn and modified from B. Alberts, D. Bray, J. Lewis, M. Raff, K. Roberts and J.D. Watson. *Molecular Biology of the Cell.* Garland Publishing, New York, 1983)

ligand and receptor are *sorted*, and the ligand may be targeted to lysosomes for degradation. The receptor is either recycled back to the plasma membrane or degraded. Lysosomal enzymes hydrolyze the cholesteryl esters in the LDL particles, freeing cholesterol to move into the cytoplasm for use in making new membrane. If too much free cholesterol accumulates, the cell shuts down cholesterol synthesis and the synthesis of LDL receptor proteins.

ORGANELLES

The eukaryotic cell is enclosed by a plasma membrane that may have various structural specializations. The nuclear envelope consists of two membrances interrupted by pore complexes and provides a selective barrier between the nucleus and cytoplasm. The cytoplasm or cytosol consists of a variety of membranes that enclose specific regions and separate them from other regions, thus defining a collection of subcellular components called *organelles.* By one definition, an organelle is a structure that can be isolated by centrifugation. Organelles of eukaryotic animal cells include mitochondria, smooth- and rough-surfaced endoplasmic reticulum, Golgi complexes, lysosomes, and peroxisomes. The cytosol also contains cytoskeletal elements including microtubules,

microfilaments, intermediate filaments, and inclusion bodies (e.g., glycogen, lipid).

MITOCHONDRIA

Mitochondria are large organelles that can be isolated by routine centrifugation methods and collected in the quantity necessary for biochemical analysis. Mitochondria are observed easily in living cells by phase contrast microscopy. The internal details of mitochondrial structures became evident only with the advent of suitable TEM techniques in the early 1950s. Mitochondria commonly range from 1 to 10 μm in length and from about 0.25 to 1 μm wide; they readily move within the cytoplasm of most cells. Mitochondria utilize the terminal products of carbohydrate, protein, and fat digestion and a multitude of enzymes to *synthesize ATP.*

The mitochondrion is surrounded by an outer mitochondrial membrane that is unique because it permits entry of all molecules smaller than 10 kD. This property is due to a transmembrane protein called *porin,* which functions as an aqueous pore, coupling the cytosol and the intermembranous space. An inner mitochondrial membrane is folded such that it partially compartmentalizes the interior of the mitochondrion; the folds are called *cristae* (Fig. 2.18). Cristae increase the

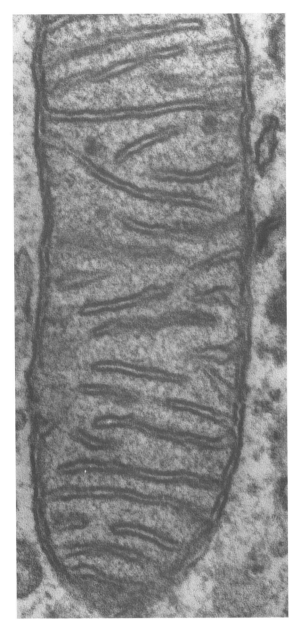

Figure 2.18. TEM of mitochondria. Elongate mitochondrion has numerous shelf-like cristae typical of a cell such as muscle with high energy requirements. ×125,000.

surface area of the inner membrane. Since the cristae contain the enzymes involved in aerobic respiration, their amplification permits more respiratory enzymes to be contained within the mitochondrion. In fact, the number of cristae in a mitochondrion is usually greatest in the more metabolically active cells such as muscle cells.

The mitochondrial *matrix* contains many *ribosomes* that can carry out protein synthesis, but they are somewhat smaller than those in the cytoplasm (Fig. 2.19). DNA is located in the mitochondrial matrix in the form of a very fine circular thread that is masked by the matrix (Fig. 2.19). The matrix also contains a variable num-

ber of electron-dense granules called *matrix granules* that contain accumulations of *divalent cations* such as Ca^{2+} (Fig. 2.19). Thus, the mitochondrion seems to store calcium ions. The mitochondrial matrix also contains many *citric acid cycle* (Kreb's cycle) enzymes, as well as glutamate dehydrogenase, pyruvate dehydrogenase, and enzymes for protein synthesis and for lipid breakdown. The cristae, in contrast, possess *respiratory enzymes* (flavoproteins and cytochromes) that are involved in *oxidative phosphorylation*, as well as coenzyme Q and some dehydrogenases. While the mitochondrion can carry out protein synthesis, there is apparently not enough DNA in the mitochondrion to code for all mitochondrial proteins; thus some mitochondrial proteins are synthesized in the cytoplasm and enter the mitochondrion.

When an isolated mitochondrion is negatively stained and examined in the TEM, many stalked knobs ("lollipops") are seen side by side in the inner mitochondrial membrane of the cristae (Fig. 2.19). Each of these structures (also called *inner membrane subunits, elementary particles, F_0F_1 complex,* or *respiratory stalks*) contains enzymes (F_1 *enzyme*) that in the intact mitochondrion are involved in *phosphorylating ADP to ATP,* that is, the production of ATP, which is the major function of the mitochondrion. The phosphorylation of ADP is important because there are approximately 7300 calories of stored energy in a single phosphate bond. The ATP formed in the mitochondrion is available for various energy-requiring activites such as motility, active transport, biosynthesis, and movement of contractile filaments.

POLYRIBOSOMES

Intracellular proteins are synthesized at groups of ribosomes called *polyribosomes* or *polysomes,* which include a messenger RNA (mRNA) strand that holds a variable number of ribosomes. The number of ribosomes in a polyribosome is directly related to the length of the mRNA transcript (Fig. 2.20). Many cells contain free or unbound polyribosomes that are not attached to membranous components of the endoplasmic reticulum. Cells may also contain elements of the rough-surfaced endoplasmic reticulum (rER) in which polyribosomes are attached to the outer surface of the endoplasmic reticulum (i.e., the side of the membrane facing the cytoplasmic matrix) (Fig. 2.20). Cells that synthesize proteins for use mainly within cells have large numbers of free polyribosomes. The basophilic erythroblast contains the complement of polyribosomes necessary to synthesize hemoglobin, which fills the mature erythrocyte. Cells that synthesize proteins for export contain abundant rER.

Cytoplasmic ribosomes in eukaryotic cells are characterized by their S value, which is 80S; the S stands for

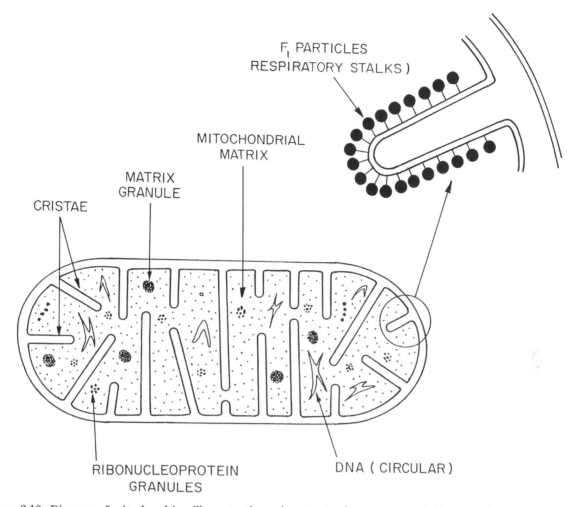

F₁ PARTICLES
RESPIRATORY STALKS)

MITOCHONDRIAL
MATRIX

MATRIX
GRANULE

CRISTAE

RIBONUCLEOPROTEIN
GRANULES

DNA (CIRCULAR)

Figure 2.19. Diagram of mitochondrion illustrates the major structural components of this organelle.

Svedberg units and refers to the speed with which they sediment in a centrifugal field. The ribosome consists of a small and a large subunit, both of which contain ribonucleic acid (RNA) and protein (about 3 or 4 RNA molecules and some 50–80 different proteins) (Fig. 2.21). The small subunit is 40S and the large subunit is 60S. The small subunit of the eukaryotic cell has a single RNA molecule, an 18S RNA molecule. The large subunit is more variable but typically includes one 28S RNA molecule, a 5S RNA, and another kind of RNA that is associated with the 28S RNA molecule (Fig. 2.21).

Ribosomal DNA (rDNA) is located in that region of the chromosome(s) to which the nucleolus (or nucleoli) is (are) attached at the *nucleolus-organizer region*. Ribosomal RNA is synthesized at the nucleolus-organizer region. A number of important events occur in the synthesis and packaging of eukaryotic ribosomes in the nucleoplasm prior to their export into the cytoplasm. All three species of RNA are essential participants in protein synthesis. *Messenger ribonucleic acid (mRNA)* carries the genetic code from the nucleus to the cytoplasm. It has the form of a long, slender strand (about 1 to 1.5 nm in diameter) of mRNA that is attached to

each ribosome of the polyribosome near the junction between the small and large subunits. *Transfer ribonucleic acid (tRNA)* deciphers the genetic code and transfers the amino acid specified by the code to the growing peptide chain. Ribosomes have binding sites for both mRNA and tRNA and function to combine these molecules together in the proper orientation. *Ribosomes are also equipped with enzymes essential for peptide bond formation and peptide chain elongation.* Once in the cytoplasm, the assembled and functional ribosome is ready to translate the genetic message from mRNA to protein.

ROUGH-SURFACED (GRANULAR) ENDOPLASMIC RETICULUM (rER)

The rough-surfaced endoplasmic reticulum (rER) consists of a system of membranous lamellae or tubules that usually occupy the basal portion of a structurally polarized cell (Fig. 2.22). The membranes enclose a compartment, or *cisterna*, which may be small or expanded and filled with the newly synthesized protein (Fig. 2.23). Ribosomes transiently attach to the outer surface of the

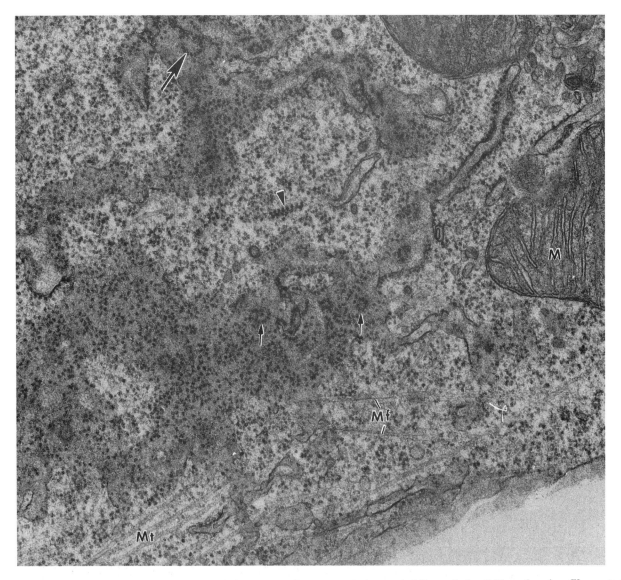

Figure 2.20. TEM of cultured cell illustrates polyribosomes that are both free in the cytosol (arrowheads) and observed en face where they are attached to membranes of the ER. (arrows). Microtubules (Mt), actin microfilaments (Mf), and mitochondria (M) are identified. ×52,000.

membranes by proteinaceous receptors called *ribophorins.* The rER is abundant in cells synthesizing protein for export.

Proteins that will be incorporated into the plasma membrane or that become functional in the Golgi, rER, or lysosome are synthesized by ribosomes on the rER. Amino acids in the bloodstream traverse the capillary endothelium and basal lamina, enter the base of the cell by active transport, and become associated with a polyribosome. Protein synthesis for export is actually initiated on free polyribosomes. The mRNA that codes for the protein to be synthesized in the rER includes an initial N-terminal sequence of bases at the 5′ end that codes for the *signal sequence* approximately 20–25 principally hydrophobic amino acids (Fig. 2.24). The signal sequence, plus a group of six different polypeptides and 7S RNA molecules, comprise a *signal recognition particle* (*SRP*) that then binds to a receptor called a *docking protein* in the rER membrane. The SRP inhibits further polypeptide elongation until the SRP-ribosome complex binds to the docking protein. When the SRP-ribosome complex has docked, the SRP, including the signal sequence, is enzymatically clipped off in the ER cisterna by a signal peptidase, and polypeptide chain elongation resumes (Fig. 2.24). As the SRP docks to the ER membrane, a *ribosome receptor* also located in the ER membrane binds to the large ribosomal subunit. The ribosome receptor consists of two integral membrane proteins, called *ribophorin I* and *ribophorin II*, located in the rER membrane. These events result in the formation of a minute pore in the rER membrane that permits the nascent polypeptide to enter the cisterna (Fig. 2.24).

In an area where the rER and the Golgi complex are closely related, ribosomes are lost on the ER adja-

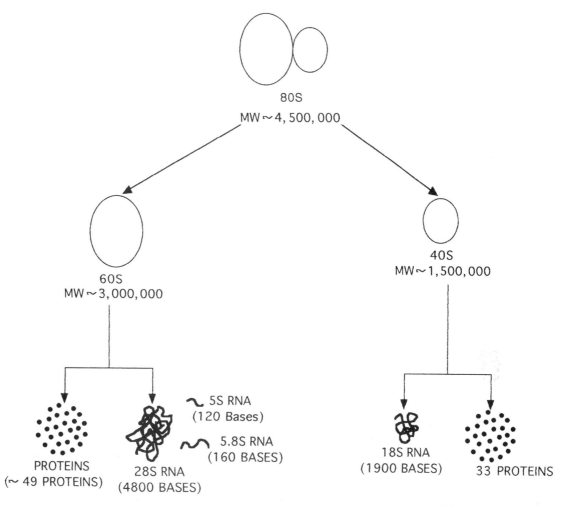

Figure 2.21. Diagram illustrates the constituents of a eukaryotic polyribosome.

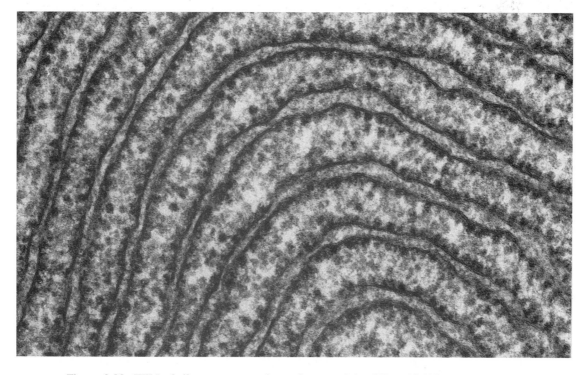

Figure 2.22. TEM of ribosome-covered membranes of the rER. ×90,000.

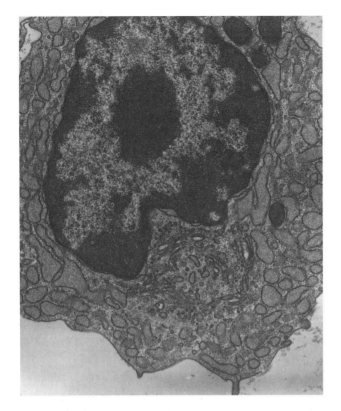

Figure 2.23. TEM of an antibody-producing plasma cell. Note that large quantities of rER cisternae are dilated with a finely granular product that represents newly synthesized antibody (protein). ×12,700.

tion vesicles involves the assembly of coat proteins. Transport of substances from the Golgi complex back to the rER can also occur. Thus, ER-resident proteins that escape to the cis Golgi network are returned to the ER by vesicular transport along microtubules.

FUNCTIONS

In addition to protein synthesis, the rER segregates the proteins for export from those that are to be used inside the cell. Multichain proteins are assembled in the rER, and posttranslational modifications of amino acids can also occur. Enzymatic clipping of the signal peptide occurs in the cisternae of the rER. The rER can function in lipid and phospholipid synthesis. Initial glycosylation of glycoproteins (N-linked oligosaccharides) occurs in the rER. It is known that a single species of oligosaccharide composed of *N-acetylglucosamine, mannose* and *glucose* (containing a total of 14 sugar residues) is *transferred* to *proteins* in the *cisternae* of the *ER*. Since they are transferred to the NH_2 *group* on the side chain of an asparagine residue of the protein, the oligosaccharide is said to be *N-linked or asparagine-linked*. The two broad classes of N-linked oligosaccharides, the *complex oligosaccharides* and *high mannose oligosaccharides*, are found in mature glycoproteins. Most membrane lipid bilayers are assembled in the ER, which produces nearly all of the lipids needed for cell membranes, including phospholipids and cholesterol. The synthesis of the major phospholipid, *phosphatidylcholine*, is catalyzed by enzymes in the ER membrane that have their active sites facing the cytoplasm, where all necessary metabolites are found.

cent to the Golgi complex. Proteins that are correctly folded and assembled in the rER are budded from the rER in transition vesicles that are delivered to the adjacent cis Golgi network. Budding of transport or transi-

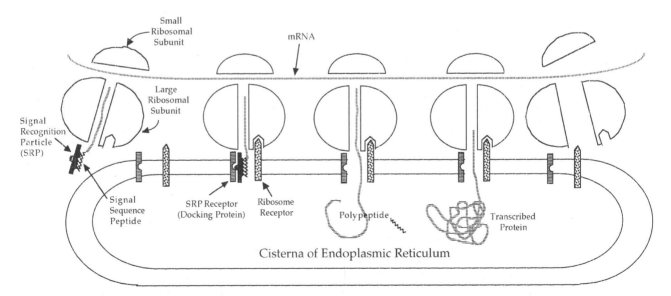

Figure 2.24. Diagram illustrates ribosome docking to ER membrane and protein translocation into ER cisterna. (Redrawn and modified from L.C. Junqueira, J. Carneiro, **and R.O. Kelley. *Basic Histology.* 7th ed. Appleton & Lange, East Norwalk, CT, ©1992 with permission) See text for additional details.**

SMOOTH (AGRANULAR) ENDOPLASMIC RETICULUM (sER)

The sER commonly takes the form of tubular and vesicular profiles in thin sections of cells examined by the TEM. The sER is an elaborate membranous lattice in which a vast array of enzymes are maintained in orderly spatial arrangement. Continuity of the rER and sER can be observed in liver cells (Fig. 2.25), and biochemical evidence suggests that the rER forms the sER. The sER is not involved in protein synthesis but is active in the *synthesis* of all classes of *lipids*, including *cholesterol, phospholipids, triglycerides,* and *steroid hormones.* In the liver, the sER contains *oxidative enzymes* involved in the *metabolism* of *lipid-soluble drugs* (e.g., phenobarbital). The sER is located in regions of the liver cell that contain extensive amounts of glycogen, and the sER appears to contain *glucose-6-phosphatase,* an enzyme that is involved in the utilization of glycogen. Glycogen that is stored in hepatocytes may be degrated to glucose, which leaves the liver cell for distribution throughout the body. Enzymes located in hepatic sER convert *water-insoluble intoxicants* into hydrophilic molecules that are easily excreted by the kidney. The sER in some cells contains enzymes involved in the *biosynthesis* of *steroids* (e.g., testosterone in the interstitial cells of Leydig in the testis).

Monoglycerides and fatty acids that result from digestion of lipids in the lumen of the digestive tract are taken into the intestinal absorptive cells, synthesized into triglycerides in the sER, and released at the base of the cells into the capillaries. The enzyme *fatty acid coenzyme A ligase* is present in the sER in the intestinal epithelial cells and is important in triglyceride synthesis.

GOLGI APPARATUS

The Golgi complex was first demonstrated by Camillo Golgi near the turn of the nineteenth century. Golgi noted that when neurons of the barn owl were impregnated with silver salts and histologic sections were then made, a fine reticular appearance was evident in the cytoplasm of the neuron. This "internal reticular apparatus" noted by Golgi now bears his name. The Golgi complex is located between the nucleus and the free or apical end of polarized secretory cells.

The Golgi complex consists of flattened or saucer-shaped, membranous sacs called *Golgi saccules.* The saccules are stacked and vary in number, usually ranging from 4 to 12. Some of the saccules at the top and bottom of the stack have perforations called *fenestrations.* The constituents of a stack of Golgi membranes or saccules include the cis Golgi network (adjacent to the ER), cis Golgi saccule, medial Golgi saccule, trans Golgi saccule, and trans Golgi network (TGN, adjacent to forming secretory vesicles). Each stack has a *forming face,* also

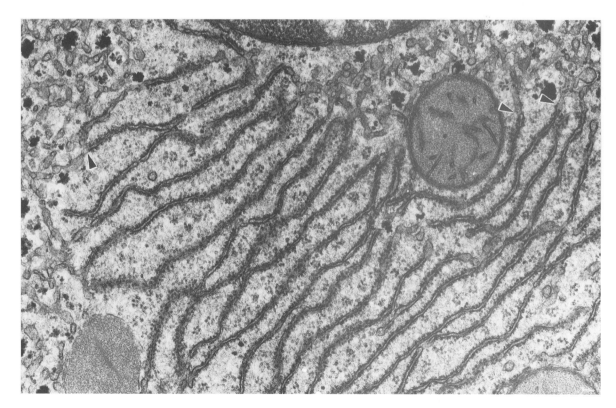

Figure 2.25. Portion of hepatocyte illustrating both sER and rER, which appear to be continuous at arrowheads. ×30,000.

called *cis* (near) *face*, which is usually convex in shape (Fig. 2.26). This is the side that receives newly synthesized protein via transition vesicles from the rER. The opposite side or face of the stack is called the *maturing* or *trans* (beyond) *face* and is typically concave (Fig. 2.26). Many rounded, membranous vesicles, the *Golgi*

vesicles, are also part of the Golgi complex (Fig. 2.27). Extensive membrane trafficking occurs between donor and target compartments inside cells. SNARE's are receptor molecules involved in the fusion of transport vesicles to target membrane. Transport vesicles contain surface markers, called v-SNAREs, that permit them to

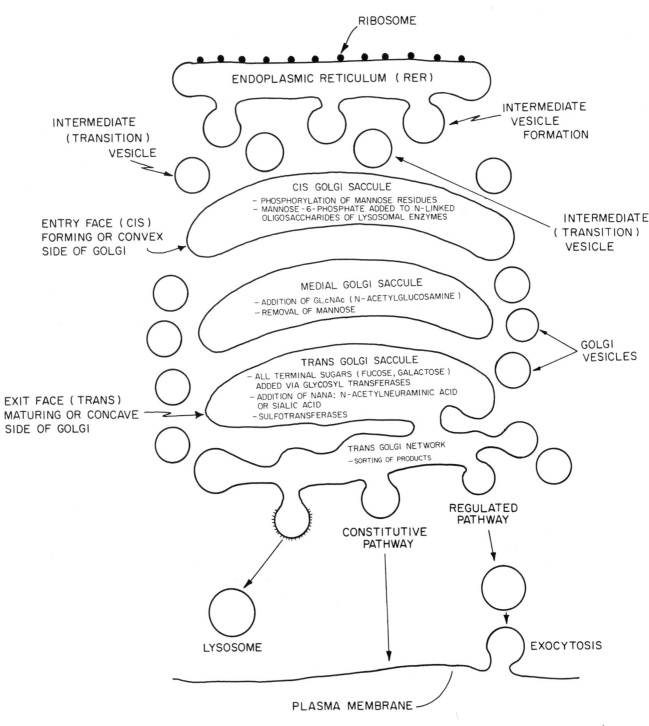

Figure 2.26. Diagram of Golgi complex and adjacent endoplasmic reticulum. Product is shuttled from rER to the cis (entry) face of the Golgi. Product moves sequentially from cis, to trans, to medial saccules, and finally to the trans Golgi network, where it may be released in membrane-bound secretion bodies of lysosomes or as secretion granules involved in regulated and constitutive secretion. The major enzymes and events that occur in each of the Golgi saccules are also indicated.

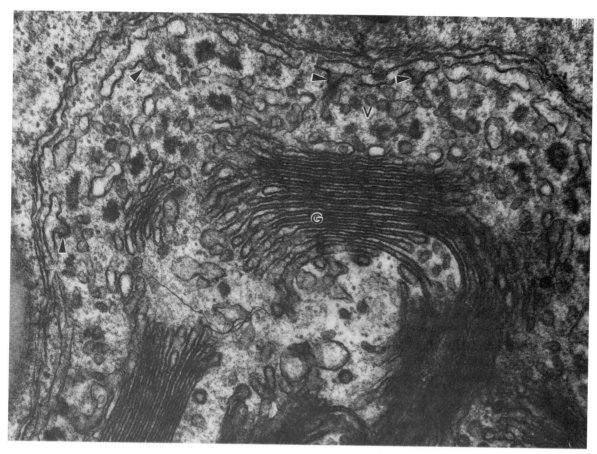

Figure 2.27. TEM of Golgi complex with Golgi saccules (G) and Golgi vesicles (V). Note the expanded regions of the ER (arrowheads), which represent a stage in the forma- **tion of intermediate vesicles (V) near the cis Golgi saccules. ×50,000.**

recognize appropriate receptors, called *t-SNAREs*, on target membranes. *Coatomer-coated vesicles* are involved in vesicular transport from the ER to the Golgi apparatus through successive Golgi saccules and from the trans Golgi network to the plasma membrane. The coatomer coats consist of seven individual coat-protein subunits called *COPs*. Coatomer coats do not self-assemble and require ATP for their formation. Both the assembly and disassembly of the coatomer coat depend on *ADP-ribosylation factor (ARF)*, one of many guanosine triphosphate (GTP)-binding proteins involved in the control of vesicular transport. A group of monomeric proteins (guanosine triphosphatases, GTPases) called *Rab proteins* are thought to play an important role in the specificity of fit between the v-SNARE and the corresponding t-SNARE, thus ensuring that the correct vesicle fuses with the appropriate target membrane. Many types of Rab proteins are present in cells, and each is involved in specific intracellular membrane trafficking. For example, Rab 1 and Rab 2 are involved in transport from the ER to the Golgi complex.

Three major classes of proteins synthesized by the rER pass through the Golgi complex for processing and sorting: secretory proteins, membrane proteins, and

lysosomal enzymes. Of the proteins that pass through the Golgi complex, nearly all are *aspargine linked (N-linked) glycoproteins*. Initial steps in glycosylation begin in the rER, but the process is not completed until inside the Golgi, for the Golgi membranes contain enzymes, called *glycosyltransferases*, necessary for final incorporation of sugars into glycoprotein (Fig. 2.26). In addition, *sulfotransferases* that sulfate secretory products are located in the Golgi complex. The Golgi complex is capable of "sorting" various secretory products, including those for *secretory granules, lysosomal enzymes,* and *cell membrane* glycoproteins; the Golgi apparatus thus receives newly synthesized proteins and lipids from the ER and distributes them to the plasma membrane, lysosomes, and secretory granules. Thiamine pyrophosphatase is a marker enzyme for the Golgi complex; ultrastructural localization of the reaction product for this enzyme is illustrated in the trans Golgi saccule and its network in Figure 2.28.

N-linked oligosaccharides on proteins are often trimmed by removal of mannose residues, and additional sugars (including *N-acetylglucosamine, galactose, fucose,* and *sialic acid residues*) are added. Some proteins have sugars added to selected *serine* or *threonine* side

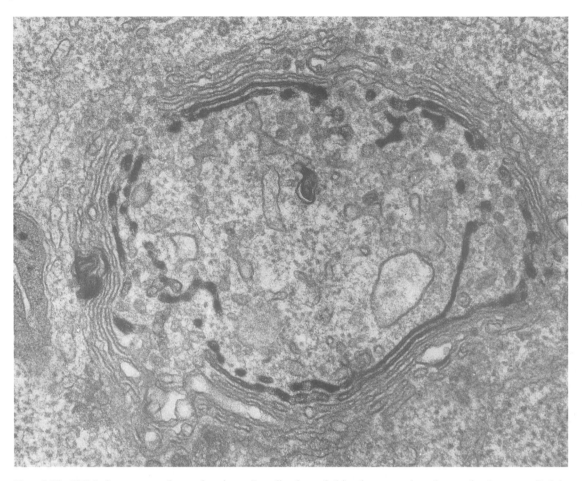

Figs. 2.28. TEM-ultrastructural cytochemistry. Localization of thiamine pyrophosphatase in the trans Golgi saccule and network is shown. ×50,000.

chains, and this *O-linked glycosylation* is catalyzed by a series of *glycosyl transferase* enzymes in the Golgi compartments. The conversion of proteoglycan core proteins to proteoglycans also occurs in the Golgi apparatus. *Sulfation of sugars* in proteoglycans and of certain tyrosines on proteins occurs in a late Golgi compartment. It is known that different saccules in a stack have different enzymes and receptors associated with them. For example, extra mannose residues are cleaved from oligosaccharide chains of glycoprotein precursors synthesized in the rER. *N-acetylglucosamine* is usually added to macromolecules in the central or *medial saccules*. Furthermore, terminal sugars such as *sialic acid* and *galactose* are added to products in the *trans Golgi saccules*. One important question is: how are secretory products for lysosomes and secretory granules separated? Lysosomal enzymes are sorted in the Golgi apparatus by a membrane-bound receptor protein that recognizes mannose-6-phosphate. Lysosomal hydrolases contain N-linked oligosaccharides that are processed in a unique way in the cis Golgi saccules so that their *mannose residues are phosphorylated.* The *mannose-6-phosphate (M6P) groups* are thus added exclusively to N-linked oligosaccharides of soluble lysosomal enzymes. M6P receptor proteins clus-

ter in the membrane of the *TGN* and become concentrated in clathrin-coated vesicles budding from the TGN (see Fig. 2.33). The receptor proteins bind the lysosomal enzymes, separate them from other proteins present, and concentrate them in coated vesicles. The vesicles lose their coats and fuse with an endolysosome (see Fig. 2.33). The M6P receptor shuttles back and forth between specific membranes. The acidification of an endosome by an ATP-dependent proton pump releases the ligand from receptor, which is then sorted (see Fig. 2.33).

LYSOSOMES

Lysosomes are membrane-bound organelles with an interior structure that varies with the organelle's physiologic state. (Figs. 2.29–2.31). Lysosomes play a variety of important roles, all involving *intracellular digestion*. Some *36 acid hydrolases* have been found in lysosomes (Fig. 2.32). Lysosomal enzymes function at acid pH, which is produced by proton pumps located in the lysosomal membrane (Fig. 2.32). Lysosomal enzymes are synthesized and packaged by the coparticipation of the ER and the Golgi apparatus and are diverted from the secretory pathway in the *TGN*. Small, membranous vesicles containing lysomal enzymes that bud from the Golgi saccules are called *primary lysosomes*. The mechanism by which lysosomal enzymes are targeted to vesicles that form from the TGN is reviewed in Figure 2.33. Cyto-

chemical tests for such lysosomal enzymes as acid phosphatase and aryl sulfatase are used to positively identify a lysosome.

Lysosomes function in the hydrolysis of exogenous macromolecules (called *heterophagy*). A bacterium ingested by a neutrophil by phagocytosis (heterophagy)

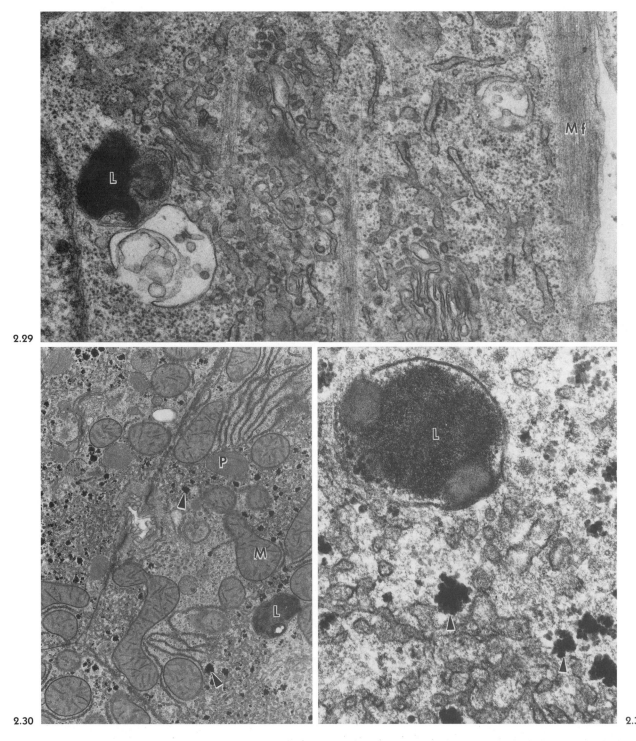

2.29

2.30

2.31

Figures 2.29–2.31. All figures are TEM of lysosomes (L) (digestive vacuoles or heterolysosomes). They appear electron dense, and the interior is heterogeneous. Actin microfilaments (Mf) of stress fiber are illustrated in Figure

2.29. Mitochondria (M) and a peroxisome (P) are identified in the hepatocyte in Figure 2.30. Glycogen deposits are denoted by arrowheads in Figures 2.30 and 2.31. Figure 2.29, ×31,000; Figure 2.30, ×17,715; Figure 2.31, ×59,650.

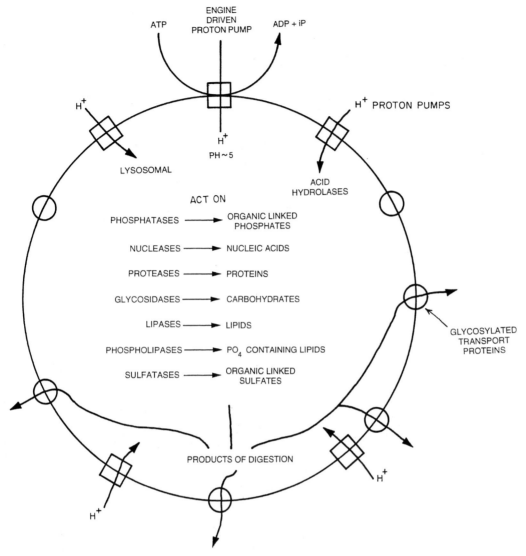

Figure 2.32. Diagram of a lysosome summarizes important events occurring in the limiting membrane and the kinds of acid hydrolases that can be present inside a lysosome.

is enclosed by a membrane and is called a *phagosome*. A lysosome containing acid hydrolases then fuses with the phagosome membrane, and digestion begins. This structure is called a *secondary lysosome, digestive vacuole, heterolysosome,* or *heterophagosome*. If the bacterium is completely digested, the soluble products enter the cell cytoplasm. In many cases, however, not all contents can be digested. In such cases, the resulting structure is called a *residual body*. It is either expelled from the cell

(exocytosis) or in some cases remains in the cell, where the residual body contents slowly transform into an "aging pigment" (also called *lipofuscin pigment*). Lysosomes can also fuse with vesicles, called *endosomes*, formed by micropinocytosis; the material incorporated into the cell by this means is also hydrolyzed. When a receptor-ligand complex is internalized, one of the first events is the uncoupling of the receptor from the ligand and the return of the receptor to the plasma membrane. The

Figure 2.33. Lysosomal precursor enzymes have mannose residues added in the rER and are transported to the cis Golgi network, where mannose-6-phosphate (M-6-P) is added. M-6-P is transported through Golgi saccules to the trans Golgi network, from where it attaches to M-6-P receptors and is budded into clathrin-coated vesicles. Clathrin coats are removed, and the vesicle fuses with a late endosome. Here the phosphate is removed, and M-6-P receptors are recycled in vesicles to trans Golgi network for reuse. Redrawn and modified from B. Alberts, D. Bray, J. Lewis, M. Raff, K. Roberts, and J. Watson. *Molecular Biology of the Cell*, 3rd ed., p. 615, Garland Publishing, New York, 1994, with permission)

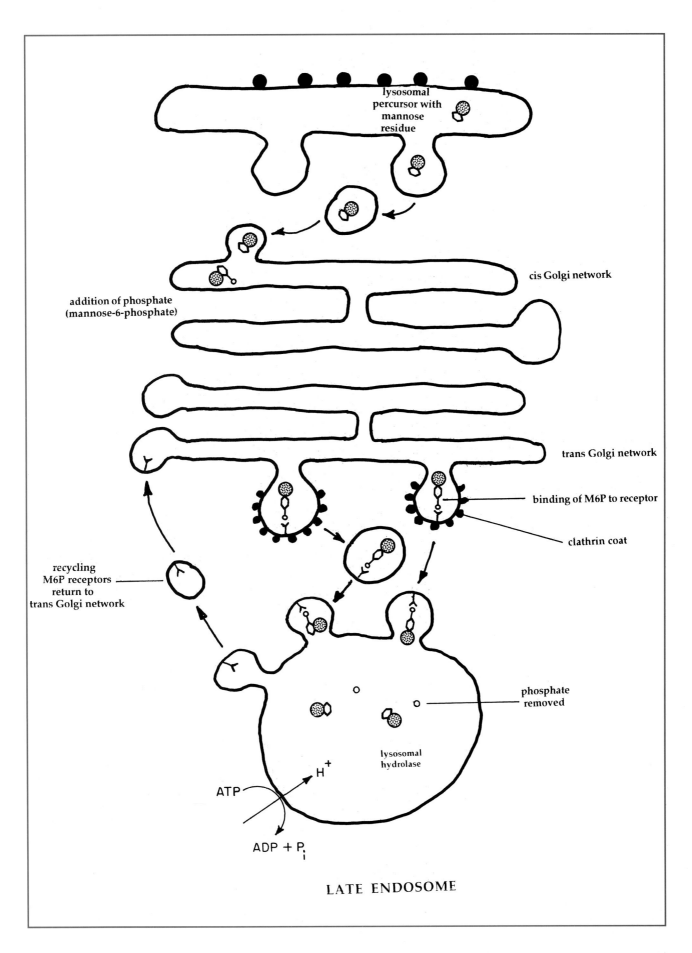

lysosomal
percursor with
mannose
residue

cis Golgi network

addition of phosphate
(mannose-6-phosphate)

trans Golgi network

binding of M6P to receptor

clathrin coat

recycling
M6P receptors
return to
trans Golgi network

phosphate
removed

lysosomal
hydrolase

ATP

H$^+$

ADP + P$_i$

LATE ENDOSOME

uncoupling occurs by the *acidification* of the vesicle by a *proton pump* in the limiting membrane. The ligand is then delivered to the lysosome.

Lysosomes have other functions; for example, organelles are not immortal and in some manner are recognized by the cell as requiring removal. The organelle to be digested is enclosed by a membrane and fuses with a lysosome, and the digestive process commences. The process by which lysosomes participate in the hydrolysis of endogeneous macromolecues is called *autophagy*.

Many lysosomal diseases are known; one, called *Pompe's disease*, occurs when a lysosomal enzyme normally present in liver cell lysosomes is absent. This enzyme is normally involved in the degradation of glycogen; thus, abnormal amounts of glycogen accumulate in liver cells. In *Tay-Sachs disease*, a lysosomal enzyme that digests a galactoside in nerve cells is lacking. As a result, residual bodies accumulate in the neuron and interfere with its function.

PEROXISOMES

Peroxisomes are membrane-bound organelles approximately 0.5–1 μm in diameter (Fig. 2.30). They were initially observed in liver and kidney cells in the 1950s with the TEM and were initially called *microbodies*. Peroxisomes can be isolated by centrifugation methods, and cytochemical techniques are available for visualizing them in the TEM. The peroxisome's interior may be finely granular and homogeneous or a central *nucleoid* may be present. The matrix surrounds the nucleoid if one is present. The central nucleoid may have a crystalline organization. Peroxisomes originate by budding from the rER. In isolated liver and kidney, several enzymes have been identified: *urate oxidase, d-amino acid oxidase,* and *α-hydroxy-acid oxidase* are enzymes involved in the production of hydrogen peroxide. Another enzyme, *catalase*, is involved in the destruction or *hydrolysis of hydrogen peroxide* and is located in the matrix. Catalase has a protective function since hydrogen peroxide is extremely toxic to cells. Peroxisomes in the liver and kidney play a role in the *breakdown of purines*; urate oxidase is the peroxisomal enzyme that appears to be involved. Purines are nitrogen-containing organic compounds such as adenine and guanine bases of nucleic acids. In plant cells, peroxisomes may play a role in converting *fat to carbohydrate*; hence the organelle is called a *glyoxysome*.

In a peroxisomal disease called *adrenoleukodystrophy*, the β-oxidation of fatty acids is impaired, resulting in abnormal lipid storage in the brain, spinal cord, and adrenal glands. This condition can result in dementia and adrenal failure.

CENTRIOLES

Although some centrioles can be observed in the LM as small, dark-staining spots near the nucleus (juxtanuclear) when stained with Heidenhain's iron hematoxylin, their structural organization was not known until the advent of the TEM. The cytoplasm containing the centrioles is called the *centrosome* or *centrosphere* (cell center). The *centrosome* is located adjacent to the nucleus and contains a pair of centrioles arranged at right angles to each other. The *centrosome* is a *major microtubule-organizing center* (*MTOC*), but not all MTOCs contain centrioles. Further, the microtubules are not *directly* nucleated by a centriole, but rather by diffuse, amorphous material of medium electron density surrounding the centriole. The *centrosome* thus includes a *centriole* and *pericentriolar material* (Fig. 2.34); although the composition of the amorphous, diffuse pericentriolar material is unknown, it does contain proteins that are similar in both plants and animal cells. The (−) ends of the microtubules are anchored in the centrosome. The (+) end can be stabilized if capped to prevent depolymerization; otherwise, if not capped, the microtubule will disassemble. The centrosome (MTOC) continually nucleates formation of new microtubules. The properties of cy-

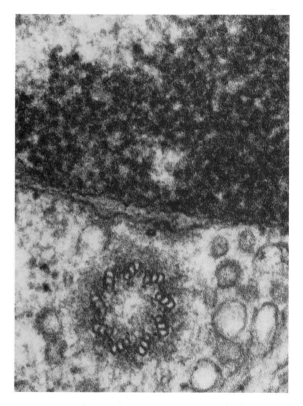

Figure 2.34. A centriole sectioned transversely displays the nine triplet tubules. A diffuse, electron-dense matrix surrounds the centriole, which is located next to the nucleus. ×100,000.

toplasmic microtubules are modified by microtubule-associated proteins (MAPs), which stabilize microtubules against disassembly and mediate their interaction with other cell components.

Centrioles are about 0.15–0.20 μm (150–200 nm) in diameter; they are usually longer than they are wide. Centrioles range from 300 to 500 nm in length. Animal (eukaryotic) cells typically contain a pair of centrioles oriented at right angles or perpendicular to each other. They are typically located in a juxtanuclear position. Although centrioles overall have the shape of a barrel or cylinder, they are open at their ends. Furthermore, the wall of the cylinder is incomplete since it is composed of nine groups of *triplet microtubules* (Fig. 2.34). The nine triplet microtubules can be discerned clearly only in a transverse section of the centriole; each tubule is about 25 nm in diameter. The tubules have also been called *subfibers*. Only one of the three triplet tubules has a complete wall. The other two tubules share part of the wall of the adjacent tubule. A lettering system has been devised to refer to the three members of the triplet microtubules of the centriole wall. The innermost tubule, which has a complete wall, is referred to as the *A subfiber* or *tubule*. The middle element is called the *B subfiber* or *tubule*, and the outermost member of the triplet is called the *C subfiber* or *tubule*. The triplet tubules are positioned at about 30° with respect to each other. Centrioles are structurally identical to the basal bodies of cilia and flagella.

The origin of centrioles is not completely understood; there is evidence that the centriole can arise de novo, but in other cells, new centrioles arise in close proximity to a preexisiting centriole. Centrioles divide in S phase. The process begins with the formation of a *procentriole* at right angles to each of the original centrioles. Initially, only a diffuse, amorphous material called the *procentriolar material* is evident. Nine single tubules are initially present in the procentriole but an additional pair forms in close relation to each of the nine original tubules, resulting in the characteristic nine triplet microtubules. After centriolar division, the two pairs of centrioles move to opposite poles and serve as the organizing centers for the mitotic spindle microtubules. The centrioles and adjacent procentriolar material constitute an *MTOC* for both the mitotic and interphase cells. While centrioles clearly exert a profound influence on the organization of the spindle apparatus during mitosis, they are not essential for spindle formation or division, since spindles can form in cells that lack centrioles.

BASAL BODIES

Basal bodies are attached to the proximal end of both cilia and flagella (Figs. 2.35, 2.36). Both cilia and fla-gella grow from centrioles that have migrated to the peripheral cytoplasm or adjacent to the plasma membrane. While new centrioles form at the proximal end of the centriole, the outgrowth of cilia or flagella occurs at the distal end only. The proximal end of the cylindrical basal body in some cells is connected to a *striated rootlet* that extends for a considerable distance into the cytoplasm. The striated basal body rootlets are not present in all ciliated cells, and they may be involved in anchoring the basal body-cilium complex into the cell.

CILIA AND FLAGELLA

Cilia and flagella are structurally quite similar, but flagella are considerably longer. Cilia are usually 5–10 μm long and may be quite numerous on a cell, as SEM images demonstrate (Fig. 2.38). Both cilia and flagella hydrolyze ATP to power their movement; cilia exhibit a whiplike power stroke, whereas flagella generate waves that originate at the base and progress toward the tip.

In the TEM, transverse sections of cilia or flagella reveal *nine peripheral* or outer *doublet microtubules* and two central microtubules (Figs. 2.37, 2.39). The peripheral doublet microtubules are actually continuous with two of the three microtubules in the connected basal body. Doublet microtubules comprise the periphery of cilia and flagella; tubule A has a complete wall, while tubule B is incomplete. Cilia and flagella microtubules consist of the protein called *tubulin*. Tubulin dimers of the microtubules make up *protofilaments*, which, in turn, comprise the subfibers or tubules of cilia and flagella. There are 13 protofilaments in each microtubule (Fig. 2.39).

Two thin hooks or fibers extend from each A tubule in the nine doublets of the cilium or flagellum (Fig. 2.39). These "arms" or "side arms" have been found to contain *dynein*. Dynein is a large protein consisting of 9–12 polypeptide chains. It is well known that ciliary and flagellar motion requires an energy source in the form of ATP. The energy is freed by the ATPase present in the dynein arms. The base of the dynein binds to the A tubule in an ATP-independent manner, but the globular dynein heads have an ATP-dependent binding site for the B microtubule. As ATP is hydrolyzed at the dynein head, movement toward the minus end of the B microtubule occurs, producing a sliding force between adjacent microtubule doublets. Actually, this protein is a *magnesium-activated ATPase*.

The two central microtubules in the cilium or flagellum are surrounded by a series of circular "hoops" called a *central sheath*. Thin structures called *radial spokes* also extend from each A tubule of the nine peripheral doublets toward the central sheath, where the spoke enlarges slightly to form the *spoke head* (Fig. 2.39). ATPase activity also resides in the spoke heads. Still another protein, *nexin*, is present in the filamentous structures in-

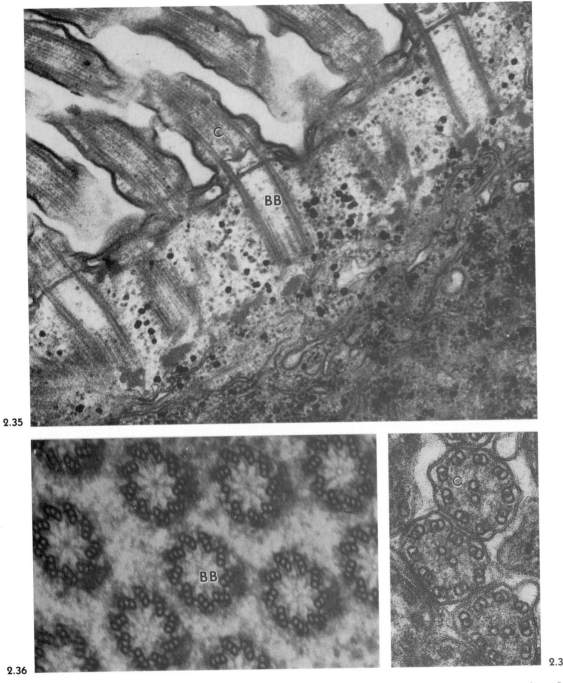

2.35

2.36

2.37

Figures 2.35–2.37. Longitudinal section of cilia (C) and basal bodies (BB). Transverse sections of basal bodies are shown in Figure 2.36. Transverse section of cilia is shown in Figure 2.37.

terconnecting the adjacent peripheral doublets. The nexin-containing links extend from tubule A of one doublet to tubule B of the next. The radial spokes extend from tubule A of each doublet to the central sheath.

ATP is the energy source for ciliary movement, and the frequency of the ciliary beat is proportional to the ATP concentration. The ATP is hydrolyzed by the ATPase in the cilium or flagellum, releasing energy re-

quired for the microtubule sliding. The movement of a cilium or flagellum involves microtubule sliding resembling the sliding of filaments in muscle contraction (see Chapter 11). The peripheral ciliary doublets slide past each other without contracting or shortening. During ATP hydrolysis, the dyneins "walk" along the adjacent B subfibers, and the radial links or spokes serve to convert the sliding of the microtubules into a bending of the axoneme.

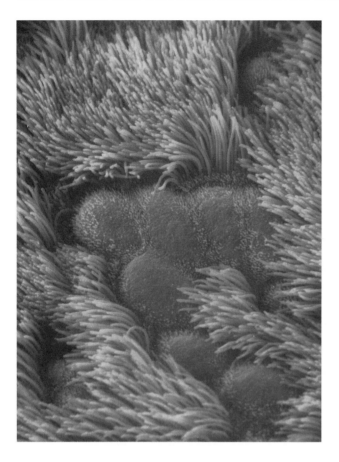

Figure 2.38. SEM of cilia. ×3100.

CYTOSKELETON

CYTOPLASMIC MICROTUBULES

Cytoplasmic microtubules are widely distributed throughout the cytoplasm. They are also used in the construction of centrioles, basal bodies, cilia, and flagella. Cytoplasmic *microtubules* are involved in *cell shape* changes, *guiding intracellular movements*, in *chromosome movements*, and in *movement* of *cilia* and *flagella*. Each microtubule is approximately *250 Å* (25 nm) in diameter but usually several micrometers in length (Figs. 2.40, 2.41). Microtubules are composed of globular protein subunits arranged as a helical wall of approximately 13 subunits. The subunits are *dimers* of a protein called *tubulin*. Assembly from tubulin dimers (α-tubulin and β-tubulin) is influenced by several structures including centrioles, basal bodies, and kinetochores. Microtubules are especially abundant in elongated cells and in the highly elongated appendages of cells; examples include axons and dendrites, axopod pseudopods in the protozoan *Actinosphaerium*, and the long cytoplasmic extensions of the melanocyte or erythrophores of fish scales. In these movements, molecular motors, such as the ATPase *dynein*, power structures along the microtubules, and the motor is fueled by *ATP hydrolysis*. Thus, in cells treated with drugs that disrupt their microtubules, mitosis is arrested, chromosomes cannot move, secretory granules cannot move to the cell surface to be exported,

Figure 2.39. Diagram illustrates the internal organization of a cilium, as seen in transverse section.

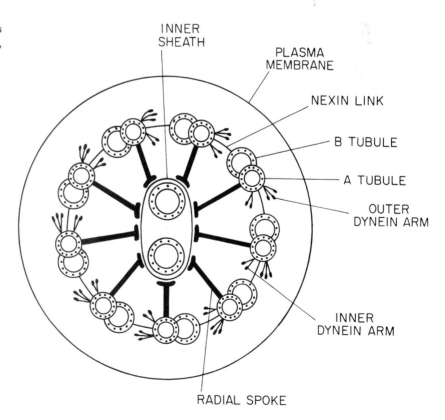

INNER SHEATH

PLASMA MEMBRANE

NEXIN LINK

B TUBULE

A TUBULE

OUTER DYNEIN ARM

INNER DYNEIN ARM

RADIAL SPOKE

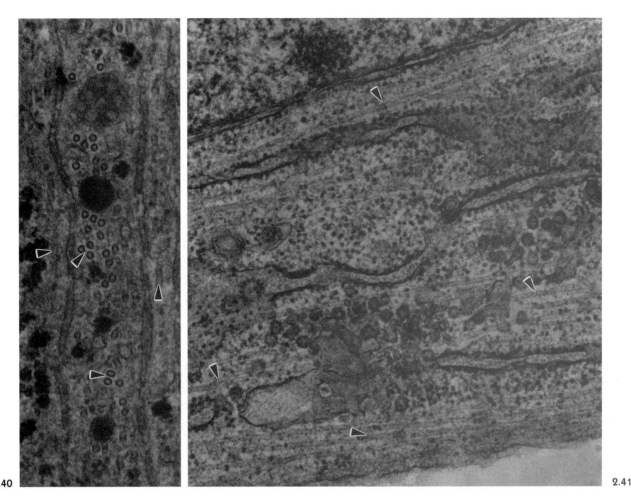

2.40

2.41

Figures 2.40, 2.41. TEM illustrates cytoplasmic microtubules (arrowheads) in longitudinal section and transverse section. ×62,250.

and the outgrowth of an axon is stopped. Microtubules are also involved in the movement of organelles in the cytoplasm. The staining of cells with immunofluorescent antibodies to tubulin conveniently displays the intracellular distribution of microtubules.

Calcium tends to inhibit tubulin polymerization in vitro. Microtubules tend to *disassemble* in the *cold* (5°C). *Hydrostatic pressure* also causes microtubule disassembly. A number of substances called *antitubulins* cause microtubule disassembly, including *colchicine, vinblastine, podophyllotoxin,* and *griseofulvine.* When cAMP is added to a container of cultured epithelial cells, the cells become elongated and fibroblastic in shape due to the assembly and orientation of microtubules in the cytoplasm. *Guanosine triphosphate (GTP)* and *magnesium ions* are important for *microtubule polymerization.* Thus, *phosphorylation* of the *tubulin monomers* in the cell by a *cAMP-dependent kinase* causes *formation* of the *microtubules.* *Taxol* is a drug that *stabilizes microtubules,* preventing further polymerization or disassembly.

Microtubules possess inherent polarity because

tubulin subunits have a specific orientation; thus, microtubules have a plus (+) end and a minus (−) end (Fig. 2.42). The fast-growing end of a microtubule is the (+) end. The (−) end of a microtubule is associated with *MTOCs.* Most microtubules grow from a centrosome (centriole) that acts as an MTOC, continually nucleating new microtubules that grow in random directions. Capping of the free (+) end stabilizes the microtubule. The transport of organelles in an axon is guided by microtubules. *Kinesin* is an *ATPase* that uses energy from ATP hydrolysis to *move vesicles* to the (+) end of microtubules in axons. In contrast, cytoplasmic *dynein* (also an ATPase) provides energy to propel *vesicles* in a *retrograde* direction, that is to the (−) end of microtubules in axons. Dynein and kinesin are examples of MAPs. MAP1C is cytoplasmic dynein that powers transport along microtubules from a nerve ending back to the cell body (retrograde transport). Kinesin is a MAP that moves particles along microtubules in a direction opposite to that of MAP1C.

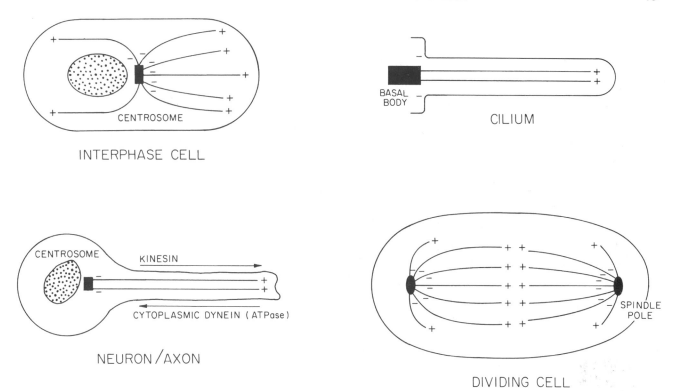

Figure 2.42. Diagram illustrates the ends of microtubules that add subunits (+) and lose subunits (−).

CYTOPLASMIC FILAMENTS

The cytoskeleton of the eukaryotic nonmuscle cell consists of four proteinaceous filament systems (actin microfilaments, intermediate filaments, microtubules, and nonmuscle myosin) that, as a dynamic intracellular system, provide for cell shape, internal organization, and motility. Some filaments play a role in cell movements and are thus contractile (e.g., actin and myosin), while some of the intermediate filaments serve a supportive function. Thus, the cytoplasmic filaments differ in their size, chemical composition and function (see the accompanying table).

Cytoskeletal Component	Approximate Diameter
Microfilaments (actin)	6–7 nm
Intermediate filaments	10–12 nm
Myosin filaments	16 nm
Microtubules	25 nm

MICROFILAMENTS

Actin-containing microfilament networks function in cell locomotion, attachment and spreading, maintenance of cell shape, and cytokinesis. Slender actin filaments are only about 7 nm in diameter, but they may

be quite long (Figs. 2.43, 2.44). Actin is located throughout the cell but is especially concentrated in a network located just inside the cell membrane, where it is a component of the *cell cortex*, a region that gives mechanical strength to the surface and permits the cell to change shape and move. Actin filaments also occur throughout the cytoplasm as *stress fibers* (Fig. 2.45). Actin microfilaments are present in *microvilli* and in motile cellular appendages such as *ruffles* or *lamellipodia*. Actin filaments form a *contractile* band or *ring* in the *cleavage furrow* and aid in constricting one cell into two during cytokinesis.

The degree to which microfilaments are organized into networks, as well as their polymerization into bundles of contractile elements, is facilitated by various actin-binding proteins. Actin filaments are linked together in a three-dimensional network by cross-linking proteins. One abundant cross-linking protein is *filamin*. Another protein, called *gelsolin*, serves to fragment actin filaments when gelsolin is activated by calcium ions. While actin, filamin, and gelsolin can undergo calcium-dependent transitions from a more firm gel to a more fluid sol, movement as in cytoplasmic streaming does not occur unless actin interacts with myosin.

The presence of actin filament bundles can be easily discerned when cells are stained with *actin antibody* using *immunofluorescent* techniques. Bundles of actin filaments can bind to the plasma membrane in a way that permits them to pull on the extracellular matrix (substratum) such as focal contacts of adhesion plaques. Many cells extend dynamic actin-containing mi-

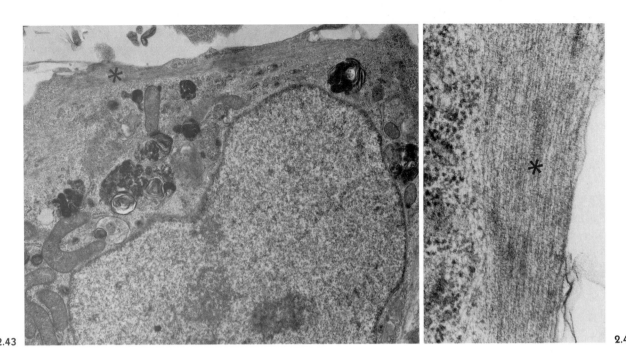

2.43   2.44

Figures 2.43, 2.44. TEM of cultured chick limb bud mesenchyme cell. The actin microfilaments of a stress fiber are denoted (*). Figure 2.43, ×9750; Figure 2.44, ×62,250.

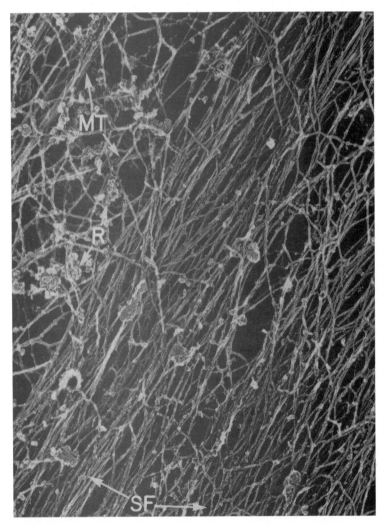

Figure 2.45. TEM of platinum replica of fibroblast cytoskeleton prepared by quick freezing and deep etching. Fibroblast was immersed in detergent to remove soluble cytoplasmic proteins and membranes. Actin microfilaments in stress fibers (SF), thicker microtubules (MT), and a more diffuse meshwork of filaments with clusters thought to be ribosomes (R) are illustrated. (Reproduced from J.E. Heuser and M. Kirschner, The *Journal of Cell Biology*, 1980, 86, 212 by copyright permission of The Rockefeller University Press)

crospikes and lamellipodia from their surface. Actin-containing extensions of the cell surface must be regulated so that they form only where needed. An example is the pseudopods of a macrophage that surround a bacterium only in the region of contact. In this case, actin assembly is controlled from the plasma membrane. Although myosin is present in filaments in muscle, myosin is not usually aggregated into distinct filaments in nonmuscle cells.

INTERMEDIATE FILAMENTS (IFS)

The components of another filamentous system are called *intermediate filaments* (*IFs*) because they are intermediate in size between actin and myosin filaments. IFs extend from the nuclear envelope to the cell periphery. They are about 10 nm in diameter. In many cells, IFs form a basket around the nucleus (Fig. 2.46) and are well developed in cells subjected to mechanical stress. IFs are present in nerve processes and extend throughout the cytoplasm of smooth muscle cells and skeletal muscle fibers. IFs are *fibrous proteins*, not globular ones such as actin and tubulin. They are classified on the basis of *amino acid sequence*. The filament types and locations of IFs are listed in the accompanying table.

assembly and disassembly during mitosis and in attaching interphase chromosomes to the inner nuclear membrane.

OTHER CELLULAR STRUCTURES

A number of cell types including germ cells, tumor or cancer cells, and embryonic cells contain stacked porous cytoplasmic membranes called *annulate lamellae* (Fig. 2.47). These membranes contain many pore complexes similar to those in the nuclear envelope. The function of these porous cytomembranes and their relationship to the nuclear envelope are presently unknown.

A nonmembranous, nonfilamentous network has been described extending throughout the cytosol among the other organelles. This system has been called the *microtrabecular meshwork* and was initially viewed in SEM images of critical point-dried cultured cells. However, there is some evidence that whether or not the proteinaceous microtrabecular meshwork is present may depend upon the degree of hydration of the cytoplasm. The nature and role of the meshwork are still under investigation.

IF Types

Type	Name	Location
Type I	Acidic keratins	Predominantly epithelial cells
	Basic keratins	
Type II	Vimentin	Cells of mesenchymal origin, fibroblasts, endothelial cells, leukocytes
	Desmin	Striated and smooth muscle
	Glial fibrillary acidic proteins	Astrocytes, oligodendroglia, microglia, Schwann cells
Type III	Neurofilaments	Axons and dendrites
Type IV	Lamins (nuclear lamina)	Inner surface of inner nuclear membrane

Cells are able to control IF assembly and disassembly by *phosphorylation* of specific residues on the IF proteins. IFs play a role in positioning the nucleus in the cell and in the mechanical integration of the intercellular space. The lamins have a role in nuclear envelope

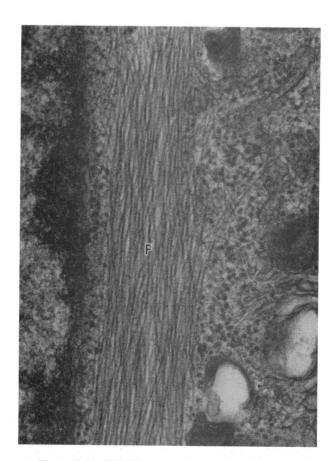

Figure 2.46. TEM illustrates intermediate filaments (F) near the cell nucleus. ×62,250.

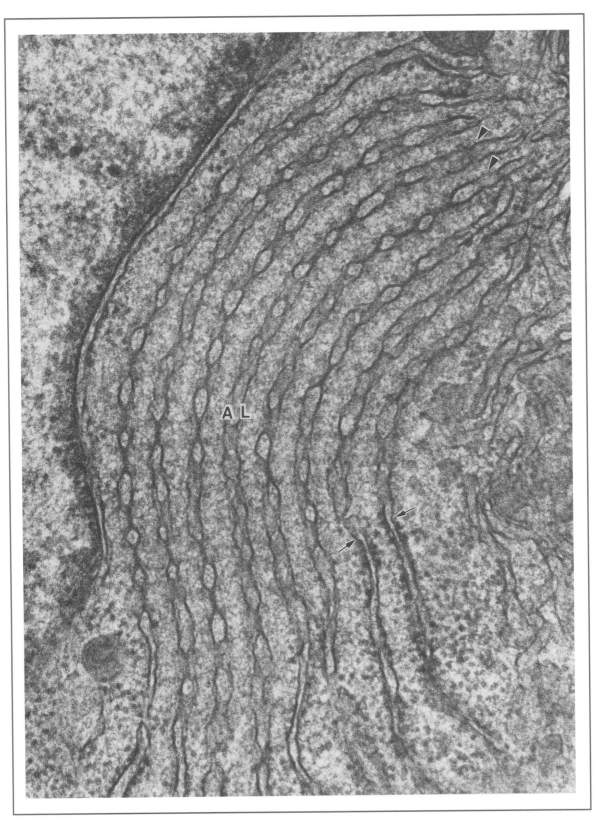

Figure 2.47. Stack of annulate lamellae (AL) are located next to the nucleus. The annulate lamellae contain many pore complexes (arrowheads) similar to those in the nuclear envelope. Note that the annulate lamellae are connected at their ends with elements of the rER (arrows) and ER (arrowheads). ×86,600.

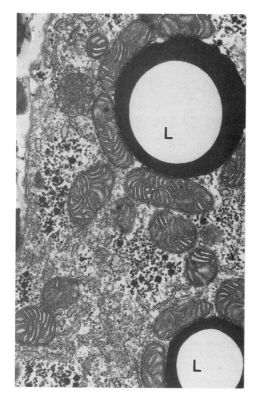

Figure 2.48. TEM of two lipid droplets (L). The droplets are closely surrounded by mitochondria. ×19,500.

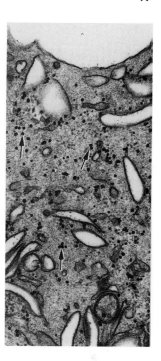

Figure 2.49. TEM of epithelial cell in urinary bladder. The small black dots (arrows) are particulate glycogen. ×40,000.

CELL INCLUSIONS

Finally, a variety of formed elements may be present in the cytoplasm, including secretory (zymogen) granules, lipid droplets, and glycogen. Secretory granules are membrane bound, while lipid bodies are not (Fig. 2.48). Glycogen may be present in two forms. Beta particles of glycogen are round, with an average diameter of 15–30 nm; beta particles can aggregate to form rosettes, called *alpha particles*, which are approximately 50–100 nm in diameter (Figs. 2.49, 2.50).

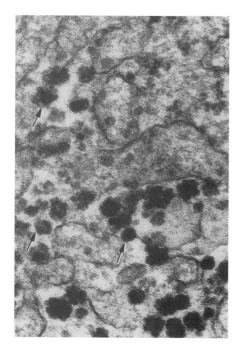

Figure 2.50. TEM of ER in hepatocyte. Rosettes of glycogen (arrows) are electron dense. ×100,000.

SELECTED BIBLIOGRAPHY

Afzelius, B.A. (1985). The immotile cilia syndrome: a microtubule-associated defect. *Crit. Rev. Biochem.* **19**, 63–87.

Amos, L.A., and Amos, W.B. (1991). *Molecules of the Cytoskeleton.* Guilford Press, New York.

Anderson, R.G., and Kaplan, J. (1983). Receptor mediated endocytosis. In *Modern Cell Biology*, Vol. 1, B.H. Satir, ed. Alan R. Liss, New York.

Attardi, G., and Schatz, G. (1988). Biogenesis of mitochondria. *Annu. Rev. Cell Biol.* **4**, 289–333.

Bornens, M., Paintrand, M., Berges, J., Marty, M.C., and Karsenti, E. (1987). Structural and chemical characterization of isolated centrioles. *Cell Motil. Cytoskeleton* **8**, 238–249.

Brown, W.J., Goodhouse, J., and Farquhar, M.G. (1986). Mannose 6-phosphate receptors for lysosomal enzymes cycle between the Golgi complex and endosomes. *J. Cell Biol.* **103**, 1235–1247.

Burgess, T.L., and Kelly, R.B. (1987). Constitutive and regulated secretion of proteins. *Annu. Rev. Cell Biol.* **3**, 243–293.

Cruetz, C.E. (1991). Membrane fusion and exocytosis. In *Membrane Dynamics and Signaling. Fundamentals of Medical Cell Biology*, Vol. 5A, E.E. Bittar, ed. JAI Press, Greenwich, CT.

Edinin, M. (1987). Rotational and lateral diffusion of membrane proteins and lipids: phenomena and function. *Curr. Top. Membr. Transp.* **29**, 91–127.

Gelfand, V.I., and Bershadsky, A.D. (1991). Microtubule dynamics: mechanism, regulation, and function. *Annu. Rev. Cell Biol.* **7**, 93–116.

Griffiths, G., Hoflack, B., Simons, K., Mellman, I., and Kornfeld, S. (1988). The mannose 6-phosphate receptor and the biogenesis of lysosomes. *Cell* **52**, 329–341.

Griffiths, G., and Simons, K. (1986). The trans-Golgi network: sorting at the exit site of the Golgi complex. *Science* **234**, 438–443.

Hortsch, M., Avossa, D., and Meyer, D.I. (1986). Characterization of secretory protein translocation: ribosome-membrane interaction in endoplasmic reticulum. *J. Cell Biol.* **103**, 241–253.

Keen, J.H. (1990). Clathrin and associated assembly and disassembly proteins. *Annu. Rev. Biochem.* **59**, 415–428.

Kelly, R.B. (1991). Secretory granule and synaptic vesicle formation. *Curr. Opin. Cell Biol.* **3**, 654–660.

Kolodny, E.H. (1976). Lysosomal storage diseases. *N. Engl. J. Med.* **294**, 1217.

Luna, E.J., and Hitt, A.L. (1992). Cytoskeleton-plasma membrane interaction. *Science* **258**, 955–964.

Mellman, I., and Simons, K. (1992). The Golgi complex: in vitro veritas? *Cell* **68**, 829–840.

Moore, P.B. (1988). The ribosome returns. *Nature* **331**, 223–227.

Munro, S., and Pelham, H.R.B. (1987). A C-terminal signal prevents secretion of luminal ER proteins. *Cell* **48**, 899–907.

Murray, J. (1994). Eukaryotic flagella. *Curr. Opin. Struct. Biol.* **4**, 180–186.

Noller, H.F. (1984). Structure of ribosomal RNA. *Annu. Rev. Biochem.* **53**, 119–162.

Pfeffer, S.R. (1992). GTP-binding proteins in intracellular transport. *Trends Cell Biol.* **2**, 41–46.

Pfeffer, S.R., and Rothman, J.E. (1987). Biosynthetic protein transport and sorting in endoplasmic reticulum. *Annu. Rev. Biochem.* **56**, 829.

Schliwa, M. (1986). *The Cytoskeleton.* Cell Biology Monographs 13. Springer-Verlag, Vienna and New York.

Stewart, M. (1990). Intermediate filaments: structure, assembly and molecular interactions. *Curr. Opin. Cell Biol.* **2**, 91–100.

Sztul, E.S., Melancon, P., and Howell, K.E. (1992). Targeting and fusion in vesicular transport. *Trends Cell Biol.* **2**, 381–386.

Vale, R.D. (1992). Microtubule motors: many new models off the assembly line. *Trends Biochem. Sci.* **17**, 300–304.

Walter, P., and Lingappa, V.R. (1986). Mechanism of protein translocation across the endoplasmic reticulum membrane. *Annu. Rev. Cell. Biol.* **2**, 499–516.

Wiedmann, M., Kurzchalia, T.V., Hartman, E., and Rapoport, T.A. (1987). A signal sequence receptor in the endoplasmic reticulum membrane. *Nature* **328**, 830–833.

Wileman, T. (1991). Membrane fusion and exocytosis. In *Membrane Dynamics and Signaling. Fundamentals of Medical Cell Biology*, Vol. 5A, E.E. Bittar, ed. JAI Press, Greenwich, CT.

Wilson, G.N. (1991). Structure-function relationships in the peroxisome: implications for human disease. *Biochem. Med. & Metab. Biol.* **46**, 288–298.

Yeagle, P., ed. (1992). *Structure of Biological Membranes.* CRC Press, Boca Raton, FL.

Summary of Eukaryotic Organelles: Structure, Organization, and Functions

Structure	Composition/Organization	Principal Functions
NUCLEUS 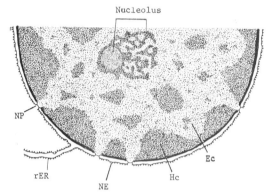	Nucleoplasm contains nucleotides, enzymes, nucleic acids (mRNA, rRNA, tRNA), proteins; nuclear matrix; chromosomes with genetic code; contains hetero-chromatin (Hc) and euchromatin (Ec).	Storing and processing of genetic information; replication, transcription; control of metabolism.
NUCLEOLUS	Ribosomal RNA processing; nucleolar genes; forms from nucleolar organizer of chromosome(s).	Site of synthesis of ribosomal subunits.
NUCLEAR ENVELOPE (NE) 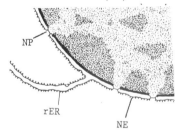	Consists of two membranes that enclose a perinuclear cisterna; interrupted by nuclear pore complexes (NP); may be continuous with rER; often contains ribosomes on outer membrane facing cytosol.	A nuclear lamina is adpressed to inner nuclear membrane and contains lamins (intermediate filaments) involved in attaching chromatin to nuclear envelope in interphase and envelope breakdown at mitosis.
NUCLEAR PORES 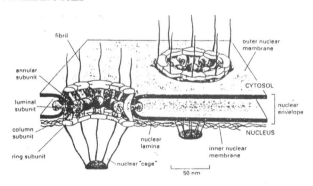	Interruptions in nuclear membranes; pore complexes with granular and filamentous subunits.	Involved in RNA translocation into cytoplasm by active transport; protein import into nucleus.

Structure	*Composition/Organization*	*Principal Functions*
PLASMA MEMBRANE 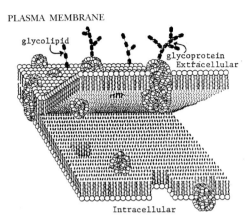	Lipid bilayer contains phospholipid, cholesterol, glycolipids, proteins, glycoproteins, oligosaccharide side chains associated with outer leaflet of bilayer.	Isolation, protection, binding, recognition, internalization; contains receptors, signaling molecules; forms communicating, sealing, and adhering intercellular junctions; couples extracellular coat and cytoskeleton.

SPECIALIZATIONS OF PLASMA MEMBRANE

Structure	*Composition/Organization*	*Principal Functions*
MICROVILLI 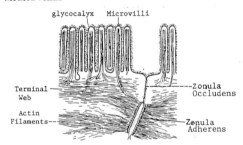	Folded lipid bilayer and extracellular coat (glycocalyx); contains actin microfilaments and other proteins.	Amplification of plasma membrane for absorption; contains enzymes, receptors; internal actin organization associated with support and primitive motility of microvilli.
CILIA, FLAGELLA 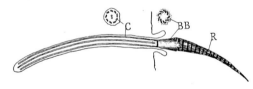	Plasma membrane extensions that contain 9 peripheral doublets and 2 central microtubules containing protein tubulin; dynein motors; attached to basal body (BB) which may have striated rootlet (Rt).	Propel material through tubular structures cavities; movement of cells (sperm).
BASAL PLASMA MEMBRANE INFOLDINGS 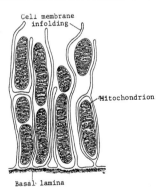	Infoldings of the plasma membrane into the basal cytoplasm.	Amplify the basal plasma membrane domain to accommodate increased numbers of membrane proteins (e.g., sodium pumps); mitochondria (M) closely associated with infoldings.

Structure	*Composition/Organization*	*Principal Functions*
JUNCTIONAL COMPLEXES 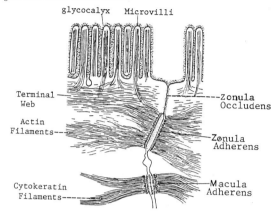 glycocalyx Microvilli Terminal Web Actin Filaments Cytokeratin Filaments Zonula Occludens Zonula Adherens Macula Adherens	Inner and outer leaflets of plasma membrane can be modified by filaments, adhesive macromolecules and integral membrane proteins.	Seal off intercellular space (zonula occludens), function in cell-cell adhesion (zonula and macula adherens) and intercellular communication (gap junctions).
COATED PITS, VESICLES 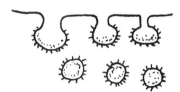	Localized pits or depressions in plasma membrane coated with clathrin—detach as coated vesicles.	Mediate selective transport of plasma membrane receptors (receptor-mediated endocytosis); transport of mannose-6-phosphate receptors from trans Golgi network.
	Coatomer-coated vesicles (no clathrin) mediate nonselective vesicular transport.	Transport from rER to Golgi, through Golgi cisternae and from trans Golgi network to plasma membrane.
PINOCYTOTIC PITS AND VESICLES 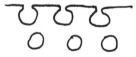	Localized vesiculation of plasma membrane—micropinocytosis—no clathrin coat, but coated with protein called caveolin; internalized as non-coated vesicles.	Involved in cellular "drinking on a small scale."
CENTROSOME 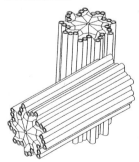	Two centrioles located at right angle, usually in juxtanuclear or supranuclear position; each centriole consists of 9 triplet tubules.	Serves as microtubule-organizing center (MTOC); involved in formation, organization and orientation of microtubules in mitotic and interphase cells; can become basal bodies and form cilia or flagella.

Structure	*Composition/Organization*	*Principal Functions*

MITOCHONDRIA

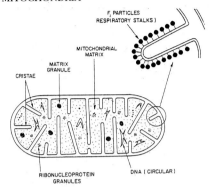

Double membrane with folded inner membrane (cristae) containing important metabolic enzymes.

Produce most of the ATP needed for energy-requiring events by cells ("powerhouses of the cell").

POLYRIBOSOMES

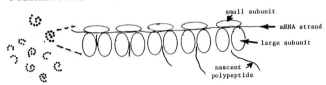

Consist of variable numbers of ribosomes joined by mRNA strand; each ribosome has small and large subunits containing RNA and protein.

Protein synthesis; polyribosomes attached to ER membrane synthesize protein largely for export; free polyribosomes synthesize protein for retention in cell.

ROUGH SURFACED ENDOPLASMIC RETICULUM (RER)

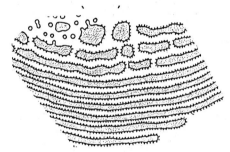

Network of branching membranous channels enclosing spaces called cisternae; outer membrane surface coated with polyribosomes.

Translation; initial glycosylation; enzymes for synthesis of diverse secretory proteins; intracellular transport and storage of nascent proteins; oligosaccharide synthesis; membrane contains receptors for signal peptides of nascent proteins.

SMOOTH (AGRANULAR) ENDOPLASMIC RETICULUM (SER)

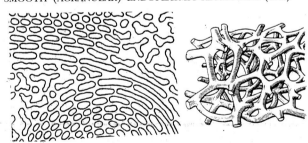

Tubular membranes that enclose cisternae (no polyribosomes).

Contains specific enzymes built into membranes; involved in lipid (steroid, cholesterol) synthesis; carbohydrate synthesis and utilization; triglyceride synthesis.

Structure	*Composition/Organization*	*Principal Functions*
GOLGI APPARATUS 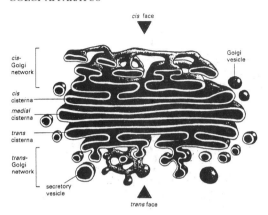	Stacks of flattened membranes (saccules) enclosing cisternae; many small membranous vesicles; different functions in different saccules; product transported from cis to trans Golgi network by shuttle vesicles.	Alteration, sorting, packaging of secretory products and lysosomes; terminal glycosylation; phosphorylation; sulfation of secretion; protein sorting.
LYSOSOME 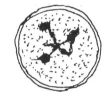 Autophagosomes Endosome, (secondary, lysosome, digestive vacuole heterolysosome).	Membrane-bound bags (vesicles) contain hydrolytic digestive enzymes.	Acid hydrolases (hydrolytic enzymes) involved in intracellular digestion (heterophagy, autophagy).
PEROXISOME 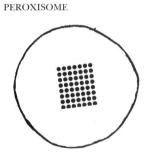	Membrane-bound organelle with an internal matrix that often contains a crystalline structure (nucleoid).	Contains enzymes in animal cells involved in formation and destruction of hydrogen peroxide; breakdown of purines; oxidation of long chain fatty acids.
CYTOSKELETON	Tubular and filamentous cytoplasmic structures.	Support, guide and move intracellular structures and materials.
MICROFILAMENTS 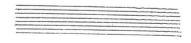 Actin subunit 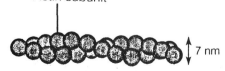 7 nm	6–7 nm diameter filaments; consist of protein actin; constituent of stress fibers; extend into cell projections; present in cleavage furrow.	Involved in movement of cells and intracellular structures; cytokinesis.

55

Structure	*Composition/Organization*	*Principal Functions*
MICROTUBULES ⌒⌒Tubulin subunit 25 nm	Long, tubular structures about 25 nm diameter containing α-, β-tubulin protein as heterodimer.	Often oriented parallel to long axis of cellular asymmetries; maintain cell shape (axons) and serve as guide to translocation of materials (e.g., synaptic vesicles, mitochondria in axons; chromosome movement).
MYOSIN-I	Nonmuscle cells contain various myosins—myosin-I is best defined; has shorter tail and reduced head compared to myosin-II in muscle.	Myosin-I tails have membrane-binding site and a binding site for second actin filament; myosin-I can move vesicle along actin filament, attach actin filament to plasma membrane or attach two closely positioned actin filaments and cause sliding of filaments.
INTERMEDIATE FILAMENTS Fibrous subunits 10 nm	Proteins arranged into fibers (keratin, desmin, vimentin) and a lamina (nuclear lamina); filaments about 10 nm in diameter.	Mechanical integration of intracellular space.
ANNULATE LAMELLAE	Stacks of flattened, porous cytoplasmic membranes that are similar in structure to nuclear envelope, but are present in the cytoplasm.	Function unknown, may represent stored or reserve pore complexes for amplification of nuclear pore functions.

Structure	*Composition/Organization*	*Principal Functions*

FORMED ELEMENTS IN THE CELL

ZYMOGEN GRANULES

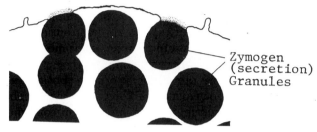

Zymogen (secretion) Granules

Membrane-bound granules that contains a moderately electron-dense matrix; usually discharged by exocytosis from apical end of secretory cell.

May contain a variety of secretory products (e.g., proteins, glycoproteins) including enzymes, hormones and other important macromolecules.

GLYCOGEN

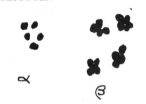

α

β

Polymers of glucose; storage form of glucose in liver and striated muscle; exists in two morphological forms, α and β, either particulate or rosette form.

A reserve food source; source of glucose.

LIPOFUSCIN GRANULES

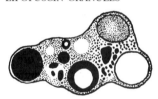

A membrane-delimited body that varies in size and may be irregular in shape; varied internal structure.

May represent a residual body with indigestible material that is not exported from the cell and that may over time transform into an "aging pigment."

LIPID DROPLETS

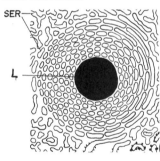

SER

L

Non-membrane-bound bodies of variable electron density; may be irregular in outline.

Contain neutral fats (triglycerides), a source of fatty acids.

Illustration of Plasma Membrane same as Figure 2-9. (From S.L. Wolfe. *Molecular and Cellular Biology*, 1993. Wadsworth, Belmont, CA.

Illustration of Golgi Apparatus and nuclear pore from B. Alberts, D. Bray, J. Lewis, M. Raff, K. Roberts, J. Watson. *Molecular Biology of the Cell*, 3rd ed. Garland Publ. Inc., New York, 1994.

The Eukaryotic Cell: The Nucleus

The eukaryotic cell is segregated into a nucleus, where DNA replication and transcription occur, and into a cytoplasm, where translation occurs. In *replication*, the two strands of a DNA double helix unwind and are duplicated. *Transcription* is the process by which RNA polymerase utilizes one DNA strand as a template for the synthesis of a complementary RNA molecule. *Translation*, which occurs on ribosomes in the cytoplasm, is the process whereby the base sequence of an mRNA molecule prescribes the amino acid sequences to be incorporated into a polypeptide chain.

Transcription is temporally and spatially separated from translation in eukaryotes by a nuclear envelope. RNA transcripts in the nucleus are processed and packaged into ribonucleoprotein (RNP) complexes, which are transported out of the nucleus through nuclear pores.

In structurally polarized cells, the nucleus is located in the basal half of the cell; in other cells, the nucleus is located in the cell center. Groups of IFs surround the nucleus and play a role in maintaining nuclear position. The nucleus can rotate in some living cells; the microfilaments and microtubules are important in this activity. Centrioles and the Golgi complex usually have a juxtanuclear (near the nucleus) or supranuclear (above the nucleus) position in the cell (Fig. 3.1).

Chromosomes are not apparent as discrete entities in the interphase cell but only during the division process. DNA is closely associated with histone proteins in the interphase nucleus as *chromatin*. In the LM and TEM, interphase nuclei show granular clumps of chromatin (Figs. 3.1, 3.5) but provide little information about its organization. Uncoiled chromosomes or chromatin in the nucleus of an interphase cells is called *euchromatin*, while chromatin that does not uncoil appreciably but remains condensed is called *heterochromatin* (Fig. 3.2). In eukaryotic chromosomes, DNA is bound to *histones* to form a repeating array of DNA-protein particles called *nucleosomes*, which are structural subunits of chromatin (see Fig. 3.6). Histones play an important role in the orderly packing of the DNA double helix and have a role in gene activity.

NUCLEAR ENVELOPE AND NUCLEAR PORES

The nuclear envelope consists of two membranes that enclose a space called a *perinuclear cisterna* (Figs. 3.1, 3.2). In some cell types the outer nuclear membrane has ribosomes attached to its cytoplasmic surface, and in a number of cell types, it is possible to observe continuities between the outer membrane of the nuclear envelope and the rER. The outer nuclear membrane contacts the cell matrix or cytoplasm, while the inner nuclear membrane is closely associated with chromatin of the nuclear matrix via a thin layer called the *nuclear lamina*. Both inner and outer membranes are interrupted by *nuclear pores*, which are connections between the nucleoplasm and cytoplasm; the nuclear pore is about 70–100 nm in diameter (Figs. 3.3–3.5). The *nuclear pore complex* (*NPC*) plays important roles in protein import into the nucleus and in the translocation of RNA species from the nucleus into the cytoplasm. By injecting particles of known molecular weight that are coated with cytoplasmic proteins, it has been determined that particles of about 17,000 D rapidly enter the nucleus, while larger particles enter more slowly and those of ~60,000 D have difficulty entering. Larger particles can pass through the nuclear pores from cytoplasm to nu-

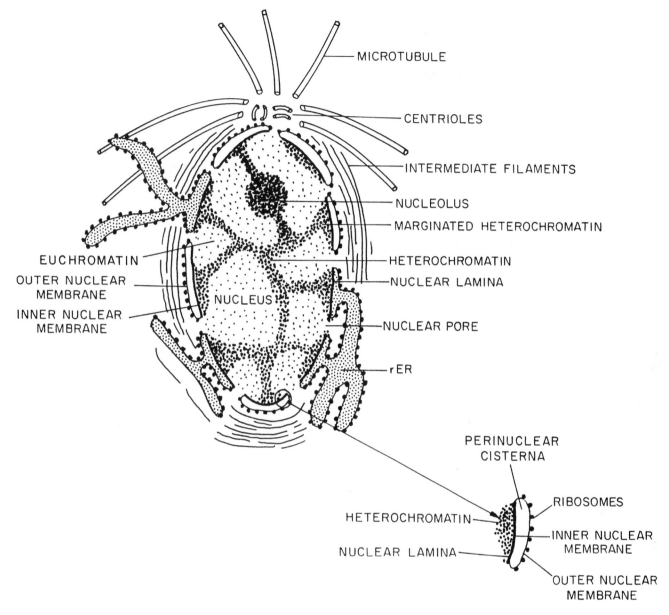

- MICROTUBULE
- CENTRIOLES
- INTERMEDIATE FILAMENTS
- NUCLEOLUS
- MARGINATED HETEROCHROMATIN
- HETEROCHROMATIN
- NUCLEAR LAMINA
- NUCLEAR PORE
- rER

EUCHROMATIN
OUTER NUCLEAR MEMBRANE
INNER NUCLEAR MEMBRANE
NUCLEUS

PERINUCLEAR CISTERNA
RIBOSOMES
HETEROCHROMATIN
INNER NUCLEAR MEMBRANE
NUCLEAR LAMINA
OUTER NUCLEAR MEMBRANE

Figure 3.1. Diagram illustrates basic structural relationships between nucleus, nuclear envelope, and surrounding organelles.

cleoplasm, but these proteins, such as DNA and RNA polymerases, interact with receptors at the pore margin and are actively transported through a narrow pore channel. A variety of proteins must be imported from the cytoplasm through the nuclear pores into the nucleoplasm, including DNA and RNA polymerases, histones, gene regulatory proteins, and RNA-processing proteins. Proteins that are actively transported into the nucleus contain short peptide sequences called *nuclear import signals*. In addition to protein import, it has been estimated that each nuclear pore in a rapidly growing cell transports approximately three ribosomes per minute to the cytoplasm. The NPC has a relative molecular mass of over 100 megadaltons, but only a few of

the molecules have been characterized. A transmembrane glycoprotein called *gp 210* extends into the lumen of the nuclear pores. It has been suggested to play a role in pore complex formation and may anchor the pore complex material in the nuclear envelope.

The exact function of the nuclear envelope for the eukaryotic cell is not completely clear. Since extensive processing of RNA molecules must occur before transcription, a nuclear compartment for these events is useful. A nuclear envelope could form a domain to protect the chromosomes from the forces of the cytoskeleton, especially the microfilaments. The nuclear envelope also keeps the nuclear compartment free of organelles and functional polyribosomes.

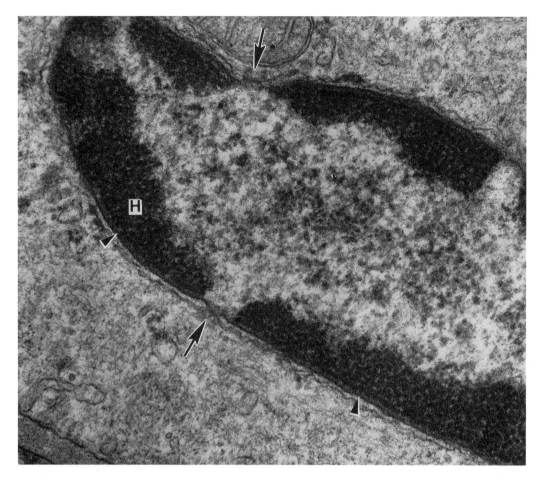

Figure 3.2. TEM of interphase nucleus illustrates heterochromatin (H), nuclear lamina (arrowheads), and nuclear pores (arrows). ×24,900.

NUCLEAR LAMINA AND LAMINS

The nuclear lamina is a thin layer attached to the inner surface of the inner nuclear membrane (Fig. 3.1). Although the layer appears homogeneous by TEM, it is a meshwork of IFs 10–20 nm thick. Although different in several respects from cytoplasmic IFs, three IF proteins comprise the nuclear lamins. The *phosphorylation* of serine residues on nuclear lamins triggers nuclear envelope breakdown during mitosis. As a cell enters interphase, the nuclear lamins are *dephosphorylated* and the nuclear envelope re-forms.

NUCLEOLUS

The nucleolus contains RNA and protein. A small amount of DNA, from the nucleolus organizer region, is also present in the nucleolus, which in TEM consists of a mass of small granular and fibrillar subunits. The nucleolus forms from a specific region of a chromosome called the *nucleolus organizer region* or *secondary constriction*. Nucleolus organizer regions are thus areas of *chromosomal DNA* that encode *ribosomal RNA* (rDNA

cistrons). Nucleoli function in the synthesis, processing, and partial assembly of ribosomal subunits. RNA polymerase I transcription occurs within the nucleolus, and the fibrillar portion of the nucleolus appears to be the rDNA transcription site. The granular region of the nucleolus contains preribosomes and both large and small ribosomal subunits. *RNP* with sedimentation coefficients of *45S, 35S,* and *28S* is present in nucleoli based on isolation and biochemical analysis. Before 45S rRNA leaves the nucleus, it is cleaved to produce 28S, 18S, and 5.8S rRNA. The 18S RNA joins with specific proteins and exits the nuclear pores into the cytoplasm, where it becomes part of the small ribosomal subunit. The 35S fragment is subsequently cleaved to a 28S RNA that, together with protein, becomes incorporated into the large ribosomal subunit.

CHROMATIN AND CHROMOSOME STRUCTURE

A more useful picture of chromatin in the interphase nucleus is obtained when the nucleus is ruptured under various conditions and the contents are placed on

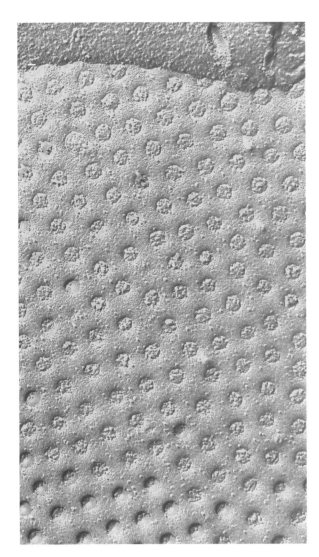

Figure 3.3. Freeze fracture of interphase nucleus illustrates numerous nuclear pores in surface view. ×62,250.

matin stains with basic dyes (e.g., hematoxylin), as well as with the *Feulgen technique* for *DNA* localization. Various Hoechst dyes and propidium iodide are fluorescent vital dyes used to localize DNA. The cell's DNA encodes information required to synthesize various proteins and other cell products. The DNA also codes for informational macromolecules such as ribosomal (rRNA), messenger (mRNA), and transfer (tRNA) ribonucleic acid that are directly responsible for the synthesis of proteins by the cell.

Human somatic cells contain *23 homologous pairs* of chromosomes (46 total). Twenty-two of the pairs are morphologically similar and are called *autosomes*. The twenty-third pair may be morphologically different and are the sex chromosomes. There are two morphologically similar XX sex chromosomes in the female gamete. There are morphologically different X and Y chromosomes in the male gametes. The *diploid* ($2n$) number of

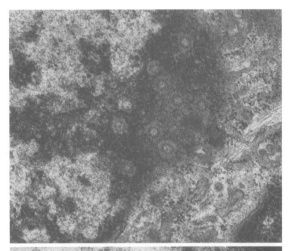

3.4

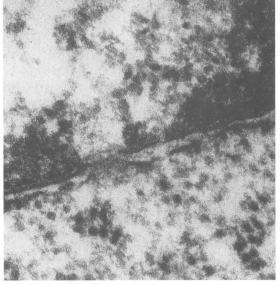

3.5

a grid for TEM observation. The chromatin appears as repeating subunits ~11 nm in diameter connected by a 4 nm thread or filament. The 4-nm filament consists of DNA, while the repeating beads, called *nucleosomes*, contain two molecules each of histones H_4, H_3, H_2A, and H_2B (Fig. 3.6). DNA, 140 base pairs in length, is coiled around each nucleosome. Spacer segments of DNA connect the nucleosomes, and histone H_1 is associated with this spacer. The small volume of the chromosome in an interphase nucleus involves its association with histones, but how this arrangement is produced and maintained remains unclear. When histones are removed from isolated chromosomes by heparin sulfate or dextran, for example, the DNA uncoils even more dramatically and shows tremendous coiling surrounding an electron-dense protein core (Fig. 3.7).

Chromatin in the interphase nucleus is attached at places to the inner nuclear membrane (Fig. 3.1). Because of the phosphate groups in DNA, heterochro-

Figures 3.4, 3.5. TEM images of nuclear pores (arrowheads) in surface view (Fig. 3.4) and side view (Fig. 3.5). Chromatin (Ch). Figure 3.4, ×36,105; Figure 3.5, ×100,000.

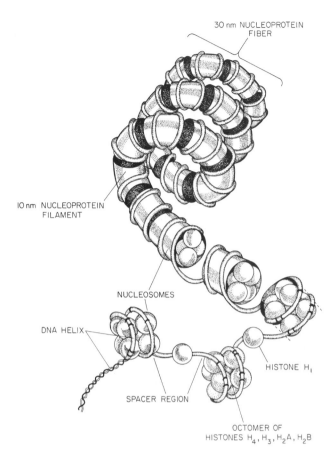

30 nm NUCLEOPROTEIN FIBER

10 nm NUCLEOPROTEIN FILAMENT

NUCLEOSOMES

DNA HELIX

HISTONE H_1

SPACER REGION

OCTOMER OF HISTONES H_4, H_3, H_2A, H_2B

Figure 3.6. Drawing illustrates a 30-nm coiled chromatin fiber. The fiber has been opened up to illustrate how the nucleosomes consist of an octaomer of histones with the DNA helix wound around them. The nucleosomes are joined by spacer DNA segments with associated histone H_1. (Redrawn from D.W. Fawcett, *A Textbook of Histology*, 11th ed., Philadephia, W.B. Saunders Company, 1986; after R. Bradbury, *La Recherche*, 9, 644, 1978 and A. Worcel and C. Benyaj, *Cell*, 88, 1978)

chromosomes in somatic cells is 46. Mature germ cells have only 23 chromosomes, which is the *haploid* or *n* number. As a result of meiosis, only one of each homologous pairs of chromosomes is present in the mature male and female gametes. When an egg with 23 chromosomes (22X) unites with a sperm also with 23 (22Y or 22X) chromosomes, the diploid chromosome number of 46 is reestablished in the resulting zygote (44XY or 44XX), which leads to more somatic cells.

The Barr body is one of the X chromosomes in the female that does not uncoil at the end of mitosis; this single X chromosome is heterochromatic and frequently appears with the LM as a dense dot on the nuclear envelope's inner surface. Interphase chromosomes may be attached to a component of the *nuclear lamina*, which is a thin layer of IF-type proteins associated with the inner nuclear membrane.

During prophase of mitosis, the chromosomes progressively shorten and thicken and become more easily

observed. If colchicine is added to the cell, the spindle microtubules are dissociated such that mitosis is blocked at metaphase. If the cells are then ruptured and stained, the entire chromosome complement of the cell, called a *karyotype*, can be observed (Fig. 3.8). When metaphase chromosomes are observed under these conditions, each chromosome appears as a double structure, split longitudinally in halves (*chromatids*) that are attached only at one site, called the *kinetochore* or *primary constriction*. In M phase (mitosis), each sister chromatid is joined and has a constricted region of condensed chromatin called the *centromere*. In late prophase, the kinetochores, consisting of specialized protein complexes, assemble on each centromere. A subset of microtubules, the chromosomal (kinetochore) spindle microtubules, binds to the kinetochore and pulls the sister chromatids toward opposite poles at anaphase. The kinetochore plays a role in controlling the assembly and disassembly of kinetochore microtubules. The numerous proteins present in mammalian kinetochores are presently under investigation. An SEM image of an isolated paired chromatid is illustrated in Figure 3.9.

GENES, REPLICATION, TRANSCRIPTION

The human haploid genome contains roughly 3×10^9 nucleotide pairs of DNA in 22 autosomes and a single sex chromosome; thus, it can code for nearly 3 million proteins of average size. However, it is estimated that any mammal could be constructed from perhaps only 60,000 proteins. Thus, coding regions of DNA appear to be interrupted by long expanses of noncoding DNA.

A *chromosome* is a very long DNA molecule containing many genes. Chromosomal DNA also contains nucleotide sequences for *replication origins*, *telomers* (that permit DNA to be replicated), and a *centromere* that attaches DNA to the mitotic spindle. A *gene* is a nucleotide sequence in a DNA molecule that produces an RNA molecule or a segment of DNA that encodes one polypeptide chain. The diversity of cell types encountered in humans and other organisms is due largely to mechanisms by which different genes are transcribed in different cells, that is, differential gene transcription.

DNA replication commences with a DNA *helicase* that is bound to the DNA by an initiator protein bound to a replication origin. The DNA helicase moves along the DNA and opens the DNA helix, forming a replication fork. Two *DNA polymerases* (α, δ) then replicate the two strands. DNA transcription is catalyzed by the enzyme *RNA polymerase* (I, II, III). Genes that code for proteins are transcribed by polymerase II. The genes that code for most structural RNAs are transcribed by polymerases I and III. DNA transcription (RNA synthesis) begins when an RNA polymerase molecule binds to a promoter sequence in the DNA double helix. The RNA chain grows in the 5′ to 3′ direction by the sequential

Figure 3.7. When histones are extracted from an isolated chromosome by treating them with dextran sulfate and heparin, the DNA undergoes a remarkable uncoiling such that an extremely long, coiled thread can be visualized in the TEM, as shown here. The region within the rectangle in the insert is enlarged in the main figure. The black material at the top represents structural protein of the chromosome. The highly coiled thread is approximately 4 nm in diameter. (From J.R. Paulsen, and U.K. Laemmli, *Cell*, 12, 817, 1977, © Cell Press, with permission; and D.W. Fawcett, *A Textbook of Histology*, 11th ed., W.B. Saunders, Philadelphia, 1986)

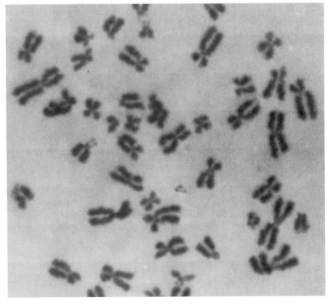

Figure 3.8. Human karyotype. Metaphase chromosomes (chromatids) were isolated from human leukocytes and stained. Whole mount preparation photographed in LM. ×2000.

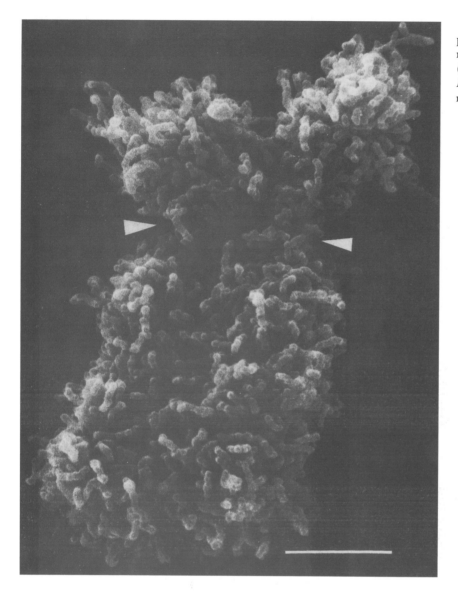

Figure 3.9. SEM image of paired chromatids with kinetochore region denoted by arrowheads. (From K. Utsumi, *Cell Structure and Function* 6, 395–401, 1981, with permission)

addition of ribonucleoside triphosphates until it reaches a stop signal or termination signal.

CELL CYCLE

The life history of the eukaryotic somatic cell consists of alternating periods of *interphase* and *mitosis* (Fig. 3.10). Interphase is divided into a G_1 (Gap 1) phase, which represents the interval from the end of mitosis to the time of DNA replication; an *S phase* in which replication of the DNA by a semiconservative method occurs; and a G_2 (Gap 2) phase is the interval from the end of DNA replication to mitosis (M phase). During DNA replication the double helix separates into its two polynucleotide strands. Each strand remains intact and acquires a new complementary partner that forms by the alignment of nucleotides along the old strand by base pairing and enzymatic linkage of the nucleotides

into a new polynucleotide chain. Some cells in G_1 pause in a resting or nonproliferative stage called G_0, which is of variable duration. Neurons and skeletal muscle do not divide, liver cells divide infrequently, and intestinal epithelial cells divide twice a day on average.

One unique and vital property of living matter is its capacity for reproduction, growth, and renewal. One type of cell division, *mitosis*, occurs in somatic cells and provides for the chromosome type and number in an organism to remain constant. Another type of cell division, *meiosis*, occurs only in male and female germ cells and reduces the chromosome number of an organism by one-half. As a consequence, the haploid chromosome set of the male and the haploid chromosome set of the female are restored to the diploid set during fertilization.

In eukaryotes, cell division includes two well-coordinated events: nuclear division (*karyokinesis*) and cytoplasmic division (*cytokinesis*) (Plate 1 A–D). Karyoki-

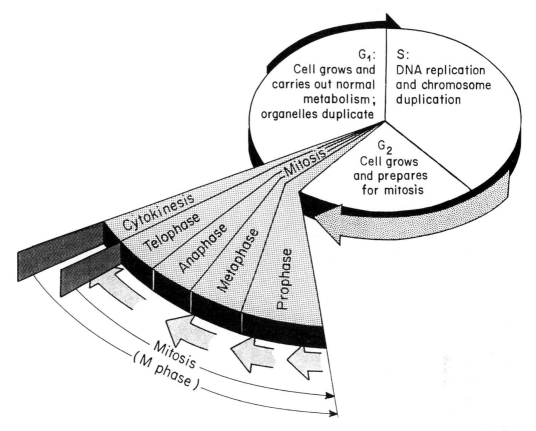

Figure 3.10. Diagram summarizing relationships between interphase and mitotic stages of the cell cycle. (Redrawn from G. Karp, *Cell and Molecular Biology*. Copyright © 1996. Reprinted by permission of John Wiley & Sons, Inc.)

nesis refers to the highly ordered process in which replicated molecules of DNA separate and are distributed to the nuclei of the two daughter cells resulting from the division process. Cytokinesis occurs after karyokinesis and involves the pinching of the cytoplasm into two distinct daughter cells or progeny (Figs. 3.11–3.16). In some instances, karyokinesis occurs without cytokinesis and results in a binucleate condition (e.g., some liver cells, some cardiac muscle cells).

MITOSIS

EVENTS AND STAGES

Mitosis results in the distribution of identical copies of a cell's genome to its offspring, which requires approximately 30–60 minutes in some mammalian cells. Stages in the process are illustrated in Plate 1 A–D. The beginning of S phase (S phase activator) and M phase (M phase promoting factor) are signaled by soluble cytoplasmic factors. In G_1 of interphase the chromosome is single and tends to be maximally uncoiled (Fig. 3.17). As indicated, replication of the DNA occurs in S phase of interphase such that each chromosome is a homologous pair of *chromatids* that are joined together at a re-

gion called the *kinetochore* (Fig. 3.17). At metaphase the DNA is intertwined in the kinetochore region. An enzyme called *topoisomerase* is concentrated in the kinetochore, and facilitates unraveling and untangling of the DNA molecules at the kinetochore so that the homologous chromosomes can move poleward to the daughter cells during anaphase and telophase. A major site of tubulin incorporation into microtubules in a mitotic cell is the kinetochores. The kinetochore is able to capture the plus end of microtubules, and more tubulin molecules are added at the kinetochore as well. Further, anaphase kinetochores move poleward along microtubules, causing a loss of tubulin subunits as they move.

In the interphase prior to prophase, the paired centrioles that are present duplicate such that two pairs of centrioles are formed, which then migrate to opposite poles of the cell (Figs. 3.18, 3.19). In the initial phase of mitosis, called *prophase*, the paired chromosomes become progressively thicker and shorter and thus more distinct. By the end of prophase, the chromatids are maximally shortened and the nuclear envelope rapidly disintegrates (Fig. 3.17). In *metaphase* the chromatids are arranged in an equatorial plane on what is called the *equatorial plate*. Metaphase requires ~30 minutes. Stages in mitosis of cultured cells are illustrated by SEM in Figures 3.11–3.16.

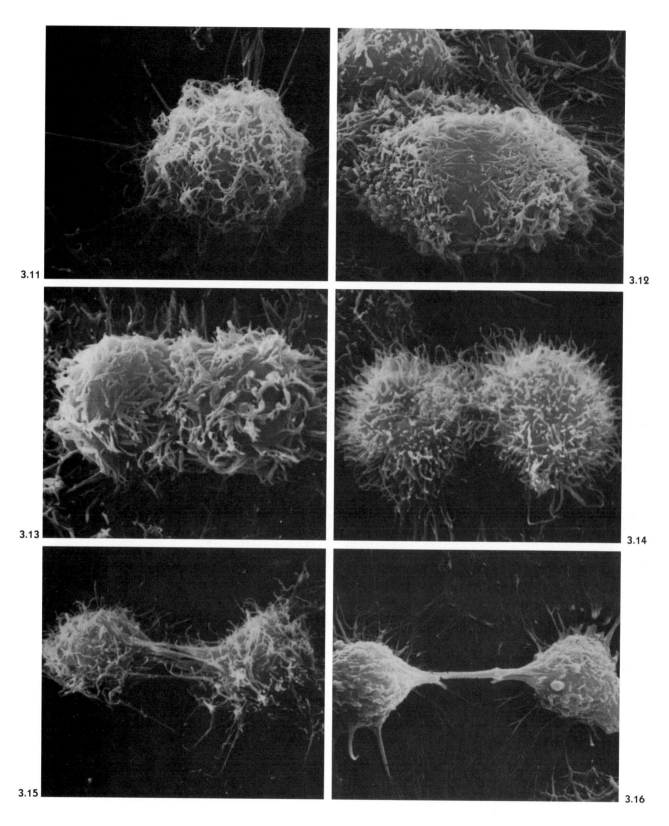

Figures 3.11–3.16. All figures are SEM images of dividing HeLa cells in culture. Note that the rounded cell (Fig. 3.11) elongates progressively and the cleavage furrow begins in Figure 3.13. The cells are pushed farther apart, but a narrow intercellular bridge (Fig. 3.16) persists for a time before complete separation occurs. Figure 3.11, ×3000; Figure 3.12, ×3280; Figure 3.13, ×3750; Figure 3.14, ×3900; Figure 3.15, ×4025; Figure 3.16, ×3300.

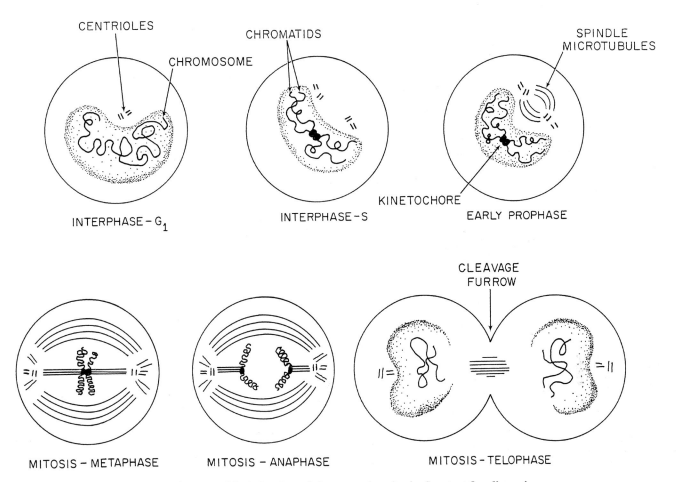

Figure 3.17 A simplified drawing of the stages in mitosis. See text for discussion.

CONTROL

A number of cell cycle regulating proteins are now known that command a cell to replicate its DNA during entry into S phase, as well as other proteins that command the cell to enter mitosis. The entry of G_2 cells into M phase involves the activity of two protein families. One is a family of *cyclin-dependent protein kinases* (*Cdk*). Cdk are enzymes (examples: Cdc2, Cdk2, Cdk4, Cdk6) that phosphorylate serine and threonine residues on other proteins, thereby either initiating or blocking activities required for progression through the cell cycle. Members of the second protein-activating family are called *cyclins*. They bind to Cdk molecules, thereby controlling their ability to phosphorylate target proteins. Cdk's are active only when bound to certain cyclins (A, B, C, D, E) to form Cdk-cyclin complexes. Cyclins are synthesized and then degraded during each cell cycle division. There are actually two main groups of cyclins: mitotic cyclins, which bind Cdk molecules during G_2 for entry into mitosis, and G_1 cyclins, which bind to different Cdk molecules during G_1 for entry into S phase. Mitotic cyclins, mainly cyclin B, gradually accumulate during G_2 and then bind to Cdk

to form a complex called *M-phase promoting factor* (*MPF*). Thus, the command to enter mitosis requires MPF, which is inactive and accumulates during G_2 phase. MPF actually consists of two subunits: Cdc2 and the mitotic protein cyclin (cyclin B). Mitotic cyclin associates with Cdc2 to form active MPF. MPF is initially inactive but is rapidly activated, thus triggering many important events that occur during mitosis. In order for a cell to exit the mitotic process as soon as it is complete, proteolytic degradation of cyclin occurs by the enzyme *ubiquitin*, which inactivates MPF. Thus, an important step in metaphase to anaphase is the destruction of cyclin by proteolysis, which switches off Cdk and stops the phosphorylation of proteins in the spindle and elsewhere in the cell.

Many molecular changes that occur in mitosis are brought about by *phosphorylation*. *MPF kinase* directly phosphorylates several substrates, in particular *histone H1*, which promotes chromosome condensation. Thus, a cascade of phosphorylations triggered by MPF is responsible for the complex events of mitosis. In somatic cells, unreplicated DNA generates an M-phase delaying signal that prevents the cytoplasmic MPF cycle from running faster than the chromosome cycle.

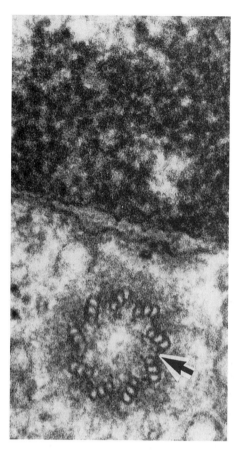

Figure 3.18. TEM of a centriole in transverse section illustrating the orientation of the paired triplet microtubules and the thin filaments (arrowhead) that extends from the A member of one triplet to the C member of the adjacent triplet. Note the diffuse material that surrounds the centriole. Cell nucleus is at top. ×125,000.

CHROMOSOME MOVEMENTS

During mitosis, microtubules pull or draw the chromosomes toward the poles at anaphase and also push the spindle poles apart. Three groups of microtubules are involved in mitosis. *Chromosomal spindle microtubules* attach to chromosomal kinetochores and extend toward the centrioles (Figs. 3.17, 3.20). *Polar microtubles* extend from the dividing cell's poles and overlap in its metaphase plate region (Fig. 3.20). *Astral microtubules* radiate from the centrioles of the centrosome or spindle pole (Fig. 3.20). The interphase eukaryotic animal cell has a single microtubule organizing center (MTOC), the centrosome, which includes the paired centrioles (Fig. 3.19). Centrioles play an important role in nucleating microtubules (MT) extending from the centrosome as astral, chromosomal and polar spindle MTs. The MTs are composed of α and β tubulin dimers. In addition, gamma tubulin is present near the MTOC and appears to be important in nucleating MT polymerization. In preparation for mitosis, phosphorylation

of microtubule-associated protein (MAP) can result in increased MT length.

During metaphase, tubulin subunits are added to the (+) end of the MT at the kinetochore and removed from the (−) end at the spindle pole. During anaphase, subunits are removed from the (+) end. Kinetochore MTs are capped and stable at metaphase, but subunits are lost during anaphase. The reason is not clear. A rapid 10-fold increase in cytosolic Ca^{2+} apparently initiates anaphase, and induces cyclin degradation and MPF inactivation. It also appears that a protein holds sister chromatids together until anaphase, when this protein must be degraded, perhaps by a cyclin protease, to permit rapid separation of the sister chromatids at anaphase. A relatively huge force of about 10^{-5} dynes per chromosome acts during early anaphase, which involves the poleward movement of chromatids and the shortening of kinetochore microtubules (*anaphase A*). Also, the polar spindle microtubules elongate (*anaphase B*). Kinetochore microtubules disassemble during anaphase A. Microtubule motor proteins appear to be involved in pushing and pulling poles apart. Plus-end-directed motor proteins (kinesin family) cross-link overlapping and antiparallel polar microtubules, causing them to slide past each other and pushing the spindle poles apart. Minus-end-directed motor proteins (dynein family) bind to astral microtubules and the cell cortex and increase the interpole distance (Fig. 3.20). The kinetochore appears to "walk" its way poleward along the MTs during anaphase. The chromosomes move at a rate of about 1 μm/min. During anaphase A, kinetochore MTs shorten as the chromosomes move closer to the poles. During anaphase B, the polar or continuous MTs elongate such that the two poles move farther apart (Fig. 3.20). Thus, two distinct processes appear to separate the chromosomes at anaphase.

It is not clear how the chromosomes move during anaphase A, although *subunits* are *lost* from the *microtubule* at the *kinetochore* end. One mechanism indicates that the kinetochore hydrolyzes ATP to move along the attached MT, followed by depolymerization of the (+) end of the MT. Another possibility is that the actual depolymerization of the MT causes the kinetochore to move passively. In the ATP-driven chromosome movement hypothesis for driving MT disassembly, an ATP-driven "walking protein," perhaps similar to kinesin or dynein, is a component of the kinetochore and uses the energy from ATP hydrolysis to pull the chromosomes along the bound MT.

The *MT motors* (dyneins and kinesins) are mechanochemical enzymes that use the energy derived from the hydrolysis of ATP to move along the surface of MTs. All known *dynein motors* move toward the (−) *ends* of the MTs. The smaller *kinesin* proteins usually move toward the (+) *ends* of MTs, but some can move toward the (−) ends. A type of dynein and a form of kinesin have been identified as constituents of the kine-

Figure 3.19. TEM of paired centrioles (longitudinal sections). Spindle microtubules (arrowheads). ×100,000.

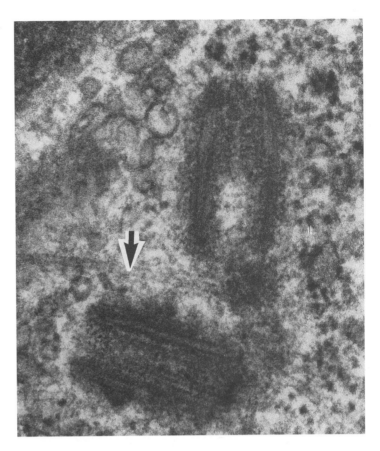

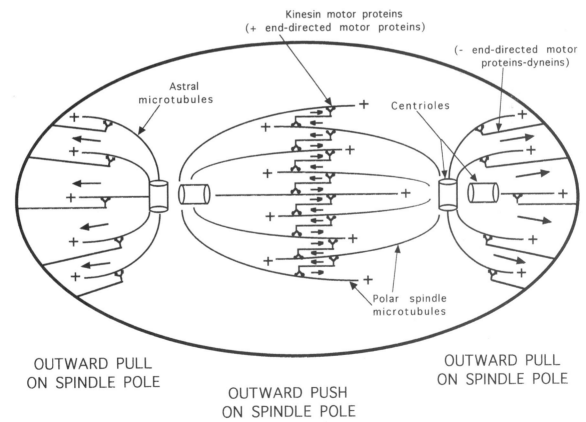

Figure 3.20. Diagram illustrates concept of how spindle poles are pushed apart by plus-end-directed motor proteins (kinesin) and how the interpole distance is increased by the action of minus-end-directed motor proteins (dynein).

(Redrawn and modified from B. Alberts, et al., *Molecular Biology of the Cell*, 3rd ed., p. 932, Garland Publishing Inc., New York, 1994, with permission)

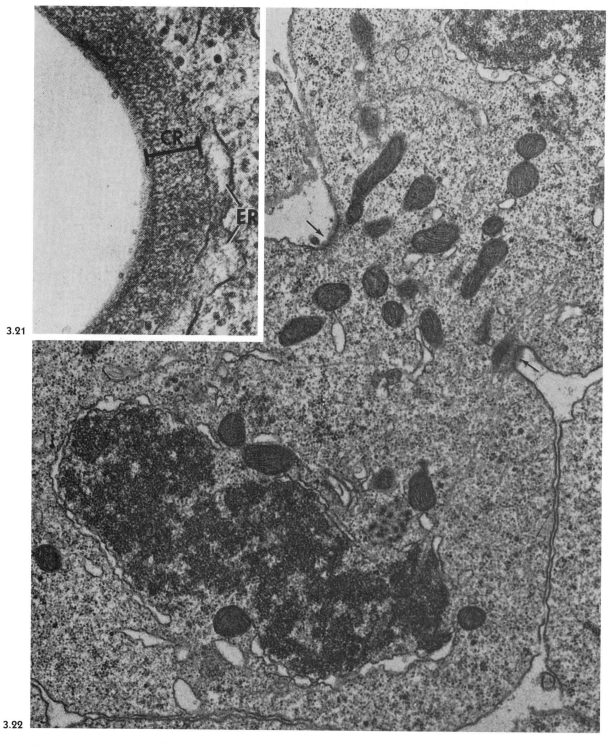

3.21

3.22

Figures 3.21, 3.22. Enlargement of cleavage furrow from the telophase stage cell in Figure 3.22. The contractile ring (CR) of actin microfilaments is located in close proximity to the cell membrane. Figure 3.22 is a low-magnification view of a telophase stage; the cleavage furrow is denoted by the arrow. Note that the nuclear envelope has begun to re-form around the decondensing chromosomes. Figure 3.21, ×100,000; Figure 3.22, ×22,600.

tochores. The presence of MT motors at the kinetochore indicates a role in chromosome movement during mitosis; perhaps they may also play a role in tethering the chromosomes to their spindle MTs.

CYTOKINESIS

Karyokinesis is followed by constriction of the cell into two separate entities (*cytokinesis*). The cleavage furrow that marks the beginning of cytokinesis occurs in the plane of the equatorial plate of metaphase (Figs. 3.21, 3.22). In this region a *subplasma membrane band* of *actin filaments* becomes associated with the cleavage furrow (Fig. 3.21). The constriction of the cell into two during telophase is related to a contractile ring of actin containing microfilaments around the cell just beneath the cell membrane where the cleavage furrow will form. The cleavage furrow deepens, and the spindle MTs become compressed by the advancing furrow. The furrow may persist for a time prior to complete separation of the daughter cells. For dividing cells in culture as well as for large eggs during cytokinesis, new plasma membrane may be inserted in the form of microvilli parallel with the cleavage furrow to provide the additional membrane required when one cell divides into two.

NUCLEAR MATRIX

The *nuclear matrix* is the insoluble structural skeleton of the nucleus that aids in the three-dimensional arrangement of DNA. The proteins comprising the nuclear matrix are currently being characterized in terms of structure and function. The chromatin and nucleolus are surrounded by the nuclear matrix, which appears in the TEM as a network of thin filaments throughout the nucleus attached to the nuclear lamina. This region was formerly called the *nucleoplasm* or *nuclear sap*. The nuclear matrix is postulated to be involved in the spatial organization of the nucleus and the assembly of different enzyme complexes; it may act as a pathway for macromolecular transport within the nucleus, and may even influence gene replication and activity.

SELECTED BIBLIOGRAPHY

Bostock, C.J., and Sumner, A.T. (1978). *The Eukaryotic Chromosome.* North-Holland, Amsterdam.

Brinkley, B.R. (1990). Toward a molecular and structural definition of the kinetochore. *Cell Motil. Cytoskeleton* **16**, 104–109.

Campbell, J. (1986). Eukaryotic DNA replication. *Annu. Rev. Biochem.* **55**, 733–772.

Cande, W.Z., and Hogan, C.J. (1989). The mechanism of anaphase spindle elongation. *BioEssays* **11**, 5–9.

Cao, L.G., and Wang, Y.L. (1990). Mechanism of the formation of contractile ring in dividing cultured animal cells. *J. Cell Biol.* **111**, 1905–1912.

Goldfarb, D.S. (1989). Nuclear transport. *Curr. Opin. Cell Biol.* **1**, 441–446.

Green, M.R. (1989). Pre-mRNA processing and mRNA nuclear export. *Curr. Opin. Cell Biol.* **1**, 519–525.

Hartwell, L.H., and Weinert, T.A. (1989). Checkpoints: controls that ensure the order of cell cycle events. *Science* **246**, 629–633.

Hyams, J.S., and Brinkley, B.R. (1989). *Mitosis. Molecules and Mechanisms.* Academic Press, San Diego, CA.

Hyman, A.A., and Mitchison, T.J. (1991). Two different microtubule-based motor activities with opposite polarities in kinetochores. *Nature* **351**, 206–211.

Jordan, E.G., and Cullis, C.A., eds. (1982). *The Nucleolus.* Cambridge University Press, Cambridge.

Kornberg, R.D., and Klug, A. (1981). The nucleosome. *Sci. Am.* **244**, 52–64.

Kornberg, R.D., and Lorch, Y. (1992). Chromatin structure and transcription. *Annu. Rev. Cell Biol.* **8**, 563–587.

Lahka, M.J. (1989). Mitotic control by metaphase-promoting factor and cdc proteins. *J. Cell Sci.* **92**, 131–135.

McIntosh, J.R., and Hering, G.E. (1991). Spindle fiber action and chromosome movement. *Annu. Rev. Cell Biol.* **7**, 403–426.

McKeon, F. (1991). Nuclear lamin proteins: domains required for nuclear targeting, assembly and cell-cycle-regulated dynamics. *Curr. Opin. Cell Biol.* **3**, 82–86.

Mitchison, T.J. (1989). Mitosis: basic concepts. *Curr. Opin. Cell Biol.* **1**, 67–74.

Moyzis, R. (1991). The human telomere. *Sci. Am.* **265**, 48–55.

Nigg, E.A. (1992). Assembly-disassembly of the nuclear lamina. *Curr. Opin. Cell Biol.* **4**, 105–109.

Satterwhite, L.L., and Pollard, T.D. (1992). Cytokinesis. *Curr. Opin. Cell Biol.* **4**, 43–52.

Warner, F.D., and McIntosh, J.R., eds. (1989). Microtubule movements during mitosis. In *Cell Movement,* Vol. 2, Section 2. Alan R. Liss, New York.

CHAPTER 4

Epithelial Tissue

NATURE OF EPITHELIUM

Epithelium is one of four basic tissue types; the others are connective tissue, muscle, and nerve. A *tissue* is an aggregation of cells that usually share a similar structure and function; often the cells are bound together by intercellular substances. Epithelium consists of closely packed sheets of cells that form *covering* and *lining layers* of the body and internal organs. For example, the entire body is covered by epithelium, but epithelium also lines the interior of the digestive, excretory, reproductive, and respiratory tracts. Therefore, epithelium functions in such important and varied activities as protection, sensory reception, and the secretion, absorption, and transport of bioactive molecules (Table 4.1). Epithelial cells can participate in regulating the ionic environment of the external and internal compartments of the body. Epithelial cells are often polarized to serve as selective permeability barriers between biological compartments; the barriers are often involved in vectorial transport by mechanisms of absorption, secretion, and transcytosis. Most of the epithelial cells originate from ectoderm and endoderm. Endothelium that lines blood vessels and mesothelium (lining body cavities, tubular cells in the kidney, and epithelium in the male and female reproductive tracts) develop from mesoderm.

THREE COMMON CHARACTERISTICS OF EPITHELIUM

There are several features common to all epithelium.

1. Epithelial cells are closely packed. Adjacent cells are separated by an intercellular or para-

cellular space that may be only ~*25 nm*. This close spatial relationship is facilitated, in part, by various cell adhesion molecules in the intercellular space.

2. Another common feature of epithelia is that an extracellular matrix is secreted at the base of the cell; the extracellular matrix is called a *basal lamina*. The basal lamina anchors the epithelium to the adjacent connective tissue. The epithelial cell-produced basal lamina and the type III collagen produced by fibroblasts in the adjacent connective tissue constitute the *basement membrane* that anchors epithelium to the underlying or adjacent connective tissue. The basal lamina also functionally integrates the extracellular coat and the cells in the external environment to a cytoskeletal system inside the cell.

3. All epithelia lack blood vessels. Because epithelium is avascular, it is necessary for the cells to obtain nutrients and oxygen by diffusion from capillaries restricted to the adjacent connective tissue. To shorten the diffusion distance from capillaries in connective tissue, the basal surface of an epithelium, especially stratified epithelium, is often folded. Metabolic waste products and carbon dioxide must also diffuse from the epithelial cells to capillaries in connective tissue.

FEATURES COMMON TO MANY EPITHELIA

1. Epithelial cells frequently exhibit a polarized morphology with specialized *apical*, *basal*, and

Table 4.1 Functions of Epithelia

Function	Example
Protection	Layered (stratified) epithelia cover surface of body, cover and line interior of organs
Absorption	Simple columnar (absorptive) cells lining small intestine and stomach absorb variety of products
Secretion	Goblet cells (unicellular mucous gland cells) in epithelial sheets; mucous and serous glands derived from epithelium; other epithelial cells in oviducts, bronchioles, type II pneumocytes, etc., secrete various products
Excretion, transport	Gallbladder and kidney tubule epithelial cells actively transport various ions, nitrogenous wastes, water, etc.
Contractility	Myoepithelial (contractile) cells around secretory units and smallest ducts of glands (e.g., salivary glands, mammary glands)
Sensory reception	Taste buds, an example of neuroepithelium on papillae in the tongue
Immunologic function	Langerhans cells in epidermis of integument, a type of antigen-presenting cell (macrophage)

lateral or *basolateral* borders or *plasma membrane domains.* The apical cellular domain faces the external compartment. The basal and lateral cellular domains face the internal compartment. The various cellular domains are functionally and biochemically distinguished by the kinds of membrane lipids, enzymes, ion transporters, receptors, and structural proteins present in the membranes. The lateral and basal cell membrane domains contain receptors and adhesion proteins that form junctional complexes and cell-substratum contacts. Associated with functions of vectorial fluid transport and directed pathways for absorption and secretion, epithelial cells have asymmetrically placed integral membrane proteins within the apical or basolateral membrane domains. Apical plasma membrane molecules such as *hydrolases* and *carrier proteins* facilitate absorption. Basolateral *hormone receptors* stimulate secretion. *Basolateral Na^+, K^+-ATPase* generates an ionic gradient causing a vectorial flow of water. Depending upon the cell type, transport between the apical and basolateral domains, or between the basolateral and apical domains, is possible and is mediated by a multistep vesicular transport pathway called *transcytosis.* The apical plasma membrane domain of a polarized epithelial cell is delineated from the basolateral plasma membrane region by tight junctions that circumnavigate the horizontal axis of the cell and seal off the intercellular space.

2. Several different kinds of specialized intercel-

lular junctions are associated with epithelium, and they function to (a) anchor the cells together, (b) seal off the intercellular space locally, or (c) permit passage of small molecules between adjacent cells. These specializations will be described in more detail subsequently.

3. The outer or free surface of many epithelial sheets of cells is kept moistened. The secretion is produced by *epithelial cells* themselves, by *goblet cells*, or by *exocrine glands* that are derived from the epithelial layers in the embryo. When the outer surface of an epithelium dries out, the cells ultimately die and slough off. Moisture permits a longer life span for epithelium.

4. Because most epithelia cover and line surfaces, the cells are subject to mechanical abrasion; therefore, it is necessary for epithelial cells to be capable of replacement. Epithelial cells are, in fact, capable of division to maintain the integrity of the cellular sheet. For example, it has been estimated that the entire epithelium lining the interior of the small intestine is replaced over a period of less than 6 days.

5. The free or apical surface of epithelial cells often possess structural specializations that may include *microvilli, stereocilia,* or *cilia.*

MICROSCOPIC FEATURES

To determine how epithelial functions are carried out, an understanding of the variability in organization is useful. The classification or identification of epithelia is

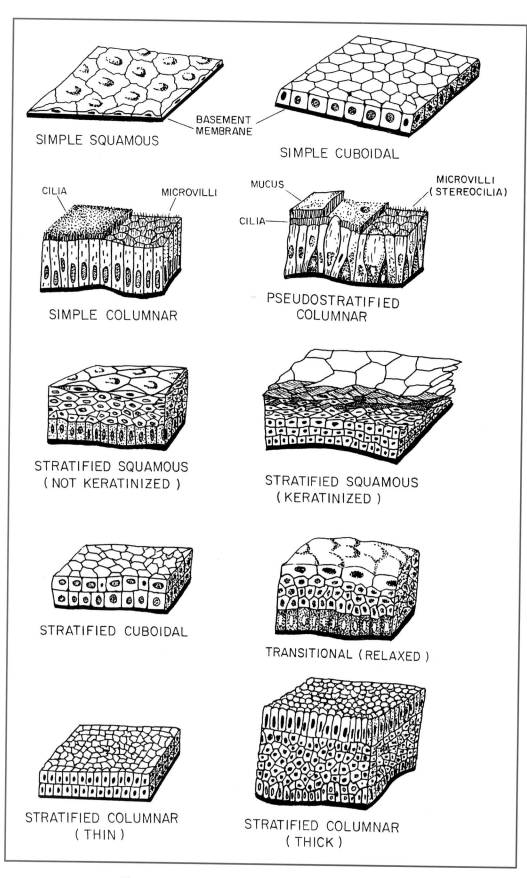

Figure 4.1. Diagrams showing all types of epithelium.

SIMPLE SQUAMOUS

BASEMENT MEMBRANE

SIMPLE CUBOIDAL

CILIA

MICROVILLI

SIMPLE COLUMNAR

MUCUS

CILIA

MICROVILLI (STEREOCILIA)

PSEUDOSTRATIFIED COLUMNAR

STRATIFIED SQUAMOUS (NOT KERATINIZED)

STRATIFIED SQUAMOUS (KERATINIZED)

STRATIFIED CUBOIDAL

TRANSITIONAL (RELAXED)

STRATIFIED COLUMNAR (THIN)

STRATIFIED COLUMNAR (THICK)

based on cell shape and number of cell layers (Fig. 4.1). An epithelial sheet that contains only a single layer of cells is called a *simple epithelium*. An epithelium two or more cells thick is designated a *stratified epithelium*. If an epithelium contains some cells that extend from the basement membrane to the free surface, but other cells that extend from the basement membrane only partially to the free surface, it is called *pseudostratified epithelium*. In addition, the shape of cells comprising the simple epithelium or the superficial layer of cells in a stratified epithelium is used in the classification. If the cells are extremely flat, they are called *squamous*; the width and depth are greater than the cell height in this case. If the length, width, and height of the cells are similar, they are called *cuboidal*. If the height of the cells exceeds the width and depth, the cell is characterized as *columnar*. The locations for different epithelial types are listed in Table 4.2.

CLASSIFICATION

SIMPLE SQUAMOUS EPITHELIUM

Simple squamous epithelium consists of cellular sheets only one cell thick. The cells are highly flattened (Plate 2A,B) Figs. 4.2–4.6) and are always associated with moist or wet surfaces. In fact, in some areas such as the alveolar (lung) epithelium, the cytoplasm is usually too thin to be distinguished with the LM. This is a delicate type of epithelium with no protective function; rather, it serves a filtering or dialyzing function because of the short diffusion distance across the cells. The location of simple squamous epithelium is indicated in Table 4.2.

The simple squamous epithelium that forms capillaries and lines the interior of all other blood vessels is called by a special name, *endothelium* (Plate 2C; Fig. 4.2). The simple squamous epithelium that forms the mesothelial layer of mesenteries is also given a special name, *mesothelium* (Fig. 4.5). Mesothelium has an adhering layer of connective tissue in a mesentery. Mesenteries can be prepared as flat mounts and stained to show surface views of the simple squamous cells.

SIMPLE CUBOIDAL EPITHELIUM

Simple cuboidal epithelium consists of a single layer of cells that are similar in height, width, and length (depth) (Plate 2D–G; Figs. 4.6–4.9). The cell nuclei appear at the same level in sections perpendicular to the epithelium. Locations of simple cuboidal epithelium are presented in Table 4.2.

SIMPLE COLUMNAR EPITHELIUM

Simple columnar epithelium consists of a single layer of cells in which the cell height exceeds the width and depth (Plate 3A–D; Fig. 4.10). It is a very widespread type of epithelium that is maintained in a moist environment. The epithelium generally functions in absorption, secretion, and protection. Various surface modifications can be associated with the apical surface of simple columnar epithelium (Table 4.3), including *microvilli*, (Figs. 4.12–4.14) which are finger-like projections of the plasma membrane, or longer, motile *cilia* (Fig. 4.11). In addition, in certain areas, some of the cells in the epithelium may be transformed from a columnar shape to a goblet (inverted flask) shape (Plate 3A). The *goblet cell* represents a *unicellular gland* that is functionally specialized to synthesize and export a glycoprotein material called *mucus*.

PSEUDOSTRATIFIED EPITHELIUM

In this epithelial type, all cells are in contact with the basement membrane, but not all the cells extend to the surface (Fig. 4.1). As a result, cell nuclei appear to be at different levels when perpendicularly sectioned and erroneously give the impression of a stratified (i.e., pseudostratified) epithelium (Plate 3E,F). The section plane markedly affects the clarity with which many epithelia can be identified. Pseudostratified epithelium may or may not contain microvilli, cilia, stereocilia, or goblet cells (Table 4.4).

STRATIFIED EPITHELIA

Stratified epithelia are sheets of cells that are two or more cells thick; therefore, this type of epithelium is more able than simple epithelia to resist wear and tear (Fig. 4.1). Because stratified epithelia are thicker, they are not as efficient in absorption or secretion. When a secretory function is required, glands are formed that connect by ducts to the lumen or surface of the epithelium.

STRATIFIED CUBOIDAL EPITHELIUM

This epithelium consists of two layers of cells, both of which are cuboidal in shape (Plate 5B). Stratified cuboidal epithelium lines the inner surface of the ciliary processes in the eye and is present in the sweat gland ducts.

Table 4.2 Location of Epithelial Tissues

Simple Squamous
- Tympanic membrane (inner surface)
- Bowman's capsule—parietal layer
- Pulmonary alveoli
- Thin loop of Henle
- Membranous labyrinth (inner surface)
- Posterior cornea
- Rete testis
- *Endothelium* of blood vessels, heart and lymph vessels, lining of sinusoids of liver
- *Mesothelium* serous membranes lining the peritoneal, pleural, and pericardial cavities
- *Mesenchymal epithelium* lining subarachnoid space, anterior eye chambers and lines perilymphatic space

Simple Cuboidal
- Thyroid
- Kidney tubules
- Some intralobular ducts of glands
- Choroid plexus
- Lens epithelium
- Pigmented layer of retina
- Liver parenchyma
- Surface of ovary

Simple Columnar
- Lines digestive tube
- Excretory ducts of glands
- Organ of Corti sensory cells
- Gallbladder
- Proximal and distal convoluted tubes of kidney
- Uterus, cervical canal (some ciliated)
- Oviduct (some ciliated)
- Bronchioles (cilia)
- Central canal spinal cord—ciliated
- Epididymus (stereocilia)
- Some paranasal sinuses (cilia)
- Stomach
- Small intestine (microvilli, goblet cells)
- Large intestine (microvilli, goblet cells)

Neuroepithelium
- Taste buds—tongue

Pseudostratified Columnar
- Parotid gland excretory duct
- Vas deferens
- Epididymis (stereocilia)

Pseudostratified Ciliated Columnar
- Trachea, bronchi (cilia, goblet cells)
- Auditory (eustachian) tube
- Tympanic cavity, membrane of middle ear
- Lacrimal sac
- Efferent ductules
- Nasopharynx
- Larynx
- Epiglottis

Transitional
- Urinary bladder
- Ureter, renal calices
- Proximal urethra

Stratified Squamous
- Esophagus
- Skin epidermis (keratinized)
- Conjunctiva
- Oral, vaginal, anal, urethral apertures
- External auditory canal
- Tear ducts, esophagus
- Mouth, pharynx
- Outer surface of cornea
- Epiglottis (parts)

Stratified Cuboidal
- Excretory ducts of sweat glands
- Lining of developing ovarian follicles
- Seminiferous tubules
- Epithelium of ciliary processes

Stratified Columnar
- Largest excretory ducts of glands
- Male urethra
- Conjunctiva of eye
- Fornix of conjunctiva (parts)
- Pharynx, epiglottis (parts)

Stratified Columnar (Ciliated)
- Nasal surface soft palate
- Larynx
- Fetal esophagus

Myoepithelium
- Surround secretory alveoli and small intralobular ducts of mammary gland, salivary glands, sweat glands

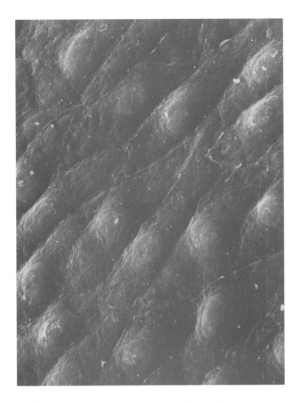

Figure 4.2. SEM of endothelium (simple squamous epithelium) lining the interior of rabbit heart (endocardium). Note the shape of the cells and bulges due to the internal location of the nucleus. ×1430.

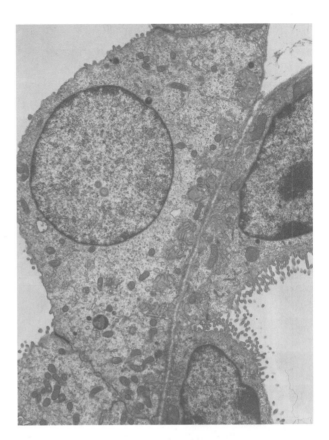

Figure 4.4. TEM of simple squamous epithelial cell in the thin limb of Henle's loop in kidney. ×6045.

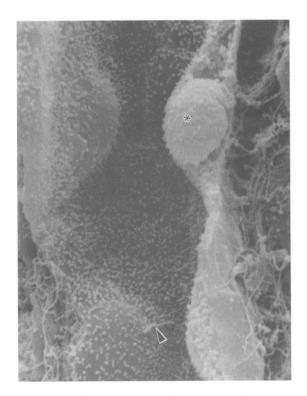

Figure 4.3. SEM of a longitudinal section of the thin limb of Henle's loop in kidney. One cell is cut open and shows the nucleus (*). Note the short, stubby microvilli on the apical surface of these simple squamous cells and a single, nonmotile cilium (arrowhead) on one cell. ×4370.

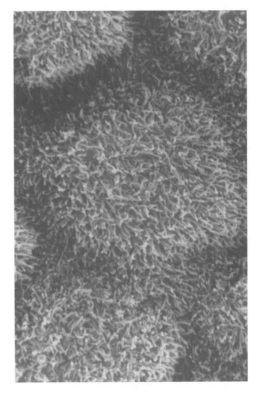

Figure 4.5. SEM of several serosal (mesothelial) cells (simple squamous epithelium) covering the outer surface of the rat spleen. Note the many long, finger-like processes (microvilli) covering the outer (free) surface of these cells. ×6500.

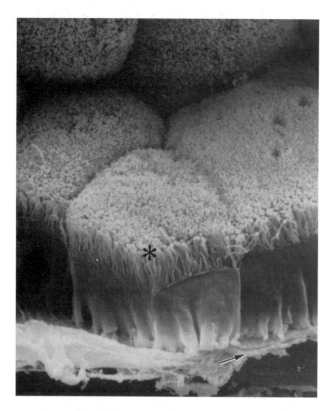

Figure 4.6. SEM of cuboidal epithelial cells in kidney. The cells have many finger-shaped microvilli (*) extending from the free surface, and the cells reside on a basement membrane (arrow). ×3575.

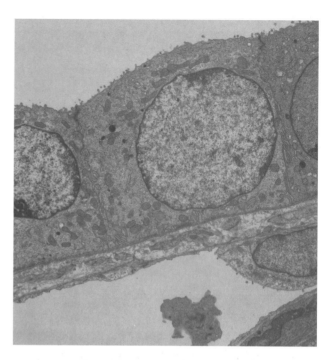

Figure 4.8. TEM of a simple cuboidal kidney tubule cell. These cells lack the prominent microvilli present on other cells. ×3875.

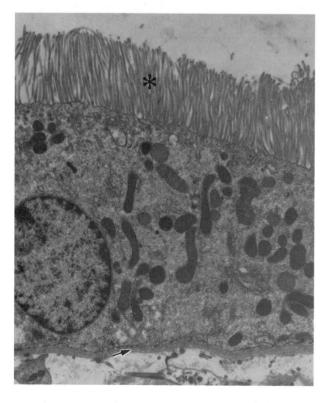

Figure 4.7. TEM of a simple cuboidal epithelial cell in kidney. Microvilli (*) on the apical surface and basement membrane (arrow) are identified. ×6045.

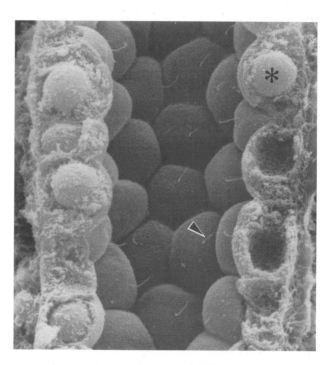

Figure 4.9. SEM of simple cuboidal epithelial cells in the collecting tubule of kidney. Note the exposed nuclei (*) and a single nonmotile cilium (arrowhead) on the apical surface of each cell. ×2170.

78

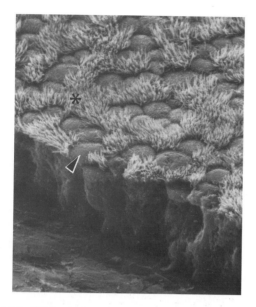

Figure 4.10. SEM of simple columnar epithelium in oviduct. Both ciliated (*) and secretory cells (arrowhead) are present in the epithelium. ×1240.

STRATIFIED COLUMNAR EPITHELIUM

This type of epithelium may consist of either a single basal layer of cells that are covered by an overlying layer of columnar-shaped cells (as in large excretory ducts of compound glands) or it may consist of several basal layers of cells that are cuboidal or polygonal in outline but covered by a single layer of columnar cells (Plate 5C,D). The thickness of this epithelium varies. Table 4.2 lists other areas where this type of epithelium can be found.

STRATIFIED SQUAMOUS (NONKERATINIZED) EPITHELIUM

Stratified squamous epithelium consists of a few to many layers of cells, but the surface cells are always squamous (Plate 4A). Two varieties exist, depending upon whether the epithelium dries out or is maintained in a moistened condition. If the epithelium is kept moist by glands associated with the epithelium, it is a nonkeratinizing type of stratified squamous epithelium (Plate 5A). In such epithelia, cells of the basal layer that are in contact with a basement membrane are columnar in shape, while several cell layers above these are polygonal in shape. The superficial cell layers, however, are squamous, hence the name of this epithelium. Locations for this epithelium are listed in Table 4.2.

Stratified squamous epithelium is highly suited for protection. Division of cells occurs in the basal layer, and the cells move toward the surface. During this time they change in shape from columnar to polygonal and then to squamous. The squamous surface cells are con-

tinually shed or lost from the epithelium; therefore, turnover or replacement of cells is required. It is the moisture or secretion from glands that keeps the surface cells in the epithelium from drying out and keratinizing.

STRATIFIED SQUAMOUS (KERATINIZED) EPITHELIUM

The surface cells of this epithelium become transformed into a tough, impermeable, nonliving layer of keratin that is attached to the underlying cells in the epithelium (Plate 4B). The keratin layer is generally waterproof, impervious to bacteria, and protects from wear and tear. This epithelium covers the body but is much thicker on the soles of the feet and palms of the hands, so these areas can withstand even greater mechanical abrasion. The keratin is continually sloughed and tends to wear away. However, the basal layer of columnar-shaped cells in the epithelium is mitotic and continually proliferates to supply new cells.

TRANSITIONAL EPITHELIUM

Transitional epithelium is a layered epithelium so named because its surface or superficial cells undergo a transition in shape, depending upon whether the epithelium is stretched (distended) or relaxed. When transitional epithelium is stretched, the surface cells are squamous or flat. When the epithelium is collapsed, however, the surface cells are more rounded or dome-shaped in appearance (Plate 4C,D). This type of epithelium is able to withstand stretching, as can be expected in organs that are distended from within, such as the urinary bladder, ureters, and renal pelvis.

NEUROEPITHELIUM

Neuroepithelium is a specialized epithelium that is exemplified by taste buds (Plate 5E; Fig. 4.15). Approximately 10,000 taste buds are present within the epithelium covering the tongue and in selected areas of the oral cavity, pharynx, and larynx. This will be described in Chapter 18.

MYOEPITHELIUM

Myoepithelial cells (formerly called *basket cells*) represent a specialized epithelial cell of limited distribution. The cells are highly branched, contain actin microfilaments, and can contract (Fig. 4.16). They are associated with the secretory avleoli and small intralobular ducts of some glands, including the mammary gland, salivary glands, and sweat glands (Fig. 4.16). In the mammary

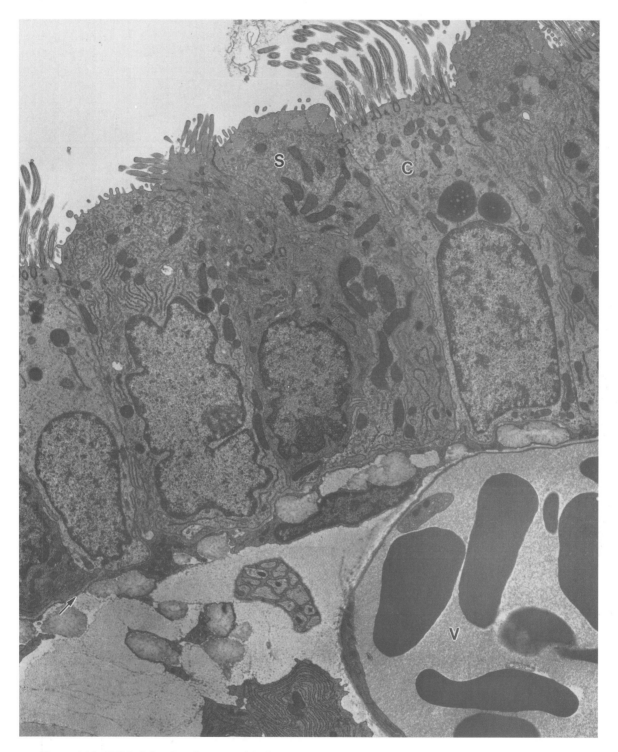

Figure 4.11. TEM of simple columnar epithelium. Both ciliated (C) cells and nonciliated, secretory (S) cells are pres- **ent. Basement membrane (arrow) and blood vessel (V) are identified. ×8100.**

gland, the hormone oxytocin causes contraction of the myoepithelial cells.

FUNCTIONS

The functions of epithelium are numerous and varied; they are summarized in Tables 4.1 and 4.5.

BASEMENT MEMBRANE

STRUCTURE

The boundary between epithelium and connective tissue is marked by a basement membrane (Figs. 4.17, 4.18). This interface was identified with the BFM as a distinct structure, which appeared as a thin line that

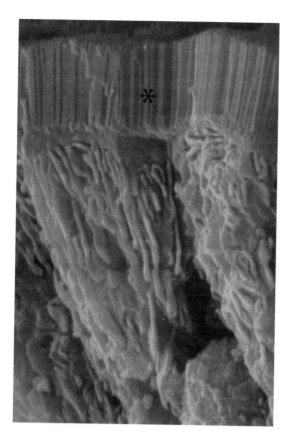

Figure 4.12. SEM of simple columnar epithelial cells showing many microvilli (*) extending from the free or apical surface. ×7190.

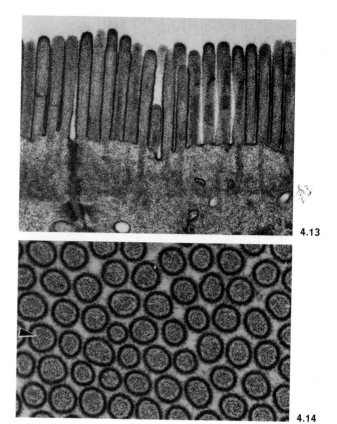

4.13

4.14

Figures 4.13, 4.14. Longitudinal (Fig. 4.13) and cross-sectional view (Fig. 4.14) of microvilli viewed in TEM. Microvilli contain many long, slender actin microfilaments (arrowhead), which are most apparent in the cross section. Figure 4.13, ×19,500; Figure 4.14, ×59,700.

stained with silver as well as the periodic acid Schiff (PAS) technique. Basement membranes are extracellular deposits at the base of epithelial sheets that are cooperatively produced by both epithelial cells and the underlying connective tissue cells. Basement membranes therefore represent a specific and regional specialization of the extracellular matrix.

The basal lamina is that portion of the basement membrane that is produced by epithelial cells. A basal lamina (basal laminae) is a continuous meshwork of specialized extracellular matrix, approximately 40–120 nm thick, that underlies all epithelial sheets and tubes (capillaries) and it also surrounds muscle cells (myocytes), fat cells (adipocytes) and Schwann cells. The basal lamina separates the cells and the adjacent connective tissue. In the TEM with conventional fixation and staining, the basal lamina consists of a *lamina lucida* adjacent to the basal plasma membrane of the cell. An electron dense *lamina densa* lies adjacent to the lamina lucida.

Type IV collagen molecules are organized into a three dimensional meshwork (Fig. 4.19) in the lamina densa. In addition, *fibronectin, laminin, heparan sulfate proteoglycan,* and *entactin* are associated with the type IV collagen. All of the aforementioned substances are produced by the epithelial cell. Type IV collagen forms a cova-

Table 4.3 Simple Columnar Epithelium

Location	Form of Simple Columnar Epithelium
Central canal—spinal cord	Many ciliated cells
Oviducts	Both ciliated and nonciliated secretory cells
Larger bronchioles	Ciliated simple columnar
Uterus	Short microvilli
Gallbladder	Stubby microvilli
Stomach	No apical modifications; cells secrete mucus directly
Cervical canal	Columnar cells secrete mucus directly; no goblet cells
Small intestine, large intestine	Prominent microvilli on absorptive cells; many goblet cells interspersed

Table 4.4 Modifications of Pseudostratified Epithelium

Variation	Possible Locations
No cilia, no microvilli, no goblet cells	Prostate gland, vas deferens, seminal vesicle, tympanic membrane
Stereocilia	Ductus epididymidis, in places in vas deferens
Cilia, no goblet cells	Eustachian tube, lacrimal sac, parts of tympanic and nasal cavities
Cilia, goblet cells	Nostrils, trachea, extrapulmonary bronchi, larger intrapulmonary bronchi

lently stabilized polygonal framework or meshwork. Laminin, a large complex consisting of three very long polypeptides, forms another polymer network in the basement membrane (Fig. 4.20). Laminin has a cross-shaped structure with a molecular weight of 900 kD. It is present throughout the basement membrane, but with a higher concentration in the lamina lucida. Laminin binds to type IV collagen; one domain binds heparin sulfate and another may bind to proteins on the cell surface. In addition laminin interacts with a laminin receptor in the epithelial cell, and aids in binding the basement membrane to the cell. Entactin/nidogen is a sulfated glycoprotein that binds to both collagen and laminin. Heparan sulfate proteoglycan is important for its charge-dependent molecular sieve properties, and binds to both laminin and type IV collagen. Heparan sulfate proteoglycan is located principally in the lamina lucida, but also in the lamina densa. Fibronectin is a high molecular weight, adhesive type of glycoprotein that is also widely distributed in basement membranes. Fibronectin is an extracellular Y-shaped molecule consisting of two similar polypeptide chains joined by two disulfide bonds (Fig. 4.23). Fibronectin attaches fibronectin receptors in the basal plasma membrane to the extracellular matrix, since each fibronectin molecule has binding sites for heparan and collagen. In addition to the lamina lucida and lamina densa of the basal lamina, the basement membrane includes a third layer, the *lamina reticularis* or *fibroreticularis*, which connects the basal lamina to the underlying connective tissue (Fig. 4.17). The reticular lamina is produced by connective tissue cells called fibroblasts and contains type III collagen (reticular fibers) (Figs. 4.17, 4.18). Fibronectin is important in attaching the lamina densa to the reticular fibers (type III collagen) of the reticular lamina. Constituents and functions of basal laminae are summarized in the table.

FUNCTIONAL ROLE

Basement membranes compartmentalize tissues, anchor cellular sheets, play a role in control of cell migration, and can act as a stimulus for cell differentiation during development. The basal laminae in the renal corpuscle play an important role as a selective filtration barrier or molecular filter. The basal laminae serve as a cellular barrier so that fibroblasts cannot touch epithelial cells. However, macrophages, lymphocytes, and nerve processes can move through the basal lamina. Basal laminae may provide a scaffolding along which cells can migrate, influence cell polarity and cell metabolism, help organize proteins in the adjacent plasma membrane, induce cell differentiation, and serve as highways for cell migration (fibronectin).

In some cases, the basement membranes are fenestrated, a condition that undoubtedly facilitates movement of cells and materials across them. For example, myofibroblasts are surrounded by an irregular and in-

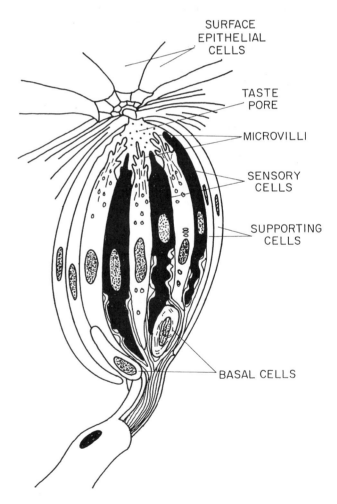

Figure 4.15. Diagram of neuroepithelial cells in the taste bud. (Redrawn from M. Ross, E. Reith and L. Romrell. *Histology, A Text and Atlas*, 2nd ed., Williams & Wilkins, Baltimore, 1989)

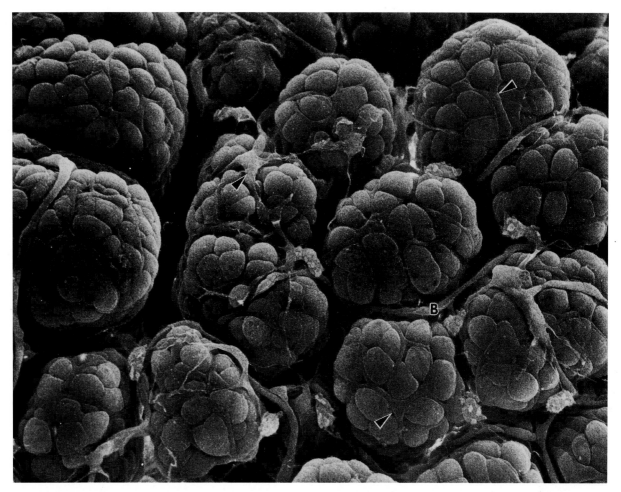

Figure 4.16. SEM illustrates outer surface of secretory alveoli (acini) in a lactating mammary gland. Most of the extracellular connective tissue was removed with enzyme-HCl digestion. Boundaries of cells are evident; blood capillaries (B); highly branched myoepithelial cells are denoted by arrowheads. (From: T. Nagato, H. Yoshida, A. Yoshida, and Y. Uehara, A scanning electron microscope study of myoepithelial cells in exocrine glands. *Cell Tissue Research* 209, 1–10, Figures 2 and 3, 1980, © Springer-Verlag, with permission)

complete basement membrane. Fenestrations occur in the basement membrane of the epithelial layer of the small intestine. Incomplete basal laminae or basement membranes are also associated with splenic sinusoids and bone marrow sinusoids. There is a discontinuous basement membrane in the extracellular spaces (space of Disse) in the liver.

MEDICAL ASPECTS

Plasminogen activator, a proteolytic enzyme that directly or indirectly degrades other proteins, permits cells to dissolve attachments and migrate through the extracellular matrix. Endothelial cells can produce plasminogen activator, which permits sprouts from capillaries to digest their way through the basal lamina of a parent capillary during angiogenesis. In invasive carcinomas, the cancer cells can apparently dissolve the ep-

ithelial basement membranes and migrate into the adjacent mesenchymal stroma. In the autoimmune skin disease bullous phemphigoid, subepidermal blisters result as dissolution of the lamina lucida occurs subsequent to deposition of autoantibodies against the bullous phemphigoid antigen. This antigen is a 220-kD polypeptide and is a component of hemidesmosomes.

EPITHELIAL CELL POLARITY, TERMINAL WEB, MICROVILLI

In epithelium, structural specializations of the apical, lateral, and basal cell surfaces are common. The cells have an internal polarity with respect to organelle distribution: the ER and mitochondria predominate in the basal cytoplasm, while the Golgi complex and secretory granules are located between the nucleus and the free

Table 4.5 Classification, Location, and Function of Epithelia

Classification		Location	Function
Simple (one cell layer)	Squamous	Mesothelium (covers and lines body cavities)	Secretion, facilitates sliding of organs
		Endothelium	Conduction, transport (active and micropinocytosis)
		Thin loop of Henle	Transport
		Alveolar sacs	Gaseous exchange
		Parietal layer of Bowman's capsule	Conduction
	Cuboidal	Lens epithelium	Formation of lens fibers and lens capsule
		Pigmented epithelium—retina	Melanin reflects light, phagocytoses rod discs
		Ovarian epithelium	Protection, forms follicle cells
		Some ducts of glands	Conduction, transport
		Some kidney tubules	Secretion, absorption
	Columnar	Stomach lining	Secretion, protection
		Gallbladder	Secretion, absorption
		Small intestine, (goblet cells, striated border)	Secretion, absorption
		Oviducts (ciliated and secretory cells)	Transport, protection secretion
Pseudostratified (nuclei at different levels; all cells touch basement membrane, not all reach surface)	Columnar	Vas deferens, excretory ducts of some glands	Conduction Conduction
	Columnar, stereocilia	Epididymis	Conduction, secretion, absorption
	Columnar, cilia, goblet cells	Nostrils (parts), trachea, large bronchi	Secretion, transport protection
Stratified (two to many layers of cells)	Squamous nonkeratinizing	Vagina, esophagus, oral cavity, conjunctivea, cornea epiglottis (parts)	Protection
	Squamous, keratinized	Skin (epidermis)	Protection, waterproofing, etc.
	Cuboidal	Ciliary processes (eye)	Secretion, zonule filament attachment, reflect light
		Ducts of sweat glands	Conduction
	Columnar	Large excretory ducts of glands	Protection, secretion, absorption
		Male urethra	Protection, secretion
	Transitional	Urinary bladder	Protection, distention
		Ureters	Protection, distention
Myoepithelium		Secretory alveoli and small ducts of large glands	Contractile, aid in movement of secretion
Neuroepithelium		Taste buds	Support for nerve ending

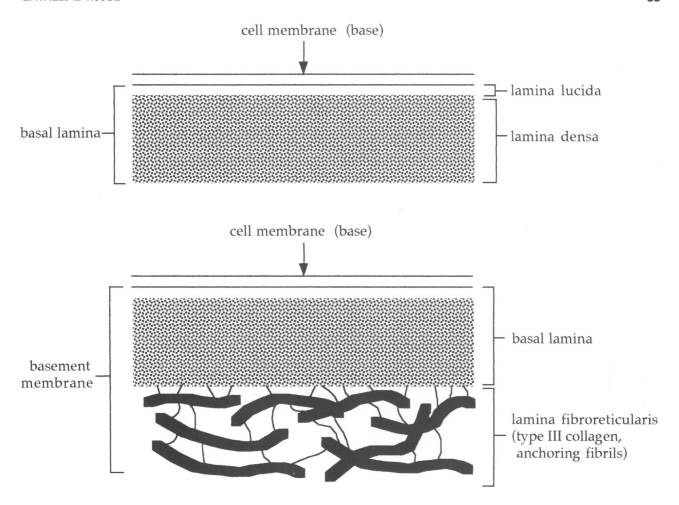

Figure 4.17. Simplified diagram illustrates layers of basal lamina and basement membrane.

or apical end of the cell (supranuclear). One structural specialization seals off a portion of the intercellular space between epithelial cells. Others promote cell adhesion and provide strength to the epithelial sheets. Still another facilitates exchange of small molecules between cells. The microvilli at the apical end of some epithelia provide for amplification of a selective part of the cell's plasma membrane. This increases the absorptive surface area or amplifies specific enzymes or macromolecules at a localized region of the cell surface. Basal infoldings of the plasma membrane are prevalent in cells with amplified transport functions (i.e., proximal tubule cells in kidney). Cilia are present on some epithelial cells and permit the cells to propel the contents of cavities lined by the epithelium.

TERMINAL WEB AND MICROVILLI

A thin, striated band was evident at the apical end of intestinal epithelial cells in early LM observations and was termed a *striated* or *brush border*. The margin at the apical end was observed to stain intensely, but the intervening region appeared homogeneous and devoid of visible structures with the LM; this area was called the *terminal web*. The striated appearance of the apical region of intestinal epithelial cells is due to the presence of many (perhaps 3000 per cell) finger-like extensions of the plasma membrane (Figs. 4.11–4.14). Each microvillus is approximately 1–5 μm long and 0.1 μm wide. Oligosaccharide side chains extend from the plasma membrane of the microvilli. The thin, polysaccharide-rich coating that covers the cell has been termed the *glycocalyx* (sweet husk) and can be identified by cytochemical staining with the PAS technique for the LM or by various polysaccharide identifying cytochemical tests for the TEM. The interior of each microvillus and the apical band of cytoplasm just beneath the microvillous border are now known to comprise a very complex domain of the cell. The core of each microvillus contains a bundle of actin filaments that extends from the tip of the microvillus into the apical terminal web region of the cell (Fig. 4.21). The *actin filaments* are oriented with their (+) ends pointing toward the tips of

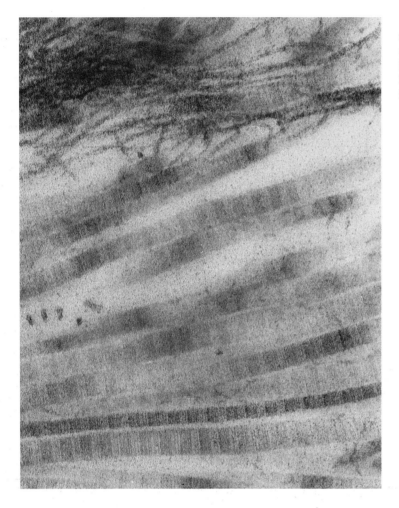

Figure 4.18. TEM of basement membrane. Thin filaments of lamina densa (top) terminate in close proximity to wider reticular fibrils (type III collagen) with an axial periodicity. ×90,000.

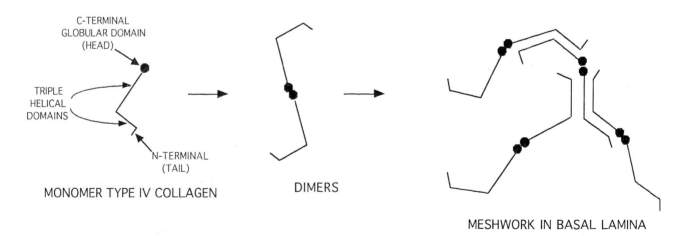

C-TERMINAL
GLOBULAR DOMAIN
(HEAD)

TRIPLE
HELICAL
DOMAINS

N-TERMINAL
(TAIL)

MONOMER TYPE IV COLLAGEN

DIMERS

MESHWORK IN BASAL LAMINA

Figure 4.19. Monomers and dimers of type IV collagen.

Figure 4.20. Structure of laminin molecule.

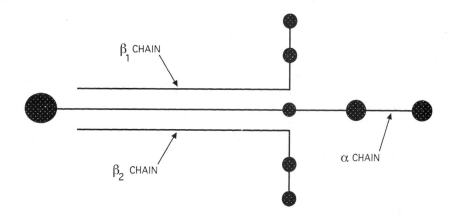

β_1 CHAIN

β_2 CHAIN

α CHAIN

the microvilli. *Villin* and *fimbrin* interconnect the actin filaments in each microvillus and bundle and cross-link the microfilaments (Fig. 4.21). Lateral sidearms extend from the plasma membrane of the microvillus to the microfilaments; these sidearms contain myosin-1 and calmodulin. The microfilaments that extend from the microvilli into the apical cytoplasm are associated with *IFs* (Figs. 4.21, 4.22) that have an overlying layer of *spectrin molecules*, an arrangement believed to stabilize and stiffen the actin microfilament bundles.

CYTOSKELETON

Epithelial cells have a cytoskeletal lattice associated with and immediately adjacent to the cell membrane. This *membrane skeleton* has been best studied in the red blood cell, where the membrane skeleton controls cell shape and restricts the lateral mobility of those membrane proteins that are anchored to the cytoskeleton (Chapter 8). In the brush border *protein 260/240* (an analog of *spectrin* in the erythrocyte) plays a structural role in associ-

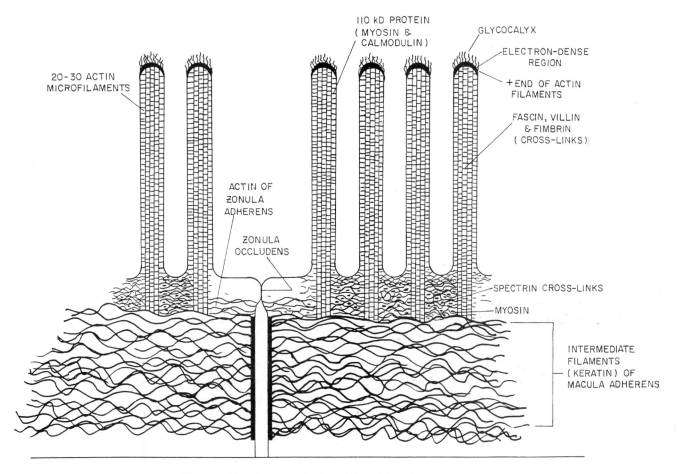

110 kD PROTEIN (MYOSIN & CALMODULIN)

GLYCOCALYX

ELECTRON-DENSE REGION

+ END OF ACTIN FILAMENTS

FASCIN, VILLIN & FIMBRIN (CROSS-LINKS)

20-30 ACTIN MICROFILAMENTS

ACTIN OF ZONULA ADHERENS

ZONULA OCCLUDENS

SPECTRIN CROSS-LINKS

MYOSIN

INTERMEDIATE FILAMENTS (KERATIN) OF MACULA ADHERENS

Figure 4.21. Diagram of microvilli and junctional complexes.

ation with myosin to interconnect adjacent microvillar core rootlets (composed of bundled actin filaments) and link them with the overlying plasma membrane. The cytoskeleton associated with the microvilli and terminal web is illustrated in Figure 4.21. Cell adhesion molecules (CAMs) like *uvomorulin* (E-cadherin) are involved in Ca^{2+}-dependent adhesion between lateral plasma membranes of epithelial cells and are located in junctional complexes.

Intracellular actin microfilaments are linked to fibronectin in the basal lamina of the extracellular matrix by way of several proteins, such as *vinculin* and *talin*. *Talin* is associated with *fibronectin receptors* in the plasma membrane, which, in turn, bind *fibronectin*. Molecules involved in linking the cytoskeleton to the extracellular matrix are illustrated in Figure 4.23.

INTERCELLULAR JUNCTIONS (JUNCTIONAL COMPLEXES)

Specialized regions of the plasma membrane called *intercellular junctions* or *junctional complexes* are present at the apical ends of contiguous epithelial cells (Fig. 4.24a–f). The intercellular junctions are named on the basis of whether they are spot-like or button-shaped (*macula*) or if the specialization completely surrounds the cells like a belt (*zonula*). The nature of the close contact between cells is also used in classification. The most frequently encountered of these junctional complexes are the tight junctions (*zonulae occludentes*), intermediate junction (*zonulae adherentes* or belt desmosomes), spot desmosomes (or *maculae adherentes*), and *gap junctions* (nexus).

ZONULA OCCLUDENS (OCCLUDING OR TIGHT JUNCTIONS)

Free diffusion of substances through the paracellular pathway between epithelial cells is prevented by a specialized region of cell-cell contact, called the *zonula occludens* (*ZO*) or *tight junction*, which encircles the cells at their apices and closes the intercellular space (Fig. 4.24f). The ZO (pl.: zonulae occludentes) is the most apically located junctional specialization and completely surrounds the cells. In thin sections viewed with the TEM, the intercellular space is obliterated due to the apparent fusion of the outer leaflets of the plasma membrane of apposed cells and the loss of the narrow intervening intercellular space (Fig. 4.25). When freeze fracture replicas of cell membranes are viewed with the TEM, the ZO is characterized by a series of thin, branching ridges on the P face and corresponding grooves on the E fracture face (Fig. 4.26). These ridges and grooves are thought to be due to the interaction of complementary intramembrane protein particles of adjacent

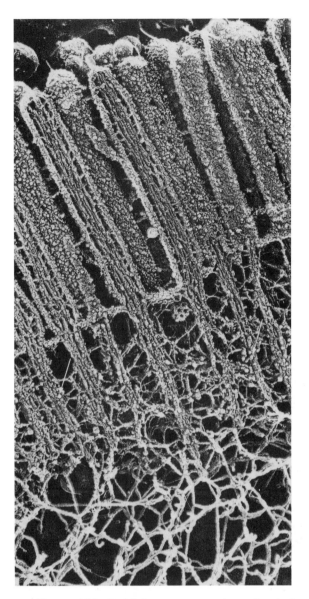

Figure 4.22. Quick-freeze preparation of apical microvilli and terminal web of intestinal epithelial cell. Actin microfilaments extend parallel to microvilli and into the terminal web as straight "rootlets." A meshwork of intermediate filaments is located at the bottom of the illustration. ×97,000. (Reproduced from N. Hirokawa, L. Tilney, K. Fujiwara, and J. Heuser, *The Journal of Cell Biology*, 1982, 94, 425 by copyright permission of The Rockefeller University Press)

and contiguous cells. The ridges comprising the network have been called *sealing strands*, and their number is variable in different epithelia. There is some evidence that the larger number of *sealing strands* is associated with more impermeable epithelia. Various markers injected into the lumen or blood vascular system, when followed by the TEM, are stopped by the ZO, thus demonstrating its role in sealing off the intercellular space. The tight junction also plays a role in epithelial cell polarity since this junction prevents the intermix-

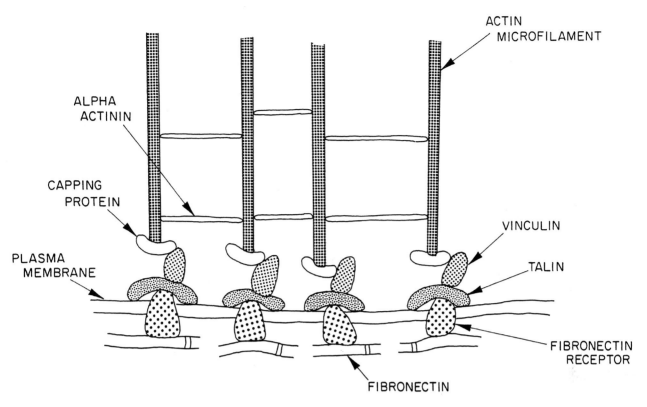

Figure 4.23. Diagram of plasma membrane and cytoskeletal interaction.

ing of membrane lipids and proteins between the apical and lateral or basolateral domains of the cell. In regions of formidable barriers like the blood brain barrier, the endothelial cells in the brain have continuous or zonular (circumferential)-type occluding junctions. The tight junction can be rapidly formed and disassembled, as occurs, for example, during leukocyte migration across endothelium and epithelium and during wound healing.

FASCIA OCCLUDENS

The fascia occludens (pl. fasciae occludentes) is band-shaped and thus does not form a continuous, belt-like differentiation around the entire cell. The endothelial cells of many blood vessels possess a fascia occludens type of junction. The fact that in many capillaries the endothelial cells have these interrupted types of junctions facilitates the formation of tissue fluid and leukocyte migration through capillary walls.

ZONULA ADHERENS (BELT DESMOSOME)

The zonula adherens (pl. zonulae adherentes) is a type of adhering junction that extends entirely around the cells, usually below the occluding junction (Figs. 4.24a, 4.25). The zonula adherens has an intercellular space

of about 20–25 nm that contains cell adhesion molecules called *cadherins*. Cadherins are Ca^{2+}-binding proteins that mediate Ca^{2+} dependent cell-cell adhesion; when calcium ions are removed, the cells dissociate and half-desmosomes and adhering junctions are internalized. A thin layer of electron-dense material is associated with the cytoplasmic side of the zonula adherens. This material contains two proteins, *α-actinin* and *vinculin*, that anchor the many actin filaments associated with this junctional complex (Fig. 4.24a). In addition, *tropomyosin* and *myosin* have been reported in the zonula adherens. The zonula adherens plays a role in support, preventing cell separation, and in producing some minor changes in apical cell shape.

DESMOSOME (MACULA ADHERENS)

A *desmosome* or *spot desmosome* is a type of adhering junction that is spot-like in its distribution (Figs. 4.24c, 4.27, 4.28). Spot desmosomes are especially numerous in the stratum spinosum layer of the epidermis. The intercellular space in the macula adherens is of the usual dimension (~25 nm). The cytoplasmic side of the cell membranes exhibits an electron-dense thickening called an *attachment plaque*. Bundles of *10-nm* filaments containing *prekeratin* are associated with the disc-like attachment plaque (Figs. 4.24c, 4.27).

Desmoglein, desmocollin I, and *desmocollin II* are Ca^{2+}-

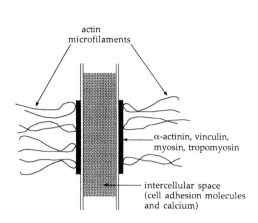

actin
microfilaments

α-actinin, vinculin,
myosin, tropomyosin

intercellular space
(cell adhesion molecules
and calcium)

(a) Adherens Junction

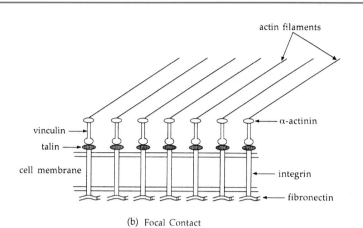

actin filaments

vinculin

α-actinin

talin

cell membrane

integrin

fibronectin

(b) Focal Contact

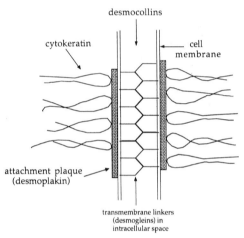

desmocollins

cytokeratin

cell
membrane

attachment plaque
(desmoplakin)

transmembrane linkers
(desmogleins) in
intracellular space

(c) Macula Adherens
(Spot Desmosome)

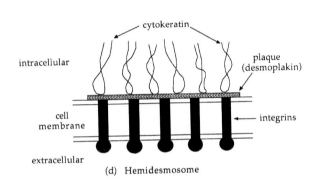

cytokeratin

intracellular

plaque
(desmoplakin)

cell
membrane

integrins

extracellular

(d) Hemidesmosome

cell membrane

pore

pore
(1.5 nm)

intercellular space
(3 nm)

(e) Gap (communicating) Junction

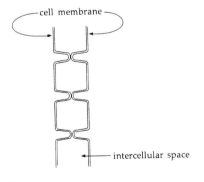

cell membrane

intercellular space

(f) Tight (occluding) Junction
(Zonula Occludens)

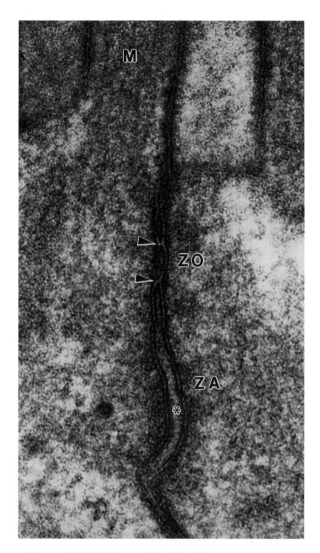

Figure 4.25. High-magnification TEM of apical end of two cells. Microvilli (M), zonula occludens (ZO), and zonula adherens (ZA) are identified. Focal fusion of outer leaflets of plasma membrane of adjacent cells is identified (arrowheads); the intercellular space (*) is obliterated in these regions. ×120,000.

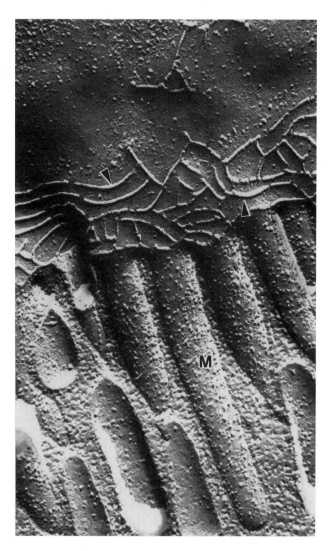

Figure 4.26. Freeze fracture replica of the apical end of epithelial cells showing the sealing strands (arrowheads) of a zonula occludens. Microvilli (M). ×81,000.

binding proteins or *glycoproteins* that mediate Ca^{2+}-dependent cell-cell adhesion; they are located primarily in the intercellular space. Desmogleins are inserted in the plasma membrane of the macula adherens, while the desmocollins are located in the intercellular space (Fig. 4.24c). Two of the largest proteins associated with the spot desmosome are *desmoplakin I* and *desmoplakin II*, which are located in the prominent *attachment plaque* just inside the plasma membrane on either side of the junction. A thin, electron-dense line also tends to bisect the intercellular space and is apparently due to a special distribution of very small transmembrane linkers that extend from cell to cell in the region of the macula adherens (Fig. 4.24c). It appears that the transmembrane linkers and associated glycoprotein material in the intercellular space perform the adhering function of this junction. In addition, the prominent system of tonofilaments appears to function in transmitting mechanical forces throughout the cells and the epithelium (Fig. 4.27). Spot desmosomes are best developed in epithelia subjected to the greatest mechanical forces.

HEMIDESMOSOME

Morphologically, the hemidesmosome appears to be one-half of a spot desmosome. It is present at the base of an

Figure 4.24a–f. Diagrams illustrate organization of adherens junction (a), focal contact (b), macula adherens (c), hemidesmosome (d), gap junction (e) and ooccluding junction (f).

TONOFILAMENTS
(INTERMEDIATE
FILAMENTS)

Figure 4.27. Diagram of macula
adherens (spot desmosome).

PLASMA
MEMBRANES

DESMOCOLLINS

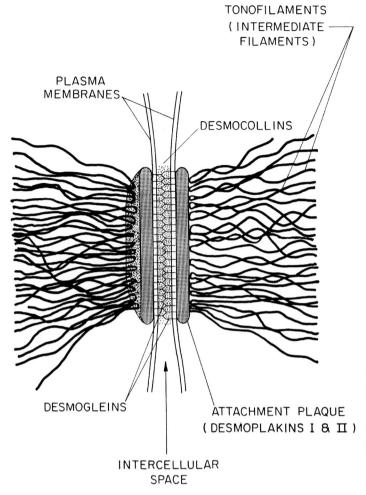

DESMOGLEINS

ATTACHMENT PLAQUE
(DESMOPLAKINS I & II)

INTERCELLULAR
SPACE

epithelial cell, as in the skin at its interface with the basement membrane and underlying connective tissue (Figs. 4.24d, 4.29). The hemidesmosome is thought to play a role in bonding epithelial cells to the underlying basement membrane and connective tissue, and anchors the cytoskeleton to the basement membrane. An attachment plaque and extensive tonofilaments are characteristic of the hemidesmosome like the macula adherens.

GAP JUNCTION (COMMUNICATING JUNCTION, NEXUS)

Gap junctions are spot-like in shape, and their name indicates that the intercellular space in this region is reduced to a small gap of 3 nm (Fig. 4.29e). Initially, in the normal staining procedure for TEM, the stain filled the intercellular gap so that it was not visible, and the junction had the appearance of a tight junction. With the use of the heavy metal marker lanthanum hydroxide, it was found that substances could move through the intercellular space in the region of the gap junc-

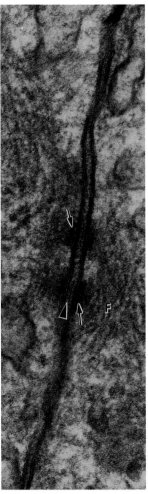

Figure 4.28. TEM of macula adherens. Central stratum (arrowhead), attachment plaque (arrows) and keratin intermediate filaments (F) are identified. ×90,000.

tion. However, the marker outlined a number of *small, hexagonal units* with a central density. Additional information from freeze fracture images showed the gap junction to consist of a patch of closely packed, intramembranous particles (Figs. 4.30, 4.31) that consist of subunits arranged in a hexagonal array. Thus, a large number of very small *tubular channels* extend between two cells in the region of the gap junction. A small channel is present inside each hexagonal array of subunits, and these units are precisely aligned, end to end, from each cell; as a result, six subunits surround a central pore ~*1.5 nm* diameter (called a *connexon*) (Fig. 4.24e). The channels are aligned between adjacent pores and are the basis for intercellular communication. With the use of fluorescent dyes, it has been determined that molecules less than *1200–1500 D* can move freely between cells through the small pores of gap junctions. Thus, small molecules such as amino acids, sugars, nucleotides, and steroids can pass from one cell to another. Cyclic AMP can move between cells and also apparently increases gap junction permeability, perhaps by incorporation of additional connexons to existing gap junctions. The concentration of intracellular *calcium* appears to regulate the opening and closing of pores in the gap junction. Normally, the concentration of intracellular calcium is less than that of tissue fluid. Under this condition, the gap junction is open. However, if the intra-

cellular calcium level rises sufficiently, gap junction channels close by a slight conformational change in the subunits.

ABNORMAL EPITHELIAL PROLIFERATION

Epithelial cells undergo extensive turnover and must therefore be able to maintain the integrity of the cellular sheets. Cells that escape the normal controls of growth and division, however, may produce a *neoplasm* or tumor. If the growth does not spread, it is classed as *benign*; if it metastasizes or spreads to other regions or organs, it is classed as *malignant*. When a malignant neoplasm is derived from epithelium, it is classed as a *carcinoma*. A carcinoma that is derived from glandular epithelium is classed as an *adenocarcinoma*.

GLANDS

CLASSIFICATION

Epithelial glands represent another form of epithelium. Glands can develop in the embryo by the localized proliferation of epithelial cells, and the resulting cells sink into the underlying connective tissue (Fig. 4.32). Those

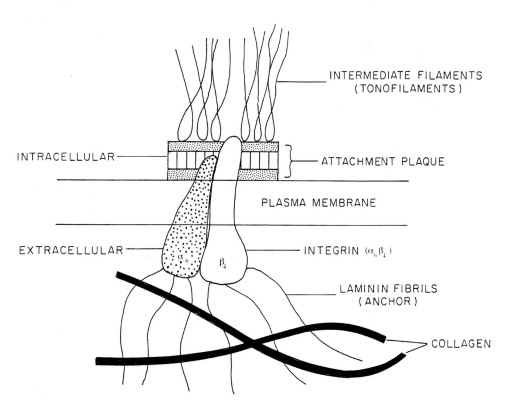

Figure 4.29. Schematic drawing of hemidesmosome that connects epithelial cell to basal lamina. The integrin ($\alpha_6\beta_4$) in the basal plasma membrane binds to intracellular attach- ment plaque proteins and to laminin in the extracellular matrix. Laminin fibrils anchor to collagen.

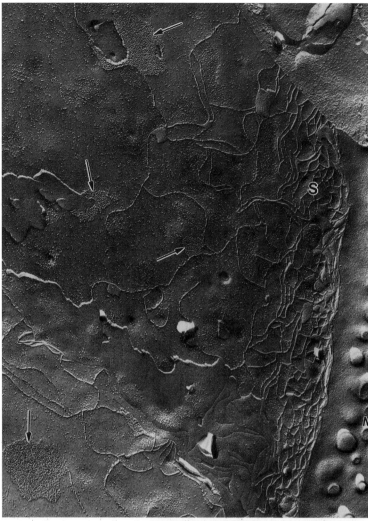

Figure 4.30 (and inset 4.31). Freeze fracture replica of apical end of a cell showing many gap junctions (arrows), one of which is enlarged in the inset to show closely packed intramembranous particles associated with the P face and a smaller region of the E face. Microvilli (M) and sealing strands (S) of the zonula occludens are also illustrated in the replica. Figure 4.30 ×39,000; Figure 4.31, ×55,000.

4.30

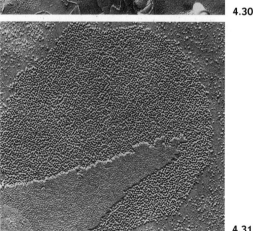

4.31

cells located deepest in the downgrowth become secretory (gland) cells, while the more superficial cells differentiate into duct cells that conduct secretions to the surface of the epithelium. Glands with a duct system are called *exocrine*. In some cases, however, the duct cells degenerate, leaving only clusters of secretory cells. These glands are called *endocrine* glands; the cell product is re-

leased into an extensive system of capillaries that surrounds these cells.

Exocrine glands may be distinguished on the basis of whether or not the duct system branches. An exocrine gland that consists of a single unbranched duct is called a *simple* gland. If the duct system branches, as it does in most larger glands, the gland is called a *compound* gland

(Fig. 4.33). The liver, pancreas, and salivary glands are examples of large compound glands. The duct system of such glands is highly branched, much like the branches from the trunk of a large tree. Examples of different gland types are summarized in Table 4.6.

Glands are also identified or classified on the basis of the morphology of their secretory units. The cells making up individual secretory units may be *tubular* in shape. In contrast, the secretory cells may take the form of grape-like or sac-like units; such secretory units are called an *acinus* (pl. acini) or *alveolus* (pl. alveoli) (Fig. 4.33). Some glands contain secretory units that are both tubular and acinar or alveolar in shape. Such glands are called *tubuloalveolar* (or *tubuloacinar*) glands. The entire classification for such a gland would include both ductal and glandular terminology, such as "compound tubuloacinar."

SECRETORY PRODUCT

The classification of glands is also based on the nature of the secretion produced. Some glands produce only a mucous secretion (glycoprotein) and are called *mucous glands*. Other glands produce a serous secretion (proteinaceous) and are called *serous glands* (e.g., parotid gland). Still other glands contain both types of cells, thus producing both mucous and serous secretions. These glands are called *seromucous* or *mixed* glands (e.g., submandibular gland). Further, some salivary glands contain mucous alveoli that are "capped" or partially surrounded by *serous demilunes* (e.g., sublingual gland) (see Chapter 19).

With the LM and hematoxylin and eosin (H&E) staining, the *mucous gland cell* stains pale since mucigen (glycoprotein) granules do not stain well. The cytoplasm of these cells often appears vacuolated, and the nuclei tend to be compressed against the cell base. In contrast, the *serous gland cell* contains well-preserved proteinaceous secretion granules and more rER; thus the cytoplasm stains basophilic. The nucleus of these cells is not compressed at the cell base. Furthermore, a distinct lumen is more likely to be evident in a mucous alveolus than in a serous alveolus.

METHOD OF SECRETION

Exocrine glands can also be classified on the basis of how the secretory product is secreted or released. In *merocrine* secretion, the secretory granules or zymogen granules in the cell are surrounded by a membrane that fuses with the apical cell membrane during discharge or *exocytosis*. In contrast, sebaceous glands secrete by a *holocrine* method. Individual cells become filled with secretion, and after moving far enough away from capillaries in the connective tissue, the cells die and then dis-

integrate. The secretion (called *sebum*) is expressed from around the hair follicles onto the surface of the skin. The mammary gland cells are believed by some to secrete by an *apocrine* method in which part of the apical end of the secretory cell is lost together with secretion granules.

Figure 4.34 illustrates other variations in the secretory process. Some cells produce a chemical messenger that combines with this cell's receptors to stimulate itself, an example of *autocrine secretion*. Secretory cells can release chemical messengers that diffuse to nearby target cells that have receptors for the particular chemical messenger; this is called *paracrine secretion*. *Synaptic secretion* is a special type of secretion occurring at the synapse between nerve cells. Finally, in *neurocrine secretion*, a nerve cell releases a neurosecretion into the bloodstream that is transported to target cells possessing appropriate receptors.

Cells communicate with each other by releasing chemical mediators that diffuse to a neighboring cell or reach more distant cells by way of the bloodstream. These chemical mediators act as messengers that interact with receptors on responsive cells and elicit a biochemical response. The importance of signaling between cells is evident when it is realized that a number of diverse diseases, including myasthenia gravis, hyperthyroidism, cholera, and certain types of diabetes, result from faulty or impaired communication among cells.

PARENCHYMA, STROMA, DUCTS

Compound glands consist of *parenchyma* and *stroma*. The parenchyma refers to both the secretory and duct cells. The stroma denotes the connective tissue components of the gland. Blood vessels, lymphatics, nerves, and ducts may be located within the stroma. The connective tissue that surrounds a gland is called a *capsule*. Some of this connective tissue extends into the interior of the gland to form *septa*. The connective tissue septa can divide the gland into *lobules* (Fig. 4.35). *Interlobular septum* (pl. septa) refers to the connective tissue located between lobules. Those ducts that are located within an interlobular septum are known as *interlobular ducts*. The connective tissue elements located within a lobule are called *intralobular septa*, and ducts located in this region are called *intralobular ducts* (Fig. 4.35). There are two major types of intralobular ducts. *Intercalated ducts* are the smallest division; their cells are low cuboidal in shape and immediately connect with the secretory units (Fig. 4.35). Larger divisions of intralobular ducts have columnar cells with basal striations due to extensive infoldings of the plasma membrane that are just evident with oil immersion in the LM. These are called *striated intralobular ducts* (Fig. 4.35).

Many glands are divided into lobules, but only a

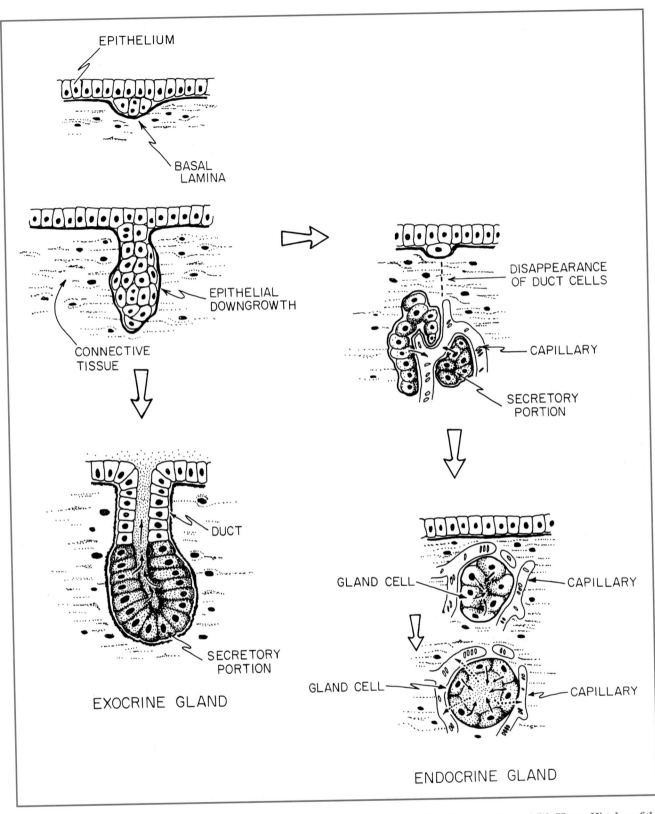

EPITHELIUM

BASAL
LAMINA

EPITHELIAL
DOWNGROWTH

CONNECTIVE
TISSUE

DISAPPEARANCE
OF DUCT CELLS

CAPILLARY

SECRETORY
PORTION

DUCT

SECRETORY
PORTION

EXOCRINE GLAND

GLAND CELL

CAPILLARY

GLAND CELL

CAPILLARY

ENDOCRINE GLAND

Figure 4.32. Diagram showing formation of exocrine and endocrine glands. (Redrawn from A.W. Ham, *Histology*, 6th ed., J.B. Lippincott, Philadephia, 1969)

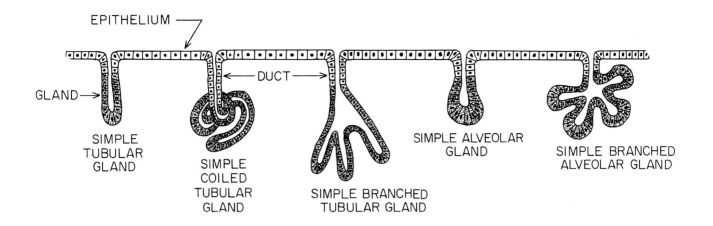

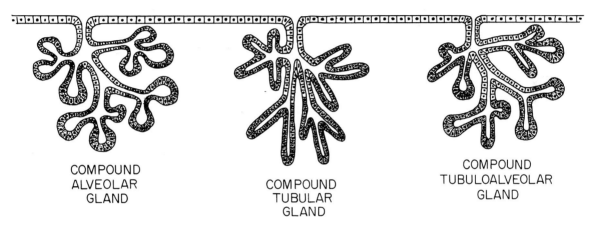

Figure 4.33. Diagram of different types of exocrine glands.

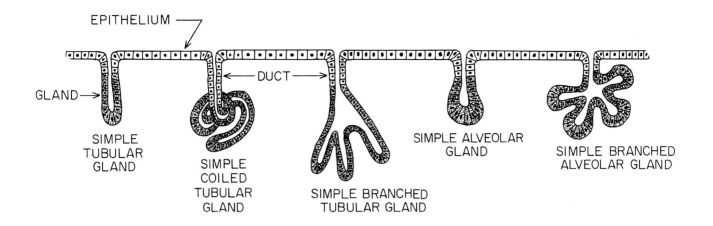

Table 4.6 Classification of Glands

Morphologic Type	Examples
Simple tubular gland	Crypts of Lieberkuhn (intestinal glands)
Simple coiled tubular gland	Eccrine sweat glands
Simple branched tubular gland	Gastric glands—stomach
Simple alveolar (acinar) gland	Some sebaceous glands
Simple branched alveolar gland	Some sebaceous glands
Compound tubular gland	Brunner's gland—duodenum
Compound tubular alveolar gland	Salivary glands, pancreas, Cowper's gland, prostate gland, ceruminous gland (ear, wax)

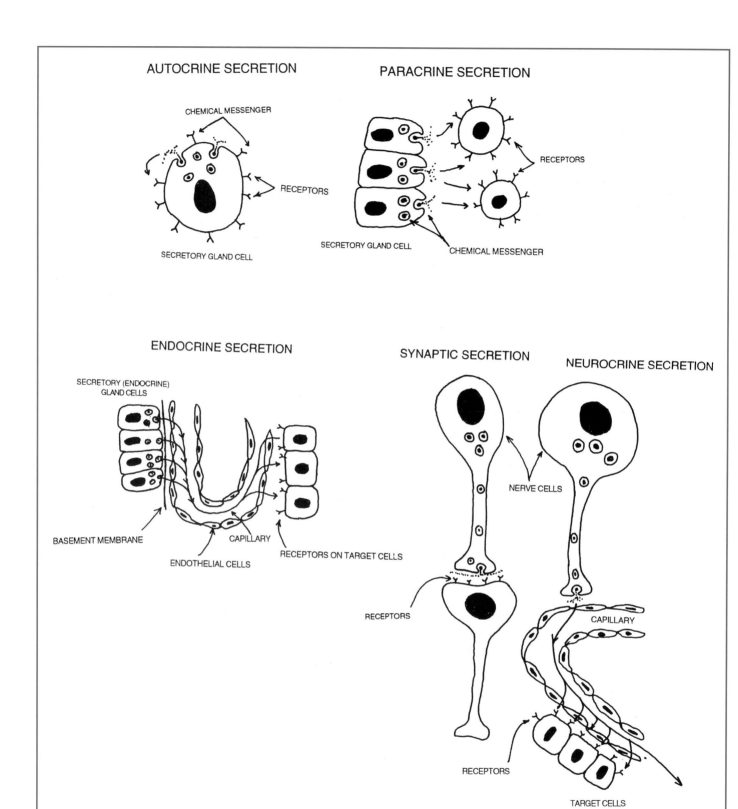

Figure 4.34. Diagram showing various types of secretion.

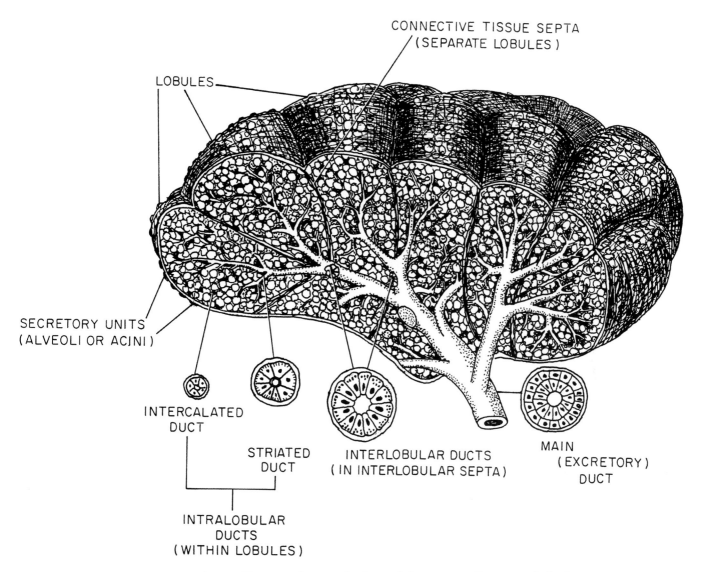

Figure 4.35. Diagram illustrates the organization and duct system of compound glands.

few glands are divided into macroscopically distinct *lobes* (e.g., liver). The connective tissue located between lobes is called *interlobar septum*. Ducts present in the interlobar septum are called *interlobar ducts*.

INNERVATION/CONTROL OF SECRETION

Secretory units of glands are innervated by both sympathetic and parasympathetic divisions of the autonomic nervous system. Thus, sweating and salivation, for example, are uncontrolled. *Parasympathetic* nervous activity usually *stimulates* secretory activity; *acetylcholine* (cholinergic) is the chemical mediator. The *sympathetic* division of the autonomic nervous system is usually *inhibitory* with respect to gland cell secretion, and the usual chemical mediator produced at these nerve endings is *epinephrine* or *adren-*

alin (adrenergic). An exception is sweat glands, where acetylcholine is released at the synapse.

SELECTED BIBLIOGRAPHY

Bosman, F.T., Cleutjens, J., Beek, C., and Havenith, M. (1989). Basement membrane heterogeneity. *Histochemistry* **21**, 629–633.

Burgess, T.L., and Kelly, R.B. (1987). Constitutive and regulated secretion of proteins. *Annu. Rev. Cell Biol.* **3**, 243–266.

Burridge, K., Fath, K., Kelly, T., Nuckolls, G., and Turner, C. (1988). Focal adhesions: transmembrane junctions between the extracellular matrix and the cytoskeleton. *Annu. Rev. Cell Biol.* **4**, 487–526.

Cereijido, M., ed. (1992). *Tight Junctions.* CRC Press, Boca Raton, FL.

Edelman, G.M., and Crossin, K.L. (1991). Cell adhesion molecules: implications for a molecular histology. *Annu. Rev. Biochem.* **60**, 155–190.

Fakuda, M. (1992). *Cell Surface Carbohydrates and Cell Development.* CRC Press, Boca Raton, FL.

Gumbiner, B. (1990). Generation and maintenance of epithelial polarity. *Curr. Opin. Cell Biol.* **2**, 881–886.

Gumbiner, B.M. (1992). Epithelial morphogenesis. *Cell* **69**, 385–387.

Heintzelman, M.B., and Mooseker, M.S. (1992). Assembly of the intestinal brush border cytoskeleton. *Curr. Top. Dev. Biol.* **26**, 93–122.

Hirokawa, N., Tilney, L.G., Fujiwara, K., and Heuser, J.E. (1982). The organization of actin, myosin and intermediate filaments in the brush border of intestinal epithelial cells. *J. Cell Biol.* **94**, 425–443.

Hynes, R. (1986). Fibronectins. *Sci. Am.* **254**, 42–51.

Hynes, R.O. (1987). Integrins: a family of cell surface receptors. *Cell* **48**, 549–554.

Madara, J.L., Parkos, C., Colgan, S., Nusrat, A., Atisook, K., and Kaoutzani, P. (1992). The movement of solutes and cells across tight junctions. *Ann. N.Y. Acad. Sci.* **664**, 47–60.

Molitoris, B.A., and Nelson, W.J. (1990). Alterations in the establishment and maintenance of epithelial cell polarity as a basis for disease processes. *J. Clin. Invest.* **85**, 3–9.

Musil, L.S., and Goodenough, D.A. (1990). Gap junctional communication and the regulation of connexin expression and function. *Curr. Opin. Cell Biol.* **2**, 875–888.

Rodriguez, E., and Nelson, W.J. (1989). Morphogenesis of the polarized epithelial cell phenotype. *Science* **245**, 718–721.

Schneeberger, E.E., and Lynch, R.D. (1992). Structure, function, and regulation of cellular tight junctions. *Am. J. Physiol.* **262**, L647–L661.

Stauffer, K.A., and Unwin, N. (1992). Structure of gap junction channels. *Semin. Cell Biol.* **3**, 17–20.

Yurchenco, P.D., and Schittny, J.C. (1990). Molecular architecture of basement membranes. *FASEB J.* **4**, 1577–1590.

CHAPTER 5

Connective Tissue: Cells, Fibers, and Amorphous Intercellular Substances

onnective tissue, a second type of tissue, consists of *cells* and products that the cells synthesize and export to the surrounding extracellular space. The products are called *intercellular* or *extracellular substances* and are of two main types: *fibers* and *amorphous jellies*. In addition, *tissue fluid* is functionally associated with connective tissues in the living state. The types of cells and the kind and amount of intercellular substances are quite variable; thus connective tissue is heterogeneous and includes such diverse examples as areolar connective tissue, ligaments, tendons, bone, cartilage, adipose tissue, blood, myeloid tissue, and lymphatic tissue (Figs. 5.1–5.4). It is not surprising that connective tissue serves a variety of functions; it connects other basic tissue types in the body and forms a supporting framework for almost all organs. The loose packing of connective tissue in organs facilitates the distribution of blood vessels, lymphatic vessels, and nerves. In addition, organs are usually surrounded by a connective tissue capsule. Tendons and ligaments represent examples of specific types of connective tissue with important supportive and connecting roles. Cartilage and bone are the most highly differentiated supporting connective tissues. In addition, macrophages have a defensive role. Plasma cells can produce humoral antibodies. Mast cells release heparin and histamine under certain conditions and are involved in allergic reactions and anaphylactic shock.

Connective tissue, with the exception of adipose connective tissue, is characterized by a relative scarcity of cells and a predominance of fibers and amorphous jellies. Unlike epithelium, mesenchyme (connective tissue) cells are not polarized and have no close spatial association with each other. It is frequently the nonliving

components, the fibrous and amorphous intercellular substances, that constitute the bulk of a specific connective tissue. Since the "jelly" components of the intercellular substances are frequently dissolved in histologic sections, it is important to remember that the spaces in such sections are filled in life with the amorphous elements and tissue fluid.

Connective tissue develops from mesenchyme (mesoderm) in the embryo; hence, *mesenchyme* represents an embryonic connective tissue type (Plate 6A). Mesenchyme initially forms a large compartment between the basal laminae of the two major epithelial surfaces, that is, between the epidermis and its derivatives and the epithelium of the digestive tract. A variety of cell types differentiates from the pluripotent mesenchymal cells, and the types of cells that differentiate reflect the particular functions served by the specific kind of connective tissue. A second type of embryonic connective tissue is *Wharton's jelly*, which is present in the embryonic umbilical cord. In both types, the cells are spindle or stellate in shape and form a loose packing in which the amorphous intercellular substances are located. The cells contain an oval, euchromatic staining nucleus with nucleoli. The mesenchyme cell is considered to be pluripotent, that is, capable of differentiating into many different cell types, including *fibroblasts, macrophages, mast cells, adipocytes, osteoblasts, chondroblasts, blood cells, mesothelial cells, endothelial cells, smooth muscle cells,* and *pericytes.* The diversity in connective tissue organization is illustrated by the scanning electron micrographs of areolar connective tissue, adipose connective tissue, cartilage and bone shown in Figures 5.1–5.4.

One method for classification of the diverse connective tissues is present in Table 5.1.

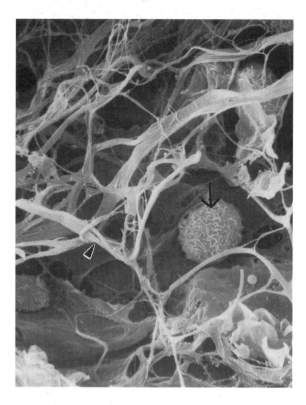

Figure 5.1. Loose connective tissue with a scarcity of cells (arrow), fibers (arrowhead), and intercellular spaces that appear empty in this preparation but that in the living organism contain the amorphous intercellular substances. ×2460. (From R. Kessel and R. Kardon, *Tissues and Organs: A Text-Atlas of Scanning Electron Microscopy*, W.H. Freeman, New York, 1979, with permission)

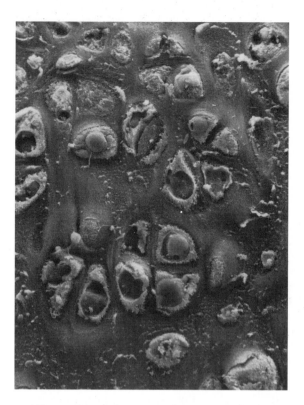

Figure 5.3. In hyaline cartilage there are cartilage cells (chondrocytes) and intercellular substance. ×815. (From R. Kessel and R. Kardon, *Tissues and Organs: A Text-Atlas of Scanning Electron Microscopy*, W.H. Freeman, New York, 1979, with permission)

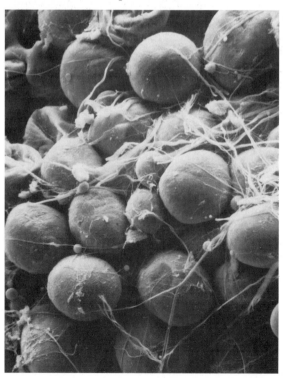

Figure 5.2. Adipose connective tissue is highly cellular and contains many closely packed adipocytes. ×450. (From R. Kessel and R. Kardon, *Tissues and Organs: A Text-Atlas of Scanning Electron Microscopy*, W.H. Freeman, New York, 1979, with permission)

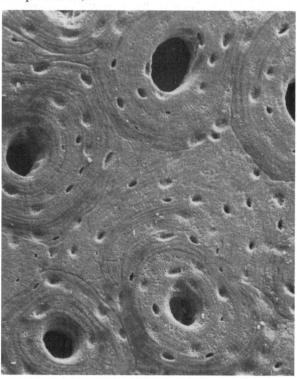

Figure 5.4. Ground bone contains mineralized organic matrix with many oval lacunae that in life contain bone cells (osteocytes) and larger channels (Haversian canals), which in life contain blood vessels and edosteum. ×815. (From R. Kessel and R. Kardon, *Tissues and Organs: A Text-Atlas of Scanning Electron Microscopy*, W.H. Freeman, New York, 1979, with permission)

Table 5.1 A Classification for Connective Tissues

I. *Embryonic Connective Tissue*

   A. *Mesenchyme*

   B. *Mucoid (mucous) connective tissue* (Wharton's jelly in umbilical cord)

II. *Adult Connective Tissues*

   A. *Loose (areolar) ordinary connective tissue*
Loosely organized, widely distributed, consists of a mixture of cells and intercellular substances; component of mesenteries, found in submucosa and lamina propria layers of organs—anchors and packs; all fiber types possible, amorphous ground substance and all possible cell types, but fibroblasts and macrophages predominate.

   B. *White adipose tissue*
Found in subcutaneous tissues, omenta, etc.; consists of unilocular fat cells arranged in lobules, with fine reticular fibers produced by fibroblasts forming a packing.

   C. *Brown adipose tissue*
Present in neck and abdomen regions of embryo. Found in hibernating bears; contains multilocular fat cells that are richly vascularized.

   D. *Reticular connective tissue*
Located in bone marrow and lymphoid organs, including the lymph nodes and spleen. Reticular fibers are produced by reticular cells in this case.

   E. *Dense, ordinary connective tissue*
Consists mainly of one of the principal fiber types; widely distributed.

     1. *Regularly arranged when the fibers are aligned and closely packed*

       a. *Dense, regularly arranged white, fibrous connective tissue (collagen fibers)*
Fiber type, in this case collagen, is closely packed into sheets, as in most tendons and some ligaments; mainly fibroblasts and collagen

       b. *Dense, regularly arranged yellow elastic connective tissue (elastic fibers)*
Two ligaments, the ligamentum nuchae and ligamentum flava, consist of yellow elastic fibers that are closely packed; also present as suspensory ligament of the penis and the elastic ligaments of Cooper in the mammary glands; mainly elastic fibers and fibroblasts.

     2. *Irregularly arranged (when fibers are more haphazard in orientation)*

       a. *Dense, irregularly arranged white, fibrous connective tissue (collagen fibers)*
Collagen fibers in various orientations; occurs in some ligaments, aponeurosis, periosteum (surrounding bone), perichondrium, (surrounding cartilage), and in certain areas of the dermis; mainly fibroblasts and collagen.

       b. *Dense, irregularly arranged yellow elastic fibers (elastic fibers)*
Yellow elastic fibers are arranged in different planes in different layers of blood vessels; also widely distributed in wall of aorta.

   F. *Supporting connective tissues*

     1. *Cartilage* (hyaline, elastic, and fibrocartilage)

     2. *Bone* (compact and cancellous bone)

   G. *Blood*

   H. *Hemopoietic connective tissue* (blood-forming connective tissue)

     1. *Myeloid connective tissue* (bone marrow)

     2. *Lymphatic (lymphoid) connective tissue* (thymus, lymph nodes, spleen, tonsils)

CONNECTIVE TISSUE FIBERS

COLLAGEN FIBERS

The connective tissue fibers are of three types: *collagen, elastic,* and *reticular.* The most abundant fiber is collagen, which comprises about 30% of all body proteins (Figs. 5.5–5.8). If a thin mesentery is examined in the fresh state with the LM, type I collagen fibers can be recognized by their wide diameter, somewhat wavy appearance, and whitish color. Collagen fibers range from *2 to 10 μm* in diameter and do not branch extensively (Figs. 5.1, 5.8–5.10). When stained in histologic sections, collagen fibers are acidophilic (Plate 6B–D); thus, they stain red or pink with eosin, green with light green of Masson's stain, and blue when stained with aniline blue of Mallory's stain. Fibers consist of smaller *fibrils* ~50 nm in width. The fibrils, in turn, are composed of smaller *microfibrils*. In the EM, the collagenic fibrils exhibit a banding pattern with an axial perodicity of *670 Å* (67 nm).

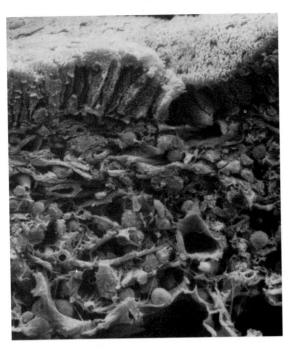

Figure 5.5. SEM of loose (areolar) connective tissue attached to a sheet of epithelial cells. The connective tissue contains cells, fibers, and spaces occupied in the living organism by the amorphous intercellular substances. ×875. (From R. Kessel and R. Kardon, *Tissues and Organs: A Text-Atlas of Scanning Electron Microscopy*, W.H. Freeman, New York, 1979, with permission)

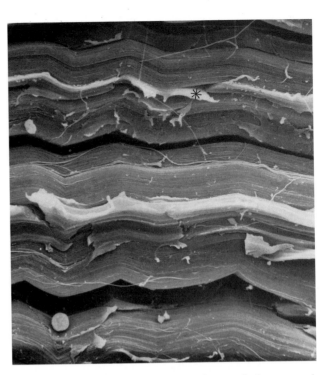

Figure 5.7. Dense connective tissue of the corneal stroma contains collagen fibers with fibroblasts (*) that are flattened between the collagen fibers. SEM. ×1000. (From R. Kessel and R. Kardon, *Tissues and Organs: A Text-Atlas of Scanning Electron Microscopy*, W.H. Freeman, New York, 1979, with permission)

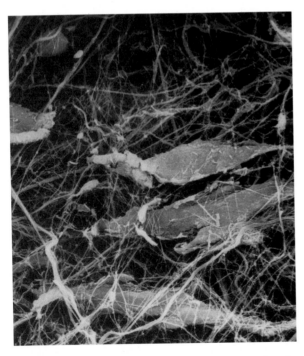

Figure 5.6. SEM of fibroblasts and connective tissue fibers. ×1005. (From R. Kessel and R. Kardon, *Tissues and Organs: A Text-Atlas of Scanning Electron Microscopy*, W.H. Freeman, 1979)

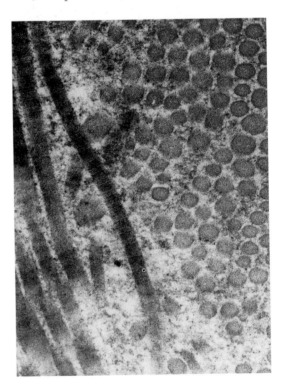

Figure 5.8. TEM of collagen fibrils, longitudinal and transverse sections. Note banding of fibrils. ×62,250. (From R. Kessel and R. Kardon, *Tissues and Organs: A Text-Atlas of Scanning Electron Microscopy*, W.H. Freeman, New York, 1979, with permission)

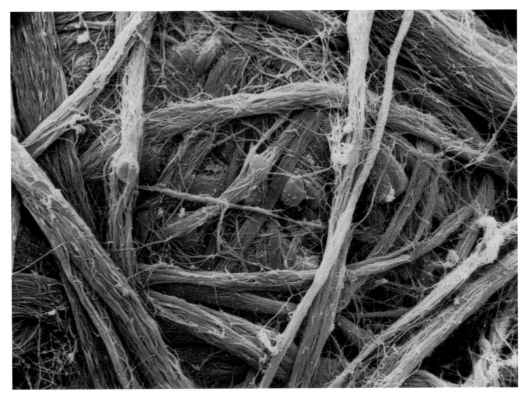

Figure 5.9. SEM illustrates dense, irregularly arranged white fibrous connective tissue. ×1495. (From R. Kessel and R. Kardon, *Tissues and Organs: A Text-Atlas of Scanning Elec-tron Microscopy*, W.H. Freeman, New York, 1979, with permission)

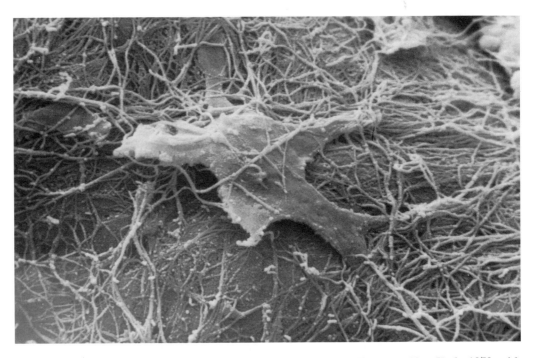

Figure 5.10. SEM of flattened, irregularly shaped fibroblasts and many collagen fibrils. ×4950. (From R. Kessel and R. Kardon, *Tissues and Organs: A Text-Atlas of Scanning Electron Microscopy*, W. H. Freeman, New York, 1979, with permission)

Collagen is a tough, fibrous protein widely distributed in all organs. Prolonged boiling of meat results in the conversion of collagen into a softer, hydrated gelatin that is easier to chew. Collagen can be made into leather. In this case, the epidermis of skin is removed and the connective tissue of the dermis, consisting of dense, irregularly arranged white fibrous connective tissue (Fig. 5.9), is treated with a tanning agent to make leather. Because collagen is white in the fresh state, tendons composed of collagen fibers are designated *dense white fibrous* connective tissue.

The protein collagen consists of three coiled polypeptide chains in a right-handed triple helix (Fig. 5.11). The polypeptide chains are called *alpha chains* (α-*chains*) and each one contains 1050 amino acids. Currently, some 20 distinct collagen α-chains have been reported; each chain is encoded by a separate gene (Table 5.2). The collagen type is given in Roman numerals. Types I, II, and III are the most abundant, are produced by fibroblasts (Figs. 5.10, 5.12), and tend to form long, thin fibrils. Collagen type I is a long (300 nm), thin (1.5 nm in diameter) protein. The different types of collagen are based on differences in segments that interrupt the triple helix. Type IV collagen is the principal constituent of the basal lamina produced by epithelial cells. Collagen alpha chains each consist of repeating sequences of three amino acids: the first amino acid is variable, the second is either *proline* or *lysine*, and the third is always *glycine* (Fig. 5.12).

Collagen is synthesized on membrane-bound ribosomes in fibroblasts and initially appears in the rER cisternae as *pro-α-chains* (Fig. 5.12). A number of posttranslational changes in polypeptide chains take place in the cisternae of the rER, including (1) cleavage of the signal peptide; (2) *hydroxylation* of *glycine, proline,* and *lysine* residues; (3) addition of O-linked and N-linked *sugar groups* (*glycosylation*) to some portions of the *hydroxylysine* residues; (4) formation of the triple helix by the three pro-α-chains; and (5) formation of *disulfide* (S-S) *bonds* that shape the molecule and provide stability. The resulting form of the molecule is called *procollagen* (Fig. 5.12). Vitamin C is important for the posttranslational changes in collagen because procollagen helix formation is inhibited in the absence of vitamin C. Procollagen is packaged into secretory vesicles in the Golgi region of the fibroblast; then secretory vesicles, assisted by actin microfilaments and microtubules, move to the plasma membrane for discharge by exocytosis into the extracellular space. When first synthesized, the α-chains have extra amino acids, called *propeptides,* at the amino- and carboxy-terminal ends of the chains. Following secretion from the fibroblast, types I, II, and III procollagen molecules have their propeptides removed by specific proteolytic enzymes called *procollagen peptidase.* As a result, the procollagen molecules become *tropocollagen* molecules (Fig. 5.12). It appears that the function of the propeptides is to prevent the formation of collagen fibers inside the cell. Therefore, fibers form

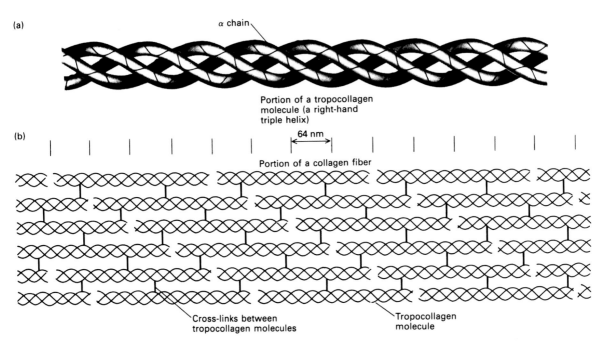

Figure 5.11. (a) The tropocollagen molecule is a right-hand triple helix. (b) Tropocollagen molecules are aligned end to end but are displaced about one-fourth of the length of a single molecule (about 67 nm). A small gap exists between the head of one tropocollagen molecule and the "tail" portion of the next, and these interactions are stabilized by cross-links between adjacent tropocollagen molecules. The packing of the tropocollagen molecules is responsible for the 67-nm cross-band pattern of the collagen fibril. (From J. Darnell, H. Lodish, and D. Baltimore, *Molecular Cell Biology*, Scientific American Books, New York, 1986, with permission)

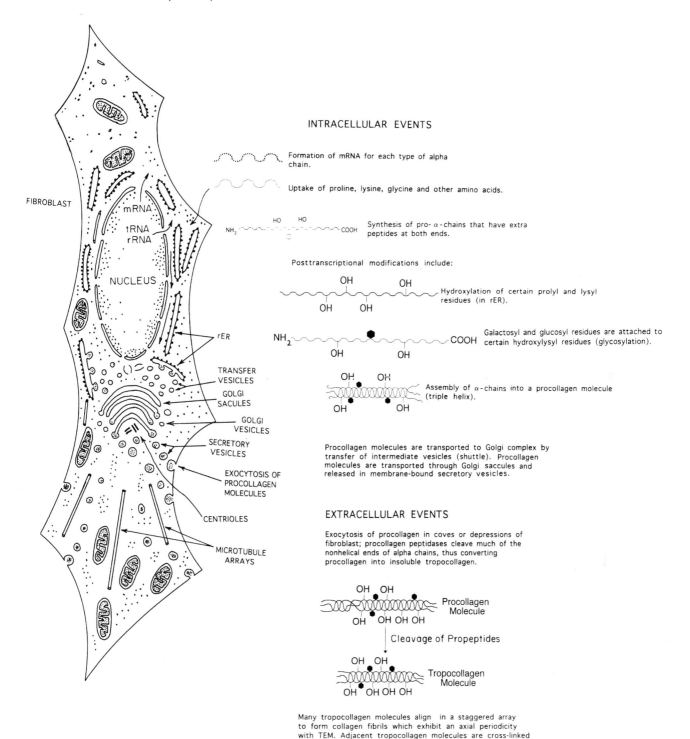

INTRACELLULAR EVENTS

Formation of mRNA for each type of alpha chain.

Uptake of proline, lysine, glycine and other amino acids.

Synthesis of pro-α-chains that have extra peptides at both ends.

Posttranscriptional modifications include:

Hydroxylation of certain prolyl and lysyl residues (in rER).

Galactosyl and glucosyl residues are attached to certain hydroxylysyl residues (glycosylation).

Assembly of α-chains into a procollagen molecule (triple helix).

Procollagen molecules are transported to Golgi complex by transfer of intermediate vesicles (shuttle). Procollagen molecules are transported through Golgi saccules and released in membrane-bound secretory vesicles.

EXTRACELLULAR EVENTS

Exocytosis of procollagen in coves or depressions of fibroblast; procollagen peptidases cleave much of the nonhelical ends of alpha chains, thus converting procollagen into insoluble tropocollagen.

Procollagen Molecule

Cleavage of Propeptides

Tropocollagen Molecule

Many tropocollagen molecules align in a staggered array to form collagen fibrils which exhibit an axial periodicity with TEM. Adjacent tropocollagen molecules are cross-linked (involves enzyme lysyl oxidase).

Figure 5.12. Diagram illustrates steps in collagen synthesis by fibroblast. (Redrawn from: L.C. funqueira, J. Carneiro, and R.O. Kelley, *Basic Histology*, 7th ed., Appleton & Lange, 1992 East Norwalk, CT, with permission)

only in the extracellular matrix after propeptide removal. The tropocollagen molecules are initially located in depressions or coves of the fibroblast surface, where tropocollagen molecules polymerize into fibrils.

Glycine, proline, and hydroxyproline are essential for formation of the triple helix. Some sugar groups may

be covalently attached to the hydroxyllysine residues; thus, collagen is properly called a glycoprotein. However, there is insufficient carbohydrate for collagen to stain with the PAS cytochemical stain. The hydroxyl groups of hydroxyproline are important in stabilizing the triple-stranded helix. Extensive cross-linking of col-

Table 5.2 Types of Collagen

Collagen Type	Location	Cells Producing	Characteristics
Type I (~90%) (composed of two types of α-chain)	Dermis of skin, tendon	Fibroblasts	Low hydroxylysine, low carbohydrate (broad fibrils)
	Loose (areolar), dense ordinary connective tissue, collagen fibers	Reticular cells and smooth muscle	
	Most widely distributed type of collagen in internal organs		
	Bone	Osteoblasts	
	Dentin (teeth)	Odontoblasts	
Type II (composed of only one type of α-chain)	Hyaline and elastic cartilage	Chondrocytes	High hydroxylysine, high carbohydrate (thinner fibrils than type I)
	Vitreous body of eye, intervertebral disc	Retina cells	
		Chondrocytes	
Type III (composed of only one type of α-chain)	Loose connective tissue; reticular fibers, papillary layer of dermis, (found early in development)	Fibroblasts and reticular cells	High hydroxyproline low hydroxylysine, low carbohydrate
	Blood vessels	Smooth muscle cells, endothelial cells	
Type IV (composed of two types of α-chain)	Basal lamina	Epithelial and endothelial cells	Very high hydroxylysine, high carbohydrate, (retains procollagen extension peptides)
	Lens capsule of eye	Lens epithelium	
Type V	Fetal membranes (placenta)	Fibroblasts	
	Basement membranes	Epithelial cells	
	Bone	Osteoblasts	
	Smooth muscle	Smooth muscle cells	

In addition, a number of other collagens have been recently identified in the following locations:

Type VI	Short triple helical segment about 100 nm long; occurs in small amounts in kidney, liver, and uterus, where type I and III collagens are found
Type VII	Basal laminae of many epithelia
Type VIII	Secretory product of endothelial cells; major component of Decemet's membrane in the cornea
Type IX	Mainly in cartilage; found with type II collagen
Type X	Confined to cartilage; in matrix surrounding hypertrophic chondrocytes
Type XI	Associated with type II collagen in cartilage; function unknown
Type XII	Tendon; properties in common with type IX collagen
Type XIII	Endothelium
Type XIV	Fetal skin and tendon

Thus far, some 25 distinct collagen α-chains, each encoded by a separate gene, have been identified.

lagen molecules during assembly gives collagen its strength. After collagen fibrils have formed in the extracellular space, they are strengthened by covalent cross-links within and between the lysine residues. Type IV collagen differs from other collagens in that the amino acid sequence of the alpha chain is interrupted in several regions so as to disrupt the triple-stranded helix. Further, the propeptides are not removed from the procollagen molecules after secretion.

Tropocollagen molecules become organized into a collagen fibril in a special manner. When secreted by a fibroblast, the tropocollagen molecules assemble into ordered polymer arrays called *fibrils* in the extracellular space. Tropocollagen molecules align end to end, with a gap of 35 nm between molecules. Adjacent tropocollagen molecules overlap their neighbors by about one-fourth of the total length of the molecule (Fig. 5.11). When collagen is negatively stained and viewed by TEM, alternating light and dark bands are evident. The light bands represent regions where there are no gaps between molecules. The dark bands result from the negative stain filling in the spaces or gaps between individual collagen molecules. The gap and the overlap are collectively responsible for the 67-nm axial periodicity that characterizes the collagenic fibrils.

RETICULAR FIBERS

Reticular fibers contain collagen but are narrower in diameter than collagen fibers and contain more sugar groups. Reticular fibers can branch and range from ~0.5 to 2 μm in diameter. With TEM, reticular fibers are made up of fibrils about 25–45 nm in diameter; the fibrils have the same axial periodicity as collagen. Reticular fibers are typically arranged into a loose meshwork in, for example, the loose areolar connective tissue of

mesenteries. Reticular fibers are present in basement membranes, are found in the liver, surround smooth muscle cells and adipocytes, and are a component of many blood vessels.

Reticular fibers do not stain with H&E, but do stain with silver. A classic way to demonstrate these fibers is by a silver impregnation technique (Plate 7A). The tissue is initially treated with a reducible silver salt and then with a reducing agent, which reduces the salt to metallic silver, which is black. Because of this response, reticular fibers are called *argyrophilic* ("liking silver"). In addition, there is sufficient glycoprotein to coat the fibers so that they stain with the PAS technique. Reticular fibers contain type III collagen. In hemopoietic tissues, reticular fibers are produced by reticular cells, but in loose connective tissues, fibroblasts appear to produce the reticular fibers. In lymph node sinuses, branched reticular cells (Figs. 5.13, 5.14) synthesize reticular fibers and export them. However, after export,

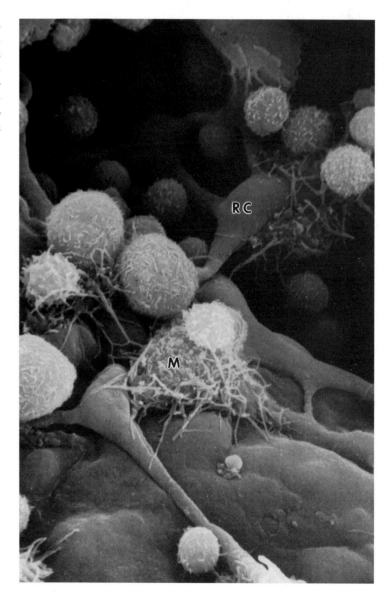

Figure 5.13. SEM of a lymph node sinus illustrates smooth, branched reticular cells (RC) and "hairy" macrophages (M). ×2600. (From: R. Kessel and R. Kardon, *Tissues and Organs: A Text-Atlas of Scanning Electron Microscopy*. W.H. Freeman, New York, 1979, with permission)

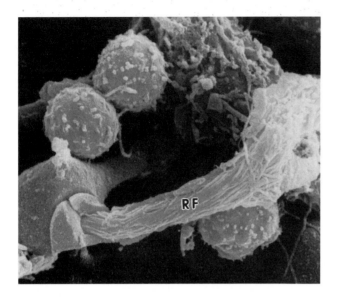

Figure 5.14. A branch of a reticular cell is broken and shows a number of reticular fibers (RF), which are normally surrounded by the reticular cell so as to be invisible in the SEM. ×5170. From: R. Kessel and R. Kordon, *Tissues and Organs: A Text-Atlas of Scanning Electron Microscopy*, W.H. Freeman, New York, 1979, with permission)

the reticular cells closely invest or enwrap the fibers, so they are not apparent unless the cell processes are removed (Figs. 5.14, 5.15). In more isolated examples, Schwann cells produce reticular fibers that are present in the endoneurium of a nerve. In addition, in another unusual case, smooth muscle cells in the walls of blood vessels can produce collagen, reticular fibers, and elastic fibers.

ELASTIC FIBERS

Elastic fibers are long and highly refractile; they are not composed of fibrils and do not possess axial periodicity. In the fresh condition, they tend to be yellow. Elastic fibers are well displayed in sections stained with *resorcin fuchsin* or *resorcin orcein* (Plate 7B,C), but they do not stain well with H&E. Among the locations of elastic fibers are loose areolar connective tissue, the matrix of elastic cartilage, walls of elastic arteries (the aorta), the elastic ligaments of Cooper of the mammary glands, the suspensory ligament of the penis, and special elastic ligaments. The major characteristics of the connective tissue fibers are described and compared in Table 5.3.

In TE micrographs the elastic fiber appears to be homogeneous, but the periphery has a glycoprotein coating in the form of microfibrils ~12 nm in diameter (Fig. 5.16). These microfibrils are secreted before the elastin molecules, so it is thought that the microfibrils play some role in orienting the extracellular elastin molecules into fibers and sheets. In older fibers, however, microfibrils are present within the fibers as

well as on the periphery; thus, during growth, some microfibrils may become trapped within the elastin. Elastic fibers are present in a few ligaments, such as *ligamentum nuchae* and *ligamentum flava*. These particular ligaments are an example of dense, yellow elastic connective tissue, in contrast to the designation of collagenic tendons as dense, white fibrous connective tissue.

Elastic fibers contain *elastin*, a nonglycosylated protein. Elastin contains *desmosine* and *isodesmosine*, which are formed from four molecules of lysine and are found only in elastin (Fig. 5.17). Desmosine and isodesmosine are isomers that cross-link the elastin (tropoelastin) chains into arrays that can be reversibly stretched in different directions. Elastin contains considerable amounts of *proline* and *glycine* but, unlike collagen, little hydroxyproline and no hydroxylysine. When secreted, elastin molecules become extensively cross-linked between the lysine molecules to form filaments and sheets. Elastin polypeptides are unfolded and exist in various random coil conformations. This arrangement permits stretching and recoiling of the elastic fibers (Fig. 5.18). Characteristics of collagen, reticular fibers, and elastic fibers are compared in Table 5.3.

TENDONS AND LIGAMENTS

Most tendons consist of closely packed bundles of collagen fibers. Rows of fibroblast nuclei are aligned between the collagen bundles, but the cytoplasm of the highly compressed cells is not usually evident in LM

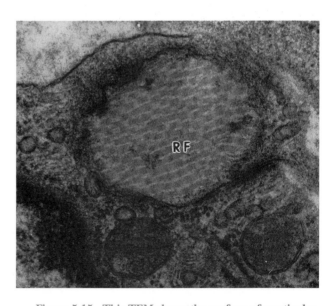

Figure 5.15. This TEM shows the surface of a reticular cell in which a number of reticular fibers (RF) appear to be completely surrounded by the cells but in fact are located in a concavity of the cell surface. ×48,000. (From R. Kessel and R. Kardon, *Tissues and Organs: A Text-Atlas of Scanning Electron Microscopy*, W.H. Freeman, New York, 1979, with permission)

Table 5.3 Comparative Characteristics of Connective Tissue Fibers

Feature	Collagen	Reticular	Elastic
Molecular organization	Triple-stranded helix; each strand ~1000 AA; molecule ~300 nm long, 1.5-nm diameter (glycine, hydroxyproline, hydroxylysine)	Type III collagen	Elastin 830 amino acid residues long; contains desmocine, isodesmocine (formed from four molecules of lysine)
Fibrillar organization	Fibers 2–10 μm in diameter (unbranched); fibrils ~50 nm in diameter; smaller microfibrils	Fibers 0.2–2 μm in diameter; fibrils 25–45 nm	Fibers 1–4 μm in diameter; fibers branch No fibrils Microfibrils ~12 nm in diameter
Axial periodicity	Fibrils 670 Å; axial periodicity	670 Å	None
Boiling water	Converts collagen to gelatin		Resistant
Weak acids and weak alkalis	Swells	Similar to collagen	Resistant to weak acids and alkalis
Strong acids and strong alkalis	Dissolved		
Staining	With acidophilic stains	Silver (argyrophilic) PAS+	Resorcin fuchsin, resorcin orcein
Enzyme effects	Pepsin and collagenase dissolve		Sensitive to elastase
Cells producing fibers	Fibroblast Smooth muscle cells in blood vessels Osteoblasts Chondroblasts Odontoblasts Type IV collagen produced by epithelial cells and endothelial cells	Reticular cells Fibroblasts Schwann cells (for endoneurium)	Fibroblast Smooth muscle cells in blood vessels

preparations. Capillaries are present between the bundles as well. Tendons attach muscles to bone. The collagenic fibers of tendons that are anchored into the bone matrix are called fibers of Sharpey. Tendons that are severed or injured can be rejoined surgically and will undergo repair. New fibroblasts from surrounding connective tissue or from the tendon sheath produce new collagen, but fibrocytes located within the tendon do not participate in the repair process.

Ligaments consist of closely packed longitudinal bundles of collagen fibers and closely packed fibrocyte nuclei. Thinner and finer collagen fibers and perhaps some elastic fibers form cross-connections with the longitudinal collagen fiber bundles. This provides some flexibility that is not usually characteristic of tendons but is functionally useful in areas of articulating joints.

AMORPHOUS INTERCELLULAR SUBSTANCES ("JELLIES")

A biochemically complex, amorphous ground substance ("jellies") surrounds fibers and cells of connective tissue and, together with tissue fluid, forms a highly hydrated, semisolid gel. This component of connective tissue is typically dissolved in most histologic preparations and thus is often overlooked. The amorphous component of connective tissue includes polysaccharide *glycosaminoglycans* (GAGs) that can be covalently linked to proteins called *proteoglycans* (Table 5.4). The GAGs and proteoglycans comprise what has been referred to as the *ground substance* and *cement substances* (bone, cartilage) of connective tissue. These macromolecules are typically highly hydrated and generally gel-like in consistency, es-

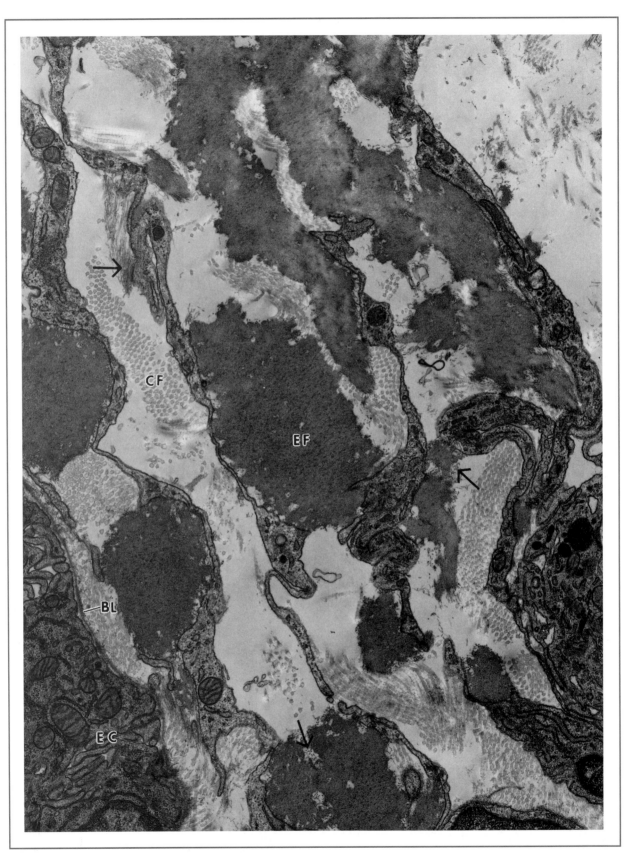

Figure 5.16. The TEM illustrates elastic fibers (EF) at the base of trachea epithelial cells (EC). The dot-like microfibrils at the periphery of the elastic fibers are denoted by arrows. Sections of irregularly shaped fibroblasts sur-round the elastic fibers. Collagenic fibrils (CF) are present in groups and lightly stained but are shown principally in transverse section. The basal lamina (BL) adjacent to the epithelial cells is identified. ×14,600.

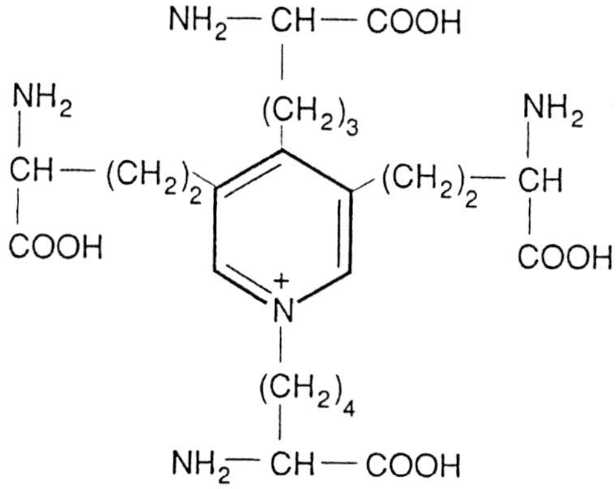

NH$_2$— CH — COOH

NH$_2$
|
CH — (CH$_2$)$_2$
|
COOH

(CH$_2$)$_3$

(CH$_2$)$_2$— CH

NH$_2$

COOH

(CH$_2$)$_4$

NH$_2$— CH — COOH

Desmosine

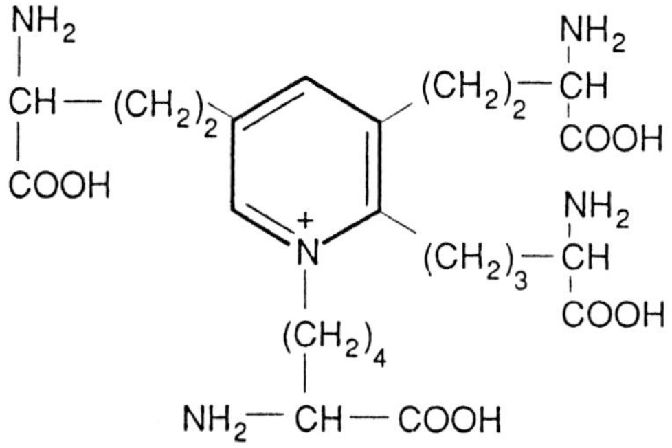

NH$_2$
|
CH — (CH$_2$)$_2$
|
COOH

NH$_2$

(CH$_2$)$_2$— CH
COOH

NH$_2$

(CH$_2$)$_3$— CH
COOH

(CH$_2$)$_4$

NH$_2$— CH — COOH

Isodesmosine

Figure 5.17. Structure of desmosine and isodesmosine.

pecially in the softer ground substances. The fibrous elements (collagen, elastin, reticular fibers) and cellular elements are embedded in the ground or cement substances.

GAGs are long, unbranched polysaccharide chains with repeating dissacharide units. One repeating sugar is always *N-acetylglucosamine* or *N-acetylgalactosamine* (hence the name *glycosaminoglycan*) (Table 5.4, Fig. 5.19). This amino sugar is often sulfated. The presence

of SO^{4-} or COOH$^-$ groups on the sugars is responsible for their strong negative charge. The second sugar is D-*glucuronic acid*, L-*iduronic acid*, or D-*galactose*. Four groups of GAGs can be distinguished by the sugar residues, the type of linkage between the residues, and the number and location of sulfate groups: (1) *hyaluronic acid* (also called *hyaluronan* or *hyaluronate*), (2) *chondroitin sulfate* and *dermatan sulfate*, (3) *heparan sulfate* and *heparin*, and (4) *keratan sulfate* (Table 5.4, Fig. 5.19).

Hyaluronic acid (also called *hyaluronan* or *hyaluronate*) is the simplest and most widespread GAG and consists of as many as 25,000 nonsulfated disaccharide units. The repeating disaccharide units of hyaluronic acid are *d-glucuronic acid* and *N-acetyl glucosamine*. Hyaluronic acid is widely distributed in many connective tissues including skin, the vitreous body of the eye, cartilage, and synovial fluid (lubricant). It is widely prevalent in embryos and in all tissues and fluids in adult organisms. It is degraded by the enzyme hyaluronidase. All other GAGs contain sulfated sugars and many different disaccharide units, have shorter chains (fewer than 300 sugar residues), and are covalently linked to protein to form proteoglycans. Some of the most common proteoglycans are listed in Table 5.5 together with information about their structure, location, and function.

GAGs such as keratan sulfate and chondroitin sulfate become covalently bound as side chains to a core protein prior to their secretion from the cell (Fig. 5.20). Many such *proteoglycan subunits* (monomers) are then covalently linked to a long, linear hyaluronic acid to form *proteoglycan aggregates* (Fig. 5.20). In the case of cartilage matrix, the proteoglycan monomers consist of a core protein to which some 80–100 chondroitin sulfate chains are attached in a manner similar to that of the bristles of a test tube brush.

The amorphous intercellular substances serve a number of important functions. They aid in maintaining the proper homeostatic environment for cells and fibers of connective tissue. They also serve a lubricative function and are involved in binding tissue fluid and

Figure 5.18. Diagram illustrates a cross-linked network of relaxed elastin molecule and stretched elastin molecules.

STRETCHED

RELAXED

CROSS-LINKED NETWORK
OF RELAXED ELASTIN
MOLECULES

CROSS-LINKED, STRETCHED
ELASTIN MOLECULES

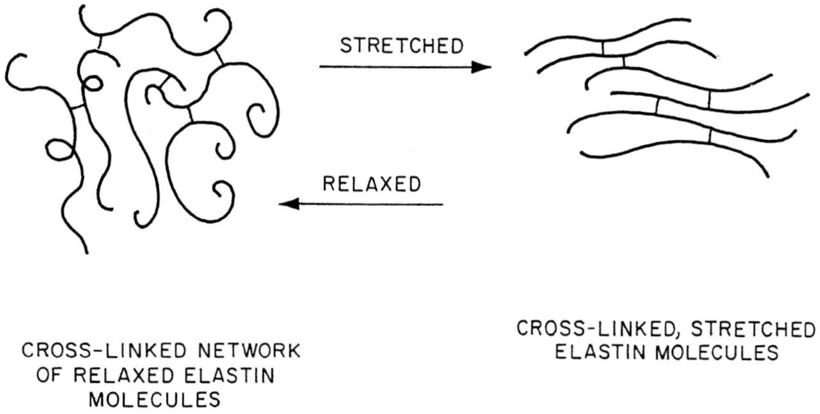

Table 5.4 Extracellular GAGs

| GAG | Repeating Disaccharide $(A\text{-}B)_n$ | | Linked to Protein | Other Sugar Components | Tissue Distribution |
	Monosaccharide A	Monosaccharide B			
Hyaluronic acid	D-Glucuronic acid	N-acetyl-D-glucosamine	—	None	Various connective tissues, skin, vitreous body, cartilage, synovial fluid
Chondroitin sulfate	D-Glucuronic acid	N-acetyl-D-galactosamine	+	D-Galactose D-Xylose	Cartilage, cornea, bone, skin, arteries
Dermatan sulfate	D-Glucuronic acid or L-Iduronic acid*	N-acetyl-D-galactosamine	+	D-Galactose D-Xylose	Skin, blood vessels, heart valves
Heparan sulfate	D-Glucuronic acid or L-Iduronic acid*	N-acetyl-D-glucosamine	+	D-Galactose D-Xylose	Lung, arteries, cell surfaces basal laminae
Heparin	D-Glucuronic acid or L-Iduronic acid*	N-acetyl-D-glucosamine	+	D-Galactose D-Xylose	Lung, liver skin, mast cells
Keratan sulfate	D-Galactose	N-acetyl-D-glucosamine	+	D-Galactosamine D-Mannose L-Fucose, siliac acid	Cartilage, cornea, skin, intervertebral disc, ligaments

*L-Iduronic acid is produced by the epimerization of D-glucuronic acid.

other macromolecules. Hydration of amorphous intercellular substances facilitates movement or diffusion of nutrients, gases, metabolites, hormones, growth factors, and other substances between the blood and resident cells in the connective tissues. Blood vessels, nerves, and lymphatic vessels are distributed throughout a particular organ in the jellies of the connective tissue. The polysaccharides are strongly hydrophilic and have a high concentration of negative charges. Thus, they tend to attract cations (e.g., Na^+) that are osmotically active and pull water into the matrix, forming hydrated gels. As a consequence, a turgor pressure is created that can withstand compressive forces. Thus, while providing mechanical support, the GAGs also permit rapid diffusion of water molecules, as well as the free movement of leukocytes, mast cells, and macrophages. While proteoglycan molecules in the extracellular matrix provide hydrated spaces around cells, the GAG chains form gels with different pore sizes and thereby regulate molecular trafficking in the extracellular matrix. Because proteoglycans bind to different signaling molecules such as growth factors, they appear to play a role in inhibiting or promoting the activity of various growth factors and other secreted proteins, including proteases and pro-

tease inhibitors. Not all proteoglycans are secreted from cells; some with relatively few GAG chains reside in the plasma membrane as integral membrane proteoglycans and may play a role in binding cells to the extracellular matrix.

CELLS OF CONNECTIVE TISSUES

A multiplicity of cell types, some transient and others more permanent, reside in the connective tissues (Table 5.6).

FIBROBLASTS

Fibroblasts are the most numerous cell type in loose or areolar connective tissue and in many tendons, ligaments, aponeuroses, and coverings of bone (periosteum) and cartilage (perichondrium) (Plate 6B; Plate 7B–D). The fibroblast can produce both the fibers and amorphous ground substances (jellies) of ordinary connective tissues. The fibroblast contains an oval, euchromatic staining nucleus with one or more prominent nu-

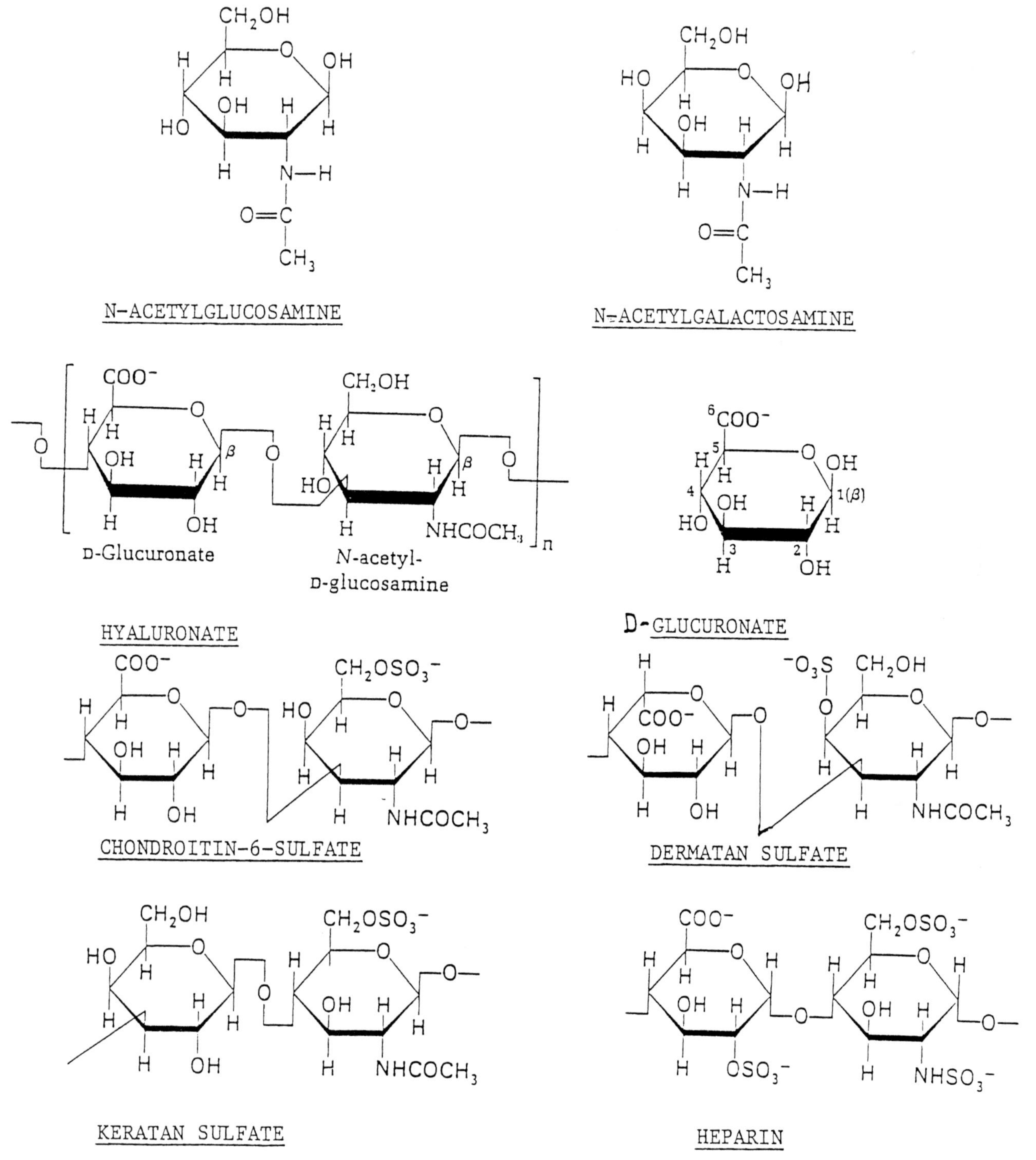

N-ACETYLGLUCOSAMINE

N-ACETYLGALACTOSAMINE

HYALURONATE

D-Glucuronate

N-acetyl-D-glucosamine

D-GLUCURONATE

CHONDROITIN-6-SULFATE

DERMATAN SULFATE

KERATAN SULFATE

HEPARIN

Figure 5.19. **Chemical structure of GAGs.**

cleoli. When the fibroblast actively synthesizes and secretes extracellular substances, its cytoplasm is more apparent and stains basophilic because of the presence of rER. The cytoplasm of inactive fibroblasts, called *fibrocytes,* is not evident with the LM. Fibroblasts tend to be flattened and irregular in shape. Since fibrocytes in adult connective tissues can incorporate radioactive proline, it has been suggested that a low level of secretion occurs in adult life.

Fibroblasts are not the only connective tissue cell that can form intercellular substances. Chondrocytes produce collagen and proteoglycan of cartilage. Osteoblasts produce collagen and proteoglycan of bone. In addition, reticular cells in lymph nodes, spleen, tonsils, and liver produce reticular fibers. Also, smooth muscle cells in blood vessels are able to produce elastic and reticular fibers. Cells other than fibroblasts that produce collagen include mesenchymal cells, odontoblasts,

Table 5.5 Common Proteoglycans

Name	Approx. Molecular Weight	Type of GAG Monomers	Approx. No. of GAG Chains	Distribution	Function
Decorin	40,000	Chondroitin sulfate, dermatan sulfate	1	Wide distribution in connective tissues	Binds type I collagen and TGF-β
Aggrecan	210,000	Chondroitin sulfate, keratan sulfate	130	Cartilage	Aggregates with hyaluronan, supportive function
Perlecan	600,000	Heparan sulfate	2–15	Basal laminae	Filtering function
Betaglycan	36,000	Chondroitin sulfate, dermatan sulfate	1	Cell surface, Extracellular matrix	Binds TGF-β
Syndecan-1	32,000	Chondroitin sulfate, heparan sulfate	1–3	Surface of fibroblast and epithelial cells	Cell adhesion, binds FGF

Abbreviations: TGF-β: transforming growth factor beta; FGF: fibroblast growth factor; GAG: glycosaminoglycans.

chondroblasts, osteoblasts, perineurial cells, myofibroblasts, cementoblasts, and some smooth muscle cells. In addition, Schwann cells, epithelial cells, muscle cells, adipocytes, and glial cells can produce type IV and type V collagen that are present in their basal laminae.

Although fibroblasts can synthesize all fiber types and intercellular materials, they appear to be the least

specialized connective tissue cell type. There is evidence that fibroblasts change into bone cells, cartilage cells, fat cells, or smooth muscle cells under appropriate conditions. During wound healing or repair of collagen-containing structures, as capillaries invade the wounded area, they bring with them cells called *pericytes* that reside at intervals on the surface of the blood vessels (Fig. 5.21). There is evidence that pericytes can differentiate into fibroblasts. Fibroblasts are also attracted to regions of injury by various growth factors such as platelet-derived growth factor. In the wound area, they divide and manufacture extracellular matrix and collagen.

Not all fibroblasts in different regions of the body apparently have the same potential or capabilities. The possibility has not been ruled out that different fibroblast lineages exist, some capable of transforming under appropriate conditions into fat cells, others into chondrocytes. It is unclear whether a fibroblast type exists with pluripotent capabilities or whether different and distinct types of fibroblasts exist with more restricted capabilities.

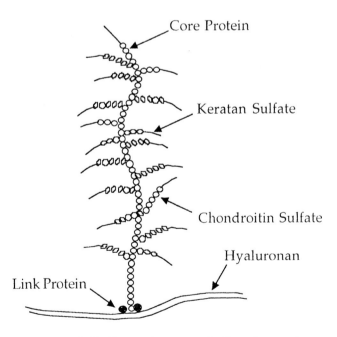

Figure 5.20. Proteoglycan organization of amorphous component of connective tissue. A core protein is linked by a link protein to hyaluronan (hyaluronic acid). Chordroitin sulfate and keratan sulfate side chains extend from the length of the core protein toward collagen fibrils.

MACROPHAGES

Macrophages in loose areolar connective tissue are rather long-lived, phagocytic cells that are remarkably active as secretory cells (Table 5.7). Macrophages are widely distributed in the body (Table 5.8). They are able to ingest or phagocytose dead cells, cellular debris, and bacteria, which are then digested by hydrolytic lysosomal enzymes. The macrophage lysosomes contain *acid hydrolase* enzymes and the microbicidal peptides *lysozyme*

Table 5.6 Cells of Connective Tissue

Cell	General Functions
Fibroblast	Produces fibers (collagen, reticular, elastin) and amorphous jellies (glycosaminoglycans, proteoglycans)
Macrophage	Phagocytic (e.g., bacteria),
	Antigen presentation
	Secretory (e.g., interleukin-1, interferon-γ)
Pericyte	Differentiate into fibroblasts, reticular cells, macrophages, smooth muscle cell in blood vessel, adipocytes
Mast cell	Secrete heparin, histamine, slow-reacting substance of anaphylaxis, eosinophilic chemotactic factor of anaphylaxis
Foreign body giant cell	Phagocytic (larger particulate material)
Reticular cell	Produce reticular fibers (type III collagen) for lymph nodes, spleen, bone marrow, etc.
Adipocytes	Fat storage, mobilization
Chondroblast (chondrocyte)	Secrete collagen or elastic fibers, as well as cartilage amorphous intercellular substances (glycosaminoglycan, proteoglycan), and other proteins
Osteoblasts	Secrete collagen, bone matrix (proteoglycans)

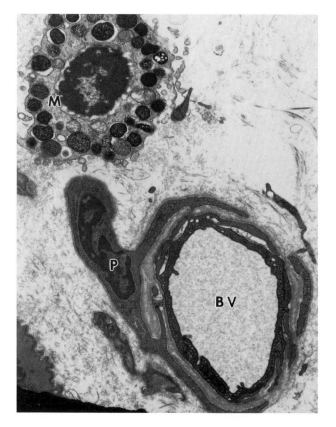

Figure 5.21. TEM of a capillary or postcapillary venule (BV) surrounded by a pericyte (P). A mast (M) cell is located nearby. ×8190.

and *myeloperoxidase.* Lysosomes fuse with phagosomes containing injested bacteria, and digestion of the bacterial cell wall is initiated. The myeloperoxidase in the lysosomes produces hydrogen peroxide (H_2O_2), oxygen, and superoxide ions. As a result of the action of these substances, the bacterium is completely digested. In loose connective tissue, the macrophage nucleus tends to be smaller, spherical, and more heterochromatic than the fibroblast nucleus (Plate 6B). The macrophage cytoplasm often contains granules that represent *lysosomal digestive vacuoles.* Monocytes are blood cells that are produced in the bone marrow. They are released into the circulation and remain for only 1–2 days; they then enter the connective tissues and become tissue macrophages. Large objects such as splinters or talcum accidentally embedded in loose connective tissues can attract macrophages and induce them to fuse and form large, multinucleated cells called *foreign body giant cells* (Plate 7E). The wide variety of macrophages located throughout the body were early identified by their ability to avidly phagocytose such vital dyes as India ink and trypan blue. Initially, macrophages were collectively considered to comprise the reticuloendothelial system. Since the cells that actively phagocytose injected dye particles are derived from monocytes, the system is now usually referred to as the *mononuclear phagocytic system.*

While macrophages (histiocytes) are numerous in connective tissue, especially the loose areolar connective tissues, they also abound in blood-forming tissues including the thymus, lymph nodes, spleen, and bone marrow. Macrophages are also abundant in the lung

Table 5.7 Functional Aspects of Macrophages

Surface receptors for:	Receptors that bind C3b component of complement
	Fc receptors, IgG
	IL-2, IL-1, IL-6
	Tumor necrosis factor (TFN)
	(Interferon)
	ATPase
	5'-Nucleotidase
Lysosome content	Acid hydrolases
	Lysozyme
	Myeloperoxidase
Macrophage activators	Lipopolysaccharide
	Interferon-γ
Interleukin effects produced	Actievates B lymphocytes
by macrophages	Chemotactic factor for neutrophils
	Increases circulating neutrophils
	Division of fibroblasts
Products phagocytosed	Dead cells
	Cellular debris
	Bacteria
Antigen presentation	Presents antigen with MHC II molecules to helper T lymphocytes (T$_H$ cells)
	IL-1 (a mitogenic protein for T lymphocytes)
	IL-6, IL-8
	TNF-α
	Interferon-α, -β; involved in fighting virus
	Colony-stimulating factors
	Macrophage-colony stimulating factor (M-CSF)
	Granulocyte-colony stimulating factor (G-CSF)
	Granulocyte-macrophage colony-stimulating factor (GM-CSF)
	Erythropoietin
	Platelet-derived growth factor (PDGF)
Selected secretory products	Fibroblast growth factor (FGF)
	Transforming growth factor-β (TGF-β)
	Protease inhibitors
	Elastase, collagenase
	Prostaglandins
	Leukotrienes
	Neutral proteases
	Coagulation factors (II, VII, IX, X, XII)
	Thrombospondin
	Plasminogen activator
	Factor inducing monocytopoiesis
	Complement componenets
	Pyrogens (mediate fever)
	Proteoglycan-degrading enzymes
	Hydrogen peroxide
	Lipases
	Superoxide

Table 5.8 Macrophage System

Name of Cell	Function(s)	Location
Macrophage	Phagocytosis, antigen presentation	Loose (areolar) connective tissue
Peritoneal or pleural macrophages	Phagocytosis	Serous cavities
Macrophage	Blood cell destruction, antigen presentation	Bone marrow
		Spleen
		Thymus
		Lymph node
Alveolar macrophage (or dust cell)	Phagocytosis	Alveoli of lung
Langerhans cell	Antigen presentation	Epidermis
Kupffer cell	Phagocytosis	Liver (perinsinusoidal macrophage)
Microglia	Phagocytosis, antigen presentation	Central nervous system
Osteoclast (multinucleate)	Bone resorption	Bone surfaces (form from fusion of monocyte-derived macrophages)
Fibroblast-derived macrophage	Phagocytosis	Intestine—lamina propria
		Uterus—endometrium
Foreign body giant cell (multinucleate)	Phagocytosis	Induced in areas of large particulate material (e.g., talc on mesentery) (fusion of monocytes, macrophages)

(*alveolar macrophages*), liver (*Kupffer cells*), epidermis (*Langerhans cell*), and central nervous system (*microglia*). Macrophages are prevalent in serous cavities, where they are called *pleural* and *peritoneal macrophages*. Macrophages can be either migratory (free) or nonmigratory (fixed). Macrophages also participate in the immune response; they can ingest and degrade certain particulate antigens. Macrophage can present antigen to lymphocytes, which, in turn, produce various protective antibodies. The macrophage plasma membrane has some 2×10^6 Fc receptors with which to bind antibodies. Among the macrophage surface receptors is one for the C3 component of complement that binds to bacteria, facilitating bacterial phagocytosis (a process called *opsinization*). Other macrophage plasma membrane receptors include those for interleukin-2 and interferon. Macrophages can also process antigen and display this antigen on their surface together with a major histocompatibility complex protein. As a consequence, a helper T cell can become activated and stimulate an appropriate B lymphocyte to respond to the antigen. Macrophages are quite sensitive to and become activated by substances (lymphokines) produced by lymphocytes. The role of macrophages in the immune system will be discussed in more detail in Chapter 10.

Macrophages can be activated by a lipopolysaccharide in the surface of gram-negative bacteria, as well as by gamma-interferon, which is produced by antigen-stimulated T lymphocytes. The interleukin produced by macrophages can stimulate and activate B lymphocytes and can also act as a chemotactic factor for neutrophils. Interleukin also causes division of fibroblasts and an increase in circulating neutrophils.

MAST CELLS

Mast cells are large, spherical, and filled with many cytoplasmic granules of rather uniform size (Plate 7B; Plate 8A,B). The mast cell contains sER, rER, mitochondria, and a Golgi complex. The centrally placed nucleus contains peripheral clumps of heterochromatin. Mast cell granules have long been known to stain *metachromatic*; thus, the color that they acquire is different from the color of the stain used. The release of mast cell granules (Figs. 5.22, 5.23), called *degranulation*, occurs if certain antigen-antibody interactions occur on the mast cell surface. Mast cells secrete or discharge granules by *compound exocytosis*, in which several granules may fuse with each other and then with the surface plasma membrane (Fig. 5.23). Mast cells are widely distributed in connective tissues of the skin and in mucous membranes of the digestive and respiratory tracts, especially near small blood vessels. Mast cell granules contain *heparin*, a sulfated GAG, as well as *histamine* and a number of other substances (Table 5.9). Heparin is an acidic GAG with a molecular weight of 12,000 to 20,000; it is an anticoagulant released in vivo from mast cells

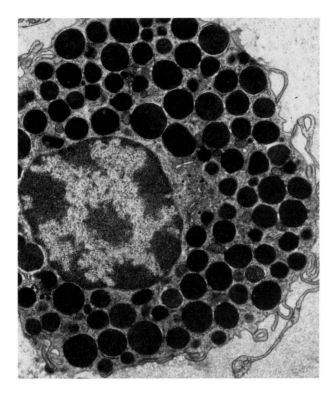

Figure 5.22. TEM of a mast cell filled with many membrane-bound secretory granules. ×12,350. (From R. Kessel and R. Kardon, *Tissues and Organs: A Text-Atlas of Scanning Electron Microscopy*, W.H. Freeman, New York, 1979, with permission)

and basophilic leukocytes during an inflammatory reaction and is responsible for the metachromatic staining of mast cell granules. Heparin has anticancer activity and may play a role in tumor regression and inhibition of tumor metastasis. It also appears to be an antiviral agent since it impairs viral replication in culture. *Histamine* is involved in certain allergic responses and acute inflammatory reactions. In rats and mice, the granules also contain serotonin, a vasoactive amine that can affect the diameter of blood vessels. In humans, *serotonin* is not present in mast cell granules but is present in platelets. Histamine, which is derived from the amino acid histidine, causes the smooth muscle in the wall of bronchioles to contract. Histamine also causes increased capillary permeability ("leakiness"). In individuals with hay fever, histamine released by mast cells into the connective tissue of the nasal mucosa causes capillaries to become leaky. Swelling occurs in the mucosa, with resultant sneezing and nasal discharge. Most substances released by mast cells are pharmacologically active locally, an example of *paracrine cellular secretion.* Mast cells, like macrophages, have receptors with an affinity for *immunoglobulin E* (*IgE*). Some individuals produce IgE when pollen or dust antigens enter their body, and the IgE molecules then attach to receptors on mast cells (or basophils). If the same antigen enters the body a second time and if it is polyvalent, it attaches to and

bridges the IgE molecules bound to the mast cell receptors formed initially. It is the second response, resulting in the polyvalent binding of the Ig, that causes mast cell degranulation. Antihistamine does not prevent histamine release by mast cells but does combine with some of the receptors on the responsive smooth muscle cells, thereby limiting the effectiveness of the histamine. Most of the IgE molecules in the body are fixed on the surface of mast cells rather than in the plasma.

Mast cells are the source of other substances, including an *eosinophil chemotactic factor of anaphylaxis* (*ECF-A*), *neutrophil chemotactic factor* (*NCF*), *lysosomal enzymes*, a *slow-reacting substance* of *anaphylaxis* (*SRS-A*; also called *leukotriene-3*), *platelet-activating factor* (*PAF*), and several *prostaglandins.* When released from mast cells, ECF-A attracts eosinophils to regions of antigen-antibody interaction, and the eosinophils can phagocytose the antigen-antibody complexes. Eosinophils release a *histaminase*, which may diminish or counteract the effect of histamine, as well as *aryl sulfatase*, which may counteract the effect of the SRS-A. The functional role of lysosomal enzymes is unclear, but they may play a role in degrading GAGs in the extracellular matrix. The leukotrienes (SRS-A) cause contraction of smooth muscle.

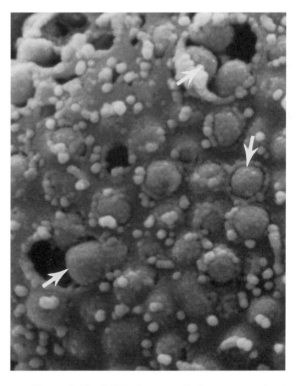

Figure 5.23. SEM of mast cell shows stages in the release of the secretory granules by exocytosis from the cell surface. Arrows denote regions of granule discharge. ×3600. (From R. Kessel and R. Kardon, *Tissues and Organs: A Text-Atlas of Scanning Electron Microscopy*, W. H. Freeman, New York, 1979, with permission)

Table 5.9 Substances Produced by Mast Cells

Heparin (acidic GAG)	Anticoagulant: binds to fibronectin, growth factors, coagulation proteins, complement compounds; has anticancer activity, causes tumor regression, inhibits tumor metastasis
Chondroitin sulfate	Sometimes present in mast cell granules rather than heparin: thus, different types of mast cells exist
Histamine	Causes contraction of smooth muscle of bronchioles: causes increased capillary permeability (leakiness)
Leukotrienes (slow-reacting substance of anaphylaxis—SRS-A)	Causes contraction of smooth muscle (not stored in cell—synthesized from membrane phospholipids)
Eosinophil chemotactic factor of anaphylaxis (ECF-A)	Attracts eosinophils to regions of antigen-antibody interaction; eosinophils phagocytize antigen-antibody complexes: eosinophils produce histaminase, which depresses histamine effects, and aryl sulfatase, which counteracts leukotrienes
Lysosomal enzymes including β-glucuronidase, hexosaminidase, aryl sulfatase	Functional role unclear: may degrade GAGs in extracellular matrix
Neutrophil chemotactic factor (NCF)	Chemoattractant for neutrophils

Other substances include *platelet-activating factor, prostaglandins* (several), and *neutral proteases* (tryptase, chymase) (most of the IgE molecules in the body are fixed on the surface of mast cells rather than in the plasma)

Anaphylaxis or shock can be demonstrated by injecting an antigen into a guinea pig. Then, about 2 weeks later, the same antigen is once again injected and the guinea pig will demonstrate anaphylactic shock. The guinea pig has difficulty breathing, has an accelerated heartbeat, and may die of asphyxiation if the smooth muscles in the wall of bronchioles contract sufficiently to shut off air.

ADIPOCYTES (FAT-STORING CELLS)

Fat-storing cells may become numerous enough to comprise a type of connective tissue called *adipose tissue.* Adipose tissue, unlike other types of connective tissue, consists principally of cells and relatively little intercellular substance. In this type of tissue, adipocytes are surrounded by fine reticular fibers, a few fibroblasts, and numerous capillaries (Figs. 5.24, 5.25). Fat serves as an efficient storage form of nutritional calories since it has twice the calorie density of carbohydrate or protein. Large numbers of adipocytes may be subdivided into lobules by fibrous septa of connective tissue. Adipose

tissue is richly vascularized, which facilitates transport of substances between the blood and adipocytes. There is a rather uniform layer of adipocytes in the connective tissue of the integument called the *panniculus adiposus.* Adipose tissue is also concentrated in the lower abdomen, axilla, thigh, and buttocks and is common in mesenteries, omentum, and bone marrow. Lipid may nearly fill the unilocular adipocyte such that only a narrow rim of cytoplasm remains and the nucleus is eccentrically placed. When the lipid is dissolved from the adipocyte, as often occurs during routine histologic preparation, these adipocytes have a "signet-ring" appearance. Lipid is retained in frozen sections of adipose tissue, and osmium tetroxide can be used to immobilize the lipid. Sudan stains (Sudan IV, V) and Oil red 0 are useful stains for lipid. Adipose connective tissue is classified as white or *unilocular* and brown or *multilocular. Multilocular* (*brown*) adipocytes contain numerous fat droplets compared to the single droplet in a unilocular adipoctye. The adipocytes of brown fat also are smaller than those of *unilocular* (*white*) fat. In humans, nearly all fat is white even though it actually has a yellowish color because of the presence of carotene. The

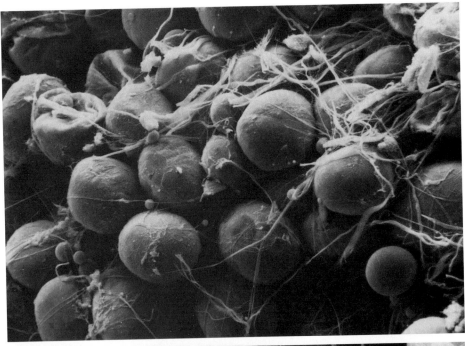

5.24

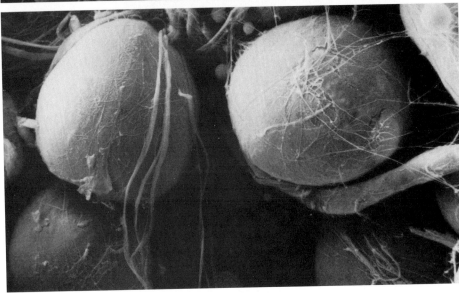

5.25

Figures 5.24, 5.25. SEMs of adipose connective tissue; individual fat cells or adipocytes are surrounded by blood vessels and fine connective tissue fibers, primarily reticular fibers. Figure 5.24, ×485; Figure 5.25, ×1145. (From R. Kessel and R. Kardon, *Tissues and Organs: A Text-Atlas of Scanning Electron Microscopy*, W.H. Freeman, New York, 1979, with permission)

multilocular adipocyte contains numerous mitochondria that are unique since they lack inner membrane subunits (elementary particles); hence the energy produced by the mitochondria of these adipocytes is dissipated in the form of heat rather than stored as ATP. Brown adipose tissue is present in hibernating animals, where it serves as a source of fuel to be used following hibernation. Multilocular fat is present in humans after birth and for several years thereafter. It then disappears from most areas of the body, although it may persist in a few areas, such as in the neck and chest and sur-

rounding the kidney and aorta. Brown fat, which is sparse in humans, has a brown color due to the presence of many capillaries in the tissue. These adipocytes are rich in mitochondria that contain cytochromes with a color similar to that of hemoglobin. Brown fat is therefore important in regulating body temperature in newborns.

The factor that triggers fat cell differentiation from a fibroblast-like precursor is growth hormone, a signaling molecule that stimulates fat cell and chondrocyte development. There is also evidence that fat precursor cells stimulated by growth hormone are also responsive to insulin-like growth factor-1 (IGF-1), causing them to proliferate and differentiate into fat cells.

Fat storage and mobilization

Fats in the digestive tract are degraded to fatty acids and glycerol by pancreatic lipase. The fatty acids and glycerol are then taken into the intestinal epithelial cell and recombined into triglycerides. The triglycerides are released from the intestinal epithelial cells into the lymphatic vessels as small bodies called *chylomicrons*. The capillaries in the adipose tissue have an enzyme, *lipoprotein lipase*, that liberates *fatty acids*, which are then taken into the adipocytes and combined with endogenous *glycerol* to form *triglycerides* (Fig. 5.26). Triglycerides can also be synthesized in adipocytes from glucose and amino acids taken up by the cells from the blood. Lipase within the adipocyte can hydrolyze the triglycerides at the lipid droplet surface, and the fatty acids thus formed are released into the circulatory system (Fig. 5.26).

The storage of fat and its liberation from the adipocyte are regulated by neural and hormonal factors. *Norepinephrine*, which is produced at the nerve endings of the sympathetic nervous system, can cause activation of an enzyme, called *lipase*, that cleaves the triglycerides in the adipocyte. Triglycerides constitute more than 90% of the lipid. During exposure to cold and during fasting, the mobilization of lipid is particularly important. Insulin, in contrast, tends to facilitate the conversion of glucose into triglycerides in the fat droplets of adipocytes. Other hormones are important in metabolic events in the adipocyte.

PLASMA CELLS

Plasma cells appear in connective tissues after birth; they result from stimulated *B lymphocytes*. Plasma cells synthesize and release *humoral antibodies*, which are immunoglobulins. The cells are oval, with an eccentrically placed nucleus that contains coarse heterochromatin distributed much like the spokes of a wheel (Plate 7D; Plate 8C). The cells contain abundant quantities of rER when the cells are synthesizing antibody, and the cytoplasm then stains basophilic (Fig. 5.27). When the Ig fills and expands the cisternae of the rER prior to release, the cytoplasm is acidophilic due to the staining property of the Ig. Plasma cells are very specific in the type of Ig they synthesize and release. Plasma cells are common in connective tissues under moist epithelial membranes, which represent imperfect barriers to the entry of foreign proteins (antigens). Plasma cells are also numerous in the lymph nodes and spleen.

When a B lymphocyte, a type of blood cell, encounters a foreign protein that it has been specifically programmed to recognize, and with the assistance of other cells of the immune system, it undergoes a marked response. The B lymphocyte enlarges and becomes mitotic. As a result, over 100 cells can be derived from a single stimulated or activated B lymphocyte. Some of the progeny of the mitosis develop an extensive system

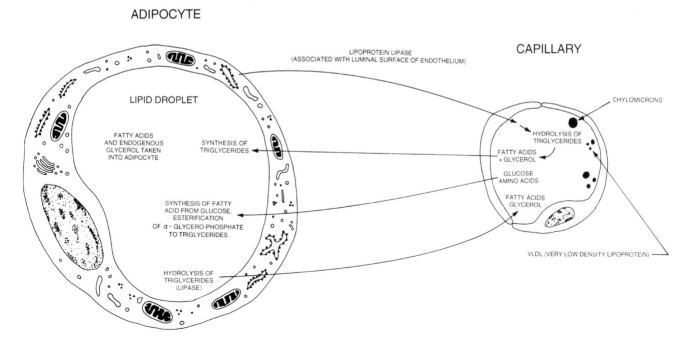

Figure 5.26. Diagrams depict the major events in the deposition of lipid in the adipocyte and the mobilization and release of triglycerides from the adipocyte.

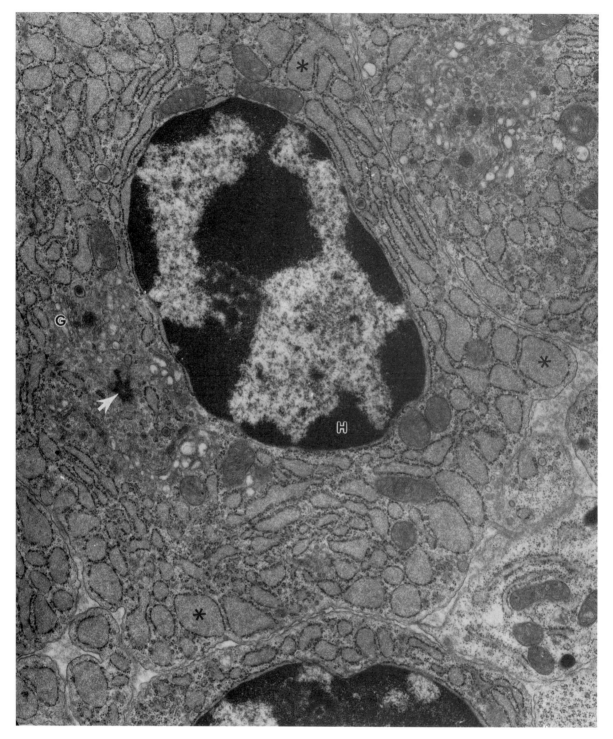

Figure 5.27. TEM of a plasma cell. Note the extensive system of rER cisternae; the cisternae, dilated in places, contain a flocculent precipitate representing Ig (*) synthesized by the cell, which will be released into the circulation. Note the nucleus with a nucleolus, heterochromatin (H), and Golgi (G) complex surrounding the centriole (arrow). ×17,000.

of rER and become *plasma cells,* which synthesize and release a specific humoral antibody capable of interacting with the specific antigen that caused the B lymphocyte to make its initial response.

PERICYTE

It has been maintained that undifferentiated mesenchyme cells persist in the adult and can give rise to differentiated cells involved in repair and regeneration. An undifferentiated cell, variously called a *pericyte*, *adventitial cell*, or *perivascular cell*, has been described that surrounds capillaries and venules (Fig. 5.21). Pericytes are surrounded by basal lamina continuous with that of the capillary endothelium, and the pericyte contains mitochondria, sparse rER, numerous free polyribosomes, and vesicles. The pericyte is branched, with processes that partially encircle the capillary. Although information is sparse, it has been postulated that pericytes have the ability to differentiate into fibroblasts, reticular cells, macrophages, smooth muscle cells, and adipocytes.

BLOOD CELLS

Most circulating blood cells are capable of entering the connective tissues; in fact, it is in this location that many blood cell functions are carried out. Thus, a rather continuous exchange of white blood cells between blood vessels and connective tissue occurs. Eosinophils and lymphocytes are most frequently encountered in connective tissue, but the number of blood cells within connective tissue markedly increases during inflammation.

BENIGN AND MALIGNANT TUMORS

A variety of benign and malignant tumors involving various connective tissue cell types can occur. The terminology used in identifying these tumors is denoted in the accompanying table.

Connective Tissue Tumors

Connective Tissue Cell Type	Benign Tumor	Malignant Tumor
Fibroblast	Fibroma	Fibrosarcoma
Myofibroblast	Fibrous histiocytoma	Malignant fibrous histiocytoma
Adipocyte	Lipoma	Liposarcoma
Chondrocyte	Chondroma	Chondrosarcoma
Osteocyte	Osteoma	Osteocarcoma

TISSUE FLUID

Tissue fluid is functionally associated with the fibers, jellies, and cells of connective tissue. The resident cells of connective tissue must receive the necessary raw materials to carry out a vast array of metabolic syntheses. These raw materials pass through the extensive network of capillaries that traverse the connective tissues and reach the cells by diffusion. Oxygen is similarly distributed to the cells of connective tissue. As the cells of connective tissue carry out their metabolic reactions, carbon dioxide and nitrogenous wastes are produced, which diffuse through the tissue fluids into capillary networks. Therefore, tissue fluid plays a major function in the distribution of cellular products. Tissue fluid is actually a filtrate of the blood and is produced at the arterial end of capillaries. Blood is a mixture of cells, parts of cells (platelets), and a fluid suspension called *plasma*. The plasma contains proteins in colloidal suspension, water, oxygen, carbon dioxide, and crystalloids that are dissolved in true solution in the plasma. The crystalloids of blood plasma include glucose, amino acids, fatty acids, and various salts. The capillary endothelium normally prevents most of the colloidal proteins from passing into the surrounding tissue spaces. However, the endothelial cells are permeable to water, crystalloids, and gases. Thus, tissue fluid consists of water, crystalloids, and gases or plasma without the colloidal blood proteins.

By the time blood passes through the arterioles and reaches the beginning of the capillary bed, there is sufficient hydrostatic pressure, due to the heart's acting as a pump on a closed system of vessels containing fluid, to cause formation of tissue fluid on the arterial side of the capillaries (Fig. 5.28) for the hydrostatic pressure here is greater than the osmotic pressure exerted by the blood proteins that remain in the blood. However, as blood progresses along the capillary bed toward the venous side of the circulation, the hydrostatic pressure gradually falls, so that the colloidal osmotic pressure of the blood becomes greater than the hydrostatic pressure. As a result, tissue fluid tends to reenter the venous end of capillaries by osmosis (Fig. 5.28). Carbon dioxide enters the capillaries because a diffusion gradient is established.

Not all tissue fluid returns immediately to the capillaries on the venous side of the circulation. Some tissue fluid enters a system of small, thin-walled tubes called *lymphatic capillary vessels*, which also permeate loose connective tissues. The tubes of the lymphatic circulatory system, which begins as blind-end tubes in the tissues, join together to produce larger vessels that ultimately connect at two places to large veins near the heart. Some of the small proteins that escape the blood capillaries can enter the lymphatic capillaries and thereby return to the bloodstream. Anything that interferes with the normal formation, circulation, and resorption of tissue fluid has adverse effects. Swelling or edema occurs because of the accumulation of fluids in the intercellular spaces of connective tissue. Edema can result from (1) lymphatic vessel obstruction in which tissue fluid or lymph cannot pass normally through these vessels; (2) increased hydrostatic pressure that does not

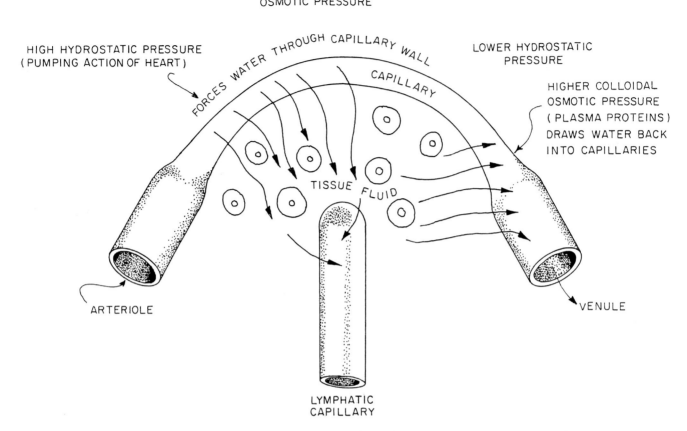

Figure 5.28. Illustration of how tissue fluid is formed at the arterial end of capillaries and resorbed into capillar- ies and venules on the venous end and into lymphatic capillaries.

fall below the osmotic pressure at the venous side of the capillary bed (as in obstruction of veins; alternatively, the heart is ineffective in returning blood from the venous side of the circulation); (3) insufficient blood protein (as in carcinoma of the liver, wherein insufficient blood proteins are made for normal colloidal osmotic pressure); and (4) increased permeability of blood capillary endothelium, which may occur with burns or other injuries to blood vessels that result in escape of the blood colloids.

CLINICAL CORRELATIONS

The connective tissue of organs except the brain contains many blood vessels. Thus, connective tissue is well suited to convey nutrients and wastes between the tissues and the blood vascular system. Connective tissue can regenerate. Surgical incisions heal because fibroblasts produce new intercellular substances. The repair of collagen in tendons is slow, but the collagen of areolar connective tissue is repaired more rapidly. Scurvy, which results from a deficiency of vitamin C, is characterized by degeneration of connective tissues since fibroblasts produce defective collagen. Adrenocorti-

cotropic hormones (cortisol, hydrocortisone) inhibit synthesis of connective tissue fibers, adversely affecting wound healing. The hormones suppress the inflammatory response by acting on connective tissue cells such as plasma cells and lymphocytes.

Connective tissue contains a number of cells that are important in inflammation, which involves a reaction to foreign substances. Inflammation can be caused by a number of substances including chemicals and pathogenic organisms; it is characterized by increased vascular permeability, increased blood flow, chemotaxis of cells in the connective tissues, and phagocytosis. Histamine, which is released by mast cells and basophils, causes increased vascularity and permeability, which result in localized swelling (edema), increased heat, and redness in the inflamed area. Various chemical mediators attract connective tissue cells and blood cells to the area of inflammation. Blood cells (neutrophils, lymphocytes, monocytes, basophils, eosinophils) can traverse the walls of capillaries and postcapillary venules to access the connective tissue. Neutrophils can produce substances to counteract the inflammatory molecules (Chapter 8). Monocytes attracted to the area transform into macrophages, which ingest and digest debris, as well as damaged cells and fibers. Immunologic reactions involve lymphocytes and macrophages, and antibodies can be produced.

Rheumatoid arthritis may involve the connective tissue throughout the body but particularly affects the synovium of joints. Osteoarthritis is a degenerative disease of the joint in which the articular cartilage wears away. Osteoporosis is a condition of reduced bone density due to a loss of bone, resulting in porous and fragile bones.

SELECTED BIBLIOGRAPHY

Auger, M.J., and Ross, J.A. (1992). The biology of the macrophage. In *The Macrophage. The Natural Immune System*, C.E. Lewis, and J. McGee, eds. IRL Press, Oxford.

Fleischmajer, R., Olsen, B., and Kuhn, K., eds. (1989). Structure, molecular biology and pathology of collagen. *Proc. N.Y. Acad. Sci.* **580**.

Galli, S.J. (1993). New concepts about the mast cell. *N. Engl. J. Med.* **328**, 257–263.

Hardingham, T.E., and Fosang, A.J. (1992). Proteoglycans: many forms and many functions. *FASEB J.* **6**, 861–870.

Larsen, G.L., and Hensen, P.M. (1993). Mediators of inflammation. *Annu. Rev. Immunol.* **1**, 335–359.

Mecham, R.P., and Heuser, J.E. (1992). The elastic fiber. In *Cell Biology of Extracellular Matrix*, 2nd ed., E.D. Hay, ed. Plenum, New York.

Rapploee, D.A., and Werb, Z. (1992). Macrophage-derived growth factors. *Curr. Top. Microbiol. Immunol.* **181**, 87–140.

Ruoslahti, R. (1988). Structure and biology of proteoglycans. *Annu. Rev. Cell Biol.* **4**, 229–255.

Van De Rest, M., and Gorrane, R. (1991). Collagen family of proteins. *FASEB J.* **5**, 2814–2823.

CHAPTER 6

Connective Tissue: Cartilage

Cartilage is a supporting connective tissue that comprises most of the temporary embryonic skeleton. Cartilage can grow rapidly enough to keep pace with embryonic and fetal growth; thus it provides a model within which most bones develop. Cartilage is important for continued growth in the length of long bones, which in juveniles is made possible by a plate of proliferating cartilage called the *epiphyseal plate*. Cartilage persists in the adult in joints where *articular cartilage* is conducive to the formation of polished surfaces (Plate 9D). The polished surfaces of articular cartilage, together with synovial membranes and synovial fluid, provide for smoothly articulating surfaces of joints. In addition, cartilage persists in the adult in a number of areas (Table 6.1).

Cartilage consists of a *matrix* or *intercellular substance* with many spaces called *lacunae* that are occupied by *chondrocytes* (cartilage cells) (Figs. 6.1–6.3). Cartilage matrix consists of *ground substance* and *collagen fibrils* (chiefly type II). The ground substance contains three *GAGs: hyaluronic acid, chondroitin sulfate,* and *keratan sulfate.* The cells that form cartilage matrix are called *chondroblasts* when they are synthetically active and *chondrocytes* when they become surrounded by their secretory product. The nature and amount of the fibers are used in classifying some types of cartilage. The types of cartilage that can be distinguished are *hyaline cartilage, elastic cartilage,* and *fibrocartilage.*

PHYSIOLOGY AND DEVELOPMENT

Cartilage has a low metabolic rate and is avascular. Cartilage is avascular because it produces substances that inhibit angiogenesis or blood vessel development. Since cartilage has no direct blood supply, chondrocyte viability is dependent upon diffusion of nutrients, wastes, ions, and gases through the intercellular substance from adjacent capillaries. GAGs in the cartilage matrix facilitate diffusion of substances between chondrocytes and blood vessels outside of the cartilage.

During differentiation of hyaline and elastic cartilage in the embryo, mesenchyme cells aggregate, enlarge, round up, and lose their long cytoplasmic processes. The cytoplasm stains basophilic due to the development of an extensive rER, which then synthesizes the fibrous and amorphous components of the matrix (Fig. 6.3). The cells, called *chondroblasts,* begin the synthesis, packaging, and export of the intercellular substances. The major events in the synthesis, packaging, and release of extracellular cartilage matrix by the chondroblast are summarized in Figure 6.4. Some mesenchyme cells in the embryo differentiate into fibroblasts, which produce collagen fibers for a perichondrium that invests the cartilage. In addition, mesenchyme cells proliferate to provide a pool of cells, called *chondrogenic cells,* that can subsequently differentiate into additional chondroblasts. During early periods of cartilage formation, the chondrogenic cells are able to proliferate. As the chondroblasts synthesize and release the intercellular substances of cartilage matrix, they soon become completely surrounded by the cartilage matrix and are called *chondrocytes.* The matrix immediately surrounding the chondrocytes, called the *territorial* or *capsular matrix,* tends to stain basophilic and metachromatic because of the high concentration of sulfated proteoglycans. The capsular matrix has less collagen than the *interterritorial matrix* located farther away from the chondrocytes.

Table 6.1 Distribution of Cartilage

Type of Cartilage	Locations
Hyaline cartilage	Cartilage models of future bones
	Epiphyseal plate
	Trachea, bronchi
	Knee cartilages
	Costal cartilages (ribs)
	Larynx, external auditory meatus (in places)
Elastic cartilage	Pinna of ear
	Corniculate and cuneiform laryngeal cartilages
	In places in epiglottis, external auditory canal, and eustachian tube
Fibrocartilage	Symphysis pubis
	Intervertebral discs
	Menisci of knee joint
	Articular discs of sternoclavicular and temporomandibular joints

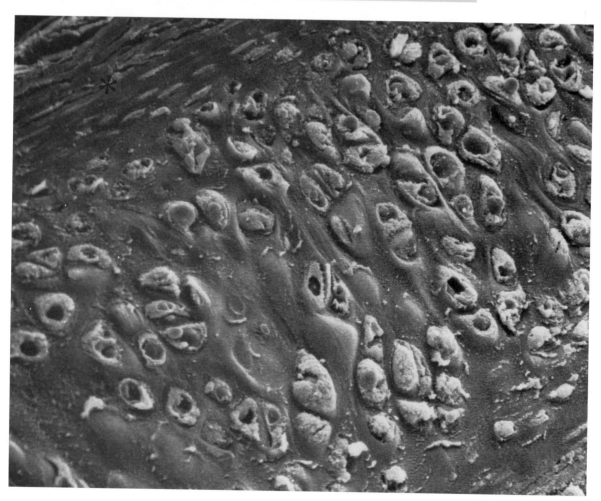

Figure 6.1. SEM of hyaline cartilage from trachea. Chondrocytes are evident in matrix, and perichondrium (*) is identified. ×755. (From R. Kessel and R. Kardon, *Tissues* *and Organs: A Text-Atlas of Scanning Electron Microscopy.* W. H. Freeman, New York, 1979, with permission)

129

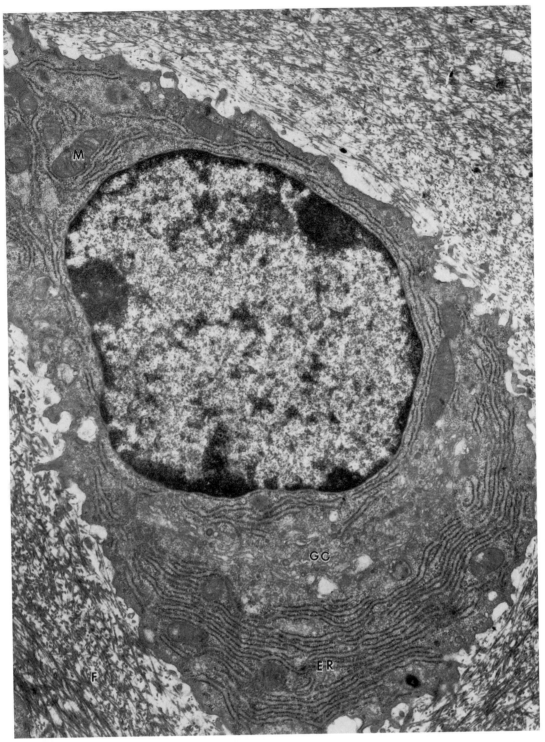

Figure 6.2. TEM of chondroblast. Golgi complex (GC), rough endoplasmic reticulum (ER), and mitochondria (M) are identified. Note the fine collagenic fibrils (F) in the matrix. ×16,740.

GROWTH

Cartilage is enclosed by a perichondrium consisting of two layers (Plate 9A,C; Fig. 6.1). The outer fibrous layer of the perichondrium consists of the collagen fibers and cells (fibroblasts, fibrocytes) that formed them. A thin internal chondrogenic layer of the perichondrium consists of chondrogenic cells, which have the capacity to divide and the potential to become chondroblasts and actively secrete new cartilage matrix on the surface of preexisting cartilage. This method of growth is called *appositional growth*, that is, growth from the surface. The

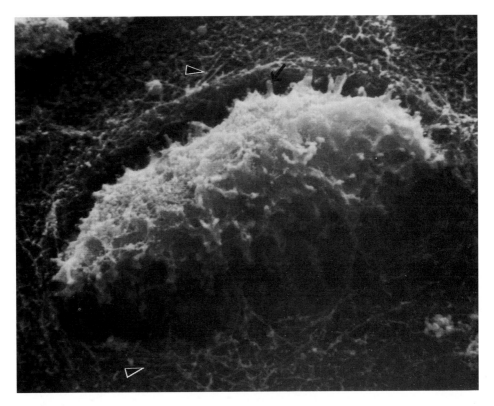

Figure 6.3. SEM of a chondrocyte in a lacuna. Note the small projections from the chondrocyte (arrow) and fibrils (arrowheads) in the matrix. ×10,565. (From R. Kessel and R. Kardon, *Tissues and Organs: A Text-Atlas of Scanning Electron Microscopy*, W. H. Freeman, New York, 1979, with permission)

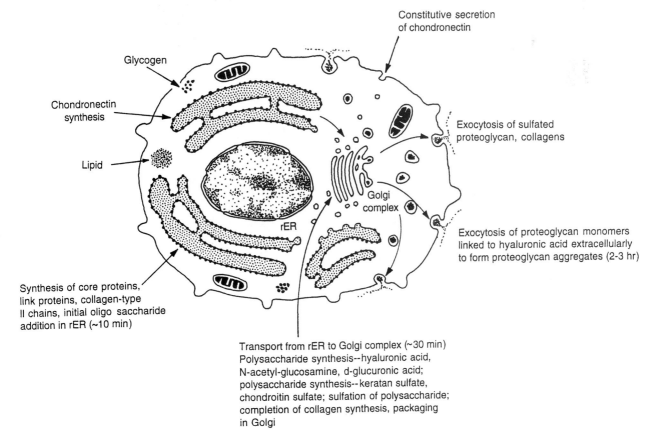

Figure 6.4. Diagram of the synthesis of cartilage extracellular matrix.

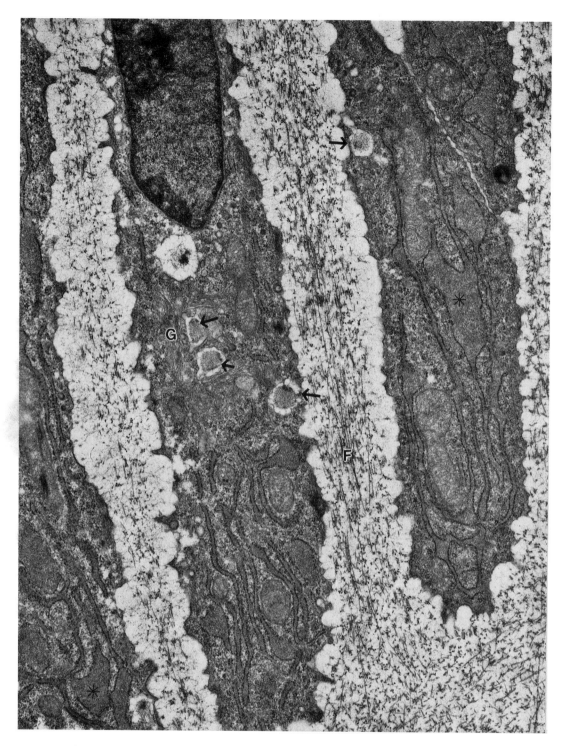

Figure 6.5. Shows several flattened chondrocytes from the epiphyseal cartilage plate in a developing long bone. Note the extensive profiles of rER, whose cisternae are di- lated (*) with secretory product. Arrows denote secretory granules and sites of granule discharge. Note the fine col- lagenic fibrils (F) in the matrix. Golgi region (G). ×20,280.

chondrogenic cells in the perichondrium also have the ability to divide and maintain a pool of cells capable of becoming chondroblasts. A perichondrium is never pre- sent at the articular surfaces of cartilage models that will become bones. In addition, some fibrocartilage lacks a perichondrium. Cartilage not only produces provisional models of future bones but also plays the leading role

in the elongation of bones during their growth. This is due to the proliferation and secretion of matrix by chon- drocytes in the epiphyseal plate or disc (Fig. 6.5).

Although a chondrocyte eventually becomes sur- rounded by matrix, it can continue to produce addi- tional matrix. Thus, cartilage can grow from within by a process called *interstitial growth*. Interstitial growth is possible because the matrix is sufficiently soft, pliable, and compressible. Since chondrocytes can divide and produce matrix for a limited time, clusters of closely packed cartilage cells may be present within the matrix (Plate 9B) of young cartilage. These cell clusters are called *isogenous cell nests* because their origin is from a single cell. The potential space in cartilage matrix occupied by the chondrocyte is called a *lacuna* (Fig. 6.3). While a lacuna is not evident in living cartilage, it is usually visible in preserved material because chondrocytes frequently shrink during fixation and dehydration. While isogenous cell nests of two, four, or eight chondrocytes may initially share a lacuna, each of the cells continues to synthesize and export cartilage matrix, and the cells separate from each other.

ORGANIZATION OF CHONDROCYTES

Young chondrocytes tend to be flattened, while mature chondrocytes are larger and rounded (Plate 9A), with a spherical nucleus containing a nucleolus. The cytoplasm of young chondroblasts contains prominent rER, a robust Golgi apparatus (Fig. 6.2), secretory granules, vesicles, IFs, actin filaments, and microtubules. Older chondrocytes tend to have abundant quantities of both lipid and glycogen. Since the glycogen and lipid tend

to be dissolved from histologic sections, chondrocytes often appear to be vacuolated (Plate 9A,C).

Synthetically active chondrocytes contain abundant rER, and the cisternae may be dilated with a moderately electron-dense product (Figs. 6.2, 6.5). The ER synthesizes the *core proteins* and *link proteins* of the *proteoglycans*, as well as *type II collagen*. Initial oligosaccharides of cartilage matrix are added in the rER. The secretory products are transferred by budding of transition vesicles in the region of the prominent juxtanuclear Golgi complex (Fig. 6.4). In the Golgi complex, collagen synthesis is completed and packaged for secretion; polysaccharide synthesis for *hyaluronic acid* (*N*-acetylglucosamine and *d*-glucuronic acid) and for *chondroitin sulfate* and *keratan sulfate* also occurs. This stage of the secretory events is completed in approximately 30 minutes, and the product is packaged in preparation for export from the cell, which occurs approximately 3–6 hours following initial matrix synthesis (Fig. 6.4). After exocytosis of the sulfated proteoglycans, hyaluronic acid, and collagen, the proteoglycan monomers are linked to hyaluronic acid outside the cell to form proteoglycan aggregates. Stages in the synthesis, packaging, and discharge of the cartilage matrix are diagrammed in Figure 6.4, and the structure of the proteoglycan aggregates is shown schematically in Figure 6.6. Chondrocytes also synthesize *chondronectin*, a glycoprotein

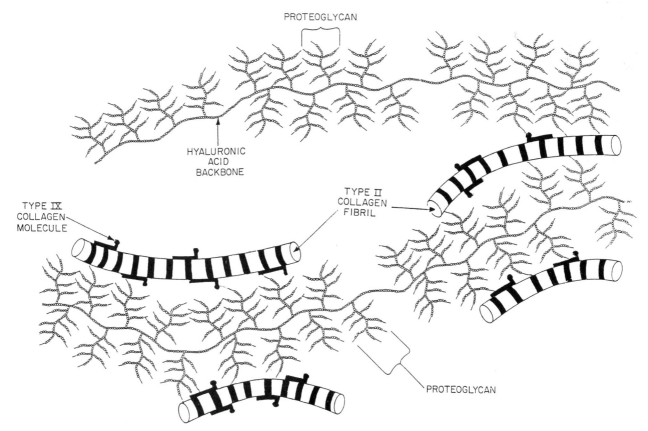

Figure 6.6. Diagram illustrates the organization of cartilage matrix. Many proteoglycans are linked to a long hyaluronic acid (hyaluronan) backbone. Many of these sub- unit aggregates are present in cartilage matrix and are closely related to type II collagen fibrils.

somewhat similar to fibronectin. Chondronectin is inserted into the surface of the chondrocyte in a process of constitutive secretion, where it binds specifically to type II collagen and GAGs. Chondrocytes can give rise to a benign tumor called a *chondroma* or to a malignant tumor called a *chondrosarcoma*.

CARTILAGE MATRIX

Cartilage matrix is predominantly a gelled proteoglycan, but other proteins and glycoproteins are also present in addition to the fibrous components. The matrix of the most widespread type of cartilage, hyaline, contains fine collagen fibrils ~20 nm diameter that contain *type II collagen*. The fibrils are too small to be observed in the LM, but they can be resolved by SEM and TEM (Figs. 6.2, 6.3). The small fibrils do not usually display an axial periodicity. Some 60–78% of cartilage matrix by net weight is water. Figure 6.7 is an electron micrograph of the interterritorial matrix after processing by high-pressure freezing, freeze substitution, and low-temperature embedding. Many points of contact between the type II collagen and components of the proteoglycan network are illustrated. *Aggrecan* is the major proteoglycan of cartilage. It consists of GAG monomers containing chondroitin sulfate and keratan sulfate covalently linked to a core protein. Many of these units are, in turn, linked to long linear molecules of *hyaluronan* (hyaluronic acid). These relationships are illustrated diagrammatically in Figure 6.6. A single hyaluronic acid molecule may have as many as 100 proteoglycan molecules linked to it (Fig. 6.6). Thus, cartilage proteoglycans contain chondroitin 4-sulfate and keratin sulfate covalently linked to core proteins, which are noncovalently associated with a long hyaluronic acid

molecule (Fig. 6.6). The chondroitin sulfate side chains bind electrostatically to collagenic fibrils in the cartilage matrix (Fig. 6.7).

The hyaluronic acid molecule is a very large molecule made up of approximately 500 disaccharide units in a long chain. Proteoglycans have a molecular mass of up to 3.5×10^6 D. The proteoglycan molecules are bound at globular heads by a link protein to the long hyaluronic acid molecule at intervals of approximately 30 nm. A glycoprotein, chondronectin, appears to promote adhesion between chondroblasts or chondrocytes and collagen.

A fibril-associated collagen called *type IX collagen* binds to type II collagen containing fibrils in cartilage matrix (Fig. 6.6) Type IX fibril-associated collagen molecules do not aggregate with each other to form fibrils but instead bind to the surface of type II collagen fibrils. Type IX molecules are more flexible than fibrillar collagen, retain their propeptides, and do not aggregate. The fibril-associated type IX collagen molecules are believed to play a role in mediating the interaction of collagen fibrils and other cartilage matrix molecules.

Tissue fluid binds the hydrophilic GAGs in cartilage matrix; there is also free fluid, which contains nutrients and gases that circulate through the ground substance. The fibrillar scaffolding formed by the collagen fibrils in cartilage matrix and the intervening hydrated proteoglycan aggregates are suited to resist tensile forces and to absorb some degree of compression. The large number of COO^- and SO_4^{2-} groups provide negative charges in the matrix, where considerable amounts of interstitial water are trapped. This condition provides some resistance to compressive forces.

Viability of chondrocytes requires the diffusion of nutrients, gases, and wastes through the matrix from capillaries adjacent to the cartilage. Therefore, anything

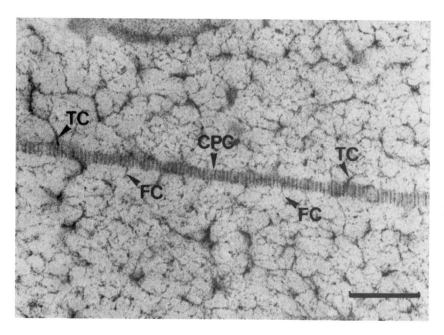

Figure 6.7. EM of interterritorial matrix processing by high-pressure freezing, freeze substitution, and low-temperature embedding. Cross-banding of type II collagen (CPG) shows many points of contact between it and thick (TC) and thin (FC) components of the proteoglycan network (bar = 0.2 μm). (Reproduced From E.B. Hunziker, and R.K. Schenk, *The Journal of Cell Biology*, 1984, 98, 277–282, by copyright permission of the Rockefeller University Press)

that interferes with the normal movement of materials through the matrix can result in chondrocyte death; this occurs when the matrix becomes calcified during intracartilaginous ossification. The calcification of cartilage results in chondrocyte death, and the calcified matrix slowly erodes away.

HYALINE CARTILAGE

Hyaline cartilage is named because in the living organism it appears "glassy" due to the translucent intercellular substance (matrix) (Plate 9A). It is the most common type of cartilage and is used to form small models of future bones-to-be in the fetus. Some permanent structures made of hyaline cartilage are listed in Table 6.1. Hyaline cartilage is also present at the junction of the sternum and the ventral ends of ribs. These forms are called *costal cartilages* and are important in permitting changes in the volume of the rib cage during inspiration and expiration. Hyaline cartilage that persists at the articular ends of long bones in adult mammals is called *articular cartilage* (Plate 9D). The surface of articular cartilage is extremely smooth, lacks a perichondrium, and forms the articular cartilage in joints. Young or newly formed hyaline cartilage is sometimes called *precartilage*. It contains smaller but more numerous and closely packed chondrocytes, including isogenous cell nests, and comparatively less matrix than older cartilage (Plate 9B).

FIBROCARTILAGE

Fibrocartilage is found in places where collagen fibers of tendons insert into hyaline cartilage; therefore, the matrix contains large type I collagen bundles. Fibrocartilage is not only located in regions of tendon insertions, but is also present in the symphysis pubis and intervertebral discs. Fibrocartilage does not differentiate from mesenchyme; rather, it differentiates in dense connective tissue involved in weight bearing. The matrix stains acidophilic because it contains an unusually large number of type I collagen fibers. The presence of many long, wide collagen fibers in the matrix also tends to induce a linear alignment of chondrocytes (Plate 9E). Fibrocartilage typically does not exist alone, but merges into hyaline cartilage. Fibrocartilage has greater tensile strength than hyaline cartilage, and it lacks a distinct perichondrium.

ELASTIC CARTILAGE

Elastic cartilage is resilient and capable of bending because of the presence of many elastic fibers in the matrix. It is located in the *pinna* of the ear, in various places in the wall of the external auditory canal, and in the Eustachian tube. It is also present in some laryngeal cartilages (corniculate and cuneiform) and in the epiglottis. The elastic fibers can be displayed by staining with resorcin fuchsin or resorcin orcein (Plate 9C). The matrix of elastic cartilage does not undergo calcification.

NUTRITION AND REPAIR

Injuries to cartilage are repaired by the perichondrium. The cells of the perichondrium tend to fill a gap or defect, and the chondrogenic cells in the perichondrium proliferate and differentiate into chondroblasts that secrete new matrix. Cartilage is affected by deficiencies in proteins, minerals, and vitamins. For example, proper levels of vitamins A, C, D, and calcium, as well as phosphorus, are required for normal development of cartilage. Growth-stimulating hormone and other hormones affect development of cartilage, as summarized in Table 6.2.

CARTILAGE GRAFTS

Epidermis and cartilage are both avascular and frequently can be transplanted successfully. Cartilage can be transplanted within an individual (an autograft). Cartilage grafting between individuals (a homograft) can also be successful, such as in the repair of nasal and ear cartilages. The grafted cartilage must continue to live because dead cartilage will be resorbed by the host. The graft must be well vascularized to supply the required nourishment. There are probably several reasons why cartilage grafts are not usually rejected. Cartilage matrix does not appear to be a very potent antigen. The chondrocytes are more potent antigenically, but they are "hidden" by the matrix from the host cells that might

Table 6.2 Hormonal Effects on Chondrocyte Synthesis	
Hormone	*Effect*
Growth hormone	Increased rate of synthesis of sulfated GAGs
Thyroxine	
Testosterone	
Cortisone	Decreased rate of synthesis of sulfated GAGs
Hydrocortisone	
Estradiol	
Somatomedin C (liver) (synthesis stimulated by somatotropin)	Growth of chondrocytes

recognize them as foreign or antigenic. Antibodies and lymphocytes do not move easily through the intercellular matrix of cartilage.

CALCIFICATION OF CARTILAGE

Calcification always occurs in cartilage that is destined to be replaced by bone at precise times in the growth of an individual. In addition, the portion of articular cartilage that is in contact with bone also becomes calcified. Further, some calcification of hyaline cartilage in the body can occur as part of the aging process.

While most future bones begin as cartilage models and grow rapidly in the fetus, it is necessary to replace the cartilage at the proper time with bone. This is achieved rather slowly by calcifying the matrix of cartilage, which leads to chondrocyte death and the slow erosion of cartilage matrix.

There are several important requirements for cartilage matrix calcification. Calcium and phosphate ions must be present in sufficient concentration within the matrix. Sunlight and vitamin D are important as well, for insufficient sunlight and vitamin D in children can cause calcium and phosphate levels to fall below a critical point and rickets may result. The pH is an important factor in calcification of cartilage matrix. At an *alkaline pH, calcium phosphate* ($Ca_3(PO_4)_2$), which is quite insoluble, precipitates. Conversely, at *acid pH, calcium hydrogen phosphate* ($CaHPO_4$), which is more soluble, precipitates. Thus, alkalinity favors calcification, while acidity hinders calcification. A protein called *chondrocalcin* plays a role in cartilage matrix calcification. An

initial sign of cartilage matrix calcification is the enlargement or *hypertrophy* that occurs in the chondrocyte. Hypertrophy is associated with the production of the enzyme *alkaline phosphatase* by the chondrocyte. Alkaline phosphatase can hydrolyze a wide range of organic phosphate-containing substrates; the enzyme can cause the release of Ca^{2+} ions as well as P_i from calcium β-glycerophosphate. The enzyme appears to be important in locally elevating the level of calcium and phosphate ions sufficiently for calcium crystals to form. Mitochondria of chondrocytes can store calcium ions for release during calcification of the matrix. Sulfated GAGs and proteoglycans are able to bind calcium ions and thereby participate in calcification, and the protein *chondrocalcin* increases in concentration in cartilage matrix prior to calcification. Chondrocalcin binds Ca^{2+} with considerable affinity. When cartilage matrix calcification begins, the lipid and glycogen stored in the local chondrocytes are lost. Thus, utilization of lipid and carbohydrate appears to be an important event in producing a suitable substrate for alkaline phosphatase. The calcification of cartilage is an important early step in endochondral or intracartilaginous ossification, to be described in Chapter 7.

In order for calcification of cartilage matrix to occur, a localized increase in calcium and phosphate ions is required. When local factors are conducive to a rise in ions, microcrystals of *hydroxyapatite* appear. Once the microcrystals begin to form, they not only continue to grow but also catalyze further crystallization of calcium phosphate. It has been observed with the TEM that in the region of calcification of cartilage matrix, there are membrane-bound matrix vesicles (Fig. 6.8), which are

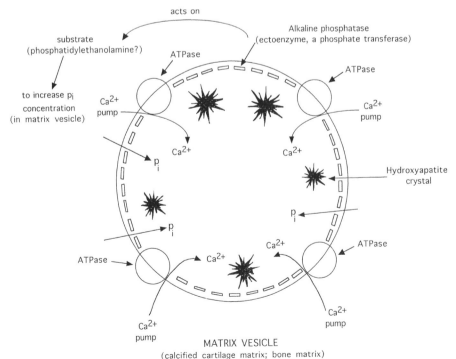

Figure 6.8. Diagram of a matrix vesicle depicts mechanisms by which calcification of cartilage matrix is initiated. Alkaline phosphatase acts on a substrate (e.g., phosphatidylethanolamine), which serves to increase the concentration of P_i inside the vesicle. Calcium pumps in the membrane elevate the concentration of Ca^{2+} inside the vesicle (energy-requiring transport). Crystals of hydroxyapatite appear inside the matrix vesicle.

acts on

substrate (phosphatidylethanolamine?)

Alkaline phosphatase (ectoenzyme, a phosphate transferase)

ATPase

ATPase

to increase p_i concentration (in matrix vesicle)

Ca^{2+} pump

Ca^{2+} pump

Ca^{2+}

Ca^{2+}

p_i

Hydroxyapatite crystal

p_i

p_i

ATPase

Ca^{2+}

Ca^{2+}

ATPase

Ca^{2+} pump

Ca^{2+} pump

MATRIX VESICLE
(calcified cartilage matrix; bone matrix)

thought to form by budding from the surface of hypertrophic chondrocytes. Crystals of hydroxyapatite form in close association with these matrix vesicles, which are also released from osteoblasts and odontoblasts during calcification. Matrix vesicles appear to be initial sites of calcium phosphate formation during calcification. Isolated matrix vesicles contain *alkaline phosphatase* and high levels of *ATPase*. The alkaline phosphatase is an ectoenzyme in the matrix vesicle membrane and apparently acts as a *phosphate transferase* on an appropriate substrate, possibly *phosphatidylethanolamine*, to increase the concentration of P_i inside the vesicle. The ATPase present in the vesicles appears to be active in the operation of a *calcium pump* in the vesicle membrane (Fig. 6.8). Hypertrophic chondrocytes form matrix vesicles containing alkaline phosphatase under in vitro conditions as well.

SELECTED BIBLIOGRAPHY

Caplan, A.I. (1984). Cartilage. *Sci. Am.* **251**(4), 84–94.

Hall, B.K., ed. (1983). *Cartilage: Structure, Function, and Biochemistry*, Vol. 1. Academic Press, San Diego, CA.

Reddy, A.H., ed. (1985). *Extracellular Matrix Structure and Functions*. Alan R. Liss, New York.

Stockwell, R.A. (1979) *Biology of Cartilage Cells*. Cambridge University Press, Cambridge.

Stuart, J., Watson, W., and Kang, A. (1988). Collagen autoimmunity and arthritis. *FASEB J.* **2**, 2950–2956.

CHAPTER 7

Connective Tissue: Bone and Bone Formation

GENERAL ORGANIZATION

Bone is a supporting connective tissue consisting of cells, called *osteoblasts*, that synthesize and export a product called *intercellular substance, extracellular substance,* or *bone matrix*. Bone matrix contains *collagen* fibers and an amorphous component with a high concentration of *sulfated proteoglycans*. In addition, bone matrix becomes calcified following secretion, and the calcium salts take the form of hydroxyapatite crystals. As osteoblasts become surrounded by their secretory product, they develop long, slender extensions, cease the secretion of bone matrix, and are called *osteocytes*. Large multinucleated cells called *osteoclasts* are able to erode bone matrix, and are important in bone remodeling and regulating plasma calcium levels. Finally, *osteogenic* or *osteoprogenitor cells* derived from embryonic *mesenchyme cells* persist in certain regions and have the capacity to differentiate into osteoblasts.

FUNCTIONS

Bone intercellular (cement) substance secreted by osteoblasts becomes calcified for added strength; as a result, bone is the most highly developed of the supporting connective tissues. Since metabolites and gases are unable to diffuse through calcified bone matrix, a direct blood supply is necessary. Bone functions as a supporting endoskeleton and for the attachment of tendons and ligaments necessary for locomotion. Bone encloses and protects the brain and spinal cord. The interior of some bones serves as the site of bone marrow and hematopoiesis (blood cell formation). In addition,

bone is a storage depot for calcium, which can be mobilized to enter the blood when levels fall below normal. Bone is very hard yet has some elasticity, can be compressed, and has considerable tensile strength. Bone responds to changing stresses and external forces by modifying its organization.

MACROSCOPIC STRUCTURE

Bones exist in a variety of shapes and sizes. Genetic factors primarily, but also hormonal, environmental, and nutritional factors, all influence bone size. Long bones such as the femur and humerus have thick-walled, tubular diaphyses or shafts that expand at each end into a metaphysis and an epiphysis. Articular cartilage covers the epiphysis at the synovial joint. Two forms of bone tissue can be distinguished from gross observation. *Compact bone* appears solid but actually contains microscopic canals and channels (Fig. 7.1). In a fully developed bone such as the femur, compact bone is external in position and is prevalent in the shaft or diaphysis. *Cancellous bone* refers to bone that exists as a latticework or scaffolding of bone spicules or trabeculae (Fig. 7.1–7.3). *Trabeculae* is a term that refers to beams of bone that are joined together in much the same way that beams of wood are joined together to form a scaffolding. Cancellous bone usually exists with compact bone, but cancellous bone is located within the shaft of a long bone and predominates at the ends (epiphyses) of bones (Fig. 7.2). Cancellous bone can be converted into compact bone directly by the continued secretion of layers of bone matrix by osteoblasts onto the surface of cancellous bone, but blood vessels must be brought into the interior of compact bone by the formation of *osteons* or

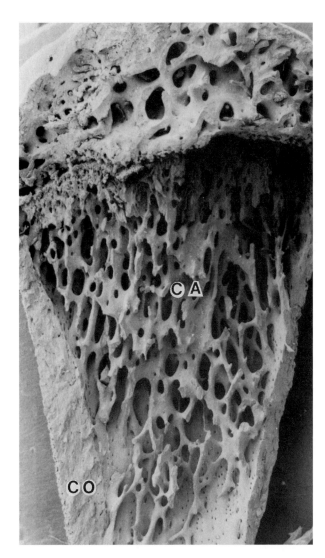

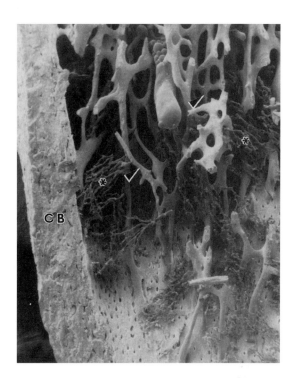

Figure 7.2. SEM (low magnification) of diaphysis (shaft) of compact bone (CB) and internally located cancellous bone (arrowheads) and replicated vessels (*) in the marrow cavity. ×30. (From R. Kessel and R.H. Kardon, *Tissues and Organs: A Text-Atlas of Scanning Electron Microscopy*, W. H. Freeman, New York, 1979, with permission)

Figure 7.1. SEM illustrates a section through long bone to show the epiphysis (at top) and diaphysis (toward bottom). Internally located cancellous (CA) bone and externally located compact (CO) bone are denoted. ×17. (From R. Kessel and R.H. Kardon, *Tissues and Organs: A Text-Atlas of Scanning Electron Microscopy*, W.H. Freeman, New York, 1979, with permission)

haversian systems. Both compact and cancellous bone undergo remodeling in response to tension or applied loads, the degree of activity or inactivity, and hormonal influences. To some extent, it is possible to change the form, strength, and mass of the skeleton. For example, bone responds to changes in loading. When an eccentrically loaded long bone bends, cells deposit new bone on the concave or compression side, but the cells resorb bone on the convex or tension side in response.

PERIOSTEUM AND ENDOSTEUM

Except at articular surfaces, bone possesses a fibrocellular sheath called a *periosteum* (Plate 11D). It consists

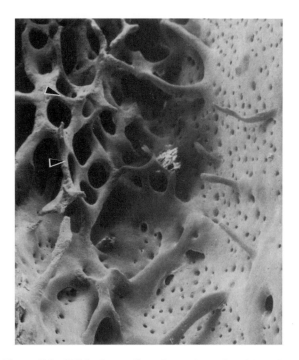

Figure 7.3. SEM of cancellous bone (arrowheads) and inner surface of compact bone in the shaft; openings represent entrances to Volkmann canals. ×65. (From R. Kessel and R.H. Kardon, *Tissues and Organs: A Text-Atlas of Scanning Electron Microscopy*, W.H. Freeman, New York, 1979, with permission)

of an outer *fibrous layer* containing collagen fibers and fibroblasts (fibrocytes) that form the collagen fibers and an inner layer called the *osteogenic layer*. This name is derived from the fact that the cells (osteogenic or osteoprogenitor cells) have the potential to become osteoblasts and secrete additional bone matrix. Bone can grow only from the surface, that is by *appositional growth*. Bone cannot grow by interstitial means because osteocytes cannot divide and, once trapped by bone matrix, cease the synthesis and export of bone matrix. Under certain conditions, as in healing of fractures, cells in the osteogenic layer produce hyaline cartilage and participate in the formation of an extraosseous callus. The periosteum becomes thinner with advancing age. *Endosteum* consists of osteogenic or osteoprogenitor cells and fine reticular fibers. Endosteum lines both haversian and Volkmann's canals and is continuous with the periosteum (see Fig. 7.6).

WOVEN AND LAMELLAR BONE

There are two forms of mineralized bone: woven (immature) and lamellar (mature). Woven bone is initially formed in the embryonic skeleton, but with continued development it is replaced by mature bone. Woven bone forms on the calcified cartilage during endochondral ossification. Subsequently, osteoclasts and chondro-

clasts erode the woven bone and calcified cartilage matrix, which are replaced by mature lamellar bone. Woven bone is not generally present in humans after about 5 years of age, but it may be formed in certain diseases and during healing of fractures. Woven bone has a higher rate of formation and turnover, a more random pattern of collagen fibril orientation, and more numerous osteocytes per unit volume compared to lamellar bone. Further, mineralization of woven bone is more irregular than that of lamellar bone. Woven bone is more easily deformed and flexible but weaker than mature bone.

MICROSCOPIC ORGANIZATION

Osteons are cylinders of bone consisting of concentric lamellae (layers) of bone matrix around a central canal called a *haversian canal*, named by Havers in 1691, that contains blood vessels, lymphatic vessels, endosteum, and an occasional nerve (Plate 10B–D; Figs. 7.4–7.6). Osteons comprise most of the mature diaphyseal compact bone. The collagen fibrils in adjacent lamellae run in different directions (Fig. 7.6), which confers additional strength. Many osteons range from 3 to 5 mm in length, are approximately 0.3 mm in diameter, and have up to six bone lamellae. Osteons can branch and anastomose. Transverse or oblique vessel channels called

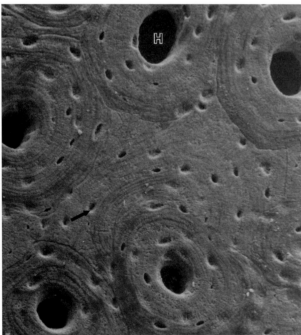

7.4

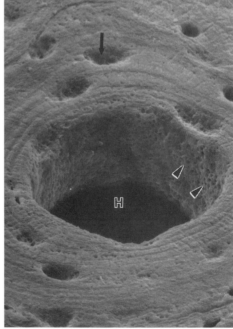

7.5

Figures 7.4, 7.5. SEM of polished specimen of ground compact bone from which cells and organic material are removed. A number of Haversian canals (H) are illustrated, surrounded by concentric layers of mineralized bone matrix. Lacunae (arrows). In Figure 7.5, the wall of the Haversian canal (H) is riddled with many small canaliculi (arrow- **heads), which also radiate through the Haversian system and connect with lacunae. Figure 7.4, ×315; Figure 7.5, ×845. (From R. Kessel and R.H. Kardon, *Tissues and Organs: A Text-Atlas of Scanning Electron Microscopy*, W.H. Freeman, New York, 1979, with permission)**

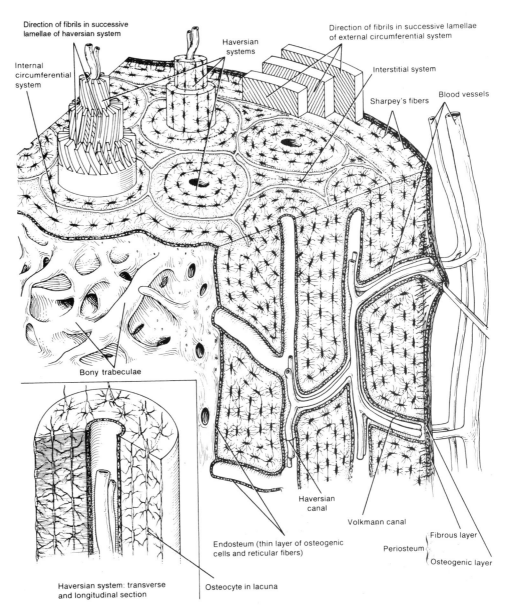

Figure 7.6. Diagram illustrates the microanatomy of compact bone. (From R. Kessel and R.H. Kardon, *Tissues and Organs: A Text-Atlas of Scanning Electron Microscopy*, W.H. Freeman, New York, 1979, with permission)

Volkmann's canals interconnect the haversian canals (Fig. 7.6). The vascular channels also communicate with both periosteal and endosteal surfaces (Fig. 7.6).

The cell bodies of bone cells (osteocytes) reside in spaces of bone matrix called *lacunae*. Many long, finger-like extensions of the osteocyte cell body extend into narrow channels called *canaliculi* (Fig. 7.7). Canaliculi radiate from the haversian canal and interconnect this canal with all the osteocytes in the osteonal lamellae (Figs. 7.6–7.8). Canaliculi do not usually cross the cement lines that mark the outer extent of osteons (Fig. 7.4). The organization of compact, cancellous, and trabecular bone is illustrated in Figure 7.6. The lamellar bone consists mainly of haversian systems containing osteonal lamellae. The outer and inner circumferential lamellae, as well as interstitial lamellae, complete the regional differenti-

ation of compact bone lamellae. The intraosseous vascular system extends through the haversian and Volkmann canals and supplies the osteocytes that reside within lacunae and canaliculi of the bone matrix. The blood vessels in the haversian and Volkmann canals are continuous with periosteal and medullary vessels; thus the vascular channels of bone communicate with both the periosteal and endosteal surfaces.

BONE CELLS

Osteoblasts

Osteoblasts arise from mesenchyme cells and are responsible for bone formation (osteogenesis). The principle tissues that are capable of giving rise to osteoblasts

Secretory Products of Osteoblasts

Substance	Action/Function or Postulated Role
Alkaline phosphatase	Associated with P_i in bone matrix calcification.
Collagen I	Organic component of bone matrix
Hyaluronic acid	Organic constituents of bone matrix
Chrondroitin sulfate	
Keratan sulfate	
Link protein	
Core protein	
Biglycan	Small glycoprotein; consists of core protein and one or two GAG chains; function unknown; possible role in cell-matrix interaction and control of cell proliferation
Decorin	Small glycoprotein; consists of core proteins and one or two GAG chains; binds type I and II collagen; implicated in regulation of collagen formation.
Osteopontin	Present in osteoid at mineralization front; role in mineralization process; plays role in anchoring osteoclast to bone surface
Osteonectin	Binds Ca^{2+} ions, hydroxyapatite, type I collagen, thrombospondin, and other matrix components
Bone scialoprotein	May play role in mineralizing process in bone
Bone morphogenetic proteins	Bone inductive activity; normal maintenance of bone; important in repair processes
Procollagenase (enzyme)	Collagenase released from procollagenase by plasmin
	Both enzymes play a role in depolymerizing osteoid
Plasminogen activator (enzyme)	Converts serum plasminogen to the neutral protease plasmin; plasmin releases collagenase from proenzyme procollagenase

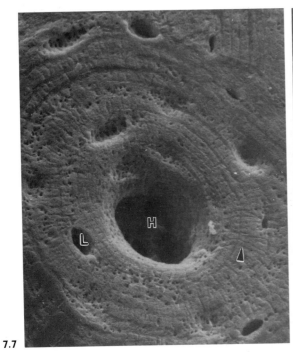

7.7

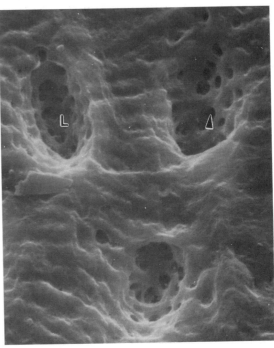

7.8

Figures 7.7, 7.8. Both figures illustrate by SEM the Haversian canal (H), lacunae (L) and canaliculi (arrowheads). Figure 7.6, ×860; Figure 7.8, ×3120. (From R. Kessel and R.H. Kardon, *Tissues and Organs: A Text-Atlas of Scanning Electron Microscopy*, W.H. Freeman, New York, 1979, with permission)

are bone marrow, periosteum, endosteum, and the periodontal membrane. Some agents that stimulate bone formation act by inducing proliferation and differentiation of osteoblast precursor cells rather than by direct stimulation of mature osteoblasts. Bone cell formation and bone deposition appear to include the production of osteoblast-derived growth factors that are involved in both autocrine and paracrine regulation. There is some evidence that bone cells can produce growth/proliferating factors and perhaps inhibitory factors as well, but the evidence is incomplete.

Osteoblasts line bone surfaces; they synthesize, package, and export the organic constituents of bone matrix including type I collagen and sulfated proteoglycans. Recent studies indicate that the secretory products of osteoblasts are quite diverse; some of them are listed in the accompanying table.

When active, osteoblasts are usually elongated or columnar, and the nucleus is located in that part of the cell farthest from the bone matrix (Plate 11A–C). The cytoplasm stains basophilic because of the extensive rER. A large juxtanuclear Golgi apparatus is usually dissolved in LM preparations, resulting in a clear area. The osteoblast secretes in a polarized fashion. Once bone matrix secretion has been initiated, additional bone matrix is secreted on preexisting bone surfaces. Some new matrix comes to surround the osteoblast. The ultimate fate of osteoblasts is to become enclosed and trapped by their secretory products. However, the osteoblast undergoes a pronounced shape change as it becomes surrounded by bone matrix. Osteoblasts that are inactive in bone matrix secretion tend to be smaller and more flattened or oval in shape than actively secreting osteoblasts.

Osteoblasts are responsive to *parathyroid hormone (PTH)*. Among the markers for osteoblasts are *alkaline phosphatase, prostaglandin E2 (PGE-2), collagenase and collagenase inhibitor, transforming growth factor-β,* and matrix components such as *type I collagen, osteonectin,* and *osteocalcin.* Receptors that have been identified in the plasma membrane of osteoblasts are listed in the accompanying table.

The microenvironment of bone cells is important in their differentiation. Among the molecules that are suggested to be osteoinductive are *fibronectin, collagen, procollagen peptides,* and larger *proteoglycans.* Osteoblast activity is affected by a number of substances; examples are listed in the accompanying table.

Some Substances Affecting Osteoblasts

Substances Affecting Osteoblast Activity	Osteoblast Activity Affected
Transforming growth factor-β (TGF-β); insulin-like growth factor (IGF)	Osteoblast proliferation; alkaline phosphatase production and matrix synthesis by osteoblast
Prostaglandin E₂	Osteoblast division; collagen synthesis by osteoblast; plasminogen activator synthesis
Interleukin-1 (IL-1)	Prostaglandin E₂ synthesis by osteoblast
Tumor necrosis factor (TNF-α)	Activates osteoblasts to produce cytokines (IL-6, granulocyte-macrophage colony-stimulating factor (GM-CSF), macrophage colony-stimulating factor (M-CSF)

Osteoblast Receptors

1, 25 Dihydroxyvitamin D₃

Retinoic acid

Parathyroid hormone

Glucocorticoids

Growth factors (transforming growth factor-β; Insulin-like growth factor)

Osteocytes

When osteoblasts deposit bone on preexisting surfaces, they eventually become surrounded by bone matrix (Plate 12C) and are called *osteocytes.* Osteocyte cell bodies reside in spaces called *lacunae,* which are especially evident in ground bone preparations in which the osteocytes are removed (Fig. 7.7). As osteoblasts become surrounded by intercellular matrix, they extend many long, slender, finger-like extensions (Figs. 7.9, 7.10, 7.11) or tendrils that contact those of nearby osteocytes (Figs. 7.12, 7.13). This results in many small channels, called *canaliculi,* that extend throughout the bone matrix and create a *canalicular circulatory system* that provides nourishment for osteocytes. The extensions of one osteocyte touch those extending from other nearby osteocytes, and *gap* or *communicating junctions* are formed. Osteocytes are electrically coupled by gap junctions, permitting small molecules and ions to pass from one osteocyte to another. The canalicular system is not completely satisfactory for the distribution of nutrients, gases, and wastes in bone since it is estimated that an osteocyte cannot survive if more than *0.20 mm* away from a capillary. If this occurs, then new haversian systems are required to bring blood vessels into closer proximity to the osteoctyes (Fig. 7.14). During formation, bone surfaces have ridges and grooves with blood vessels running in the grooves. By the localized transformation of the osteogenic cells in the periosteum to osteoblasts, bone is deposited on the ridges so that they become higher and eventually fuse completely to form a tunnel (haversian canal) containing the central blood vessels. The osteogenic cells proliferate and differentiate into more osteoblasts to deposit bone in the tunnel from its periphery toward the centrally located blood vessels; thus, a new haversian system or osteon is formed. Throughout life, slow remodeling of osteons occurs in response to changing stresses in bone. Haversian systems are not only slowly remodeled, parts of them can be converted into interstitial lamellae. *Cement lines* are regions where bone resorption ceased and new bone formation commenced (Fig. 7.4). Cement lines are apparent around osteons and contain little collagen. Collagen fibrils do not cross cement lines. Fractures tend to follow cement lines rather than crossing osteons.

Osteoprogenitor cells

A population of mesenchyme-derived cells, called *osteoprogenitor cells*, can proliferate and differentiate into osteoblasts and chondroblasts in some cases. The osteoprogenitor cells are present throughout postnatal life and can be found on bone surfaces. The cells become

activated during bone fractures and are involved in repair.

BONE MATRIX (INTERCELLULAR SUBSTANCE)

Organic

The unique mechanical qualities that permit bone to serve as a supporting connective tissue are due to the nature of the intercellular or extracellular substance, which contains both inorganic and organic components. The inorganic portion is about 65% of bone dry weight, and the organic component comprises about 32% of the dry weight. Nearly 90% of the organic matrix of bone is collagen, principally *type I collagen*, which causes acidophilic staining. Collagen fibers are not evident in routine histologic bone sections because they are masked by the mineralized bone matrix. Roughly 10% of the organic content consists of proteins and glycoproteins, as well as heparan sulfate, keratan sulfate, chondroitin sulfate, and hyaluronic acid, largely in the form of *proteoglycan aggregates*. The organic component, collagen, enables bone to resist tension, while the mineral component permits bone to resist compression. The various calcium salts in bone matrix provide hardness and rigidity. The initial organic matrix that is secreted is called *osteoid*. As osteoid becomes mineralized, it is then converted into bone. The osteoid matrix contains molecules that bind both collagen and mineral. Collagen contains regions that stimulate or catalyze the nucleation of mineral crystals.

Mineral

The final mineral product in bone matrix is similar to crystalline *hydroxyapatite* ($Ca_5(PO_4)_3OH$), and the mineral deposits form in close spatial relation to *matrix vesicles* and collagen fibrils. Noncrystalline calcium phosphate is also present in bone matrix. Bone mineral also contains citrate and bicarbonate ions, as well as fluoride, magnesium, potassium, and sodium ions. Bone matrix can be decalcified by steeping in dilute acids or ethylenediaminetetra-acetic acid (EDTA), a chelating agent that has a great affinity for Ca^{2+}. Sections can then be prepared and stained with H&E. Demineralized bone is flexible and pliable. When the organic matrix is removed, bone becomes rigid, hard, and brittle. Chalk results when the organic components of bone are removed, as in burning. Relatively little water is present in bone (~8–9%) compared to cartilage (~75%). It is also possible to study the overall organization of bone matrix, including osteons, interstitial lamellae, circumferential lamellae, and the canalicular system, by grinding bone to a very thin piece on a grinding wheel. The cellular elements are removed in such a preparation but the thinly ground bone is placed on a slide, mounted with permount and a coverslip placed over the bone

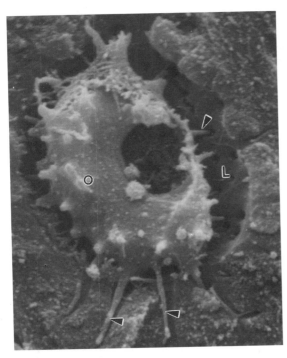

Figure 7.9. SEM of an osteocyte (O) in a lacuna (L). Note the many long processes (arrowheads) of the osteocyte, which extend into canaliculi (arrowheads). ×7435. (From R. Kessel and R.H. Kardon, *Tissues and Organs: A Text-Atlas of Scanning Electron Microscopy*, W.H. Freeman, New York, 1979, with permission)

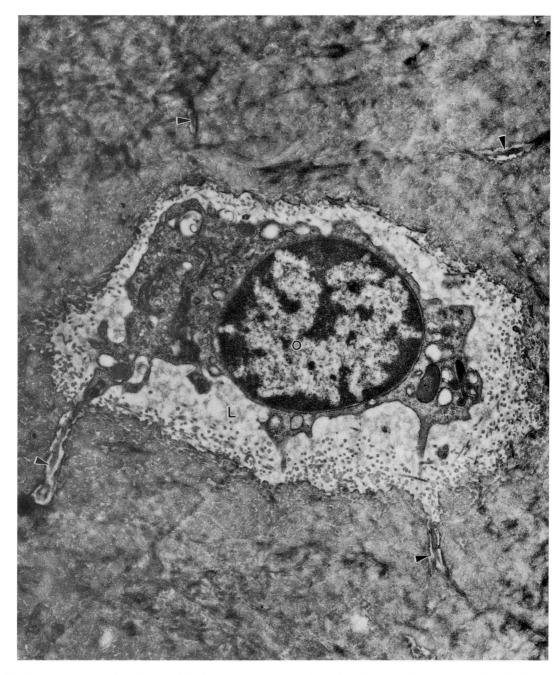

Figure 7.10. TEM of an osteocyte in a lacuna (L). Osteocyte processes (arrowheads) extend into the canaliculi in bone matrix. ×16,305.

pieces. The fine channels, including Volkmann canals, haversian canals, lacunae, and canaliculi, appear opaque in such preparations (Fig. 7.6; Plate 10D).

Immature bone is the first bone to develop in the embryo or in the repair of fractures. It has proportionately more cells and collagen and less cement substance and mineral than mature bone. *Mature bone* can be distinguished from immature bone in that it stains evenly, by the regularity of the lamellae, and by the fact that the orientation of collagen fibrils in adjacent lamellae is different. There are fewer osteocytes, and they are more

regularly arranged and in flatter lacunae in mature bone compared to immature bone.

Calcification

Calcification of bone matrix is required for its proper function but limits diffusion. Chondrocytes respond to matrix calcification by dying; osteocytes adapt by forming connections via canaliculi to a blood supply. Although many details about bone matrix calcification are unclear, several important events are associated with the

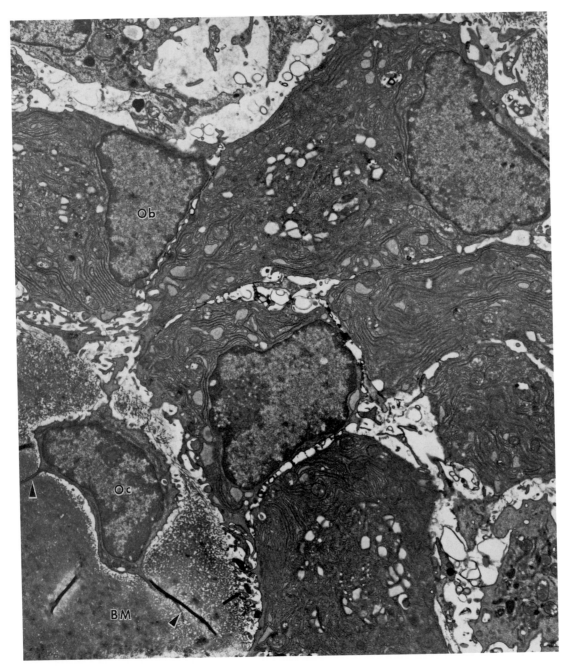

Figure 7.11. Several osteoblasts (Ob) with extensive rER occupy most of the field. An osteocyte (Oc) (apparently recently trapped by bone matrix) has a number of long, slender processes (arrowheads). Bone matrix (BM) and some calcium salts (arrows) are seen. ×6575.

process. The proteins *osteocalcin* and *osteonectin* bind extracellular Ca^{2+} ions to produce a locally high concentration of these ions. Osteopontin is present in osteoid at the mineralizing front and appears to play a role in the mineralization process. Osteoblasts elaborate *matrix vesicles* (described in Chapter 6) by budding from the plasma membrane and are involved in initial stages of hydroxyapatite formation.

Collagen fibers in bone matrix may also be important for the precipitation of calcium and phosphate into an insoluble salt. Under certain conditions, solutions of calcium and phosphate form apatite crystals in the presence of collagen. In addition, early calcium phosphate deposits appear at the periphery of staggered procollagen molecules in TEM. However, calcification does not occur in other tissues that have considerable amounts of collagen. While initial stages of crystalline calcium deposits in bone matrix are closely associated with collagen fibrils, their precise role in the calcification process remains unclear. Many questions remain about mechanisms involved in the calcification of bone.

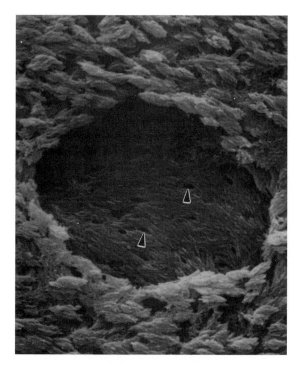

Figure 7.12. A lacuna in bone was exposed by fracturing the shaft and the organic constituents were removed by acid treatment, revealing a pattern of collagen fibrils. Small canalicular openings (arrowheads) extend from the back wall of the lacuna. ×5400. (From R. Kessel and R.H. Kardon, *Tissues and Organs: A Text-Atlas of Scanning Electron Microscopy*, W.H. Freeman, New York, 1979, with permission)

OSTEOCLASTS

Large, multinucleated cells called *osteoclasts* are present on the surfaces of bone where resorption occurs. Osteoclasts reside in depressions or recesses called *Howship's lacunae* or *resorption bays* (Plate 12A–C). Resorption bays therefore denote the eroded bone surfaces. Osteoclasts appear to be capable of moving on bone surfaces. Multincleated osteoclasts are found only in mineralized tissues. The source of osteoclasts is not completely clear, but one possibility is that they form from the fusion of monocytes that come in contact with bone matrix. Another possibility, illustrated in the accompanying figure, is that osteoclasts can develop from mesenchyme cells through a "pro-osteoclast" intermediate. The figure also indicates other details of bone lineage.

Secretory Products of Osteoclasts	
Lysosomal enzymes	β-Glycerophosphate, aryl sulfatase, β-glucuronidase, cathepsins B, C, L
Nonlysosomal enzymes	Collagenase, Plasminogen activator, Lysozyme, Stromelysin
Other proteins	Osteopontin, Transforming growth factor-β, Bone scialoproteins
Cytokine	Interleukin-6

The osteoclast is morphologically and functionally polarized. Its membrane has an apical (resorbing compartment) and a basolateral (vascular) surface. Osteoclasts contain mitochondria, lysosomes, and free polyribosomes. The striated or *ruffled border* is due to the folded plasma membrane adjacent to the surface of bone (Plate 12B). The osteoclast is able to produce a variety of secretory products; major ones are listed in the accompanying table.

Na^+/K^+-*ATPase* is present in the osteoclast ruffled border and may act as a sodium or calcium exchanger for hydrogen ions in regulating the acidity of this region. *Carbonic anhydrase*, an enzyme that may also participate in acidification adjacent to the ruffled border, has been localized within the osteoclast. Hydrogen ion transport by ATPase across the ruffled border is important in the production of an acidic environment for resorption (Fig. 7.15).

CALCIUM IN BONE

Newly deposited calcium is somewhat labile; thus calcium can be mobilized to enter an adjacent capillary or it can be removed from the blood and deposited in bone matrix as needed. Labeling studies indicate that during every minute in the life of an adult human, one of every four calcium ions present in blood exchanges with calcium ions in bone; thus, some interchange of calcium ions between blood and bone matrix occurs without osteoclast intervention. Bone resorption is important in remodeling bones and making them stronger and serves as a reservoir of calcium. A stable concentration of cal-

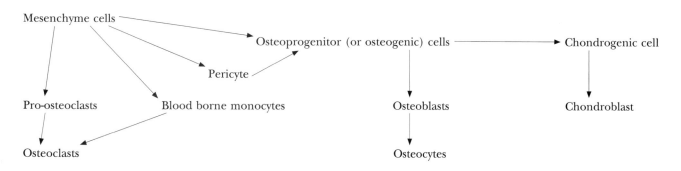

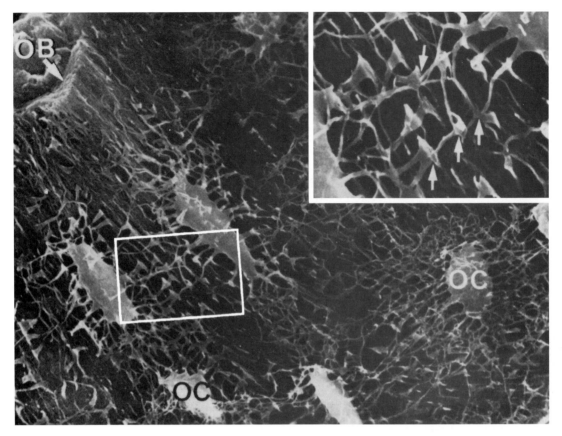

Figure 7.13. SEM illustrates osteoblasts (OB) and osteocytes (OC), with their many thin cytoplasmic extensions. Region in the square is enlarged to show the connections between the osteocytes. The bone matrix has been removed to illustrate the highly branched form of the osteocytes. (From S. Ejiri and H. Ozawa, *Archivum Histologicum Japonicum* 45, 402, 1982, by permission of the Archives of Histology and Cytology)

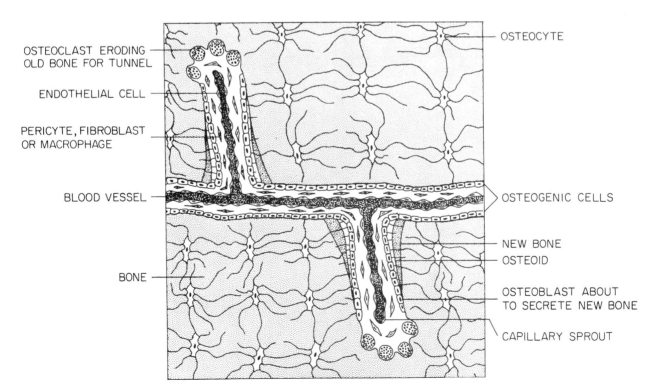

Figure 7.14. Diagram illustrates the formation of haversian canals in compact bone.

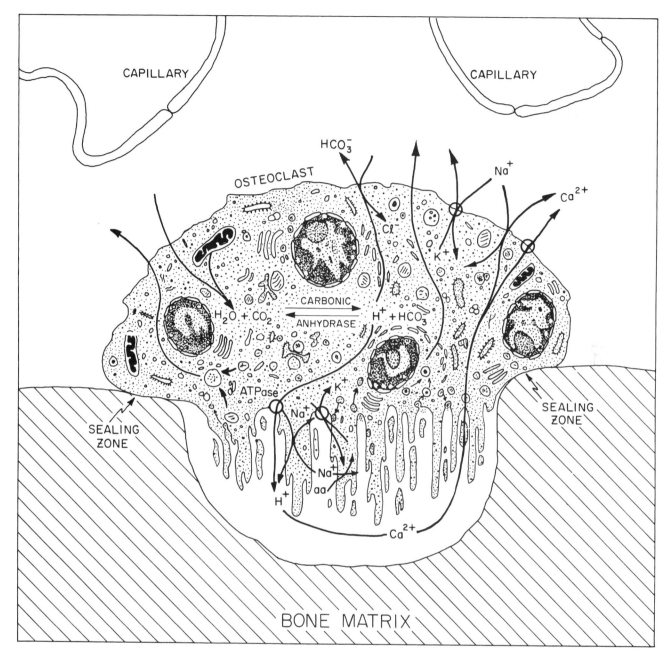

Figure 7.15. Diagram illustrates the organization of an osteoclast and major physiologic events associated with this cell.

cium ions in the blood is extremely important. The normal calcium concentration is about *10 mg/100 ml* of blood plasma. Bone matrix serves as a reservoir for excess calcium ions or as a source of calcium ions, if needed.

BONE RESORPTION

Osteoclasts actively acidify the extracellular space in a resorption bay. The intracellular source of the protons results from the carbonic anhydrase-dependent hydration of CO_2 to H_2CO_3. The hydrogen ions resulting from the dissociation are secreted into the resorbing compartment by a *proton pump* (Fig. 7.15). The bicarbonate (HCO_3^-) leaves the cell by the Cl^-/HCO_3^- exchanger located in the basolateral membrane. The basolateral membrane also contains Na^+/K^+-ATPase as well a Ca^{2+}-ATPase.

Located at the periphery of the ruffled border is a region called the *clear zone*, which contains principally actin microfilaments, vinculin, and talin. This region completely encircles the ruffled border. It is an area where the osteoclast firmly adheres to the adjacent substratum and may assist in sealing off the acidic compartment adjacent to the ruffled border. Vacuoles and coated and uncoated vesicles in osteoclasts are involved in both endocytosis and exocytosis.

PTH
IL-1   } Osteoblasts ⟶ Activated   —secrete→   { M-CSF
TNF-α   osteoblasts   GM-CSF   These cytokines cause osteoclast
                                                     IL-6   maturation and recruitment

Enzymes packaged in the Golgi complex move to the ruffled border, where they are released into the space adjacent to the mineralized bone. Products of resorption are taken into the cell, further digested in secondary lysosomes, and released in adjacent blood vessels. While collagen degradation seems to be confined to the extracellular compartment adjacent to the osteoclast, the sulfated extracellular matrix seems to be phagocytized by the osteoclast and degraded intracellularly. Acid phosphatase is not only localized within the osteoclast, but is secreted onto the resorbed bone surface. The osteoclast appears to be capable of absorbing the osteocytes as well as the bone matrix.

The *osteoclast* is a major target of *calcitonin* action. Calcitonin appears to inhibit osteoclastic resorption directly at extremely low concentrations. Osteoclasts are essential for the proper growth, remodeling, and repair of bone, and normally their activity is tightly coupled to bone formation by osteoblasts.

When the blood calcium level becomes elevated above normal (hypercalcemia), another hormone called *thyrocalcitonin* or *calcitonin* is produced by cells (parafollicular, C cells) scattered throughout the thyroid gland. The action of calcitonin opposes that of PTH. Calcitonin receptors are located in the osteoclast plasma membrane. When stimulated by calcitonin, osteoclasts decrease their activity and motility. Calcitonin stimulates bone deposition by osteoblasts. As new bone matrix is calcified, the blood calcium level is reduced.

Other hormones and factors that stimulate bone resorption, such as *PTH, 1,25 dihydroxy vitamin D₃ (1,25 (OH₂D)* and *interleukin-1*, do not appear to act directly on osteoclasts but rather on osteoblasts. The osteoblasts then secrete specific cytokines, which, in turn, stimulate the osteoclasts. *Receptors* for *PTH* and *1,25 (OH₂D)*, both of which cause bone resorption, are found on *osteoblasts*, not osteoclasts. Inducers of bone resorption including PTH, interleukin-1 (IL-1), and tumor necrosis factor-α (TNF-α) can activate osteoblasts to secrete specific substances such as macrophage colony-stimulating factor (M-CSF), granulocyte-macrophage colony-stimulating factor (GM-CSF), and interlukin-6 (IL-6), which are involved in osteoclast maturation and recruitment, as diagrammed above.

Cytokines produced by hematopoietic cells in the bone marrow include IL-1, TNF-α, and GM-CSF, all of which stimulate bone resorption (see the accompanying table). It appears that osteoblasts can initiate bone resorption by neutral protease digestion of the unmineralized (osteoid) surface, exposing resorption-stimulating mineralized bone to osteoclast contact.

Prostaglandins may act to reduce or terminate resorption by osteoclasts.

Some postmenopausal women suffer enchanced bone loss and skeletal fragility due to decreased production of estrogen. Estrogen tends to depress or inhibit the secretion of several potent inducers of bone resorption (IL-1, TNF-α, GM-CSF) by peripheral blood monocytes.

Substances That Directly or Indirectly Stimulate Osteoclast Recruitment, Differentiation, and Activity	*Substances That Inhibit Osteoclast Activity*
IL-1α (indirect)	Calcitonin
IL-1β	
IL-3	IL-4
IL-6	TGF-β
TNF-α (indirect)	
PTH (indirect)	
M-CSF	
GM-CSF	

OSTEOCYTIC OSTEOLYSIS

To a very limited degree, osteocytes participate in bone resorption under appropriate conditions, especially in connection with the maintenance of normal serum calcium homeostasis. In deep areas of bone, osteocytes have been observed with the scanning EM that have a ruffled surface and are sometimes covered with spherules of solubilized bone matrix (Figs. 7.16, 7.17). Exposed collagenic fibrils are observed in the walls of some of these lacunae (Figs. 7.18, 7.19). It has been suggested that these morphologic variations reflect a localized resorption process by osteocytes called *osteocytic osteolysis*.

FACTORS AFFECTING BONE RESORPTION

If the blood calcium level falls below normal (*hypocalcemia*), cells in the *parathyroid gland* sense this lowered level from the blood circulating through the gland. The cells respond by a feedback mechanism involving release of *PTH*. The elevated level of PTH tends to *stimulate monocytes* or bloodstem cells indirectly to *fuse*

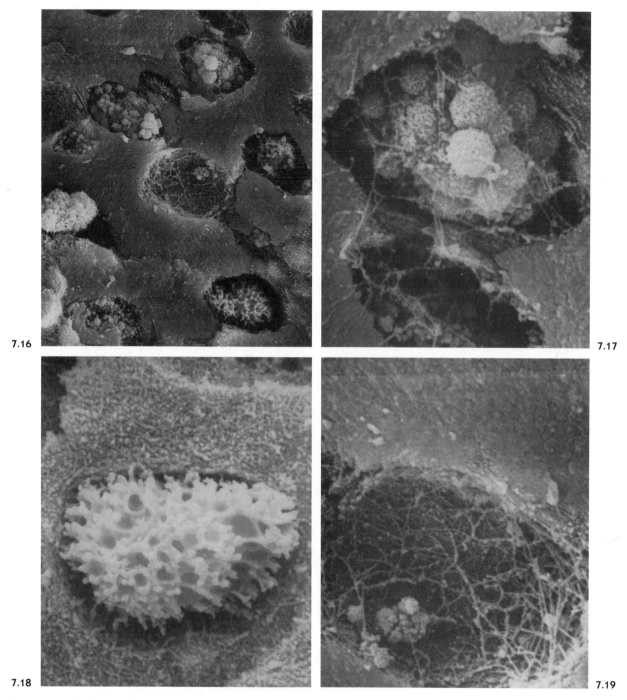

7.16

7.17

7.18

7.19

Figures 7.16–7.19. Osteocytes and lacunae exposed from deep within the temporal bone. Some osteocytes have a ruffled surface (Fig. 7.18), while others are covered with solubilized bone spherules (Figs. 7.16, 7.17). In those lacunae where osteocytes are removed, collagen fibers are ex- posed (Figs. 7.16, 7.19). Images such as these suggest that osteocytes located deep within bones might participate in limited bone erosion. Figure 7.16, ×2730; Figure 7.17, ×8,790; Figure 7.18, ×8060; Figure 7.19, ×8710.

together to form *multinucleated osteoclasts* or causes mono-cytes to differentiate into macrophages, which then fuse together to form the osteoclasts. PTH, as well as IL-1 and TNF-α, appears to act on osteoblasts, causing them to secrete cytokines that stimulate osteoclastic resorp-tion of bone.

The osteoclasts cause solubilization of calcium salts in bone matrix, and the calcium ions enter the blood-stream to elevate the blood Ca^{2+} level. Parathyroid gland cells monitor the blood calcium level; when it is elevated, the cells cease the production and release of hormone. PTH tends to promote resorption of calcium from the glomerular filtrate by the kidney tubule cells. PTH also tends to stimulate synthesis of a hydroxylated vitamin D$_3$, which promotes calcium absorption from the intestine. PTH not only increases the number of osteoclasts but also enhances ruffled border activity by the osteoclasts. In contrast, activity of the ruffled borders of osteoclasts is reduced by calcitonin (CT). Transforming growth factor-β (TGF-β) inhibits osteoclast activation.

OSSIFICATION (OSTEOGENESIS)

The process of bone formation is called *ossification* or *osteogenesis*. There are several environments in which bone can form; consequently, different names have been given to these events. It should be noted, however, that the terms refer only to the environments in which osteogenesis occurs, not to the kind of bone formed, for it is the same in all cases. The principal types of bone formation are intramembranous and endochondral (or intracartilagenous) ossification.

INTRAMEMBRANOUS OSSIFICATION

In the process of *intramembranous ossification*, bone is formed by the direct differentiation of mesenchyme cells into osteoblasts. This process may begin as early as the eighth week of gestation in the human fetus. Intramembranous ossification occurs in most of the facial bones, bones of the vault of the skull, and most of the clavicle. Two important requirements for intramembranous ossification are the presence of mesenchyme cells and an extensively vascularized area. Where bone is to form, mesenchyme cells that are typically irregular, branched, or stellate in shape lose their processes and aggregate or form clusters. Pericytes or perivascular cells are associated at intervals with the blood capillaries in the mesenchyme and provide a ready source of osteogenic cells and fibroblasts. Division of mesenchymal cells occurs and provides an increasing number of cells for subsequent differentiation. Some of the mesenchyme cells become osteoprogenitor cells. Some of the osteoprogenitor cells acquire a basophilic staining cytoplasm due to the presence of extensive rER (Plate 11A–C). A prominent Golgi complex becomes apparent as well. These events signal the osteoprogenitor cells to differentiate into osteoblasts to synthesize, package, and export bone matrix. The appearance of bone matrix surrounded by a cluster of osteoblasts results initially in a *spicule*, which increases in size by appositional growth. Soon some of the osteoblasts become surrounded or trapped in lacunae by the secreted bone matrix and become osteocytes, which no longer secrete bone matrix but possess long, slender cellular extensions that lie in canaliculi. Large, multinucleate osteoclasts can appear on the spicules of bone matrix shortly after they have

formed. The early appearance of osteoclasts indicates that bone undergoes remodeling very early. Through the action of osteoclasts, the final shape of bone is achieved and the interior may be remodeled to form a marrow cavity. As bone deposition continues, additional mesenchyme cells and pericytes differentiate into osteoblasts, which continue to become trapped; therefore, more osteocytes are present in the bone spicule. The bone spicules continue to enlarge such that beams or trabeculae are formed that interconnect or anastomose with other trabeculae, resulting in a *cancellous* or grating appearance. Osteocytes in cancellous bone receive nourishment by diffusion from marrow vessels. Osteoclasts that reside on the surface of bone trabeculae can remodel this type of bone directly. The rate of bone deposition has been estimated by various tracers to be one to several micrometers a day. The continued secretion of bone matrix and the action of osteoclasts ultimately result, in the case of flat bones of the skull, in two plates of compact bone separated by an intervening marrow cavity (diplöe). A small amount of cancellous bone may remain associated with the inner surface of compact bone. Cancellous bone that forms initially is easily converted into compact bone by the continued secretion by osteoblasts. The conversion of cancellous bone into compact bone requires the development of haversian systems (osteons) utilizing the many blood vessels that richly vascularize the centers of ossification. The center of ossification denotes the region in which initial bone deposition occurs. A periosteum is formed around the bone by fibroblasts that form collagen and pericytes, which persist as osteogenic or osteoprogenitor cells capable of producing appositional growth.

Since compact bone has a complex intraosseous circulatory system, osteoclasts must reabsorb compact bone to create tunnels for vascular sprouting in the remodeling process. Thus, groups of osteoclasts operate in concert to excavate tunnels through the old bone (Fig. 7.14). This erosion has been described to proceed at the rate of approximately 50 μm/day. Following tunnel formation, osteogenic cells migrate into the tunnel together with capillary sprouts (Fig. 7.14). The osteogenic cells become osteoblasts that synthesize and export bone matrix to fill in the tunnel with concentric layers of new bone, but a small central haversian canal containing the blood vessel remains. The blood vessel delivers the nutrients that the osteocytes require for survival. It has been estimated that perhaps 5–10% of the bone in an individual may be remodeled in this manner each year.

INTRACARTILAGINOUS (ENDOCHONDRAL) OSSIFICATION

The appendicular skeleton, the bones of the vertebral column, and the bones at the base of the skull form by endochondral or intracartilaginous ossification. Much of the clavicle forms by intramembranous ossification, but it has a secondary center of ossification and a growth plate that forms by endochondral ossification. The process of intracartilaginous ossification is preceded by the formation of small hyaline cartilage models of the future bones (see Chapter 6). In embryonic limbs, for example, mesenchyme cells cluster and organize into the shape of a future bone. The mesenchyme cells enlarge, differentiate the organelles necessary to synthesize, package, and export the cartilage matrix. In addition, cells produce a perichondrium that surrounds the forming cartilage model.

One important initial event in endochondral ossification is that the chondrocytes in the midsection of the model *hypertrophy* (*enlarge*) and then undergo *cartilage matrix calcification*, as described in Chapter 6. The calcification of cartilage matrix prevents nutrients, wastes, and gases from diffusing through the matrix to reach the chondrocytes, resulting in chondrocyte death. Chondrocyte death is marked by degenerative changes of the cytoplasm, pyknosis of the nucleus, and eventually the presence of empty lacunae. Once a chondrocyte dies, the calcified matrix that surrounded the cell slowly erodes. The hypertrophy of chondrocytes and calcification of cartilage matrix initially occurs in a region identified as the *primary center of ossification*. In a bone such as the femur, which begins as a cartilage model, these activities occur in the midsection of the future shaft (or diaphysis) of the bone, which is called a *diaphyseal center of ossification*.

As chondrocytes undergo hypertrophy and calcification in the center of the cartilage model, vascular changes occur in the adjacent perichondrium. Blood vessels grow into the perichondrium locally in the region of the primary center of ossification. The increased vascularity and elevated oxygen tension produced by the ingrowth of blood vessels exert a profound effect on the chondrogenic cells in the localized region of the perichondrium. The chondrogenic cells become osteogenic and soon differentiate into osteoblasts that secrete a thin layer of bone. Based on its new function in this region, the perichondrium actually becomes a periosteum and the bone is called *subperiosteal bone*. The blood vessels that grow into the former perichondrium and cause its conversion into a periosteum are called *periosteal vessels*. The importance of increased vascularity and increased oxygen concentration for bone formation can be demonstrated, for if the periosteal vessels are removed, the osteogenic cells in the periosteum will revert to chondrogenic cells. Considerable lability appears to exist between chondrogenic cells and osteogenic or osteoprogenitor cells, illustrating how the expression of different cell types with close affinities can be easily altered.

The hypertrophy of chondrocytes and the resulting maturation and calcification of cartilage spread from the center of the model in a wave toward both ends. The periosteal vessels that invaded the perichondrium and caused its local transformation into a periosteum continue to grow into the midsection of the model, where spaces have resulted from the eroding, calcified cartilage matrix. The growing blood vessels have osteogenic or osteoprogenitor cells on their surface, as well as pericytes that can become osteogenic cells. The *pericytes* or *perivascular cells* that arise from mesenchyme cells retain broad capabilities for differentiating into a variety of cell types, including osteoblasts (Fig. 7.20). These cells attach to the surfaces of calcified cartilage matrix, differentiate into osteoblasts, and secrete bone matrix (Figs. 7.11, 7.21). This secretory activity soon results initially in the formation of bone spicules and, with further activity, trabeculae. Initially, bone matrix covers calcified cartilage matrix. As a consequence, a cancellous bone appears in the midsection of the model. With H&E staining, the calcified cartilage stains blue (basophilic), while the forming bone matrix stains red (acidophilic). Blood monocytes enter the area and form osteoclasts to erode bone. With continued deposition of subperiosteal bone, this particular layer thickens and eventually becomes organized into compact diaphyseal bone containing haversian systems. Osteoprogenitor cells in the endosteum and periosteum can proliferate and differentiate into osteoblasts.

The fact that the maturation and calcification of cartilage proceed from the midsection to each end of the future bone results in zones or rows of activity (Plate 13A–C). A thin band or zone, one to two lacunae thick, adjacent to the region of bone matrix deposition can be denoted in which the lacunae are empty, resulting from the degeneration of the chondrocytes or the lacunae contain dying chondrocytes. The area around the lacuna is occupied by calcified cartilage. This zone is called the *zone of calcifying cartilage*. Immediately adjacent to this zone is a layer consisting of one to three rows of obviously enlarged or hypertrophied chondrocytes. This layer is called the *zone of maturing* or *hypertrophying cartilage*. Adjacent to the zone of maturing cartilage is a thicker zone or band in which the chondrocytes are more flattened and stacked in rows. This is the *zone of proliferating cartilage* and represents or reflects the persistent interstitial growth in length of the remaining hyaline cartilage. Finally, there is a zone of *resting cartilage* that is located farthest from the center of ossification. As the wave of calcification and erosion of cartilage matrix progressively extends toward the ends of the cartilage models, the periosteal vessels continue to grow into the regions and bring osteogenic cells that become attached to pieces of eroding, calcified cartilage matrix. The osteogenic cells differentiate into osteoblasts that secrete bone matrix and eventually become surrounded by bone matrix (Figs. 7.20, 7.21) that becomes calcified. Growth in the diameter of the diaphysis results from appositional growth beneath the pe-

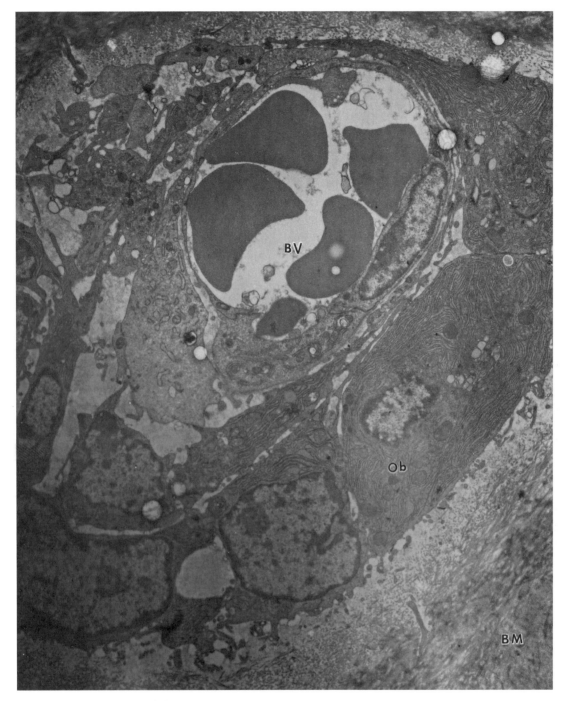

Figure 7.20. This TEM illustrates a localized area of bone deposition. The bone matrix (BM) is located in the lower right corner of the figure. Osteoblasts (Ob) are aligned in close proximity to a blood vessel (BV). ×6575.

riosteum, a process referred to as *subperiosteal intramembranous ossification* (Plate 13D). This permits the diaphysis to become stronger and wider. Osteoclasts remove bone on the inner surface of the bone to enlarge the marrow cavity, providing a site for hematopoietic (myeloid) tissue (bone marrow).

While most primary or diaphyseal centers of ossification are present and their development is well underway prior to birth, secondary centers of ossification usually appear shortly after birth in longer bones. These secondary centers of ossification at the ends of epiphyses of future bones are called *epiphyseal centers of ossification* and develop in a manner similar to that of diaphyseal centers of ossification. The appearance and development of secondary centers of ossification at the ends of long bones result in a transverse plate of proliferating cartilage between the two centers of ossification. This is called the *epiphyseal plate* and it represents the region where interstitial growth of cartilage continues. In addition, there are zones of hypertrophying or

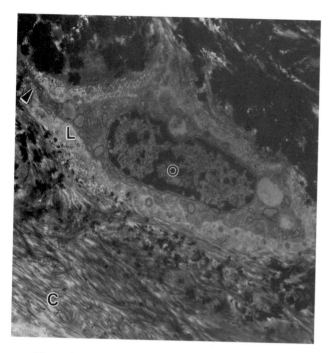

Figure 7.21. TEM of osteocyte (O) with processes (arrowheads) that extend into canaliculi. Calcified bone matrix at the top appears black. Collagen fibers (C). ×8400.

maturing and calcified cartilage still associated with either side of the proliferating epiphyseal plate. Eventually, the cartilage completely disappears except for a narrow band on the articulating surfaces of the bones. The bone of the epiphyses eventually fuses with that of the diaphysis to produce a type of joint known as a *synostosis*, that is, direct fusion of bone to bone.

MEDICAL CONSIDERATIONS

Ossification is a complex, integrated process that requires a long time and the precise coordination of many events. In addition to genetic control, the process is dependent upon the proper concentration of specific ions, hormones, vitamins, and many other factors in suitable quantity. For example, in protein-deficient diets and those lacking vitamin A, the thickness of the epiphyseal plate is rapidly decreased. In cases of rickets involving the absence of vitamin D, the epiphyseal cartilage proliferates but the matrix fails to calcify and the bones become deformed. Lack of growth hormone results in a decrease in the thickness of the epiphyseal plate and in the number of chondrocytes. It is also important to recall that bone undergoes continual remodeling during and after ossification, which permits it to respond more effectively to various stresses.

Both cartilage and bone tend to deteriorate with aging. *Osteoarthritis* is a condition in which articular cartilage becomes damaged and may completely disappear in some areas. If this occurs, the joint becomes swollen and bone may thicken, greatly restricting joint movement. This condition is most likely to involve the spine, knees, hips, and fingers. While genetic and mechanical factors are involved in osteoarthritis, the precise causative factors are presently unclear. Bone resorption tends to exceed the synthesis of bone matrix at about age 30, and osteoporosis can eventually result. *Osteoporosis* involves weakening of the bones, which become more easily fractured. Calcitonin is used as a therapeutic agent in osteoporosis because it decreases osteoclast activity and stimulates bone matrix secretion by osteoblasts. The incidence of osteoarthritis in women increases with aging due to a decrease in estrogen production after menopause.

In the disease osteopetrosis, the lack of appropriate osteoclast activity results in very dense bones, with bone replacing most of the marrow cavities. Thus, there is insufficient area for a marrow cavity. As a result of the loss of marrow, severe anemia can result. While osteoclasts fail to resorb bone and calcified cartilage in this disease, in some cases an infusion of spleen or marrow cells from an appropriate donor provides the monocytes that are able to differentiate into osteoclasts to digest some of the bone and calcified cartilage so as to produce a marrow cavity.

Heterotopic ossification is an unusual and restricted situation in which bone may appear in unusual places such as the tonsil or kidneys. It can sometimes occur if calcium is deposited in a dying tissue that may then stimulate persistent, undifferentiated mesenchymal cells and pericytes to become osteogenic and then osteoblastic in their activity.

SELECTED BIBLIOGRAPHY

Belanger, L.F. (1969). Osteocytic osteolysis. *Calcif. Tissue. Res.* **4**:1.

Bonucci, E., ed. (1992). *Calcification in Biological Systems.* CRC Press, Boca Raton, FL.

Currey, J. (1984). *The Mechanical Adaptations of Bone.* Princeton University Press, Princeton, NJ.

Hall, B. (1988). The embryonic development of bone. *Am. Sci.* **76**, 174–181.

Hall, B.K., ed. (1991). *Bone: Bone Matrix and Bone Specific Products,* Vol. 3. CRC Press, Boca Raton, FL.

Hall, B.K., ed. (1991). *Bone: The Osteoclast,* Vol. 2, CRC Press, Boca Raton, FL.

Hall, B.K., ed. (1991). *Bone: The Osteoblast and Osteocyte,* Vol. 1. Telford Press, Caldwell, NJ.

Heinegard, D., and Oldberg, A. (1989). Structure and biology of cartilage and bone matrix noncollagenous macromolecules. *FASEB J.* **3**, 2042–2051.

Holtrop, M.E. (1975). The ultrastructure of bone. *Ann. Clin. Lab. Sci.* **5**, 264.

Martin, R.B., and Burr, D.B. (1989). *Structure, Function and Adaptation of Compact Bone.* Raven Press, New York.

Noda, M., ed. (1993). *Cellular and Molecular Biology of Bone.* Academic Press, San Diego, CA.

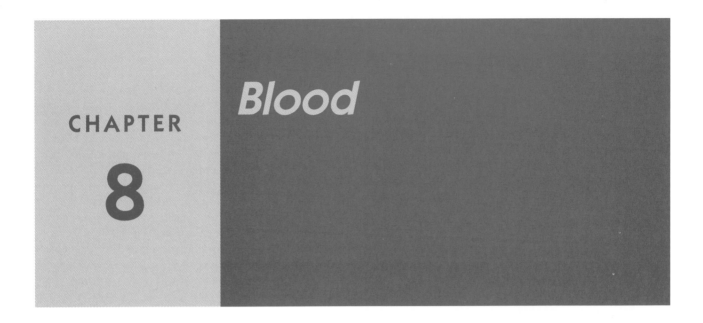

CHAPTER 8

Blood

Blood is a specialized type of connective tissue in which cells (*leukocytes* and *erythrocytes*) and fragments of cells (*platelets*) are suspended in a fluid intercellular substance called *plasma*. It is only when clotting that fibrous elements (*fibrin* threads) appear in the plasma. Blood constitutes roughly 7% of the body weight. A 70-kg human male contains ~5–6 liters of blood. Blood has a pH between 7.35 and 7.45 and is isotonic to 0.85% NaCl. The different types of cells present in blood exhibit marked structural and functional diversity. *Erythrocytes* transport life-sustaining oxygen to all cellular residents in the body and carbon dioxide to the lungs for exhaling. Small platelets arrest bleeding by promoting clotting. The leukocytes, including lymphocytes, monocytes, and neutrophils, comprise an immune system that is responsible for protecting the body against attack by foreign molecules including microorganisms, foreign cells, and viruses. Other leukocytes, the eosinophils and basophils, are also involved in a protective function. Remarkably, all of the aforementioned cells develop from a master cell called a *blood-forming* or *hematopoietic stem cell*.

Because of the enormous number of blood cells and because each has a finite life span, provision must be made for the production of new cells and the destruction of worn-out cells. These functions are carried out by hematopoietic tissues by a process called *hematopoiesis*. There are two special types of hematopoietic connective tissue: *myeloid tissue* (bone marrow) and lymphoid or *lymphatic tissue*. Myeloid tissue functions in the formation of new erythrocytes, platelets, and most leukocytes, as well as in the destruction of worn-out erythrocytes, platelets, and granular leukocytes. Lymphoid tissue, which is represented by the thymus, lymph nodes, spleen, tonsils, and solitary lymphatic nodules located

elsewhere in the body, is involved with the production of only some leukocytes (including T and B lymphocytes) and plasma cells.

PREPARATION OF BLOOD SMEARS AND STAINING

A cleansed finger is pricked with a sterile needle to obtain blood for a smear. The initial drop of blood is discarded, but the second drop is touched near the end of a clean microscope slide. Another slide, positioned at an angle of about 30° to the first slide, is pushed over the slide to spread the blood into a monolayer. This requires some skill to ensure that blood cells are evenly dispersed and are not damaged by the movement of the slide. The speed with which the drop of blood is spread can also affect the quality of the smear. The smear of cells is fixed and stained with several possible blood stains. Each blood stain consists of a single solution with several stains to stain the acidophilic, basophilic, and neutrophilic components. Wright's stain is a mixture of eosin (acidic) and methylene blue (basic). The eosin stains used include eosin Y, eosin B, erythrosin B, and phloxine B. The blood smear is covered with the stain and then rinsed with an acidic buffer (pH 6.5) to dilute the stain and to differentiate the colors. The preparation is then rinsed, dried, and observed in this manner, or a coverslip can be applied to the preparation for longer preservation. A differential white blood cell count can then be made. Giemsa's stain is a mixture of azure II-eosin, azure II, glycerin, and methanol. Romanovsky's stain for blood smears is a mixture of methylene blue (basic dye), azure (basic), and eosin (an acid dye).

PLASMA

The fluid portion of the blood, called *plasma*, consists of different *proteins* that exert *colloidal osmotic pressure*. Plasma also contains water and such crystalloids as amino acids, sugars, fatty acids, and salts. Oxygen and carbon dioxide are dissolved in the plasma as well. Plasma consists of 90–92% water and 7–8% proteins. The remainder of the plasma contains solutes and electrolytes including Na^+, K^+, Ca^{2+}, Mg^{2+}, Cl^-, HCO_3^-, PO_4^{3-}, and SO_4^{2-}. Other constituents include urea, uric acid, ammonium salts (creatinine and creatine), hormones, growth factors, enzymes, and nutrients (glucose, amino acids, and lipids), in addition to oxygen and carbon dioxide. Because plasma freely exchanges with tissue fluid, blood is exceedingly important in maintaining homeostasis for all resident cells of the body and serves as an indicator of many disease processes.

The major plasma proteins include albumin, globulins, and the blood-clotting protein *fibrinogen*. Plasma without fibrinogen is called *serum*. *Albumin*, which has a molecular weight of 59,000, is the smallest and most abundant of the plasma proteins. It is synthesized in the liver and performs the very important function of maintaining blood colloidal osmotic pressure. If the liver becomes damaged and incapable of producing enough albumin to maintain sufficient colloidal osmotic pressure, edema or swelling results because of an inability to resorb sufficient tissue fluid. The *globulins* are of several types, including gamma globulin, which includes the immunoglobulins (antibodies). Beta globulins can participate in the transport of hormones, metal ions, and lipids.

ERYTHROCYTES

NUMBER

One cubic millimeter of blood in an average human male contains some 5 to 5.5 million red blood cells (erythrocytes); in females, 1 mm^3 of blood contains 4.5 to 5 million erythrocytes. The term *erythron* refers to the total number of erythrocytes or red blood corpuscles in the body, and is 27×10^{12} in human males and 18×10^{12} in human females. However, individuals born and living at higher altitudes, such as the Andes or Himalayan mountains, have more red blood cells. The total number of red blood cells in an average individual would provide a total surface of about 4200 square yards, which is similar to that of a football field.

Blood samples can be centrifuged to separate blood cells from the plasma. The *hematocrit* is the volume occupied by the erythrocytes or packed cells, expressed as a percentage of the total volume of the blood sample. Normal hematocrit values are slightly less than 45% for females and slightly more than 45% for males. Since erythrocytes normally have a life span of 100–125 days, approximately 2.5 million new red blood cells must enter the bloodstream every second, while an equal number are lost. The task of removing worn-out erythrocytes is performed by macrophages present in the spleen, bone marrow, and liver.

HEMOGLOBIN

As a consequence of their differentiation, erythrocytes tend to lose not only their nucleus, but also polyribosomes, mitochondria, Golgi complex, and centrioles. They become essentially nonmotile bags of *hemoglobin*, which is a complex iron-containing protein synthesized during erythrocyte differentiation. Hemoglobin contains a protein moiety, *globin*, joined to a heme pigment. Only approximately 4% of hemoglobin consists of heme. The mature erythrocyte is approximately 6% water and 33% hemoglobin. In human males, there is approximately 15 g of hemoglobin per 100 ml of blood, but in females the ratio is ~13.5 g/100 ml. Hemoglobin can take up approximately 1.3 times its weight in oxygen in regions of high oxygen tension such as the lungs. In this oxygenated form, called *oxyhemoglobin*, it can be transported to the tissues, where, in response to low oxygen tension or concentration, it releases the oxygen and reversibly complexes with carbon dioxide (reduced hemoglobin). In the lungs, hemoglobin combines with an oxygen molecule and gives up a H^+ ion as follows:

$$HHb \quad + \quad O_2 \longrightarrow HbO_2 \quad + \quad H^+$$

reduced   oxygen   oxygenated   hydrogen
hemoglobin   hemoglobin   ion

The hydrogen ions released combine with bicarbonate ions in the plasma to form carbonic acid, from which carbon dioxide is released to be exhaled.

$$H^+ \quad + \quad HCO_3^- \longrightarrow H_2CO_3 \longrightarrow CO_2 + H_2O$$

hydrogen   bicarbonate   carbonic   carbon   water
ion   ion   acid   dioxide

Red blood cells contain the enzyme *carbonic anhydrase*, which functions in the following reaction:

$$\text{carbonic anhydrase}$$
$$\overset{\text{tissues}}{CO_2 + H_2O \underset{\text{lungs}}{\rightleftharpoons} H_2CO_3}$$

In the tissues where CO_2 is formed, carbonic anhydrase moves the reaction to the right. In areas of low concentrations of carbon dioxide, such as the lung, carbonic anhydrase moves the reaction to the left.

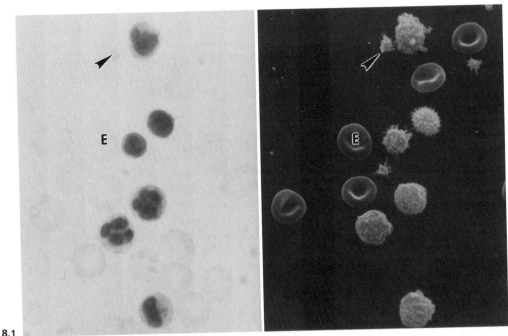

8.1

8.2

Figures 8.1, 8.2. LM of human leukocytes attached to a coverslip in a stained but wet-mount preparation. A similar preparation is illustrated by the SEM in Figure 8.2; thus, identical cells can be shown by both LM and SEM. From top to bottom in Figure 8.1, the leukocytes are a monocyte, two lymphocytes, two neutrophils, and a monocyte; these correspond to cells in Figure 8.2. Erythrocytes (E) and dendritic platelets (arrowhead) are also identified; some of which were lost during preparation and observation in the SEM. ×2260. (From R. Kessel and R. Kardon, *Tissues and Organs: A Text-Atlas of Scanning Electron Microscopy*, W.H. Freeman, New York, 1979, with permission)

SIZE AND SHAPE

Erythrocytes average ~7.2–7.5 μm in diameter and approximately 1.9 μm in width. The terms *red blood cell* and *erythrocyte* are something of a misnomer since in mammals these cells have no nuclei in the mature state; thus, the term *red blood corpuscle* is sometimes used to refer to a nonnucleated erythrocyte. In all mammals, the nucleus is discarded during a terminal phase of differentiation as a device to increase the respiratory efficiency of the erythrocyte. The extrusion of the nucleus and the presence of a cytoskeleton immediately inside the plasma membrane of the erythrocyte results in a biconcave shape (Figs. 8.1–8.3). A biconcave disc not only possesses 20–30% more surface area than a sphere, but the diffusion distance from the surface of the erythrocyte to the most internal regions is less in a biconcave disc than in a sphere. A nucleus is present in mature erythrocytes of all nonmammalian vertebrates. However, some erythrocytes may be slightly smaller than normal and are called *microcytes* (<6 μm in diameter), while others may be slightly larger than normal and are termed *macrocytes* (~9–12 μm in diameter). Erythrocytes are easily deformed and can become dumbbell-shaped when moving between endothelial cells of splenic sinusoids, for example. Erythrocytes act as osmometers since they are very sensitive to osmotic pressure changes in the plasma. Normally, plasma osmotic pressure is similar to that of the erythrocyte. If, however, the plasma becomes hypotonic or less concentrated, as might occur in response to snake venom or bile salts, then the erythrocyte swells and eventually ruptures. The process is referred to as *hemolysis*. If hemolysis is severe and prolonged, erythrocytes become leaky and lose hemoglobin into the plasma, perhaps even becoming eliminated in the urine. Such a condition is called *black water fever* in humans and *red water fever* in cattle. In contrast, if the plasma becomes too concentrated or hypertonic, as might occur under conditions of severe dessication, the erythrocyte shrinks and spiny projections extend from its surface. Such a condition is called *crenation*, and the erythrocyte is said to be *crenated* (Fig. 8.4).

CIRCULATING IMMATURE ERYTHROCYTES

When immature nucleated erythrocytes are present in the circulating blood of mammals, they are called *normoblasts* (see Chapter 9). It is sometimes possible to observe erythrocytes in the circulating blood that have a small piece of chromatin that was not eliminated with the nucleus, which is called a *Howell-Jolly body*. In addition, remnants of the nuclear envelope not extruded with the remainder of the nucleus in the process of differentiation may sometimes be present in erythrocytes

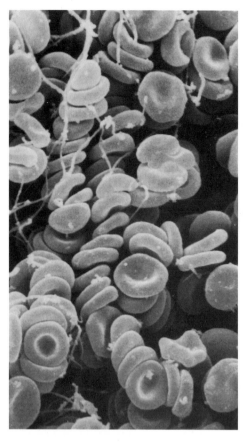

Figure 8.3. SEM of erythrocytes which are viewed end on and from their surface, so their biconcave shape is apparent. A few fibrin threads are present. ×2925. (From R. Kessel and R. Kardon, *Tissues and Organs: A Text-Atlas of Scanning Electron Microscopy*, W.H. Freeman, New York, 1979, with permission)

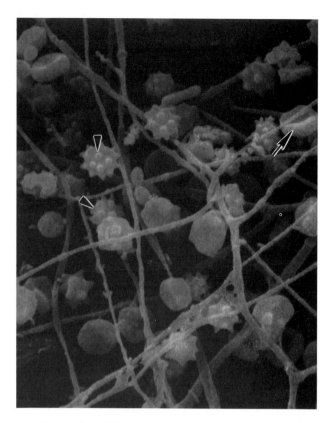

Figure 8.4 SEM of blood with fibrin threads. Crenated erythrocyte (arrowhead). ×2025 (From R. Kessel and R. Kardon, *Tissues and Organs: A Text-Atlas of Scanning Electron Microscopy*. W.H. Freeman, New York, 1979)

of circulating blood. Such remnants of the nuclear envelope are called *Cabot's rings*. Finally, it is possible to observe circulating erythrocytes that still contain some polyribosomes. When these immature erythrocytes are stained with new methylene blue, a component of some blood stains, the stain causes the polyribosomes to condense or coagulate into a fine reticulum that stains blue; such cells are called *reticulocytes*.

ERYTHROCYTE PLASMA MEMBRANE PROTEINS

Two rather well characterized integral membrane proteins, *glycophorin* and *band III*, are present in the erythrocyte plasma membrane (Fig. 8.5). Glycophorin spans the membrane only once and consists of a chain of 131 amino acids oriented such that the amino terminus is outside the cell, while the carboxyl terminus is in the cytosol. Carbohydrate moieties comprise approximately 60% of the glycophorin mass, and these carbohydrates contain many anionic sialic acid residues. The negative charge associated with glycophorin has

been suggested to prevent adhesion of the erythrocytes and surface of endothelial cells lining blood vessels.

Band III is an *anion-exchange protein* that facilitates the movement of *bicarbonate* and *chloride ions* across the erythrocyte plasma membrane. The exchange of these ions is necessary for *carbon dioxide transport*. As illustrated in Figure 8.6, the band 3 anion exchanger facilitates diffusion of HCO_3^- to the outside and the uptake of Cl^-. The process is reversed in the lungs and Cl^- is transported out of the erythrocyte, but this is coupled to the uptake of HCO_3^-, which is converted to carbon dioxide and exhaled. Band III traverses the membrane several times and is arranged such that an aqueous pore is formed to traverse the membrane. This pore permits anions to cross the membrane without exposure to the hydrophobic membrane interior.

RED BLOOD CELL CYTOSKELETON

The erythrocyte plasma membrane, like the plasma membranes of many other cell types, is closely associated with elements of the cytoskeleton, an arrangement that permits a degree of membrane rigidity compatible

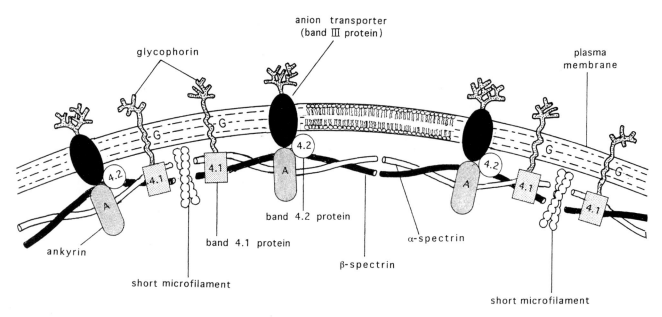

Figure 8.5. Diagram depicts the red blood cell cytoskeleton. Band III dimers are coupled to spectrin tetramers, and this association is mediated by ankyrin molecules. Spectrin tetramers are linked to short microactin filaments, and band 4.1 (squares) mediates this association. (From S.L. Wolfe, Molecular and Cellular Biology, 1993, Wadsworth Publishing Co., Belmont California).

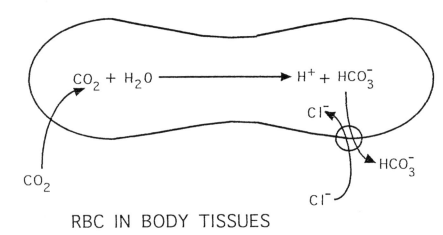

RBC IN BODY TISSUES

Figure 8.6. The band III protein in the RBC membrane (circle) is an anion exchanger that is involved in transporting carbon dioxide. Carbon dioxide produced by cells in tissues and organs diffuses into the RBC, where it is converted into bicarbonate and hydrogen ions by carbonic anhydrase, an enzyme in the RBC. Band III facilitates the diffusion of bicarbonate ions out of the RBC and the uptake of chloride ions. In the lung, the process is reversed. Chloride ions are transported out of the RBC, and the bicarbonate ions are taken into the RBC and then converted to carbon dioxide, which is exhaled.

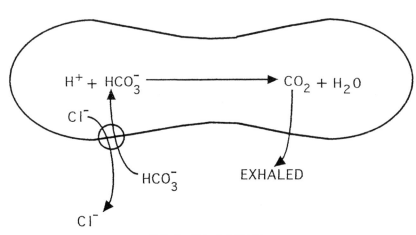

RBC IN LUNG

with maintaining a stable shape. The proteins comprising the erythrocyte cytoskeleton include ankyrin, spectrin, band 4.1, and actin filaments (Fig. 8.5). Actin and spectrin are both filamentous proteins, and they form a meshwork that is closely associated with the cytoplasmic surface of the plasma membrane. Band 4.1 connects actin and spectrin so as to produce an extensive filamentous network. Ankyrin anchors this filamentous meshwork by specific associations with both band III in the membrane and spectrin in the cytoskeleton, thereby restricting the movement of band III in the plane of the membrane. Figure 8.5 illustrates the nature and position of the spectrin-based cytoskeleton on the cytoplasmic side of the erythrocyte cell membrane.

BLOOD GROUPS

The blood group antigens (A, B, and O) are carbohydrates linked to membrane lipids and proteins of red blood cell membranes. They are genetically determined. The *O antigen* is a chain of *fucose, galactose, N-acetylglucosamine,* and *glucose* that may be linked to either protein or lipid (Fig. 8.7). The *A antigen* is identical to the O antigen except for an *N-acetylgalactosamine* residue attached to the terminal galactose residue. The *B antigen* is identical to the O antigen except for an additional *galactose* residue attached to the outer galactose

of the O antigen. All individuals have enzymes that synthesize the O antigen. Individuals with *type A* blood possess the enzyme to add the extra *N-acetylgalactosamine.* Individuals with *type B* blood possess the enzyme to add the extra *galactose.* Individuals with type AB blood have enzymes that synthesize both A and B antigens. Individuals with type O blood can synthesize only the O antigen. The genes specifying the enzymes are inherited in a simple Mendelian manner. Since the carbohydrates are genetically determined, if an individual receives a mismatched blood transfusion, the foreign carbohydrates stimulate the production of an immune response. For example, if either B or AB type blood were injected into an individual with either A or O type blood, the anti-B antibodies would bind to the injected cells and initiate agglutination and lysis of donor cells and their destruction by phagocytic cells. Likewise, A or AB type blood cannot be injected into individuals with B or O blood type. Type O blood can, however, be injected into individuals with O, A, B, or AB blood types. Individuals with type AB blood lack both anti-A and anti-B antibodies and can therefore receive injections of any blood type. Rh is another blood group antigen of clinical importance. If, for example, an Rh-negative mother were carrying an Rh-positive fetus, the mother might produce antibody to Rh antigen, and this maternal antibody could cross the placenta to cause lysis of fetal erythrocytes.

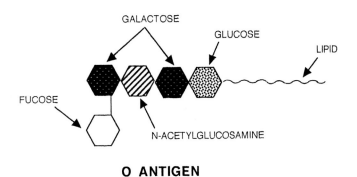

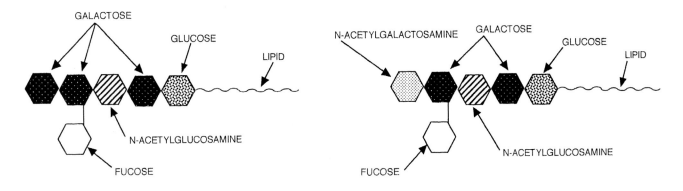

Figure 8.7. Differences in the O, B and A antigen. Note the position of the terminal sugars in the different blood types.

PLATELETS

NUMBER, SIZE, ORGANIZATION

In humans, there are some 250,000 to 300,000 platelets per cubic millimeter of blood. Platelets are oval, biconvex discs about 2–3 μm in diameter (Figs. 8.8, 8.9). They are colorless and anucleate. With radioactive tracers it has been determined that their life span in the circulating blood is about 5–9 days. Old

platelets are probably removed by macrophages in the spleen, liver, and bone marrow. The platelets are produced by giant cells in the bone marrow known as *megakaryocytes.*

In stained blood smears viewed with oil immersion lens, the platelet can be observed to contain a central stained region called a *granulomere.* This region appears to consist of several red- to purple-stained granules (Plate 14E,F). In contrast, a peripheral pale-staining region is called a *hyalomere.*

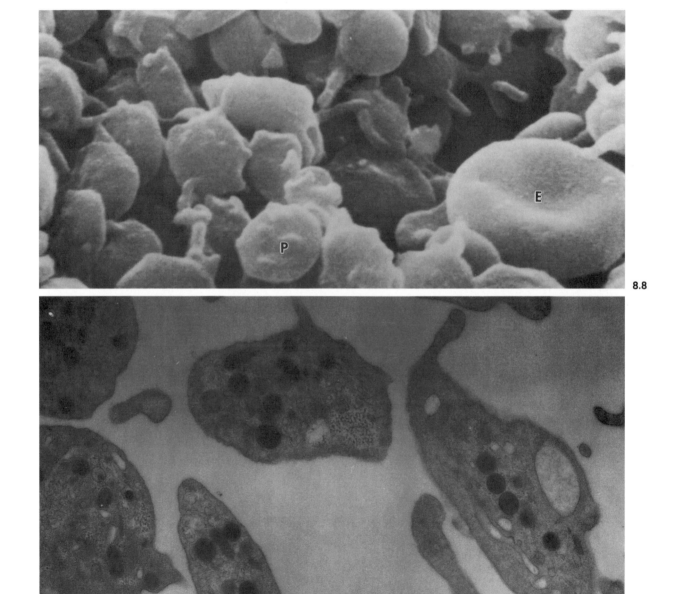

8.8

8.9

Figures 8.8, 8.9. SEM of biconvex platelets (P) is shown in Figure 8.8 as well as in erythrocyte (E). TEM of platelets (Fig. 8.9) shows dense granules (electron dense) and α-granules (less electron dense). Figure 8.8, ×7200; Figure 8.9, ×19,500.

In TEM micrographs, the constituents of platelets include *alpha granules*, very *dense granules*, *mitochondria*, *polyribosomes*, *glycogen*, *microtubules*, and *microfilaments* (Figs. 8.9, 8.10). In addition, there is a *surface conducting system* and a dense *tubular system* that serve to store and release Ca^{2+} ions. The microtubules tend to completely surround the platelet just inside the plasma membrane in what has been termed a *marginal band* of microtubules. *Alpha granules* are more numerous than *dense granules*. The *alpha granules* contain a variety of proteins (Table 8.1). Those proteins, which are needed for normal blood clotting, include platelet factor IV (an anticoagulant), platelet-derived growth factor (which stimulates growth of arterial smooth muscle cells), fibrinogen, and the blood clotting factor V, which is called proaccelerin. *Alpha granules* also contain *lysosomal enzymes* including acid phosphatase, β-glucuronidase, and cathepsin. Platelet factor 3 or platelet thromboplastin is formed during platelet disintegration. The *very dense*

granules are so named because they are extremely electron dense in the electron microscope. They contain *serotonin* or *5′-hydroxytryptamine*, which causes smooth muscles in the wall of blood vessels to contract; they also contain *calcium*, *ATP*, and *ADP* (Table 8.1).

CLOTTING

Platelets are involved in both *agglutination* and *clotting*, complicated events that are summarized in Figures 8.11 and 8.12. *Agglutination* refers to the tendency for activated or dendritic platelets to stick together at the site of injury to a blood vessel. The adhesion of platelets to collagen in a cut or damaged blood vessel wall causes platelets to secrete adenosine diphosphate (ADP), which results in platelet aggregation. Other platelets adhere to those already bound to collagen. ADP is a potent aggregating agent, and its release from dense gran-

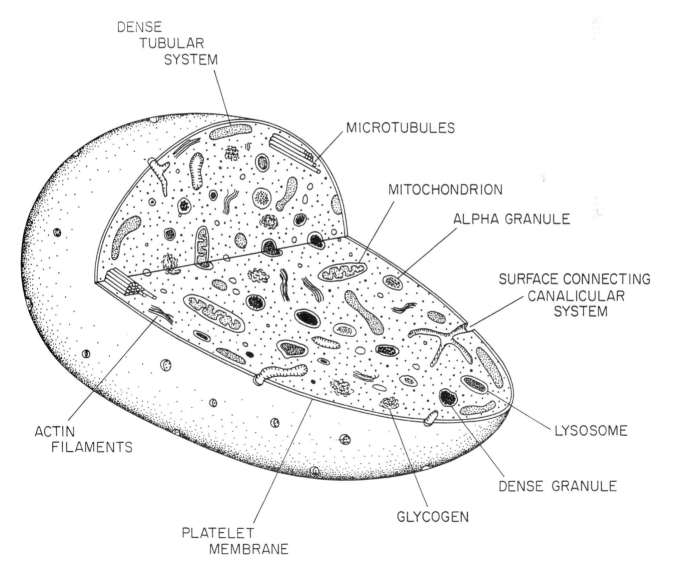

Figure 8.10. Diagram of a platelet illustrating the major constituents of these small, biconvex disks.

Table 8.1 Constituents of Platelet Granules

Dense Granules	Serotonin, Ca²⁺, ADP, ATP
α-Granules	Platelet factor 4 (counteracts anticoagulant heparin)
	Factor 5 (involved in converting prothrombin to thrombin)
	Platelet-derived growth factor (PDG-F)—a potent growth-stimulating factor
	Fibrinogen
Lysosomes	Various hydrolytic enzymes

ules appears to be responsible for platelet aggregation when exposed to collagen. Platelets stimulated by ADP become irregular or dendritic in shape and express fibrinogen receptors on their platelet surface. Both actin and myosin are also present in platelets and appear to be involved in the shape change that occurs during platelet activation, in which the platelet changes from a disc-shaped structure to one with short projections or pseudopods (Fig. 8.13). Serotonin, which is present in

platelet-dense granules, is a vasoconstrictor that locally narrows the blood vessel to reduce blood loss. Thrombin also stimulates platelet aggregation and causes them to secrete. Platelet stimulation by either collagen or thrombin liberates arachidonic acid from the platelet membrane. The arachidonic acid is quickly converted to enteroperoxides, which are converted into thromboxane A₂, a stimulus for platelet secretion. Aspirin can block the conversion of arachidonic acid to thromboxane A₂.

When a blood vessel is damaged sufficiently that a platelet plug is unable to stop bleeding, the *coagulation phase* of blood clotting is initiated. This phase involves the following events:

1. In the presence of a plasma globulin called *antihemophilic factor*, blood platelets disintegrate and release the enzyme called *thromboplastinogenase* and *platelet factor 3*.
2. Thromboplastinogenase combines with antihemophilic factor, and this complex converts the plasma globulin thromboplastinogen into the enzyme thromboplastin.
3. Thromboplastin combines with calcium ions and converts the inactive plasma protein prothrombin into the active enzyme thrombin.

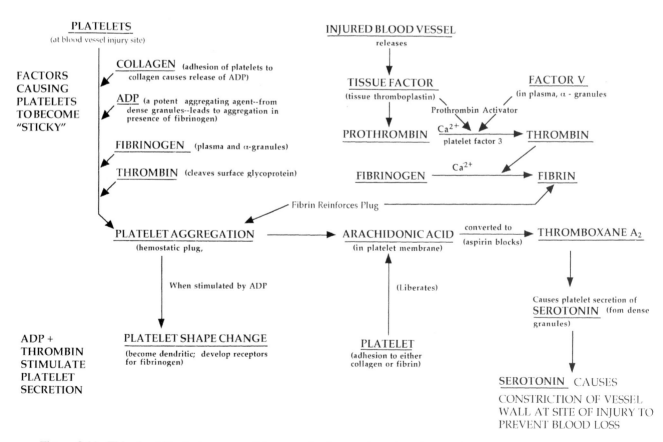

Figure 8.11. This chart illustrates some of the complex interactions that characterize the role of platelets in agglutination and blood clotting.

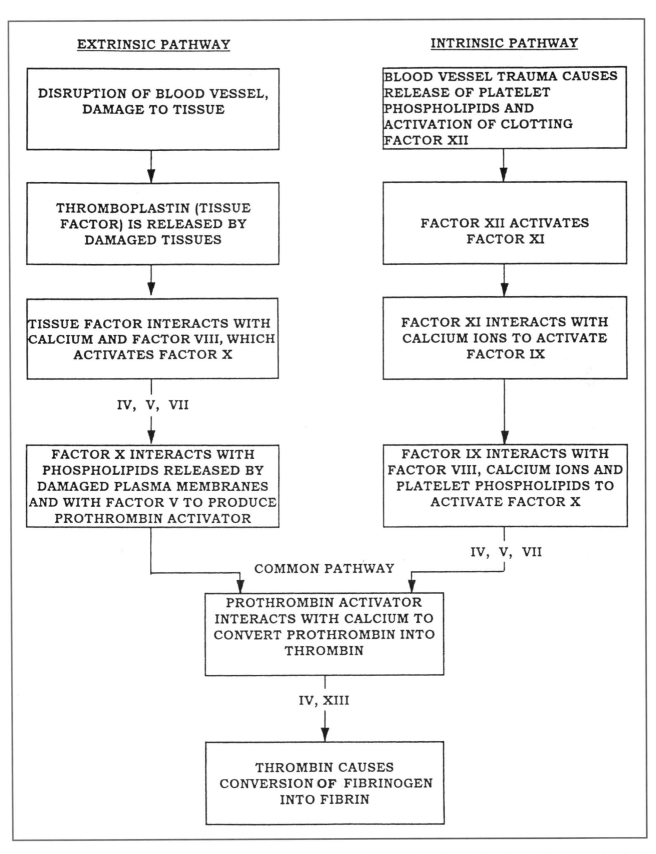

Figure 8.12. The extrinsic and intrinsic pathways of blood clotting are outlined, as well as the clotting factors involved at the various steps.

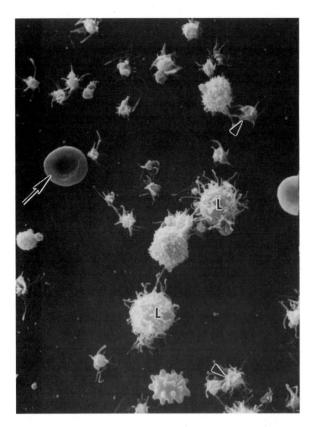

Figure 8.13. SEM of blood. Erythrocytes (arrow), activated dendritic platelets (arrowheads) and leukocyte (Lo) are shown. ×2655. (From R. Kessel and R. Kardon, *Tissues and Organs: A Text-Atlas of Scanning Electron Microscopy*. W.H. Freeman, New York, 1979)

4. Thrombin acts as a catalyst to convert the soluble plasma protein fibrinogen into the insoluble threads made of the protein fibrin, which assist in trapping the blood cells and clot formation (Fig. 8.4).

While details of the conversions of prothrombin into thrombin and of fibrinogen into fibrin are rather well understood, the means by which prothrombin is initially activated is less clear. The *extrinsic pathway* of blood clotting is one that permits rapid clotting when blood vessels are ruptured and tissue damage occurs (see Fig. 8.12). The *intrinsic pathway* of blood clotting occurs when the inner layers of blood vessels become damaged. In the extrinsic pathway, damaged tissues release *thromboplastin* (called *tissue factor*), which initiates blood clotting. Tissue factor combines with several *enzymes* and the *phospholipids* of damaged cell membranes in the region of the injured tissue, resulting in the production of *prothrombin activator*. It is at this point that the extrinsic pathway merges with the intrinsic pathway to form a common pathway. The *intrinsic pathway* involves substances present in the blood that are called *clotting factors*. When an injury occurs to the inner wall of a blood vessel, clotting factor XII is activated and trig-

gers a cascade of rapid chemical reactions, resulting in the production of *prothrombin activator*. Following the formation of prothrombin activator, the extrinsic and intrinsic pathways merge and proceed through the common pathway. The extrinsic pathway can produce a clot in only 15 seconds. The intrinsic pathway usually requires 2–6 minutes to produce a clot. The fibrin threads that form around the injury site are observed in the TEM to have an axial periodicity or banding pattern that has a precise 230-Å spacing.

HEMOSTASIS AND COAGULATION

Damage to blood vessels often leads to blood loss. In the case of minor damage, there are several mechanisms to arrest bleeding (hemostasis). Initially, constriction occurs in the smooth muscle of the vessel wall. Additional vasoconstriction occurs as serotonin is released from platelet granules. Platelets in the region adhere to the damaged elements of the vessel, and these platelets aggregate to form a temporary plug in the region. When platelets adhere to collagen that is exposed in regions of blood vessel injury, the platelets respond by releasing calcium and ADP, which facilitates their adhesion to the exposed collagen. Blood clotting then occurs, with the appearance of fibrin threads. Finally, in clot retraction, serum is squeezed from the fibrin clot and a plug is formed in the wound area that seals the area and constitutes a framework for repair processes. Substances needed for blood coagulation are also present in blood as inactive precursors. There are a number of these coagulation factors, and they are typically referred to by Roman numerals in order of their discovery. These coagulation factors are listed in Figure 8.12.

In blood clotting, during phase 1, tissue damage results in tissue thromboplastin, which interacts with plasma coagulation factors (IV, V, VII, X) to produce what is called *extrinsic thromboplastin*. Vascular damage results in platelet adherence and production of platelet factors that interact with various plasma coagulation factors (IV, V, VII, IX, X, XI, XII) to produce *intrinsic thromboplastin*. The *thromboplastins*, together with *coagulation factors IV, V, VII*, and *X*, are involved in the conversion of *prothrombin* (normally present in blood; coagulation factor II) into *thrombin*. *Fibrinogen* (factor I, normally present in blood) is converted into *fibrin* threads of a clot by *thrombin* and *coagulation factors IV* and *XIII*. These steps in blood clotting are summarized in Figures 8.11 and 8.12.

ENDOTHELIAL CELLS

The endothelial cells of the vascular system produce plasma factors; some of them are involved in preventing blood loss, while others prevent inappropriate blood

Table 8.2 Some Characteristics of Human Blood Cells

Cell/Constituent	Size/Diameter	Life Span	Normal Number	Cytoplasmic Granules	Function	Concentration (Cells/Liter)
Platelets (thrombocytes)	2–3 μm (smear)	5–9 days	200,000–300,000/mm^3 (150,000–400,000)	Granulomere (α-granules, dense granules)	Initiate blood clotting	3×10^{11}
Erythrocytes (red blood corpuscles)	7.5 μm (smear)	120 days	5–5.5 million/mm^3 ($\male$) 4.5–5 million/mm^3 ($\female$)	No granules	Transport $O_2 + CO_2$	5×10^{12}
White blood cells (leucocytes)						
A. Granulocytes 1. *Neutrophils*	10–12 μm (smear) 7–9 μm (living)	10 hr in blood, then 1–2 days in conn. tissue	55–65% leukocytes (3,000–6,000/mm^3)	Neutrophilic (specific) and azurophilic (nonspecific) granules	Phagocytose and digest bacteria	5×10^9
2. *Eosinophils*	10–15 μm (smear) ~9 μm (living)	8 hr in blood, several days in conn. tissue	1–4% (120–450/mm^3)	Eosinophilic granules; azurophilic granules possible	Destroy parasites; involved in allergy, inflammation	2×10^8
3. *Basophils*	10–12 μm (smear) ~9 μ (living)	Several days	0.5–1% (50–80/mm^3)	Basophilic granules; azurophilic possible	IgE receptors, release histamine in some reactions	4×10^7
B. Agranulocytes 1. *Lymphocytes*	6–9 μm ~8% to 15 μm	Months to years	20–30% 1,500–4,000/mm^3	No specific granules; ~10% have azurophilic granules	Produce humoral antibodies; cell-mediated immune reactions	
B cells					Produce humoral antibodies	2×10^9
T cells					Kill virus-infected cells and some tumors	1×10^9
NK cells					Kill virus-infected cells and some tumors	1×10^8
2. *Monocytes*	12–15 μm (smear) 9–12 μm (living)	Several days in circulation; then to tissues as macrophages	3–8% 200–600/mm^3	No specific granules; some may have azurophilic granules	Become tissue macrophages to phagocytose foreign material, present antigen	4×10^8

clotting. Rod-shaped granules in the cytoplasm of endothelial cells, called *Weibel-Palade granules*, contain a protein involved in blood coagulation. This protein is known as *von Willebrand factor* or *factor VIII*. A deficiency in this protein results in excessive bleeding, a cause of *hemophilia*. Endothelial cells also produce *antithrombin III*, which blocks the action of thrombin, and *plasminogen activator*, which triggers clot dissolution and *prostacyclin*, a vasodilator and an inhibitor of platelet aggregation.

PLATELET-DERIVED GROWTH FACTOR

If a wound results in disruption of both epidermis and an adjacent blood vessel in the connective tissue, platelet-derived growth factor (PDGF) is released by platelets in the wound area, as well as perhaps macrophages, endothelial cells, and smooth muscle in the blood vessel wall. PDGF causes proliferation of fibroblasts and smooth muscle and stimulates fibroblasts to produce more extracellular matrix. PDGF acts as a chemotactic signal for fibroblasts and macrophages but is only one of a number of factors that are involved in wound healing.

LEUKOCYTES

Nucleated cells in the circulating blood number 5000 to 9000 per cubic millimeter of blood under normal conditions. The term *leukocytosis* refers to an increase in the number of white blood cells, which may indicate a pathologic or disease condition. A decrease below normal in the number of white blood cells is termed *leukopenia*. Some causes of abnormal leukocyte counts are indicated in the table (Table 8.3).

In a single individual, the total number of leukocytes ranges from 18 to 36 billion. The cells are motile to varying degrees and are capable of leaving the blood capillaries and entering the connective tissues; some of them are phagocytic. Leukocytes are separated into two types, called *granulocytes* or *agranulocytes*, based on the presence or absence of universally present, specific staining cytoplasmic granules. The granulocytes include *neutrophilic granular leukocytes, eosinophilic granular leuko-*

Table 8.3 Some Causes of Abnormal Leukocyte Counts

Leukocytosis (increase in leukocytes)	
Neutrophilia	Acute infections such as certain bacterial, fungal, and viral infections
	Toxemia (such as uremia, diabetic acidosis, eclampsia); also acute hemorrhage
	Tumors of the bone marrow, liver, gastrointestinal tract and in Hodgkin's disease
	Granulocytic leukemia
Eosinophilia	Allergies such as hay fever, bronchial asthma
	Parasitic infections
	Hodgkin's disease
	Granulocytic leukemia
Lymphocytosis	Acute infections (pertussis, mumps, German measles)
	Infectious mononucleosis
	Chronic infections (tuberculosis, infectious hepatitis)
	Lymphatic leukemia
Monocytosis	Bacterial infections (tuberculosis)
	Protozoan infections (malaria)
	Rickettsial infections (Rocky Mountain spotted fever, typhus)
	Hodgkin's disease
	Monocytic leukemia
Leukopenia (decrease in leukocytes)	Bacterial infections (typhoid, paratyphoid)
	Viral infections (influenza, measles, German measles)
	Protozoan infections (malaria)
	Agranulocytosis
	Drugs, such as antithyroidals, anticonvulsants, antihistamines, sulfonamide, adrenocorticotropic hormone (ACTH), cortisol

cytes, and *basophilic granular leukocytes*. This designation refers to the characteristic staining qualities of their specific granules. Characteristically, the nucleus of neutrophilic and eosinophilic granulocytes is lobated. The *agranulocytes* are those leukocytes that do not possess specific staining cytoplasmic granules and include both *lymphocytes* and *monocytes*. However, a small percentage of each cell type may contain some cytoplasmic azurophilic granules.

NEUTROPHILIC (OR HETEROPHILIC) GRANULAR LEUKOCYTE (NEUTROPHIL, POLYMORPHONUCLEAR LEUKOCYTE)

Structure, number, appearance

Neutrophils are the most numerous of the blood leukocytes, ranging from 60% to 70% of the total leukocytes under normal conditions (Fig. 8.14). Their life span varies from 1 day to several days. They are migratory and phagocytic. The ingestion and digestion of bacteria by neutrophils is more efficient during subsequent infections for which antibodies exist for bacterial surface antigen. In this case, IgG binds to the surface of the bacterium, and a component of complement C3b binds to the antigen-antibody complex on the bacterium. The neutrophil has receptors for IgG and C3b, which facilitates the binding of the bacterium for phagocytosis. Like most leukocytes, they tend to be somewhat larger in diameter in stained blood smears compared

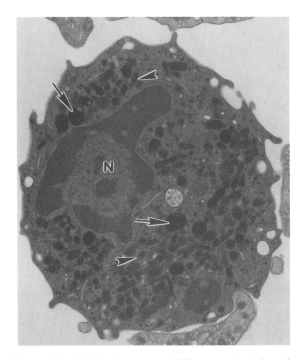

Figure 8.14. TEM of a neutrophil illustrates the lobated nucleus (N) and the azurophilic (arrows) and neutrophilic (arrowheads) granules. ×12,090.

to living cells. The nucleus tends to be lobated, with three to five lobes being common (Plate 14A–D). Older neutrophils tend to have more lobes. A stalked knob, called the *drumstick*, extends from the nucleus; this is the *Barr body*, which represents a single heterochromatic X chromosome in the female (Plate 14B).

Neutrophilic granules

The cytoplasm contains a number of small, dust-like granules that stain a lilac color in well-stained blood smears. Since the granules are only slightly larger than the resolution of the LM and since the granules are difficult to stain, they are not always apparent in all neutrophils. The specific neutrophilic granules were once thought to contain both alkaline phosphatase and antibacterial (bactericidal) substances. However, alkaline phosphatase has recently been described to be located in a novel intracellular compartment (a phosphasome), and not in either specific or azurophil granules. One antibacterial substance present in neutrophilic granules is called *phagocytin*. Components recently described in specific neutrophilic granules include lactoferrin, vitamin B_{12} binding protein, b-cytochrome, complement receptor CR3, and some extracellular matrix receptors.

Azurophilic granules

In addition to the more numerous and smaller neutrophilic granules, neutrophils contain larger but usually less numerous granules called *azurophilic granules* because they stain with methylene azure, which is a component of some blood stains. Among the substances present in azurophil granules is myeloperoxidase, which acts with hydrogen peroxide in microbicidal activity. Other polypeptides in azurophil granules include defensins, cationic proteins, and the typical array of lysosomal enzymes. The azurophilic granules are primary lysosomes because they contain acid hydrolase enzymes, but they also contain peroxidase. The hydrolytic enzymes present in the azurophilic granules include acid phosphatase, aryl sulfatase, esterase, β-glucuronidase, β-galactosidase, and nucleotidase. When immature neutrophils are still in the marrow, cytoplasmic azurophilic granules are much more numerous and they appear prior to the specific neutrophilic granules. Since the number of azurophilic granules decreases prior to complete neutrophil maturity and release into the bloodstream, a circulating neutrophil with many azurophilic granules would indicate a slightly immature cell released prematurely into the bloodstream, as might occur during infection. Immature neutrophils also appear in the circulation before the nucleus has undergone extensive constriction into lobes. For example, a juvenile neutrophil, also an example of a neutrophilic metamyelocyte, may possess a sightly indented nucleus. Band or stab neutrophils, which are also examples of neu-

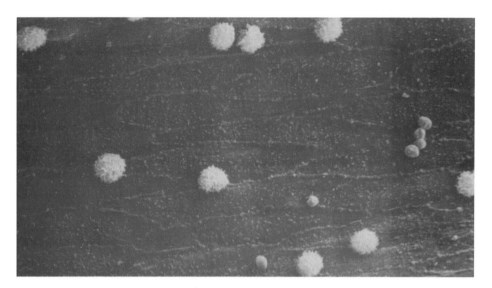

Figure 8.15. SEM of an endothelium lining blood vessel. Note that leukocytes adhere to the endothelium and resist being dislodged during tissue preparation ×1700.

trophilic metamyelocytes, have a horseshoe-shaped nucleus. Both cells represent stages in the extensive constriction of the nucleus into distinct lobes during final maturation. If distinct nuclear lobes are apparent, the neutrophil is segmented.

Inflammation and neutrophils

Inflammation is a physiologic response of the body to tissue injury; it involves dilation of blood vessels, especially postcapillary venules, and increased blood vessel permeability. Neutrophils enter the inflammatory site and engage in active phagocytosis of bacteria and passive phagocytosis of damaged connective tissue cells, erythrocytes, and fibrin. Monocytes also enter the connective tissue during inflammation and transform into macrophages that phacocytose cell and tissue debris.

Lymphocytes, eosinophils, and basophils are more involved in immunologic aspects of inflammation; eosinophils and lymphocytes are more likely to be involved in chronic inflammation.

Although many leukocytes are suspended and rapidly swept along by the rapid flow of blood around them, they are also able to attach to the endothelium and migrate along its surface without being dislodged by the blood flow (Figs. 8.15, 8.16). This activity may be followed by the movement of leukocytes across the endothelium into the surrounding tissue spaces. Neutrophils are especially responsive to various cytokines and mediators that are formed and released in areas of inflammation. They are attracted into connective tissues from the bloodstream in areas of inflammation and bacterial infections. Various components of the complement system and some cytokines present in regions of

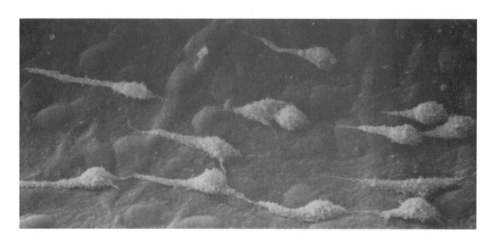

Figure 8.16. SEM of a blood vessel interior showing a number of leukocytes that were preserved in the process of migrating along the endothelial lining at the time of preservation. ×2125

bacterial infection stimulate endothelial cells to produce a surface glycoprotein called *endothelial cell adhesion molecule 1* (*ELAM-1*), which causes the lumen surface to be sticky. Neutrophils can produce a *leukocyte adhesion molecule* (*LeuCAM*) that causes leukocytes to adhere to endothelial surfaces preparatory to their migration through the endothelial capillaries into the connective tissues.

Phagocytic cells including neutrophils can synthesize a group of compounds called *leukotrienes* from arachidonic acid in their plasma membrane. The various leukotrienes promote neutrophil adhesion to endothelium and movement into the connective tissues, and attract eosinophils, monocytes, and other neutrophils. Leukotrienes increase the permeability of postcapillary venules, which results in edema or swelling at sites of inflammation. Since the leukotrienes act as vasoconstrictors, they may make breathing difficult. Neutrophils function in the phagocytosis of bacteria and dead cells, and they can digest bacteria by means of substances in neutrophilic and azurophilic granules. During microbicidal function, the neutrophil generates such toxic oxygen species as superoxide and hydrogen peroxide. After the bacterium is internalized in a phagocytic vacuole, neutrophilic granules fuse with the phagosome, followed by fusion of the azurophilic granules with the phagosome, resulting in a digestive vacuole or secondary lysosome. The enzymes in these granules then digest the bacteria. Neutrophils often die following phagocytosis, which is an energy-dependent event. When neutrophils die, the lysosomal enzymes are released into the extracellular space. The dead neutrophils, adjacent tissue fluid, and other cellular debris are collectively called *pus*.

EOSINOPHILIC (ACIDOPHILIC) GRANULAR LEUKOCYTES (OR EOSINOPHILS)

Number, size, structure

Eosinophils comprise approximately 1–4% of the total leukocytes (Fig. 8.17; Plate 14F–G). Therefore, they number about 150–450 per cubic millimeter of blood. Eosinophils appear to circulate in the blood for less than a day. They then move into the connective tissues, where they survive for several days. Eosinophils are approximately 9 μm in diameter in the living organism but 12–17 μm in diameter in blood smears. The nucleus is commonly constricted into two or three lobes, with only a thin segment of chromatin connecting the lobes. The cytoplasm is typically filled with specific granules that stain acidophilic (orange) and are all approximately similar in size (~1 μm). The eosinophilic staining granules contain *peroxidase*, as well as several *lysosomal enzymes*.

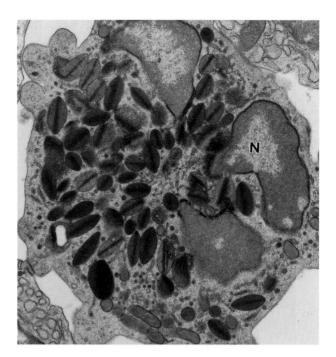

Figure 8.17. TEM of an eosinophil. Note the lobated nucleus (N) and characteristic eosinophilic granules in the cytoplasm. ×12,090.

Granule composition and function

It has been recognized for some time that the eosinophil plays a role in allergic reactions and stress phenomena. Although the mechanisms involved were previously unknown, some information is now available. Eosinophils are attracted to regions of antigen-antibody interaction because of the release of an *eosinophilic chemotactic factor* of *anaphylaxis* contained in *mast cell* granules that are discharged during appropriate immunologic encounters. Eosinophils then phagocytize the antigen-antibody complexes at the site of the interaction. Eosinophils have also been found to produce a *histaminase*, which could reduce the deleterious effects of allergic reactions where histamine is produced. One of the enzymes present in the eosinophilic granules, *aryl sulfatase*, may neutralize the *slow-reacting substance* of *anaphalaxis* that is released by *mast cells* under the appropriate stimulation. Both histaminase and aryl sulfatase would diminish the deleterious effects of these vasoactive agents. Hydrocortisone is a steroid produced by the adrenal cortex. When it is injected into the body, it tends to depress allergic reactions and causes many of the circulating eosinophils to leave the bloodstream and enter the connective tissues, where many immunologic battles occur. In parasitic infections, the number of eosinophils is greatly elevated, and it is thought that eosinophils may be involved in the *destruction* of certain *larger parasites*. Interleukin 4 (IL-4) is a substance with potent antitumor activity and appears to be released by eosinophils at sites of tumor cell death.

BASOPHILIC GRANULAR LEUKOCYTES (BASOPHILS)

Basophils comprise 0.5% to 1% of the circulating blood leukocytes and range from 10 to 15 μm in diameter in blood smears (Plate 14H,I). The nucleus may be bent, lobated, or even S-shaped. Specific granules stain basophilic, but they are somewhat water soluble in humans (Fig. 8.18); as a result, the concentration of the basophilic granules can vary with the preparatory conditions. Granules of basophils, like those in mast cells, stain *metachromatically*, and contain *heparin*, *histamine*, and perhaps other *vasoactive substances*. Sulfated proteoglycans, chondroitin sulfate, and leukotriene-3 have also been described in basophil granules. The basophil granules in humans have a central crystalline structure when viewed in the TEM. It has been known for some time that the basophils and mast cells share certain similarities; in fact, in the past, mast cells were called *tissue basophils*. Granule contents in the two cells are similar, and both mast cells and basophils have *IgE* molecules

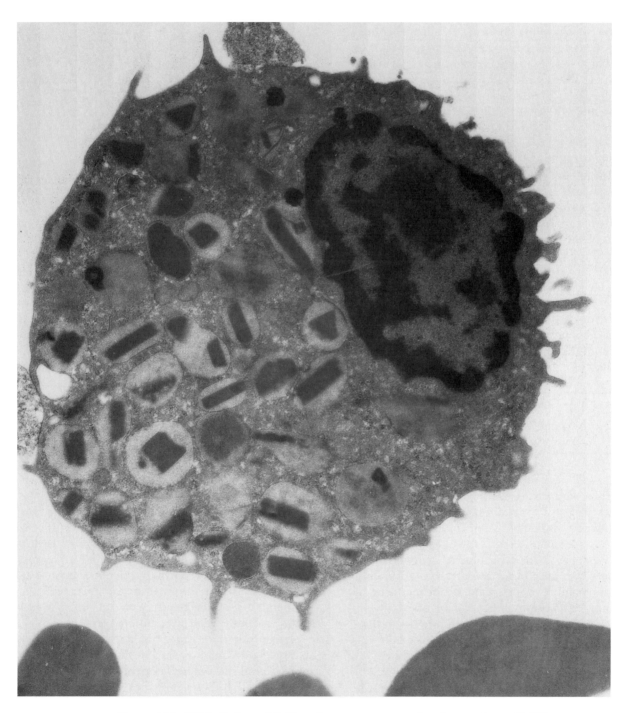

Figure 8.18. TEM of a basophil. Note the numerous cytoplasmic granules. ×20,250.

on their surfaces. IgE can bind antigen and, upon subsequent exposure to the antigen, will cause release or degranulation of the vasoactive cytoplasmic substances, resulting in vascular changes associated with hypersensitivity and anaphylaxis.

LYMPHOCYTES

Structure, size, number

Lymphocytes are the second most abundant leukocyte, reportedly ranging from 20% to 50% of the circulating white blood cells (Plate 14J–L). Lymphocytes are motile, and many are 6–9 μm in diameter. Lymphocytes are not only found in blood, they are also present in lymph, lymphoid organs (Chapter 10), and some connective tissues (Chapter 5). While most circulating lymphocytes are small, approximately 8% range up to 15 μm in diameter (Fig. 8.19) and probably represent activated B lymphoblasts. As a consequence, small, medium-sized, and large lymphocytes have been described. The lymphocyte nucleus is typically spherical, and the chromatin is often highly condensed; therefore, these nuclei stain dark blue or purple with blood stains (Plate 14J–L). Frequently, a narrow rim of moderately basophilic staining cytoplasm is apparent in localized regions, but it may not form a complete band around the nucleus. Perhaps only 10% or less of the circulating lymphocytes have a few reddish-purple-staining (azurophilic) granules in the cytoplasm. When lymphocytes are studied in the TEM, the cytoplasm contains mitochondria, free polyribosomes, and a Golgi complex (Fig. 8.19). The rER is rather sparse, and a lysosome is sometimes present.

Lymphocyte and immunity

About 40 years ago, lymphocytes were considered to be "dead end" cells of unknown function. It is now evident that lymphocytes constitute the cellular basis of many immunologic reactions. It is possible for many proteins to enter the body that are different from those present in the body itself. The foreign proteins are called *antigens*, and when they enter the body, immunologic cells called *B lymphocytes* respond directly and indirectly to produce substances called *antibodies* (see Chapter 10, Fig. 10.2) to counteract or fight the invading foreign proteins. Lymphocytes represent a vast population of cells with many different genetic capabilities for recognizing specific foreign molecules. Lymphocytes that can recognize an antigen as foreign respond to an initial encounter with the antigen by undergoing certain changes that endow them with a specific memory for that particular antigen. The recognition of antigen by antibody is a very specific and precise event.

The antibody molecule (immunoglobulins)

An important feature of the immune system is that B cells are endowed with the capacity to synthesize specific antibody molecules that can be inserted into the plasma membrane of these cells. Plasma cells synthesize

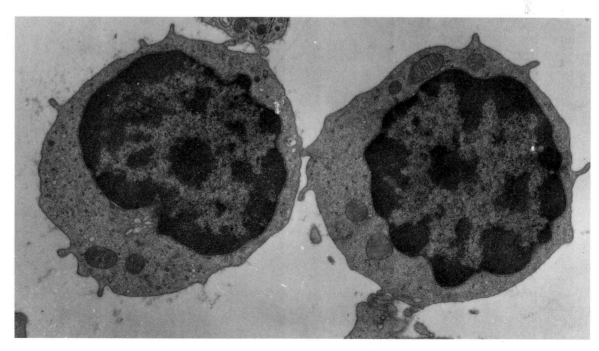

Figure 8.19. TEM of two lymphocytes. The nucleus contains abundant heterochromatin; the cytoplasm contains polyribosomes, mitochondria, and a single Golgi complex. ×12,250.

antibodies for secretion. Therefore, knowledge of the structure and diversity of antibody molecules is basic to understanding the immune system. The simplest antibodies are Y-shaped molecules with two identical antigen-binding sites, one at each tip of the Y. Each antibody molecule consists of four polypeptide chains: two identical light (L) chains (each consisting of approximately 214 amino acids) and two identical heavy (H) chains (each consisting of approximately 440 amino acids). Both L and H chains have variable and constant regions. It is the variable regions of the molecule that determine the recognition and binding of antibody to antigens (See Chapt. 10). The constant regions do not affect the specificity of an antibody for an antigen. The antigen-binding sites are formed by amino-terminal regions of both L and H chains. The tail of the Y-shaped antibody molecule determines what occurs after antigen is bound to the antibody, including the ability to activate complement and bind to phagocytic cells.

In higher vertebrates there are five classes of antibody H chains: IgA, IgD, IgE, IgG, and IgM, and each one has its own class of H chain (α, δ, ϵ, σ, and γ). Further, there are several subclasses of IgG and IgA immunoglobulins. Four human IgG subclasses, denoted IgG1, IgG2, IgG3, and IgG4, have γ_1, γ_2, γ_3, and γ_4 H chains, respectively. In addition to five classes of H chains, higher vertebrates have two types of L chains, either (κ) or (λ), but not both. Some properties of the major classes of human antibodies are denoted in the Table 10.1.

Antibody diversity

An individual can generate enormous genetic diversity in antibodies to specifically recognize a vast array of foreign antigens. It is important to emphasize that each lymphocyte or population of lymphocytes has a different specificity for molecular recognition and that lymphocytes are preprogrammed with this specificity prior to their first encounter with antigen. The extensive diversity apparent in the different families of lymphocytes is due to changes in the variable regions of the L and H chains of the Y-shaped Ig molecule. According to the *clonal selection theory*, each lymphocyte during its development becomes committed to recognize and react with only one specific antigen before it ever encounters this antigen. This occurs by the acquisition of cell surface receptors that specifically recognize or "fit" the antigen. When an antigen binds to a receptor that it recognizes, the lymphocyte proliferates and matures. The evidence is substantial that lymphocytes are committed to respond to a specific antigen before they are ever exposed to the antigen, and the recognition is based on specific receptors in the lymphocyte plasma membrane for a single specific antigen. The specific antigen receptors on the lymphocyte are encoded by genes that are assembled from gene segments through a type of genetic re-

combination very early in the development of the lymphocyte.

If the human genome contains $\sim 10^5$ genes and a human can make $\sim 10^{15}$ different antibodies, how can an individual make more antibodies than there are genes? Both the L and H chains participate in forming an antibody site. An individual with 1000 genes encoding L chains and 1000 genes encoding H chains could combine these to generate 10^6 different antigen-binding sites (1000 × 1000). An enormous number of different L and H chains can be produced by joining separate gene segments together before they are transcribed.

B Lymphocytes (B cells).   While many lymphocytes look the same in blood smears, there are many populations of lymphocytes with diverse genetic codes that are specifically capable of recognizing a vast array of possible foreign proteins or other molecules. Approximately 25% of the circulating lymphocytes are B cells. The B lymphocyte or B cell develops in the bone marrow in humans and, when suitably stimulated by the appropriate antigen, has the capacity to proliferate and then differentiate into two populations of cells. The stimulated B lymphocyte, called a *B lymphoblast*, divides repeatedly and some of the cells differentiate into *plasma cells*. The plasma cells acquire extensive rER, and they synthesize and release *humoral* (circulating) *antibody* that binds to and destroys the specific antigen that caused its production. Some progeny of the dividing B lymphoblast remain as "memory" B lymphocytes with information to interact with the specific antigen should it again appear. B lymphocytes thus recognize antigen by the antigen-specific Ig receptor molecules on these cells. Another type of lymphocyte, the *helper T lymphocyte*, is required for most B cells to respond to an antigen; this subject will be discussed in Chapter 10. When B lymphocytes are formed in the bone marrow, they travel to and settle in such lymphatic tissues or organs as the lymph nodes, spleen, and solitary lymphatic nodules comprising the tonsils and Peyer's patches in the ileum.

T lymphocytes (T cells).   T cells develop from stem cells that migrate to and colonize the *thymus* in the fetus. T cells participate in *cell-mediated immunity*, and play an important role in the destruction of foreign cells and infected cells, including virus-infected cells. There are several kinds of T cells, including *helper, inducer, suppressor, killer,* and *memory* cells. T killer cells are the only cells that can destroy foreign or virus-infected cells directly. Unlike the B-cell receptor, the T-cell receptor is not an antibody molecule. In the fetus and after birth but prior to puberty, the thymus is a place where large, specific populations of lymphocytes are produced and differentiate. Following their formation and maturation in the thymus, the mature T lymphocytes become distributed to other lymphatic tissues (e.g., lymph nodes

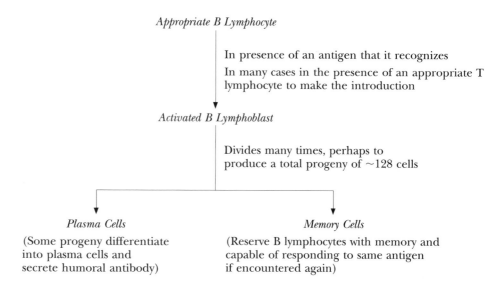

Appropriate B Lymphocyte

In presence of an antigen that it recognizes

In many cases in the presence of an appropriate T lymphocyte to make the introduction

Activated B Lymphoblast

Divides many times, perhaps to produce a total progeny of ~128 cells

Plasma Cells
(Some progeny differentiate into plasma cells and secrete humoral antibody)

Memory Cells
(Reserve B lymphocytes with memory and capable of responding to same antigen if encountered again)

and spleen), where they populate *thymus-dependent regions.*

Most T cells do not directly recognize circulating antigens, but require that the antigen or fragments be presented to lymphocyte receptors in conjunction with a major histocompatibility complex (MHC) protein; these are a family of cell surface glycoproteins encoded by a gene complex and will be discribed in more detail in Chapter 10. The MHC molecule and antigen fragment complex is used to "show" the specific T cell that the complex is "altered self" molecules and therefore should be destroyed. The altered self molecules are usually associated with virus-infected cells or cells that have become cancerous. This aspect of T-cell activity will also be discussed in more detail in Chapter 10.

What occurs when the appropriate T lymphocyte encounters a foreign protein (antigen) that it is programmed to recognize? Although the mechanism is complex and is discussed in more detail in Chapter 10, it is briefly described here. This stimulated T lymphocyte enlarges and becomes a mitotic cell called a *T lymphoblast.* The T lymphoblast proliferates and the progeny (perhaps 128 cells or more) can differentiate into

several different cell lines, as noted in the following diagram. T-lymphocyte progeny can never form plasma cells; only appropriately stimulated B lymphocytes can do this.

MONOCYTES

Monocytes are usually the largest of the leukocytes; they are 12–15 μm in diameter in stained blood smears but only 9–12 μm in diameter in living preparations (Plate 14M–O). Monocytes normally comprise 3–8% of the leukocytes. The main function of monocytes is to serve as precursors for macrophages. After their formation, they usually remain in the bloodstream for only 2 or 3 days and then move into the extravascular tissue spaces, where they may live for perhaps 2 months or longer. The monocyte nucleus is usually oval or kidney-shaped and eccentrically placed in the cell (Fig. 8.20). Some monocytes may initially be confused with large lymphocytes in stained blood smears. However, the monocyte has more cytoplasm than does a lymphocyte. A few azurophilic staining granules may be present in the

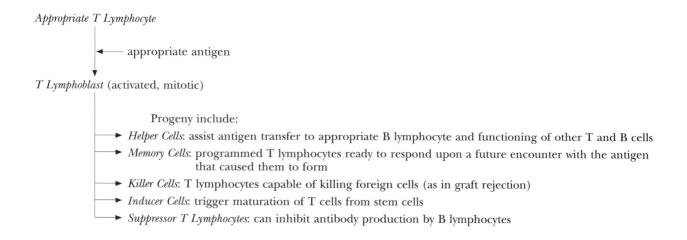

Appropriate T Lymphocyte

appropriate antigen

T Lymphoblast (activated, mitotic)

Progeny include:

Helper Cells: assist antigen transfer to appropriate B lymphocyte and functioning of other T and B cells

Memory Cells: programmed T lymphocytes ready to respond upon a future encounter with the antigen that caused them to form

Killer Cells: T lymphocytes capable of killing foreign cells (as in graft rejection)

Inducer Cells: trigger maturation of T cells from stem cells

Suppressor T Lymphocytes: can inhibit antibody production by B lymphocytes

monocyte cytoplasm (Fig. 8.20). In addition, the cytoplasm of a monocyte is generally less basophilic than that of a lymphocyte. Furthermore, the monocyte nucleus is frequently not as heterochromatic and thus not as darkly stained as a lymphocyte nucleus.

Monocytes and tissue macrophages, which comprise the mononuclear phagocyte system, are very active cells that respond to hormonal and cellular signals and participate in a variety of physiologic and pathologic events. Macrophages are important for their role in internalizing antigen and in processing and presenting antigen together with MHC molecules.

LYMPHOKINES AND MONOKINES

It is known that certain cells of the immune system are able to secrete small amounts of very potent hormones called *cytokines*, which are of two types: *lymphokines* and *monokines* produced by lymphocytes and monocyte/macrophages. These cytokines act locally and do not circulate in the bloodstream. Lymphocytes not only synthesize antibodies, they produce low molecular weight substances called *lymphokines* that act as messengers to signal various responses in the immune system, such as

lymphocyte proliferation, lymphocyte migration, macrophage activation, and target cell death. Cytokines will be discussed in more detail in the following chapter.

Important characteristics of human blood cells are compared and summarized in Table 8.2. Causes of abnormal elevated leukocyte counts are listed in Table 8.3.

CLINICAL CORRELATIONS

ANEMIA

An erythrocyte count below normal is called *anemia.* Anemia can result from an increased rate of destruction of the erythrocyte or a deficient rate of production. A slight change in the chemical composition of hemoglobin may result in altered erythrocyte shape. Thus, in the disease known as *sickle-cell anemia,* the erythrocytes assume the shape of sickles and, as a consequence, are more readily destroyed during circulation. In this disease, an alteration of a base sequence in DNA results in the substitution of one amino acid, valine, for the usual or normal one, glutamic acid, in the hemoglobin molecule. Since erythrocytes with the altered hemoglobulin are destroyed faster than they are replaced, the re-

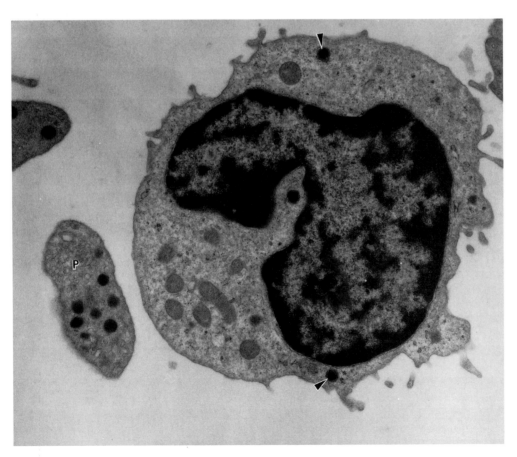

Figure 8.20. TEM of a monocyte. Note the indented nucleus. The cytoplasm contains polyribosomes, mitochon- dria, and a few azurophilic granules (arrowheads). A platelet (P) is present adjacent to the monocyte. ×15,500.

sulting reduced number of erythrocytes produces anemia.

SELECTED BIBLIOGRAPHY

Blackman, L. (1986). Shape control in the human red cell. *J. Cell Biol.* **80**, 281–288.

Boxer, L.A., and Smolen, J.E. (1988). Neutrophil granule constituents and their release in health and disease. *Hematol./Oncol. Clin. North Am.* **2**, 101–134.

Colman, R.W. (1990). Aggregin: a platelet ADP receptor that mediates activation. *FASEB J.* **4**, 1425–1435.

Crosier, P.S., and Clark, S.C. (1992). Basic biology of the hematopoietic growth factors. *Semin. Oncol.* **19**, 349–361.

Dvorak, H.F., and Dvorak, A.M. (1975). Basophilic leukocytes: structure, function, and role in disease. *Clin. Hematol.* **4**, 651–660.

Escolar, G., and White, J.G. (1991). The platelet open canalicular system: a final common pathway. *Blood Cells* **17**, 467–485.

Huber, A.R., Kunkel, S.L., Todd, R.E., and Weiss, S. (1991). Regulation of transendothelial neutrophil migration by endogenous interleukin-8. *Science* **254**, 99.

Ikuta, K., Uchida, N., Friedman, J., and Weissman, I.L. (1992). Lymphocyte development from stem cells. *Annu. Rev. Immunol.* **10**, 759–783.

Jay, D., and Cantely, L. (1986). Structural aspects of the red cell anion exchange protein. *Annu. Rev. Biochem.* **55**, 511–538.

Lisiewicz, J. (1980). *Human Neutrophils.* Charles Press, Bowie, MD.

Makino, S., and Fukuda, T., eds. (1993). *Eosinophils: Biological and Clinical Aspects.* CRC Press, Boca Raton, FL.

Movat, H.Z. (1985). *The Inflammatory Reaction.* Elsevier Press, Amsterdam.

Oates, J.A., Hawiger, J., and Ross, R. (eds.). (1985). *Interaction of Platelets with the Vessel Wall.* Williams & Wilkins, Baltimore.

Patek, J., and Lux, S.E. (1988). Red cell membrane skeleton defects in hereditary and acquired hemolytic anemias. *Semin. Hematol.* **20**, 189–198.

Stenberg, P.E., and Levin, J. (1989) Mechanisms of platelet production. *Blood Cells* **15**, 23–47.

Weller, P.F. (1992). Cytokine regulation of eosinophil function. *Clin. Immunol. Immunopathol.* **62**, S55–S59.

Wintrobe, M.M., et al. (1981). *Clinical Hematology,* 8th ed. Lea & Febiger, Philadelphia.

Ziegler-Heitbrock, H.W. (1989). The biology of the monocyte system. *Eur. J. Cell Biol.* **49**, 1–12.

Zipori, D. (1992). The renewal and differentiation of hemopoietic stem cells. *FASEB J.* **6**, 2691–2697.

Zucker-Franklin, D., et al. (1981). *Atlas of Blood Cells: Function and Pathology,* Vols. 1 and 2. Lea & Febiger, Philadelphia.

Hematopoietic Tissue: Myeloid Tissue

Initially, blood cells are formed by mesoderm cells of the yolk sac. Later, the liver and speen serve as temporary sites of blood cell formation. Bone marrow assumes the blood-forming function (hematopoiesis) as ossification of the skeleton occurs. After birth, granular leukocytes, monocytes, and platelets are derived from stem cells located in the bone marrow. Bone marrow also produces stem cells that migrate to lymphoid organs (tissues) and develop into different types of lymphocytes (Chapter 10).

The task of replacing blood cells is enormous. Billions of cells must be added to the circulation each day because circulating blood cells have a finite life span. Because erythrocytes survive for ~120 days, platelets for 5–9 days, and granular leukocytes for a matter of days or weeks, and because of the large number of cells that must be replaced, a specialized type of connective tissue called *hematopoietic tissue* is necessary. *Hematopoiesis* is the process in which worn-out blood cells are removed and new ones are added to the circulation. The blood-producing myeloid tissue responds to these needs. For example, during infections, stem cells proliferate to provide additional leukocytes to fight infectious bacteria or other organisms. Stem cells proliferate at high altitudes to provide more red blood cells to carry additional oxygen. Most circulating blood cells are unable to divide. Lymphocytes, if appropriately stimulated by an antigen that is recognized, enlarge into lymphoblasts that are mitotic and produce many additional cells of different subtypes.

ORGANIZATION

Myeloid tissue (bone marrow) consists of blood-forming cells and connective tissue stroma. Myeloid tissue is located in some bone marrow cavities in humans where erythrocytes, granular leukocytes, megakaryocytes and platelets, B lymphocytes, and monocytes are produced. Several names have been given to the cell that represents the ultimate source of all blood cells, including *hemocytoblast, stem cell* and *colony-forming unit* (*CFU*) *cell*. In addition to the blood-forming cells, pericytes (or perivascular cells) are present in marrow. These cells are derived from mesenchyme, are highly branched, and are relatively undifferentiated. They have the capacity to differentiate into several other cells types in marrow, including fibroblasts, reticular cells, macrophages, adipocytes, smooth muscle cells, and endothelial cells. Fibroblasts form the collagen necessary for the support of arteries, arterioles, venules, and sinusoids located in the marrow stroma. Reticular cells differentiate from mesenchyme cells or perivascular cells and provide a network of delicate fibers in which blood cell formation occurs. Macrophages are common in marrow, where they play phagocytic and other roles. Adipocytes are relatively scarce in red marrow but constitute the bulk of the cell population in yellow marrow. Smooth muscle cells are the major constituent of the larger blood vessels of the myeloid stroma and endothelial cells line the sinusoids. When examined grossly, marrow is found to be either red (Fig 9.1) or yellow (Fig 9.2). Yellow marrow is inactive in hematopoiesis, and the yellow color is due to the presence of large numbers of fat cells or adipocytes. Red marrow indicates active hematopoiesis and contains relatively few adipocytes. Many bones in the body may contain active red marrow at some period in development, but in adult humans, red marrow is largely restricted to the flat bones of the skull, clavicles, vertebrae, ribs, sternum, and pelvis. When examined histologically, bone marrow is found to be filled with many vessels called *si-*

Figure 9.1. SEM of bone marrow. Note the high concentration of cells and many large sinusoids (S). ×465. (From R. Kessel and R. Kardon, *Tissues and Organs: A Text-Atlas of Scanning Electron Microscopy*, W.H. Freeman, New York, 1979, with permission)

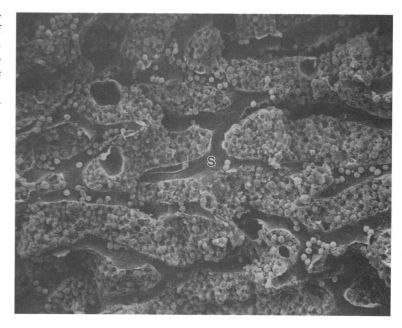

nusoids. The sinusoids in marrow are wide, thin-walled blood channels; thus newly formed blood cells move easily through the walls of these vessels to enter the bloodstream. Blood cells can move between sinusoidal endothelial cells since there are no junctional complexes to seal off these intercellular spaces. In addition, however, cellular elements of the marrow are able to move through temporary perforations within the endothelial cells. *Diapedesis* is a term used to denote the migration of blood cells between the endothelial cells of the marrow sinusoids. The release of mature blood cells from the marrow has been described to be due to "releasing" factors including a component of complement called *C3.* Glucocorticoids and androgens, as well as some bacterial toxins, also have a role in this event. Sinusoidal lining or endothelial cells are supported by delicate

reticular fibers, have a larger lumen than regular capillaries, and have an incomplete basal lamina. The delicate walls of sinusoids are protected from inward collapse by the many surrounding cells and because the nutrient vein of the bone is smaller than its companion artery. Thus, a sufficiently high hydrostatic pressure can be generated in the sinusoids to prevent their collapse.

STROMA

The connective tissue framework within bone marrow, called the *stroma,* consists of a meshwork of *reticular fibers* that are synthesized and exported by *reticular cells.* Macrophages abound in the marrow. Massive numbers of hematopoietic cells are crowded into the interstices

Figure 9.2. SEM of marrow in which numerous adipocytes filled with lipid (A) are scattered among the blood-forming cellular elements. ×450. (From R. Kessel and R. Kardon, *Tissues and Organs: A Text-Atlas of Scanning Electron Microscopy*, W.H. Freeman, New York, 1979, with permission)

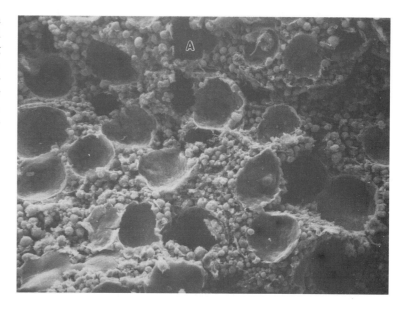

of the stromal network (Plate 17A–C). Some of the molecules present in marrow matrix include *types I and III collagen, fibronectin, laminin,* and *proteoglycan.* Another molecule, called *hemonectin,* has been reported to interact with receptors on the marrow cells to secure them in the matrix. Laminin and fibronectin have also been described to have this function. The stem cell of blood is able to replicate repeatedly and then differentiate into different kinds of secondary cells capable of further differentiation. The earliest stem cell is described as pluripotent since it can differentiate into any cell type in the blood or immune system; this is followed by multipotential (multipotent) cells somewhat more restricted in their capacities. Thus, a single stem cell in the marrow can differentiate into all types of blood cells. The stem cells proliferate, and one lineage forms the myeloid cells that develop in the bone marrow, including granular leukocytes, monocyes, erythrocytes and megakaryocytes. Another stem cell lineage proliferates and forms lymphoid cells (lymophocytes). Early in development, lymphoid cells migrate to the lymph nodes, spleen, and thymus, where further lymphocyte differentiation occurs. Cells become progressively more committed to a specific terminal cell as differentiation continues.

CELL DIFFERENTIATION

Erythrocytes and granular leukocytes evolve from a stem cell through a series of gradual cytologic transformations that were previously studied by making bone marrow smears and using one of several stains (Wright's, Giemsa's, or Romanovsky's) to study an array of cell types and to arrange them in a sequence reflecting the progressive differentiation in the cell lines. These studies were laborious and sometimes difficult to follow, for the cells do not undergo abrupt changes from an unspecialized cell to a terminally differentiated one.

Older studies of blood cell differentiation were based on making bone marrow smears, followed by staining and study in the LM. Hematologists early described a cell called a *hemocytoblast* that was able to differentiate through a series of developmental sequences into blood cells. In stained bone marrow smears the hemocytoblast was described as a rather large cell, some 15–20 μm in diameter, with a large, ovoid nucleus containing one or more nucleoli and a relatively undifferentiated nucleus with dispersed chromatin (euchromatin) so that the nucleus stained a light pink or red, sometimes with a purple tinge. This staining condition indicated a relatively euchromatic nucleus. In addition, the cytoplasm of this cell was lightly basophilic or clear, reflecting the fact that little or no endoplasmic reticulum (or polyribosomes) had been formed to begin synthetic activities. More recently, other types of studies have been used to investigate blood cell differentiation.

One of these methods, called the *spleen colony technique,* involves the use of tissue culture, chromosomal markers, irradiation, and density gradient centrifugation. In 1961, Till and McCulloch exposed mice to lethal doses of irradiation to kill cells in the hematopoietic tissues. The mice were then injected with bone marrow from a healthy, genetically compatible donor mouse. Somewhat over a week later, they removed the spleens from the irradiated mice and found numerous colonies of blood-producing cells growing in the spleen. These spleens were found to contain a great deal of irradiation-induced destruction but also a number of grossly visible nodules that represented small colonies of proliferating hematopoietic cells. In these nodules, it was determined that precursors of all the blood cells normally found in the circulating blood, as well as macrophages, were represented. Evidence from use of chromosomal markers indicated that each of the colonies was a *clone,* that is, derived from a single cell. The cell was called a *CFU cell* or *CFU-S* (S = spleen) and was believed to represent the stem blood cell. The term *CFU-C* was used to characterize the stem cell in experiments using cell culture. It is now possible to identify specific cells in the marrow by using a series of *monoclonal antibodies* that bind only to antigens on specific cell types in the marrow. It has been determined that the stem cells of bone marrow that are capable of reconstituting the blood cells comprise only about *0.1%* of the cells in the marrow.

HEMATOPOIETIC GROWTH FACTORS

A major limitation of cell culture techniques for the study of bone marrow cells outside of the body is the fact that marrow stroma cells produce substances necessary for stem cell viability. Several growth factors have now been identified and isolated, and the development of recombinant DNA techniques has permitted mass production of these growth factors in the laboratory.

Some success has been achieved in creating a culture system to permit hematopoiesis in the laboratory. The growth of marrow cells in culture conditions requires an environment as similar to that in the marrow as possible: this includes the presence of fibroblasts, fat cells, endothelial cells, macrophages, and various cell matrix proteins (collagens, fibronectins, laminin) since cells of the marrow appear to be capable of producing various *cytokines* or hormones that are important in the differentiation process. Based on such studies, another growth factor, called *stem cell factor (SCF), c-kit Ligand (KL),* or *mast cell growth factor (MGF),* has been isolated. It is a potent hematopoietic peptide growth factor or *cytokine* and has been shown to have broad effects on hematopoiesis, especially in combination with growth factors and cytokines, as summarized in Figure 9.3. This cytokine is able to stimulate early progenitor or stem

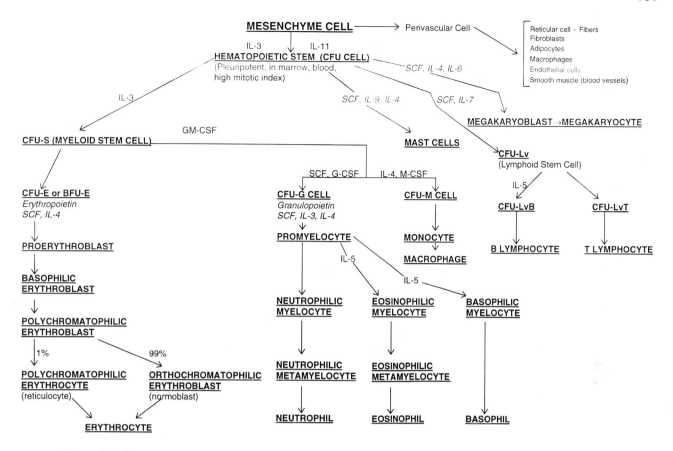

Figure 9.3. Flow chart of the stages in blood cell differentiation and some factors involved in the process.

cells in hematopoiesis and to also stimulate the proliferation and survival of mast cells as well as melanocytes and germ cells. Thus, SCF is able to stimulate colony formation from immature hematopoietic progenitors and it is known to act synergistically with other growth factors. SCF also stimulates megakaryoblasts. A number of cytokines that are important in blood cell growth and differentiation and their principal functions are listed in Table 9.1.

ERYTHROPOIESIS

MAJOR EVENTS

Erythropoiesis essentially involves the synthesis of ribonucleotides and then the synthesis of hemoglobin, followed by the loss of organelles and the nucleus. The general events that occur during erythropoiesis include (1) a gradual decrease in the size of cells as mitosis occurs, (2) a decrease in the size of the nucleus and then removal, (3) an increase in staining intensity of the nucleus from pink to dark purple, reflecting the transition from euchromatin to more heterochromatin, and (4) an initial increase in cytoplasmic basophilia followed by a progressive decrease in basophilic staining because of

the progressive increase in acidophilic staining due to increasing amounts of hemoglobin.

STAGES

The pluripotent stem cells comprise only ~0.1% of the nucleated marrow cells. They proliferate but more slowly than "committed" cells that are responsive to a variety of growth or colony-stimulating factors now known to affect blood cell differentiation. The stem cells of blood, either CFU-S or CFU-C cells, differentiate into cells committed to undergo a series of developmental sequences leading to an erythrocyte called an *erythropoietic burst-forming unit* (*BFU-E*) or *erythropoietic colony-forming unit* (*CFU-E*) cells. Some investigators have identified a BFU-E cell, which is described as smaller than the CFU-E, but with a much greater capacity for proliferation. The CFU-E cell is described as being 7–10 μm in diameter and to have mitochondria, free polyribosomes, and a euchromatic staining nucleus. Early progenitors of the erythroid series are also classified on the basis of their response to two growth factors: interleukin-3 (IL-3) and erythropoietin (Ep). Ep is a 166-amino acid glycoprotein (~70,000 MW) that is produced in modified smooth muscle cells in the wall of

Table 9.1 Factors Affecting Blood Cell Proliferation and Differentiation

Cytokine	Actions
Stem cell factor (SCF), c-kit ligand, or mast cell growth factor	Stimulates poliferation of hemtopoietic cells, mast cells, melanocytes, and germ cells
Interleukin-1 (IL-1)	Induces IL-2 production by T_H cells; regulates B-cell differentiation; stimulates cytotoxic T-cell development; stimulates prostaglandin and collagenase release from macrophages, fibroblasts
Interleukin-2 (IL-2)	Activates T_H cells, NK cells, and antibody-producing B cells
Interleukin-3 (IL-3)	Acts on multipotent hematopoietic stem cells; causes colony formation of macrophages, neutrophils, mast cells, megakaryocytes
Interleukin-4 (IL-4)	Causes proliferation and differentiation of T and B cells, erythroid cells, macrophages, megakaryocytes, mast cells, and monocyte precursors
Interleukin-5 (IL-5)	Stimulates maturation and differentiation of eosinophils and basophils; induces B-lymphocyte antibody production; acts with IL-2, causing cytotoxic T-cell development.
Interleukin-6 (IL-6)	Affects B and T lymphocytes
Interleukin-11 (IL-11)	Controls speed with which human stem cells proliferate and differentiate
Granulocyte colony-stimulating factor (G-CSF)	Stimulates proliferation of progenitor cells committed to granulocyte lineages
Granulocyte-macrophage colony-stimulating factor (GM-CSF)	Promotes proliferation and differentiation of progenitors to neutrophils, macrophages, eosinophils, erythrocytes, and megakaryocytes
Macrophage colony stimulating factor (M-CSF)	Involved in activation and survival of monocytes and macrophages

afferent arterioles in the kidney in response to hypoxic stress. It acts by binding to specific surface receptors on BFU-E and CFU-E cells. The CFU-E and BFU-E cells require IL-3 and Ep for growth. The BFU-E and CFU-E cells undergo additional proliferation prior to terminal differentiation. The proerythroblasts no longer require Ep to complete erythroid differentiation. The CFU-E cells develop into the proerythroblast, followed by the basophilic erythroblast, polychromatophilic erythroblast, normoblast, reticulocyte, and erythrocyte. This developmental sequence requires 2 to 3 days.

The major difference between the proerythroblast (pronormoblast) and the stem cell or CFU-E cell is that the cytoplasm stains somewhat more basophilic since it has begun to acquire polyribosomes, which increase markedly in number and eventually begin to synthesize the protein hemoglobin (Plate 15A). The *proerythroblast* stage is followed by a *basophilic erythroblast* (basophilic normoblast) stage in which the cytoplasm now stains intensely basophilic or dark blue in color in stained bone marrow smears (Plate 15B–D). The basophilic erythroblast has the full complement of polyribosomes necessary for the synthesis of hemoglobin. Since the ba-

sophilic erythroblast synthesizes hemoglobin, which will be retained inside the cell, the synthesis is accomplished primarily by free polyribosomes. When the basophilic erythroblast begins hemoglobin synthesis, a number of small, localized areas appear in the cytoplasm that have a pink color due to the acidophilic staining of the hemoglobin. These cells are called *polychromatophilic* or *polychromatic erythroblasts* (Figs. 9.4, 9.5). *Polychromatophilic* is a term meaning "likes many colors." The "many" colors are two: reddish due to hemoglobin acidophilic staining and blue due to polyribosomes basophilic staining. Frequently, the acidophilic or reddish and basophilic or bluish colors are mixed, producing a bluish-gray color (Plate 15D,E). All stages, including the proerythroblast, basophilic erythroblast, and polychromatophilic erythroblast, are able to divide, thereby increasing the pool of differentiating cells. In approximately 99% of the cases, the polychromatophilic erythroblast is followed by the *orthochromatophilic* (or *orthochromatic*) *erythroblast*, also called the *normoblast* (Plate 16A–C). The cytoplasmic basophilia is lost because the ribosomes are extruded or degenerate and the cytoplasm is completely filled with hemoglobin. All other

Figures 9.4, 9.5. Both figures illustrate polychromatophilic erythroblasts (pyknotic nucleus and
polyribosomes) and mature erythrocytes. ×14,000.

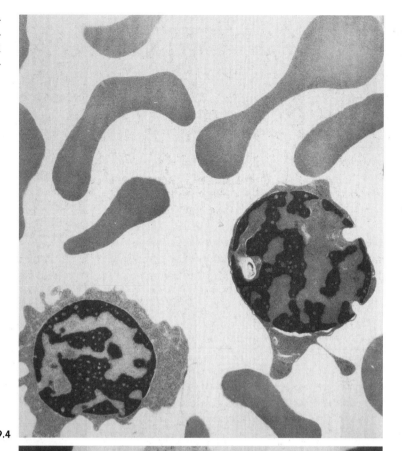

9.4

9.5

organelles are absent, and only an extremely hete-rochromatic, pyknotic nucleus remains. The extrusion of the nucleus is the final event in the transition to an erythrocyte and its entry into the circulation (Plate 16B–D). In limited cases, pieces of chromatin may remain in the erythrocyte; these are called *Howell-Jollie bodies* (Plate 16E). In 1% of the cases, the nucleus is extruded prior to the loss of the polyribosomes; the resulting cell is called a *polychromatophilic* or polychromatic *erythrocyte* or a *reticulocyte* (Plate 16F). When these cells are stained with a supravital dye, the polyribosomes that remain precipitate into a fine, basophilic-stained reticulum, hence the name *reticulocyte*. The polyribosomes are then lost before the erythrocyte enters the circulation. During the course of its development the mammalian erythrocyte is reduced to a membrane-bound bag of proteins, some 90% or more of which is hemoglobin.

FACTORS AFFECTING ERYTHROPOIESIS

The factors presently thought to regulate the survival, proliferation and differentiation of erythroid precursor cells are identified in the table. In addition to erythropoietin several other growth factors, mainly secreted by nonerythroid bone marrow cells, are also important in stimulating growth and differentiation of erythroid precursor cells. Although the information is still incomplete, the effects appear to be mediated by second messenger signaling systems. Still other hematopoietic growth factors are produced locally by cells (*e.g.* T cells, monocytes or fibroid stroma cells) in the bone marrow.

Factors Affecting Erythropoiesis

Factors	Effects
Erythropoietin, IL-1, IL-3, IL-4, GM-CSF	All enhance proliferation and survival of BFU-E cells
IGF-I, PDGF	Stimulate BFU-E and CFU-E cells by enhancing effect of erythropoietin
Activin-A, TGF-β	Peptide growth factors; stimulate growth and differentiation of erythroid cells

Erythropoiesis involves the synthesis of nucleotides followed by the synthesis of hemoglobin. The major stages in differentiation are reviewed in the following chart.

TRANSFERRIN RECEPTOR

Transferrin is a protein that carries iron in the blood. The differentiating erythroblast acquires plasma membrane transferrin receptors that are involved in the uptake of the transferrin-bound iron. Many membrane functions are then lost in the reticulocyte, including the transferrin receptor. Transferrin receptors appear to be internalized in reticulocytes and packaged into multivesicular bodies. The vesicular contents are then externalized by exocytosis.

CONTROL OF ERYTHROPOIESIS

In addition to *Ep* and various growth factors, there are other factors that influence red blood cell differentiation. *Oxygen deficiency* encountered at higher elevations serves as a stimulus for increased erythropoiesis. *Increased temperature* also appears to influence erythropoiesis, for if the tail bones of a rat are transplanted into the body cavity (i.e., increased temperature), the rate of erythrocyte production is elevated. Anemia occurs if there is insufficient vitamin B_{12}. *Vitamin B_{12}* is a coenzyme in the biosynthesis of RNAs. In order for vitamin B_{12} to be absorbed in the digestive tract, an intrinsic factor must be produced by the fundic stomach. If intrinsic factor is not produced, anemia results. The larger than normal erythrocytes that develop during vitamin B_{12} deficiency are termed *megalocytes* or *macrocytes* and have a decreased life span. Since the number of circulating erythrocytes tends to be constant and their normal life span is about 120 days, it is possible to calculate that in a 70-kg man with a turnover rate of 0.83–1.00% daily, 17.9–21.6×10^{10} erythrocytes are produced each day and the same number are destroyed. The changes that trigger the destruction of an erythrocyte are not well understood.

GRANULOPOIESIS

DEVELOPMENTAL STAGES

The differentiation of granular leukocytes is called *granulopoiesis*. The stem cell of blood (CFU cell) differentiates into a CFU-G cell (colony-forming unit-granulocyte) under the stimulation of a postulated hormone called *granulopoietin*. The term *CFU-G* indicates that the cell is committed to differentiate into a granulocyte but cannot be identified cytologically. The CFU-G cell becomes a myeloblast that has dispersed chromatin and nucleoli. However, some texts do not distinguish between the CFU-G cell and the myeloblast. The myeloblast is followed by a *promyelocyte*, which is readily identified cytologically because it synthesizes many primary granules that stain with methylene azure of blood

---

Summary Chart: Erythropoiesis

HEMATOPOIETIC STEM CELL
↓

CFU-E CELL (erythropoietin sensitive; SCF, IL-4)
↓

BFU-E (burst-forming unit-erythroid)
↓

PROERYTHROBLAST
- 12–15 μm in diameter
- Coarse chromatin pattern; nucleus stains pink to red
- Scanty cytoplasm; stains somewhat basophilic (some cytoplasmic polyribosomes)

↓

BASOPHILIC ERYTHROBLAST
- Usually smaller than proerythroblast
- Chromatin more heterochromatic; often clumped, so stains more purple (darker)
- Cytoplasm intensely basophilic (polyribosomes completely synthesized)
- Develops transferrin receptors

↓

POLYCHROMATOPHILIC ERYTHROBLAST
- Smaller than basophilic erythroblast
- Hemoglobin synthesis begins
- Cytoplasm "loves many colors" (polychromatophilic) because polyribosomes stain with basic components of blood stains but hemoglobin stains with acid components of blood stains
- Nucleus is smaller, more heterochromatic, clumped chromatin, so stains very basophilic (deep purple or black) with blood stains
- No nucleoli
- Last cell in erythrocyte series capable of mitosis—about 1 in 100 cases (1% of the time)

↓ ↓

ORTHOCHROMATIC ERYTHROBLAST
- (also called *normoblast*)
- Cytoplasmic basophilia lost (polyribosomes no longer present)
- Cytoplasm acidophilic due to large quantity of hemoglobin
- Cytoplasmic organelles lost
- Spherical, darkly stained, pyknotic nucleus

POLYCHROMATOPHILIC ERYTHROCYTE
- (also called *reticulocyte*)
- Nucleus extruded
- Polyribosomes not lost, but when stained with supravital stains, polyribosomes precipitate into a reticulum

↓ ↓

ERYTHROCYTE
- Nucleus extruded
- Any other organelles extruded

ERYTHROCYTE
- Loss of polyribosomes and other cytoplasmic organelles

---

stains (Plate 15F,G); hence, the granules are called *azurophilic* ("liking azure"). Actually, the development of granulocytes involves the synthesis and packaging of two types of cytoplasmic granules called *primary* and *secondary granules*. The promyelocyte (progranulocyte) may enlarge and acquire an extensive population of cytoplasmic azurophilic granules. These *azurophilic* (primary) *granules* are approximately 0.4 μm in diameter and are lysosomes. They contain histochemically demonstrable peroxidase, acid phosphatase, aryl sulfatase, esterase, β-glucuronidase, β-galactosidase, and 5′-nucleotidase. The specific (secondary) granules appear slightly later in differentiation; thus, it is not possible at this stage to distinguish different types of promyelocytes. The promyelocyte nucleus tends to be spherical and relatively euchromatic; that is, it stains more pink than purple with blood stains. Subsequent changes during differentiation involve a decrease in the size of cells, a decrease in the size of the nuclei, and the appearance of specific secondary granules (i.e., neutrophilic, eosinophilic, or basophilic granules). The nuclei also become more heterochromatic (more purple, less red in their staining), flattened, indented, and then lobated. The promyelocyte transforms into myelocytes of different types, depending upon which specific granules appear in the cytoplasm. There are neutrophilic myelocytes (Plate 15G), eosinophilic myelocytes (Plate 15H,I), and basophilic myelocytes; early in development, a few azurophilic granules may persist. The nuclei of the myelocyte stages are spherical, but they become indented and lobated in the metamyelocyte stage. Neutrophilic metamyelocytes in the circulation are called *band* or *stab neutrophils*.

FACTORS AFFECTING GRANULOPOIESIS

A number of substances are now known to influence differentiation of granulocytes. The *granulocyte-macrophage colony-stimulating factors* (*GM-CSF*) are humoral glycoproteins that stimulate the proliferation of these cells. GM-CSF are present in a variety of tissues and are produced from cells such as endothelial cells, fibroblasts, macrophages, and lymphocytes. While the factors are continuously produced, they increase markedly in emergency conditions such as infections. The GM-CS factors stimulate phagocytosis and the production of metabolically active products synthesized by mature cells. The GM-CSFs also appear to stimulate proliferation of hematopoietic cells of other lineages.

CELL DIFFERENTIATION DURING GRANULOPOIESIS

The stages of granulocyte development are illustrated in the accompanying diagram. The undifferentiated stem cell lacks granules but contains polyribosomes and rER for protein synthesis, a Golgi apparatus, and mitochondria. Primary azurophilic granules are packaged in the Golgi region of the promyelocyte. Secondary or neutrophilic granules are synthesized in the myelocyte stage. Constriction and lobation of the nucleus and increased heterochromatin are characteristic of the metamyelocyte (band and stab stages).

MEGAKARYOCYTES AND PLATELET FORMATION

Megakaryocytes are giant (35–150 μm in diameter) polyploid cells distributed throughout bone marrow (Plate 17A–C). Platelets that circulate in the blood form as excrescences of the megakaryocyte cytoplasm. While the cell body of the megakaryocyte is located in the marrow, long, slender extensions of these cells have been

described to extend through the sinusoidal lining and into the lumen of the venous sinuses. The tendrils that extend from the megakaryocyte cell body can be usefully illustrated in the SEM (Fig. 9.6). The cellular extensions of the megakaryocyte often terminate as rounded tips that are similar in size to nearby isolated platelets, and small but periodic expansions of the megakaryocyte process can be observed (Fig. 9.7). These observations have led to the view that platelets form by the successive pinching off and detachment of segments of the megakaryocyte processes. How the constituents of each platelet might be prepackaged, and details of platelet detachment are unclear. Previously, before the long, slender extensions of the megakaryocyte cell body were observed, it was believed that the platelets originated by a fragmentation process of the megakaryocyte cell body within the marrow. Stem cell factor, IL-3, and IL-6 are all involved in megakaryocyte differentiation from hematopoietic stem cells.

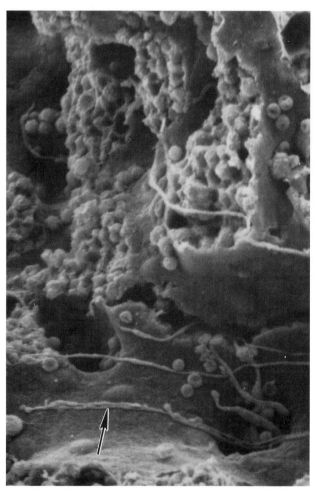

Figure 9.6. SEM of bone marrow showing long, slender processes (arrows) in the lumen of the sinusoids. These projections are from megakaryocytes located in the surrounding marrow. (From R. Kessel and R. Kardon, *Tissues and Organs: A Text-Atlas of Scanning Electron Microscopy*, W.H. Freeman, New York, 1979, with permission)

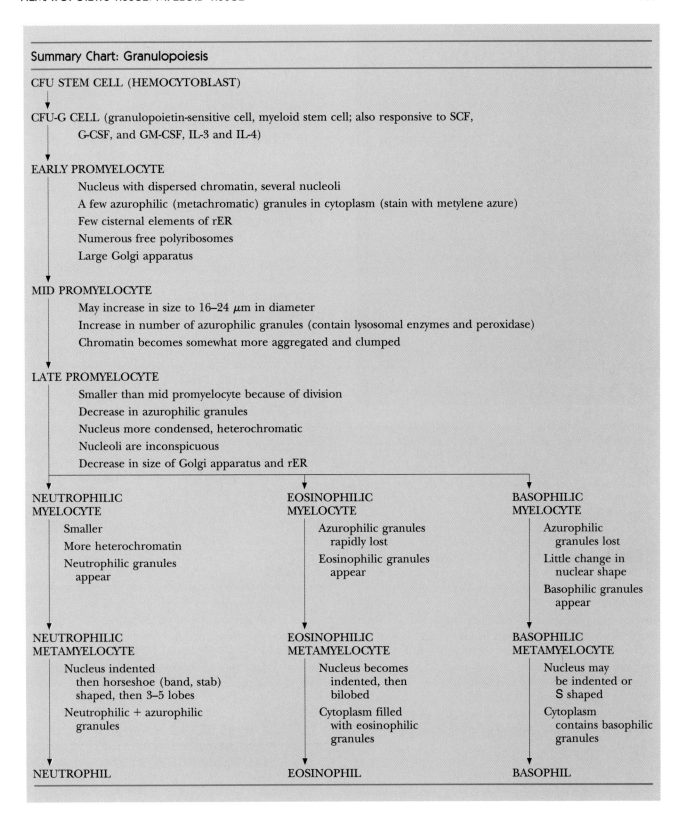

Summary Chart: Granulopoiesis

CFU STEM CELL (HEMOCYTOBLAST)

CFU-G CELL (granulopoietin-sensitive cell, myeloid stem cell; also responsive to SCF,
     G-CSF, and GM-CSF, IL-3 and IL-4)

EARLY PROMYELOCYTE
     Nucleus with dispersed chromatin, several nucleoli
     A few azurophilic (metachromatic) granules in cytoplasm (stain with metylene azure)
     Few cisternal elements of rER
     Numerous free polyribosomes
     Large Golgi apparatus

MID PROMYELOCYTE
     May increase in size to 16–24 μm in diameter
     Increase in number of azurophilic granules (contain lysosomal enzymes and peroxidase)
     Chromatin becomes somewhat more aggregated and clumped

LATE PROMYELOCYTE
     Smaller than mid promyelocyte because of division
     Decrease in azurophilic granules
     Nucleus more condensed, heterochromatic
     Nucleoli are inconspicuous
     Decrease in size of Golgi apparatus and rER

NEUTROPHILIC   EOSINOPHILIC   BASOPHILIC
MYELOCYTE   MYELOCYTE   MYELOCYTE
   Smaller   Azurophilic granules   Azurophilic
   More heterochromatin   rapidly lost   granules lost
   Neutrophilic granules   Eosinophilic granules   Little change in
      appear   appear   nuclear shape
                                                                           Basophilic granules
                                                                              appear

NEUTROPHILIC   EOSINOPHILIC   BASOPHILIC
METAMYELOCYTE   METAMYELOCYTE   METAMYELOCYTE
   Nucleus indented   Nucleus becomes   Nucleus may
      then horseshoe (band, stab)   indented, then   be indented or
      shaped, then 3–5 lobes   bilobed   S shaped
   Neutrophilic + azurophilic   Cytoplasm filled   Cytoplasm
      granules   with eosinophilic   contains basophilic
                                         granules   granules

NEUTROPHIL   EOSINOPHIL   BASOPHIL

PROGRAMMED CELL DEATH

The amount of programmed cell death during hematopoiesis is considerable. The dying cells undergo a change called *apoptosis*. The cell and nucleus shrink, the chromatin condenses, and the nucleus often fragments. Cells that die by accident or injury swell and burst, a process called *necrosis*, and the cellular debris generated can elicit an inflammatory response. Apoptotic cells, in contrast, tend to be rapidly phagocytosed

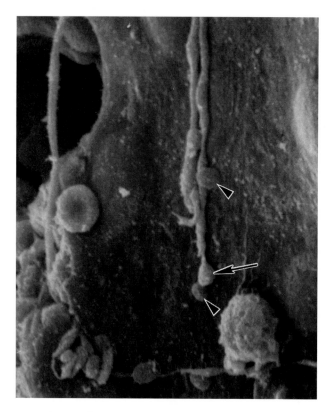

Figure 9.7. SEM of megakaryocyte processes in sinusoids of bone marrow. Note that the tips of the megakaryocyte process (arrow) are rounded and similar in size to
nearby isolated platelets (arrowhead). ×2710. (From R.
Kessel and R. Kardon, *Tissues and Organs: A Text-Atlas of Scanning Electron Microscopy*, W.H. Freeman, New York, 1979,
with permission)

by macrophages so that an inflammatory response is not
generated. Macrophages appear to recognize, by their
surface lectin, altered sugar groups on the apoptotic cell
surface. In other cases, an integrin on the macrophage
surface recognizes an extracellular matrix protein called
thrombospondin, which is secreted by the macrophage
and which seems to act as a bridge between it and the
apoptotic cell. In still other cases, the macrophage apparently recognizes *phosphatidylserine*, a negatively
charged phospholipid normally found in the cytosolic
leaflet of the plasma membrane, which moves to the extracellular leaflet in some apoptotic blood cells.

BLOOD DISORDERS

There are many known blood disorders such as
leukemias, hemophilia, and lymphomas. In addition,
there are several clotting disorders and various diseases
caused by alterations in hemoglobin. The techniques of
gene therapy are currently being used to correct various blood disorders. In such therapy, foreign genes are
introduced into cells of a patient with a disorder in order to correct a problem. Blood is particularly well

suited for gene therapy because the bone marrow can
be removed, genetically altered, and then reintroduced
into the individual. In leukemia, a cancer of the blood,
too many blood cells are produced. In chronic myel-
ogenous leukemia, the marrow stem cells are overactive
and a white blood cell tends to grow out of control at
the expense of other blood cell types. One such cancer
of the blood involves a chromosomal translocation; a
portion of chromosome 22 breaks off and comes to rest
at the tip of chromosome 9, while a piece of chromosome 9 migrates to the tip of the shortened chromosome 22. This is one example of how specific chromosomal translocations are related to different leukemias.

BONE MARROW TRANSPLANTATION

Since various injuries can occur to the stem cells in bone
marrow as a result of certain diseases, or from radiation
therapy or chemotherapy, severe impairment of the immune response may result. In some cases, it is now possible to transplant bone marrow to repopulate the marrow with stem cells. This has had an important impact
in treating cases of certain anemias, autoimmune disorders, and cancers, for example. It is now possible in
certain cases to remove an individual's bone marrow
and subsequently replace it, a procedure called *auto-
transplantation*. Further, the bone marrow of one individual can be injected into another individual with sufficient genetic similarity. This is called *allogenic
transplantation*. Bone marrow can be removed, frozen,
and maintained in the frozen state until required for
future transplantation.

Ep is the principal hormone that regulates proliferation and differentiation of immature erythroid cells.
In mammals, Ep is produced in fetal liver and adult kidney in response to hypoxia. It circulates in the bloodstream to target receptors on progenitor cells in the
bone marrow. Recombinant human erythropoietin is
widely used in the treatment of patients with anemia
due to renal failure, cancer chemotherapy, and azi-
dothymidine treatment.

SELECTED BIBLIOGRAPHY

Becker, R.P., and DeBruyn, P.P. (1976). The transmural passage of blood cells into myeloid sinusoids and the entry of platelets into the sinusoidal circulation. *Am. J.
Anat.* **145**, 183–197.

Campbell, A.D., and Wicha, M.S. (1988). Extracellular matrix and the haemopoietic microenvironment. *J. Lab.
Clin. Med.* **112**, 140–156.

Cannistra, S.A., and Griffin, J.D. (1988). Regulation of production and function of granulocytes and monocytes.
Semin. Hematol. **25**, 173–189.

Clark, S.C., and Kamen, R. (1987). The hemopoietic colony
stimulation factors. *Science* **236**, 1229–1232.

Dexter, T.M., and Spooncer, E. (1987). Growth and differentiation in the hemopoietic system. *Annu. Rev. Cell Biol.* **3**, 423–441.

Evatt, B.L., Levine, R.F., and Williams, N.T. (1981). *Megakaryocyte Biology and Precursors: In Vitro Cloning and Cellular Properties.* Amsterdam, Elsevier/North-Holland.

Golde, D. (1991). The stem cell. *Sci. Am.* **265**, 86–93.

Metcalf, D. (1984). *The Hemopoietic Colony-Stimulating Factors.* Elsevier, Amsterdam.

Metcalf, D. (1985). The granulocyte-macrophage colony stimulation factors. *Science* **229**, 16–21.

Porzig, H. (1991). Signaling mechanisms in erythropoiesis: new insights. *News Physiol. Sci.* **6**, 247–254.

Tavassoli, M., and Yoffey, J.M. (1983). *Bone Marrow Structure and Function.* Alan R. Liss, New York.

Till, J.E., and McCulloch, E.A. (1961). A direct measurement of the radiation sensitivity of normal mouse bone marrow cells. *Radiat. Res.* **14**, 213–222.

Till, T.E., and McCulloch, E.A. (1980). Hemopoietic stem cell differentiation. *Biochem. Biophys. Acta* **605**, 431–439.

Williams, W.J., et al., eds. (1990). *Hematology*, 4th ed. McGraw-Hill, New York.

Wintrobe, M.M. (1980). *Blood, Pure and Eloquent.* McGraw-Hill, New York.

Zucker, M. (1980). The functioning of blood platelets. *Sci. Am.* **242**, 86–103.

Hematopoietic Connective Tissue: Immunity and Lymphatic Tissue

IMMUNITY

INTRODUCTION

All vertebrates possess an immune system that through genetic diversity provides a protective response to nearly any foreign cell or substance. Virtually any macromolecule, if it is perceived as foreign to the host, can induce an immune response. Furthermore, the immune system is able to distinguish proteinaceous antigens that differ in only a single amino acid. Substances that bind to antibody and cause production of antibody are called *antigens*. Thus, an antigen is a substance that can be recognized and bound to receptors on cells of the immune system. The antigen may be an entire organism, such as a bacterium, or individual molecules.

General characteristics

The term *antigen* is derived from "antibody generation" because when antigens enter the body they elicit an immune response. Immune responses are specific. The parts of an antigen that combine with the antigen-binding site of an antibody molecule or lymphocyte receptor are called *antigenic determinants* or *epitopes*. The specificity of the immune response is based on specific receptors in the lymphocyte plasma membrane that are able to distinguish or detect slight differences in antigens. It has been estimated that an individual immune system can recognize and discriminate 10^9 or more distinct antigenic determinants because of the great variability in antigen-binding sites of lymphocyte receptors; *diversity* is thus a characteristic of the immune system. The immune system also has a *memory*. Exposure to an antigen makes it easier to respond once again to the same antigen; this *secondary immune response* is usually more rapid than the *primary immune response*. The immune system is capable of self-regulation so that a response to an antigen is eventually terminated. Finally, the immune system can discriminate between self and non-self molecules. Although the immune system is genetically capable of responding to self-antigens, it is normally unresponsive to its own macromolecules. The process leading to *acquired immunologic tolerance* (self-tolerance) may involve killing any lymphocytes that might be self-reactive cells in a process called *clonal anergy*.

Kinds of immunity

Natural immunity refers to devices that prevent antigen from entering the body such as the integument (Table 10.1). *Acquired immunity* refers to the elimination of antigen in the body. The acquired immunity system has two types of responses: (1) the *humoral immune response*, which is based on the presence of *antibodies* (Figs. 10.1, 10.2) in the blood plasma, and (2) the *cell-mediated response*, which is dependent upon lymphocytes. In the humoral immune response, plasma cells that have differentiated from appropriately stimulated B lymphocytes release antibody into the blood and body fluids. In cell-mediated responses, activated cytotoxic (killer) T lymphocytes destroy defective cells, either foreign or virus-infected cells.

Kinds of T lymphocytes

There are two important types of T lymphocytes (Table 10.2) based on specific plasma membrane receptors: (1) *cytotoxic T cells*, which kill virus-infected cells, and (2)

Table 10.1 Characteristics of Natural and Acquired Immunity

	Natural Immunity	*Specific (Acquired) Immunity*
Cells	Phagocytes, including macrophages, neutrophils, and NK cells	T and B lymphocytes
Circulating molecules	Complement	Antibodies
Soluble mediators	Macrophages produce cytokines (α- and β-interferons, TNF)	Lymphocytes produce cytokines such as γ-interferon
Barrier	Integument and mucous membranes	Immune cells in integument and mucous membranes (antibodies in mucous membrane secretions)

helper T cells, which mediate many immune responses by releasing substances called *cytokines* (Table 10.3) (sometimes called *lymphokines*). There are two types of helper T cells, T_H1 and T_H2. Type I helper cells produce mainly *IL-2* and *interferon-γ* (Table 10.4), which are involved in delayed hypersensitivity reactions and macrophage activation. Type II helper cells produce *IL-4*, *IL-5*, and *IL-10*, which cause a humoral immune response by activating B lymphocytes that produce antibodies after transforming into plasma cells. T_H2 cells also produce *IL-2*, which is involved in all types of T-cell proliferation.

T-cell receptor and co-receptors

The *T-cell receptor* (TCR) consists of several subunits that are involved in antigen binding (Fig. 10.3). The $\alpha\beta$ subunits of the TCR have constant (C) and variable (V) regions. In addition to the TCR, there are two co-receptors, *CD4* and *CD8* (Figs. 10.4, 10.5). T cells are unique in that they require a co-receptor to become active. The *co-receptor* binds the *TCR* to a *major histocompatibility complex (MHC)-peptide complex* (Fig. 10.3). CD4 and CD8 are important in recognizing self MHC complexes and will not bind to non-self MHC. Thus a determination of self and non-self depends on the T-cell–MHC interaction.

T cells involved in helper and inducer functions are classified as *T4 (CD4$^+$)* cells, while T cells with cytotoxic and suppressor functions are classified as *T8 (CD8$^+$)* cells. In the peripheral blood, approximately 60% of the T cells are CD4$^+$ and approximately 40% are CD8$^+$. CD4$^+$ T cells (helper and inducer T cells) respond to antigen that is associated with *class II MHC proteins* and stimulate antibody production by B cells (plasma cells) (Fig. 10.4). In contrast, CD8$^+$ T lymphocytes recognize antigen in association with *class I MHC proteins* and include *cytotoxic T* cells that kill virus-infected cells (Fig. 10.5) or foreign cells and *suppressor T cells*, which assist in regulating the immune response. These molecules and their functional roles are summarized in Table 10.2.

Immune responses may be turned off by expression of CTLA-4, a surface molecule that has an inhibitory role in T-cell activation. Another method of turning off the immune response is through death (apoptosis) of T cells.

Major histocompatibility complex

T cells cannot recognize free antigens, but the antigens must be presented to a T cell after being attached to an *MHC* molecule. MHC are of two types. *Class I MHCs* are expressed on virtually *all nucleated body* cells (Fig. 10.3). *Class II MHCs* are expressed only on *antigen-presenting cells (APC)* such as macrophages (Fig. 10.3). To be activated, a T cell must be presented with an antigen attached to an MHC complex and then a co-stimulatory signal. APCs ingest the antigen, break it into smaller peptides, bind the peptides to the MHC, and present this complex on the surface of an APC; this process is called *antigen processing* (Fig. 10.4). The TCR recognizes the MHC-peptide complex, but it must also be presented with a co-stimulatory signal. The best studied co-stimulatory signal of the T lymphocyte is the *CD28-B7 complex* (Fig. 10.4). *CD28* is a surface glycoprotein expressd by all *CD4+ T cells*, but approximately 50% of the CD8+ T cells express CD28. If CD28 is lacking, T cells presented with a peptide-MHC complex do not become activated. In order for *CD28* to be activated, a complementary structure, called *B7*, must be present on the APC to which the T cell can bind (Fig. 10.4).

DIVERSITY OF THE IMMUNE SYSTEM AND CLONAL SELECTION

The immune system operates by clonal selection. Thus, during development, a lymphocyte becomes committed or programmed to react with a particular antigen prior to exposure to it. This programming induces the for-

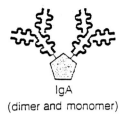

IgA present in limited quantity as a monomer in plasma; dimer (called secretory IgA) is present in body secretions (sweat, milk, saliva); serves to decrease chances of pathogens (e.g., bacteria) adhering to epithelial membranes

IgA
(dimer and monomer)

IgD is bound to external surface of B lymphocytes; functions as antigen receptor and is important in B-cell activation.

IgD
(monomer)

IgE secreted by plasma cells in skin and moist epithelial membranes; stem (constant) region of molecule is bound to surfaces of mast cell and basophil; when receptor end interacts appropriately with antigen, cells release content of secretory granules; little IgE in plasma, but amounts increase with severe parasitic infections or allergic reaction

IgE
(monomer)

IgG comprises about 80% of circulating antibodies in plasma; protective against bacteria, viruses, and toxins in blood and lymph; fixes complement; is principal antibody of the primary and secondary immune responses; crosses placenta--confers passive immunity from mother to fetus.

IgG
(monomer)

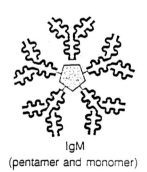

IgM exists in both monomer and pentamer forms: monomer is attached to surface of B cells and acts as antigen receptors; pentamer is the first Ig to be released by plasma cells during primary response; circulates in plasma; able to cause agglutination; activates and fixes complement because of the many antigen-biding sites in this molecule.

IgM
(pentamer and monomer)

Figure 10.1. Important characteristics of the major Ig classes and the general morphology of antibodies.

mation of cell-surface receptor proteins that specifically fit the antigen, and the binding of antigen to the receptor causes the cell to proliferate and mature. By variously combining inherited gene segments that code for the variable regions of the L and H chains of an Ig molecule, an animal can produce thousands of different L and H chains that can associate to form millions of different antigen-binding sites. Variability is further achieved by loss or gain of nucleotides during gene-segment joining and also by somatic mutations.

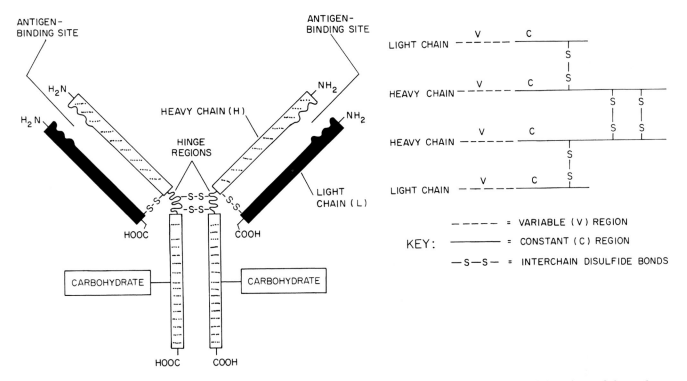

Figure 10.2. Diagram of the antibody (Ig) molecule, including the L and H chains and the V and C regions of the molecule.

Name of Cell	Cluster of Differentiation Determinants (CD Molecules)	HLA (Human Leukocyte Antigen) and MHC (Major Histocompatibility Complex) Molecules	Cytokines Produced	Functions
T$_H$ (T-helper cell)	CD4+	Type II	IL-2, IL-4, IL-5, IL-6, IFN-γ interferon-γ	Interact with antigen-presenting cells (APCs); Induce B cells to respond to antigens; induce differentiation and activation of T$_C$ cells
T$_C$ (T-cytotoxic cells)	CD8+	Type I	Interferon-γ	Produce perforins that lyse foreign cells and virus-infected cells
T$_S$ (T-suppressor cells)	CD8+			Suppress T$_H$ cell activity
T$_M$ (T-memory cells)	CD4+ (T$_H$) CD8+ (T$_C$)			Persist as immunocompetent in circulation and other areas for more rapid secondary immune response

Table 10.2 Types of T Lymphocytes

Table 10.3 Source of Cytokines and Their Actions

Interleukins	Source	Target of Action/Functions
IL-1	Macrophages (antigen-presenting cells)	Activates T helper (T_H) cell; makes T cells responsive to signals; activates fibroblasts, granulocytes, osteoclasts (via osteoblasts)
IL-2	T_H cells	Proliferation of T cells, B cells, and NK cells
IL-3	T_H cells	Stimulates development of hematopoietic cells
IL-4	T_H cells	Activates T cells, mast cells, erythroid cells, macrophages, megakaryocytes, monocytes; B-cell isotype switching to IgG_1 and IgE
IL-5	T cells, macrophages B cells (?)	Stimulates proliferation and differentiation of B cells, eosinophils, basophils; IgA production; acts with IL-2 to cause cytotoxic T cell production
IL-6	T_H cells, macrophages, fibroblasts	Activates T cells; stimulates secretion of IgG by B cells
IL-7	Bone marrow, some T_H cells, macrophages	Differentiation and maturation of B cells
IL-8	Keratinocytes, fibroblasts, monocytes	Neutrophil chemotaxis, activation
IL-9	T cells	Proliferation of T cells, thymocytes, mast cells
IL-10	T cells, mast cells	Proliferation of mast cells; inhibition of cytokine synthesis

Table 10.4A Interferons

Interferon	Origins	Some Functions
INF-α	Produced by leukocytes	Decreases viral replication; antiproliferative
INF-β	Produced by fibroblasts and epithelial cells	Decreases viral replication; antiproliferative
INF-γ	Produced by activated T cells	Activates macrophages; induces class II MHC expression on cells; antagonistic to IL-4

Table 10.4B Colony-Stimulating Factors

	Origins	Some Functions
Granulocyte CSF	Produced by T cells (involved in regulating inflammatory response)	Regulates production of neutrophils, eosinophils, basophils
Granulocyte-monocyte CSF	Produced by T cells (involved in regulating inflammatory response)	Regulates production of monocytes

Notes: Tumor necrosis factor-α (TNF-α) and tumor necrosis factor-β (TNF-β) involved in inflammation, wound healing, tumor defense. Transforming growth factor-β involved in inflammation, wound healing, tumor defense.

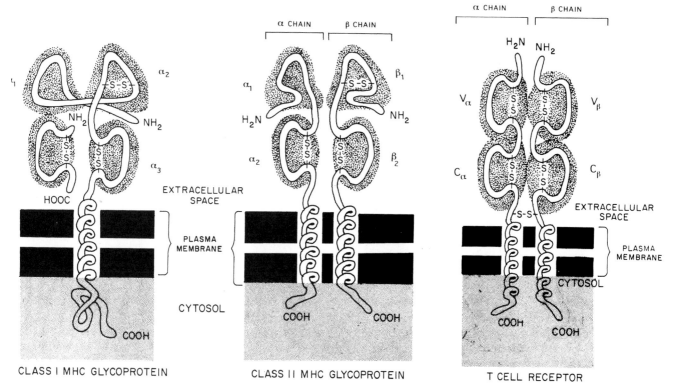

Figure 10.3. Diagrams of TCR, class I and class II MHC glycoproteins. (Redrawn from B. Alberts, D. Bray, F. Lewis, M. Raff, K. Roberts, and F. Watson, *Molecular Biology of the Cell.* 3rd ed., pp. 1228, Garland Publishing Inc., New York, 1994, with permission)

B-CELL FUNCTION

Some stem cells in the bone marrow give rise to B lymphocytes (B cells), which are subsequently released to circulate in the blood and lymph. Contact of these B cells with appropriate and specific antigen presented in conjunction with helper T4 lymphocytes and macrophages causes them to proliferate and differentiate into *plasma cells*, which secrete *humoral antibody*, and *memory cells*, which are responsible for prolonged immunity.

The first antibodies made by a newly formed B cell are not secreted but are inserted into the plasma membrane, where they serve as receptors for antigen. Each B cell has approximately 10^5 antibody molecules in its plasma membrane. Antibodies defend the body from infections by inactivating virus and bacterial toxins, as well as by involving the complement system and activating leukocytes to kill foreign microorganisms and parasites. The humoral antibodies are called *immunoglobulins (Ig)* and comprise about 20% of the blood plasma proteins. When antigen is bound to B cell Ig receptors, it activates *tyrosine protein kinases*, which, in turn, initiate a number of phosphorylation reactions in the B cell, resulting in its activation. The B cell can recognize an antigen because many receptors of a single kind are present in its plasma membrane. The B cell is then stimulated or activated when its receptors come in contact

with the corresponding specific antigen, which may be circulating in the blood or present on the surface of an infected cell. *Helper T cells* are required for most B cells to respond to antigen (Fig. 10.4). Helper T cells help activate B cells by secreting *ILs*. IL-2 is a hormone that promotes proliferation of antigen-activated B cells. Some of the progeny of these activated B cells become plasma cells and actively synthesize antibody that is specific in recognizing the antigen that caused the plasma cell to form. The plasma cell contains extensive quantities of rER. The antibody is released from the cell, and this circulating, or humoral, antibody is distributed in the blood and lymph, where it can bind to the antigen and aid in its removal or destruction. Other progeny of the activated or stimulated B cells do not become plasma cells, but remain with the memory of the antigen that caused the initial activation of the maternal B lymphocyte. These persisting memory B cells, which may circulate in the body for years, permit a more rapid response to a future encounter with the same antigen.

IgM is initially produced by a developing B cell, which then may switch to making other classes (IgA, IgE) of antibody. As IgM is secreted from a B lymphocyte during a primary antibody response, it has five four-chain units that provide a total of 10 antigen-binding sites. The binding of antigen such as the surface of a microorganism to parts of the secreted IgM can activate the first component of the complement system. *Com-*

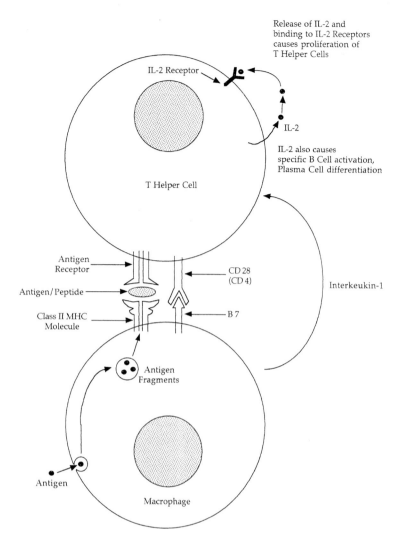

Release of IL-2 and
binding to IL-2 Receptors
causes proliferation of
T Helper Cells

IL-2 Receptor

IL-2

IL-2 also causes
specific B Cell activation,
Plasma Cell differentiation

T Helper Cell

Antigen
Receptor

CD 28
(CD 4)

Antigen/Peptide

Class II MHC
Molecule

B 7

Interkeukin-1

Antigen
Fragments

Antigen

Macrophage

Figure 10.4. Interaction of macrophage and helper T Lymphocyte.

plement involves a complex series of some 20 circulating soluble enzymatic proteins that are present in normal serum and which interact to combine with antigen-antibody complexes, resulting in cell lysis when the antigen is a foreign cell.

IgG is produced in considerable quantity during the secondary immune response. It can activate the complement system. In addition, the Fc region of an IgG molecule binds to receptors on macrophages and neutrophils, causing them to bind to, ingest, and destroy the microorganism. Thus, when a bacterium becomes coated with IgG antibody, since the macrophage or neutrophil has receptors in its plasma membrane that are able to bind the Fc region of IgG molecules, the bacterium can be phagocytized and destroyed.

The B lymphocytes are widely distributed in lymphatic nodules present in lymph nodes, spleen, digestive tract, and tonsils. Solitary lymphatic nodules are also distributed under moist epithelial membranes; they are imperfect barriers to the entry of foreign antigens and microorganisms. B lymphocytes are also widely distributed in loose connective tissues.

The ends of both L and H chains of an antibody molecule contribute to the antigen-binding site. The antigen-binding sites of the antibody bind to specific parts of the antigen molecule called *antigenic determinants*. If two or more of these antigenic determinants are identical, the antigen is called *multivalent*. Only multivalent antigen molecules can stimulate B cells by themselves, without the intervention of helper T cells. A number of microbial polysaccharides can directly stimulate B lymphocytes to proliferate and mature without assistance from T helper cells. These are called *T-cell-independent antigens*. They are typically large polymers with repeating, identical antigenic determinants.

MACROPHAGES AND NATURAL KILLER CELLS

Other important cells in the immune system are the APCs and natural killer (NK) cells. The major APC is the macrophage. Macrophages abound in the lymph nodes, spleen, and thymus. Macrophages in the spleen and lymph nodes assist in the presentation of antigen

Figure 10.5. Interaction of cytotoxic T lymphocytes and virus-infected cell.

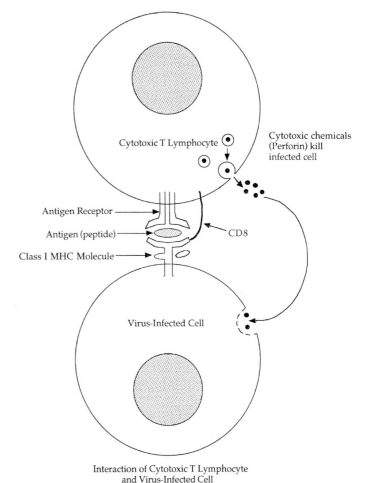

Interaction of Cytotoxic T Lymphocyte and Virus-Infected Cell

to T and B lymphocytes that might circulate through these organs and thus be recognized as foreign. These cells are scavengers that develop from blood monocytes and can phagocytize virus or other particulate material. Once the macrophage ingests and digests the virus, for example, the resulting antigenic fragments are displayed, along with the class II MHC proteins, on the macrophage surface membrane so that T4 cells can recognize the antigen. Some helper T cells activate macrophages by secreting interferon-γ. Macrophages secrete substances such as *interferon-γ* and *IL-1*, which cause the fever and malaise associated with many viral infections. Cellular interactions in immune responses are summarized in Figure 10.6.

The proliferation of T cells is controlled by IL-2 after an antigen that has been ingested and presented by a macrophage activates individual T cells. The antigen stimulates the T cells to secrete IL-2 and to make IL-2 receptors. The binding of IL-2 to its receptors is the cue that signals the T cells to divide, resulting in a clone of identical antigen-specific T cells that eliminate the antigen from the body. Antibodies that block the binding of IL-2 to its receptor completely inhibit the antigen-specific proliferation of T cells in tissue culture.

NK cells originate and differentiate from precursor bone marrow cells; they are especially prevalent in the spleen. NK cells have a relatively short life span. Approximately 9–10% of the peripheral blood lymphocytes have NK activity. The ability of the NK cell to lyse Ig-coated targets is due to the expression of a receptor for the constant (Fc) portion of Ig on NK cells. When a variety of receptors on NK cell surfaces are activated, intracellular signals are generated that result in exocytosis of granule contents, lysis of targets, alteration of gene expression, and/or proliferation of NK cells.

NK cells are able to destroy virus-infected cells and tumor or cancer cells directly, without interacting with lymphocytes or being able to recognize a particular antigen. Thus, *NK cells are not antigen-specific*, but rather attack any foreign molecule. They comprise about 10% of the total circulating lymphocyte population and are stimulated by *IL-2*.

INTERLEUKINS AND INTERFERONS

Cytokines are soluble polypeptide and glycoproteins that are similar to hormones but may not be endocrine-de-

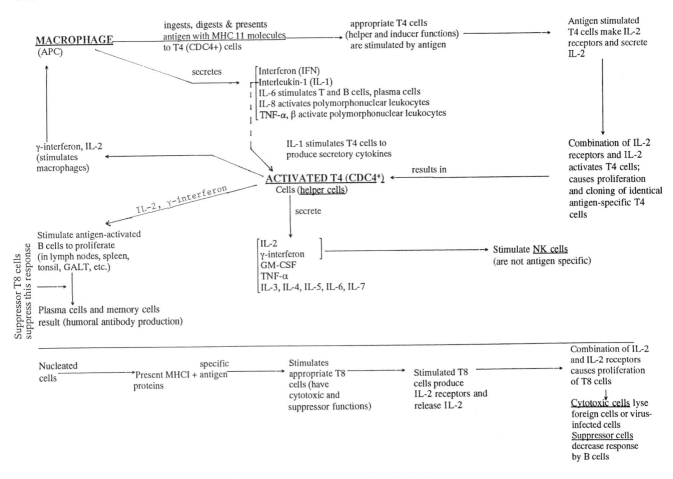

Figure 10.6. Summary of cellular interactions in the immune response.

rived. Cytokines often act locally, usually in an autocrine or paracrine fashion. They regulate cellular activity (including growth, differentiation, and function) by binding to receptors and are extremely effective at low concentrations. Initial terms used included *lymphokine* and *monokine*, depending upon whether the substances were produced by lymphocytes or monocytes/macrophages. The term *interleukin* was later introduced together with an identifying number (e.g., IL-1, IL-2). Since ILs affect other cell types in addition to leukocytes, the term *cytokine* is now more widely used.

The interactions between immune and inflammatory cells are in large measure mediated by IL, which are proteins. Some 10 ILs have been described. They originate from cell types such as macrophages, keratinocytes, T cells, mast cells, B cells, and monocytes. Some of the functions of ILs overlap. For example, IL-1, IL-6, and IL-8 are described as proinflammatory. IL-2 and IL-9 are potent lymphocyte growth factors. IL-4 and IL-5 are involved in Ig isotype switching. IL-3 causes proliferation of hematopoietic stem cells. IL-10 appears to depress cytokine synthesis, thus participating in a negative feedback effect. IL-1 and IL-6 are produced by macrophages and play important roles in immunity and inflammation. T cells produce IL-2 through IL-6.

IL-1 and IL-6 induce fever. IL-2 markedly enhances proliferation of T cells, *NK cells*, and lymphokine-activated killer cells. IL-4 through IL-6 enhance B-cell proliferation and antibody production. Differentiation of eosinophils is markedly enhanced by IL-5. The properties of some selected ILs are summarized in the accompanying table.

Still another group of cytokines are the *interferons* (*IFNs*). Three major classes of IFN are presently known: IFN-α, IFN-β, and IFN-γ. IFN-α is produced by leukocytes. IFN-β is produced by both fibroblasts and epithelial cells. IFN-α and IFN-β tend to suppress viral replication and proliferation in a number of cell types. IFN-γ is produced by activated T cells and is an important activator of macrophages. Finally, various CSFs, as indicated in Table 10.4, are examples of cytokines.

IMMUNE RESPONSE TO MEASLES VIRUS INFECTION

The interplay of cells and events in an immune response can be reviewed by briefly analyzing the body's response to a viral infection such as measles. Cells infected with measles virus secrete IFNs, which stimulate activity by NK cells within 1 or 2 days of infection. Then

Properties of Selected Interleukins

Interleukin	Source	Principal Target	Principal Action in Immune Response
IL-1	Antigen-presenting cells	T_H cells; also B cells, cytotoxic T cells	Involved in T_H cell activation and induces IL-2 production; regulates B-cell differentiation, cytotoxic T-cell development.
IL-2	Some T_H cells	All activated T and B cells	Stimulates proliferation of T and B cells; activates NK cells, antibody-reproducing B cells.
IL-3	Some T_H cells	Some hematopoietic cells	Stimulates hematopoietic cell proliferation (including macrophages, neutrophils, mast cells, megakaryocytes)
IL-4	Some T_H cells	B cells	Stimulates proliferation and maturation of B cells (and switching to IgE and IgG1); also stimulates differentiation erythroid cells, macrophages, monocytes, mast cells, monocytes
IL-5	T_H cells that also produce IL-4	B cells, eosinophils	Stimulates proliferation and maturation of B cells, eosinophils, basophils; with IL-2 stimulates cytotoxic T-cell production
IL-6	Some T_H cells and macrophages	Activated B cells, T cells	Stimulate B cells to secrete Ig; assist in T-cell activation
Interferon-γ	T_H cells that also produce IL-2	B cells, macrophages, endothelial cells	Activates macrophages: Activates certain MHC genes (induces class II MHC molecules)

macrophages ingest and degrade the virus. The viral proteins, the antigens, are displayed together with class II MHC proteins on the surface of macrophages. Activated T cells produce soluble factors called lymphokines. IL-2 is a lymphokine secreted by T4 and T8 cells. In response to IL-2, the antigen stimulates T cells to proliferate into expanded clones of mature cells including cytotoxic, suppressor, and helper T cells. In approximately a week, cytotoxic T cells lyse the measles virus-infected cells. The number of suppressor T cells formed after several weeks of infection is then sufficient to reduce or suppress the cytotoxic T-cell response. Helper and inducer T4 cells act by direct contact or by producing and releasing lymphokines, and are necessary for the action of cytotoxic and suppressor T cells. Helper and inducer T cells also produce IL-2, which stimulates macrophages to ingest virus and present surface antigen. Memory T cells persist from a reaction to measles virus, and they may persist for life. In addition, helper T cells cause antigen-specific B cells to multiply into populations of antibody-secreting plasma cells and memory B cells. The helper T cells act on B cells either by direct contact or by the elaboration of lymphokines such as interferon-γ. The plasma cells then release humoral antibody that can degrade the measles virus. Eventually the B-cell response is decreased due to suppressor T8 cell activity.

ANTIGEN-ANTIBODY COMPLEXES AND COMPLEMENT

The complexes resulting from the binding of antigen and antibody can facilitate phagocytosis of the antigen or activate a system of blood proteins called *complement* that kills the antigen. Complement consists of a number of serum proteins that can be activated either by antigen-antibody complexes or by microorganisms. The complement system consists of about 20 interactive, soluble proteins that are synthesized in the liver and circulate in the blood and tissue fluids. When activated, the proteins undergo a number of proteolytic reactions that ultimately result in the formation of membrane attack complexes. Such complexes can form small holes in the microorganisms so as to destroy them. Complement also improves on the ability of phagocytic cells to bind to, ingest, and destroy the microorganisms under attack. Complement *complements* and amplifies the antibody action, and the complement system is involved in defense against most bacterial infections.

LYMPHATIC TISSUE

INTRODUCTION

Lymphatic or lymphoid tissue is an important specialized hematopoietic connective tissue. This tissue actually consists of discrete organs including the thymus, lymph nodes, and spleen, as well as nonencapsulated lymphatic nodules comprising the tonsils and Peyer's patches in the ileum. The lymphatic tissues or organs play a central role in immunity and in the generation of an immune response. The circulation of lymphocytes in both blood and lymph is important, allowing the cells to contact the specific antigens that they recognize. Further, the circulation permits lymphocytes to come into contact with each other, which is necessary for an immune response. Lymphocytes are highly migratory within lymphatic tissues and in the bloodstream. They have surface adhesion proteins that cause the cells to adhere to endothelial cells of postcapillary venules and, to a less extent, other en-

dothelial cells. The lymphocyte surface also has stronger adhesion molecules whose activity is preliminary to exiting the blood vessel into, for example, a lymph node. Because of these functions, lymphocyte receptors have been referred to as *homing* receptors.

THYMUS

Organization and cell types

The thymus is a pinkish-gray, bilobed, H-shaped structure located immediately below the superior portion of the sternum and below the thyroid gland. The thymus is large in the fetus and juveniles, but it tends to undergo involution in response to the sex hormones produced in puberty. The thymus develops embryologically as paired outgrowths of the endodermal epithelium of the third pharyngeal pouches. The epithelial outgrowths detach from the embryonic pharynx and are pulled into the upper part of the thorax.

Each lobe of the thymus is subdivided either completely or incompletely into lobules, and each lobule is surrounded by a small amount of connective tissue (Fig. 10.7). Each of the numerous lobules contains an outer

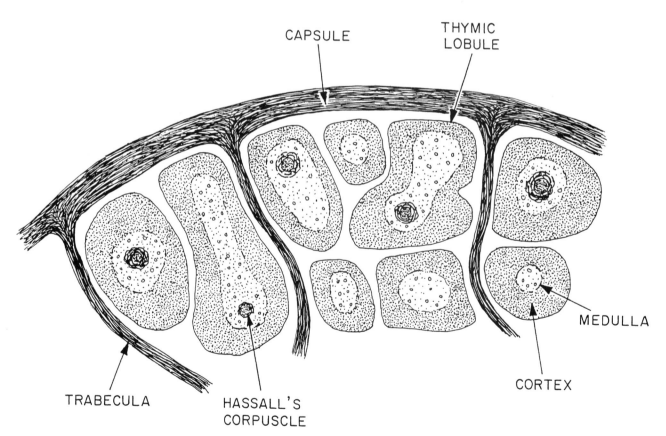

Figure 10.7. Diagram illustrates several thymic lobules. The cortex is densely packed with T lymphocytes and T lymphoblasts. The cortex contains macrophages and highly branched or stellate epithelial reticular cells (derived from endoderm). The medulla contains many more epithelial reticular cells, some of which are flattened and concentrically arranged around keratin or keratohyalin (collectively called *thymic corpuscles* or *Hassall's corpuscles*). The capsule and trabeculae contain connective tissue and blood vessels.

cortex and an inner medulla. The cortex stains darker than the medulla because of the presence of many closely packed cells with heterochromatic-staining nuclei (Plate 18A–D). The cells present in the cortex include *epithelial reticular cells, macrophages, T lymphoblasts,* and *T lymphocytes* (Fig. 10.8). The epithelial reticular cells are derived from endoderm and are highly branched (Fig. 10.9). Branches of adjacent epithelial reticular cells touch, and desmosomes are located in these regions such that many epithelial reticular cells form a cytoreticulum, or cellular reticulum, in the interstices of which are packed many T lymphoblasts and T lymphocytes, as well as macrophages (Figs. 10.9–10.12). There are no reticular fibers in the thymus

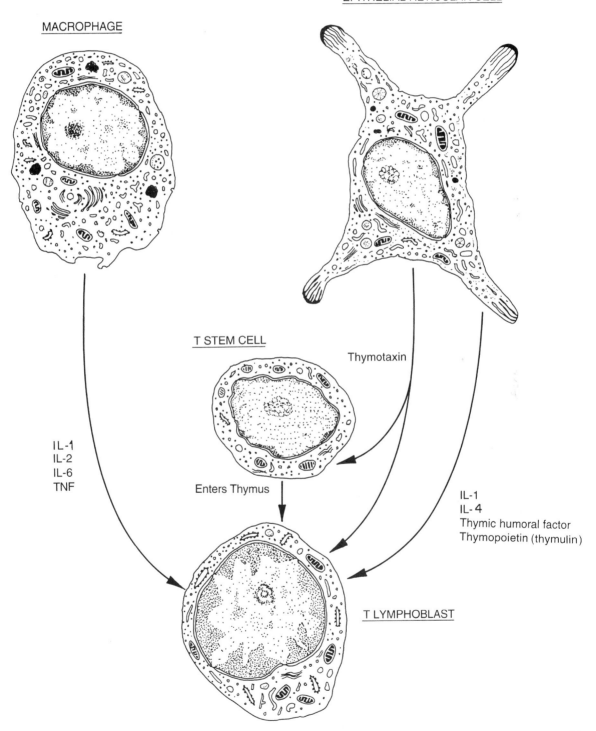

Figure 10.8. Diagram of cells in the thymus (macrophage, epithelial-reticular cell, T stem cell, and T lymphoblast) and some of the important molecules participating in T-cell differentiation.

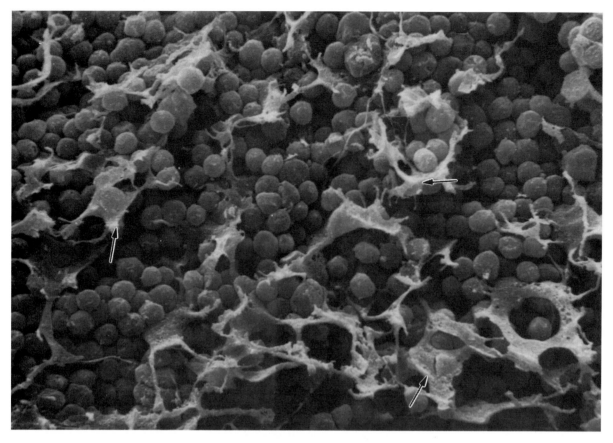

Figure 10.9. SEM of thymus cortex. Pieces of epithelial-reticular cells (arrows) are surrounded by many T lymphoblasts and lymphocytes. ×1420. (From R. Kessel and R. Kardon, *Tissues and Organs: A Text-Atlas of Scanning Electron Microscopy*. W.H. Freeman, New York, 1979)

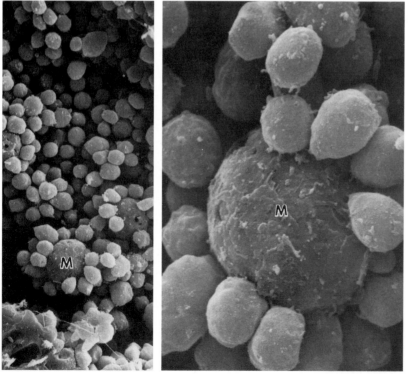

Figures 10.10, 10.11. SEM of thymus cortex. The large, round cells are macrophages (M). Note how T lymphocytes cluster and seem to stick to the macrophage. Figure 10.10, ×1100; Figure 10.11, ×2860. (From R. Kessel and R. Kardon, *Tissues and Organs: A Text-Atlas of Scanning Electron Microscopy*. W.H. Freeman, New York, 1979)

10.10

10.11

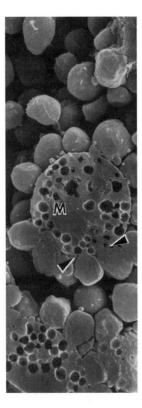

Figure 10.12. SEM of fractured preparation of thymus cortex. The macrophage (M) has a number of vacuolated areas, and a lymphocyte (arrowheads) appears to be in the initial stage of being ingested. ×2200. (From R. Kessel and R. Kardon, *Tissues and Organs: A Text-Atlas of Scanning Electron Microscopy.* W.H. Freeman, New York, 1979)

because mesoderm-derived reticular cells are not present there. Both macrophages and epithelial-reticular cells serve as APCs.

General function

Precursor T cells arise in the bone marrow and move to the thymus early in embryonic development. In the thymic cortex the thymocytes divide, mature, and undergo a selection process. Early T-cell development in the thymus involves a number of coordinated interactions between thymocytes and a protein on the surface of stromal cells. The stem cells that colonize the thymus are eventually committed to express either $\gamma\delta$ or $\alpha\beta$ T-cell antigen receptors. The thymocytes that emerge from the thymus are either CD4+ or CD8+.

The stem cells (a type of CFU cell) develop into T lymphoblasts and undergo extensive proliferation, forming many T lymphocytes packed in the cortex. The differentiated and preprogrammed T lymphocytes constitute a diverse genetic population capable of recognizing a vast array of foreign proteins. There appear to be several hundred immunoglobulin receptor molecules in the plasma membrane of the programmed T lymphocyte. For about 15 years, the thymus continues

to produce a large population of T lymphocytes with enormous genetic variability for recognizing many different foreign proteins. Many of these programmed T lymphocytes are delivered via the circulatory system to specific regions of the lymph nodes and spleen, where they colonize specific regions called *thymus-dependent areas.* During their release from the thymus, the T lymphocytes move into the medulla region of the lobules and apparently migrate through walls of postcapillary venules.

T-cell formation

The T lymphocytes that originate in and become programmed in the thymus are long-lived, persisting for years in some cases. They can circulate between the blood and lymph, so they are likely to be exposed to any antigen that might gain access to the body.

Stem cells for the generation of T lymphocytes arise in the yolk sac and embryonic liver and travel in the bloodstream to the thymus, where they are induced to enter the thymus by a chemotactic peptide called *thymotaxin* (Fig. 10.8). Thymotaxin is secreted by epithelial reticular cells near the capsule. An enormous number of T cells result from the proliferation of T lymphoblasts that form from the stem cells. Initially, the T cells are immature and unable to take part in an immune reaction or response, but during their differentiation and maturation in the thymic cortex, the cells acquire distinctive surface marker molecules (CD4+ or CD8+) that determine the specificity to MHC molecules (either MHC I or MHC II). In addition, T cells synthesize plasma membrane receptors that recognize foreign antigens and determine the specificity for MHC molecules. The genes for the α- and β-receptor chains undergo extensive rearrangement to produce a large variety of genetic sequences. If sequences are produced that recognize self-MHC molecules, they normally undergo programmed cell death (apoptosis). This selection process results in an enormous amount of cell death in the thymus. Those T cells that cannot react to self-molecules undergo clonal expansion. The immunologically competent T cells enter the circulation through the walls of postcapillary venules at the corticomedullary junction. Lymphocytes are therefore much less numerous in the medulla than in the cortex. Many T lymphocytes undergo cell death in the cortex, where they are disposed of by macrophages (Fig. 10.13).

Hassall's corpuscles

Several different types of epithelial reticular cells have been described in the thymus based on different antigenic properties. For example epithelial reticular cells in Hassall's corpuscles react with anti-epidermal antibodies, but other epithelial reticular cells do not. Hassall's corpuscles are characteristic elements of the thy-

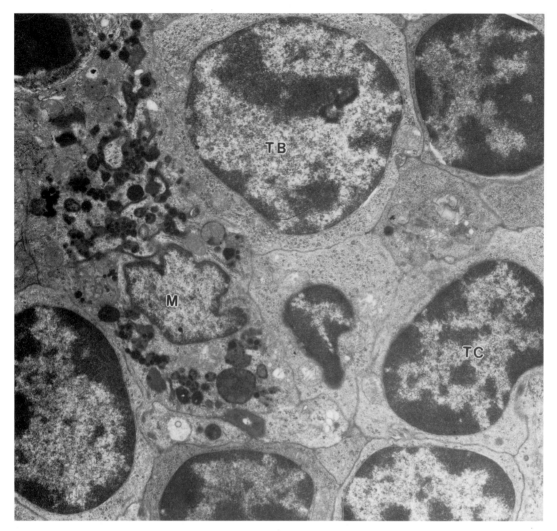

Figure 10.13. TEM of thymus cortex. The macrophage (M) contains many secondary lysosomes or digestive vacuoles. T lymphoblasts (TB) and T lymphocytes (TC) are also present. ×9750. (From R. Kessel and R. Kardon, *Tissues and Organs: A Text-Atlas of Scanning Electron Microscopy.* W.H. Freeman, New York, 1979)

mus medulla. They consist of concentric arrays of flattened cells with desmosomes and prominent bundles of tonofilaments that indicate the epithelial nature of these cells. Keratin and keratohyalin are often present (Plate 19A,B). Although the function of Hassall's corpuscles is unclear, they do not appear to be static structures since antigenic stimulation and irradiation both cause sequential changes in the corpuscles characterized by an increase in size and number, disappearance, and reconstitution. In some animals at least, Hassall's corpuscles may be broken down by macrophages shortly after birth and replaced by newly formed corpuscles.

Epithelial-reticular cells

Epithelial-reticular cells appear to secrete peptides that act locally on cells in the thymus (Fig. 10.8). *Thymulin* (thymopoietin) or thymic humoral factor appears to have an effect on the synthesis of T-cell markers and to play an important role in T-cell clonal expansion and differentiation. Various subtypes of epithelial-reticular cells have been described based primarily on slight ultrastructural differences. Some of the cortical epithelial reticular cells have been shown to have *MHC molecules* on their surface. Therefore, these cells appear to be important in the development of self-tolerance and the MHC–T-cell immune response. Epithelial-reticular cells in the thymus secrete the cytokines *IL-1* and *IL-4*, which affect T-lymphocyte differentiation. The *macrophages* in the thymus can also secrete cytokines (*IL-1, IL-2, IL-6,* and *TNF*) that are important in T-cell clonal proliferation and maturation.

Circulation

Arteries in the thymus are branches of the internal thoracic arteries. Arterioles near the cortical-medullary junction give off capillaries that loop into the cortex. Some of these cortical capillary loops are connected by collateral anastomoses. The capillaries are continuous with postcapillary venules at the cortical-medullary boundary. Thus, the cortex of the thymic lobules are supplied exclusively by capillaries. When electron-opaque tracers were used to assess the vascular permeability of the thymic cortex, very little transendothelial movement of tracer from the blood into the thymic cortex occurred. Medullary vessels, in contrast, are much more permeable to marker or tracer molecules in the blood plasma.

T-cell maturation and thymus-blood barrier

During the early stages of T-lymphocyte formation in the thymus, the cells are susceptible to a "premature encounter" with an antigen they are programmed to recognize. In fact, a premature encounter with the antigen before the lymphocyte is mature could be fatal to the lymphocyte. It is also important to note that none of these T cells should recognize any of the host's own cells as foreign during fetal life, when many T lymphocytes are being produced. For if this occurred, an immunologic reaction to self-proteins would result. In fact, a number of autoimmune diseases are known in which the T cells for some reason believe that certain of the body's cells or proteins are foreign, and they attempt to reject or destroy them. It appears that the reason

wrongly programmed T lymphocytes are not formed in the fetus is that blood flows freely through all parts of the thymus, exposing the differentiating and maturing T cells to all host proteins. Since this occurs before T lymphocytes become mature, any T lymphocytes that might recognize its host's body proteins as foreign would be killed by a premature encounter with the antigen. This would likely cause extensive cell death in the thymus during fetal life, and there does, in fact, appear to be an enormous amount of cell death during this time. Macrophages can injest these dying T lymphocytes.

What then prevents foreign proteins that enter the body after birth from killing by a premature encounter those T lymphocytes being produced in the thymus that might recognize these proteins as foreign? The basis for this selectivity seems to be a change in the nature of the blood circulation in the thymus at birth by the development of a *thymic-blood barrier* (Figs. 10.14, 10.15). In fetal life, there are no circumferential tight or occluding junctions between endothelial cells of capillaries in the thymic cortex. Therefore, cells and substances circulating in the blood can circulate freely in the thymus. However, after birth, extensive *circumferential tight junctions* are present between endothelial cells of the capillaries in the thymic cortex. In addition to the endothelial cell tight junctions, the endothelium is surrounded

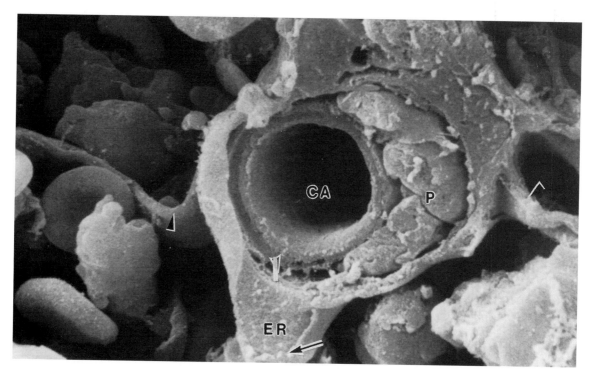

Figure 10.14. SEM of thymus cortex. Branches of an epithelial-reticular cell (ER) are denoted by arrowheads. Capillary (CA), basal laminae of endothelium and epithelial-reticular cells (arrows), possible pericyte or macrophage (P) in the perivascular space. Capillaries in the thymus cortex are ensheathed by basal laminae and the branched epithelial-reticular cells. After birth there are circumferential

tight junctions associated with these capillary endothelial cells; collectively, these components comprise the thymus-blood barrier for protecting developing T lymphoblasts from a premature encounter with an antigen. ×5670. (From R. Kessel and R. Kardon, *Tissues and Organs: A Text-Atlas of Scanning Electron Microscopy*. W.H. Freeman, New York, 1979)

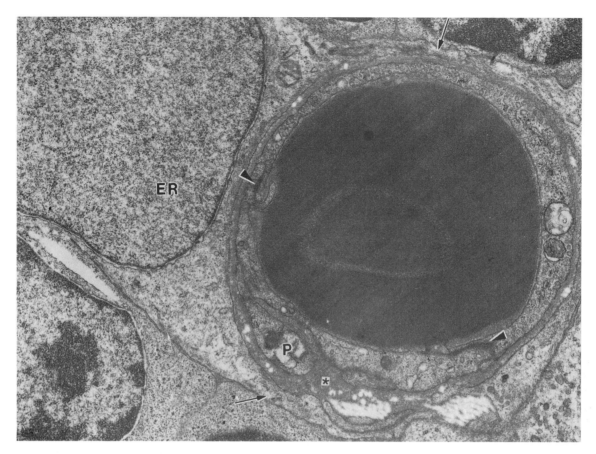

Figure 10.15. TEM of a capillary (with erythrocyte) in thymus cortex. Junctions between endothelial cells are denoted by the arrowhead. Cytoplasm of a macrophage or pericyte (P), basal laminae (*), and epithelial-reticular (ER) cell that ensheathes (arrows) the capillary. ×17,400. (From R. Kessel and R. Kardon, *Tissues and Organs: A Text-Atlas of Scanning Electron Microscopy.* W.H. Freeman, New York, 1979)

by a basal lamina, and both *pericytes* and *macrophages* may be located in the perivascular space. Further, the *epithelial reticular cells* completely ensheath the capillaries in the thymic cortex, and these cells are also lined with an inner basal lamina (Fig. 10.16). Therefore, under these protective conditions, it would be difficult for an antigen to traverse the endothelium, cross the endothelial basal lamina, traverse the perivascular space containing a pericyte or macrophage, and cross the basal lamina and epithelial reticular cell cytoplasm to reach the differentiating T lymphoblasts. The thymus-blood barrier, therefore, is functionally important and effective in preventing a premature encounter between a forming T lymphoblast and its specific antigen. The mature, preprogrammed T lymphocytes penetrate the blood vessel wall near the cortical-medullary junction of thymic lobules and circulate throughout the body.

Immunologic tolerance

Immunologic tolerance develops in the fetus when immature lymphocytes are exposed to self-antigens. T lymphocytes learn to distinguish between self and non-self

in the thymus; the process involves rearrangement of TCR genes. Negative selection of T lymphocytes occurs after interaction of the TCR with self-antigen and MHC molecules. T lymphocytes are positively selected by having receptors that recognize self-MHC proteins. The interaction of the self-MHC molecules and T lymphocytes occurs on epithelial-reticular cells in the thymus without any foreign peptide. Thus, whether a T cell becomes a CD4+ or CD8+ population is determined by the cell's interaction with class I or class II MHC molecules.

Immunologic tolerance to certain foreign antigens can sometimes be induced successfully, but this is easier to accomplish in immature animals than in adults. Tolerance can sometimes be produced by injecting the antigen either in a high dose or in repeated low doses. In some cases, an immunosuppressive drug must be used. Thus, binding of antigen to receptors on lymphocytes can either stimulate the lymphocyte to divide and mature or inactivate or eliminate the lymphocyte, producing tolerance. Many factors seem to determine the outcome, such as the maturity of the lymphocyte and the nature and concentration of the antigen, as well as interactions between the lymphocytes and APCs.

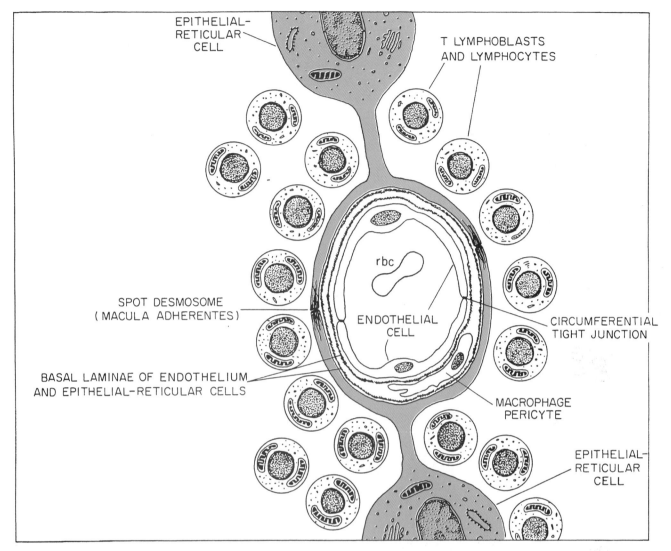

Figure 10.16. Diagram illustrates how epithelial-reticular cells ensheath the cortical capillary network in the thymic cortex and are stabilized by desmosomes. The endothelial cells of these cortical capillaries may have circumferential zonula occludentes after birth, and a macrophage or pericyte is present in the perivascular space. The basal lamina of the endothelium and epithelial reticular cells also invest the capillary.

Abnormalities in the acquisition of self-tolerance do arise, however, and can lead to potentially fatal autoimmune diseases. For example, *myasthenia gravis* is an autoimmune disease in which infected individuals make antibodies against acetylcholine receptors on their skeletal muscle fibers. The antibodies thus formed do not permit normal functioning of the receptors. It is possible for such individuals to die because of breathing difficulties due to defective motor end plates on the intercostal muscles.

Age-related changes in the immune system

The aging process typically involves a variety of changes in the immune system and its function. In addition to involution of the thymus, the number of circulating helper T cells decreases and the T cells, in general, show impaired proliferative ability. Older individuals produce fewer antibodies after immunization, and autoantibodies may increase in number. The general decline in immune surveillance in older individuals has been postulated to be one reason for the increase in cancer and infections.

LYMPH NODES

Organization

Lymph nodes are lima bean-shaped structures that are located, often in groups, in scattered areas of the body such as in the elbow, neck, armpit, knee, and groin, along the aorta, and in other regions of the body. The node is surrounded by a connective tissue capsule that extends for varying distances into the interior (Fig.

10.17). These connective tissue extensions of the capsule, called trabeculae, are variable in number. The capsule on the convex side of the node is pierced by a number of *afferent lymphatic vessels* that have valves to direct the flow of lymph into the node (Fig. 10.17). Lymph nodes, in fact, represent a type of lymphatic tissue designed to filter lymph. The lymph that flows into the node passes through a number of channels, called *sinuses*, that converge into an efferent lymph vessel at the hilus region that emerges from the concave side of the node (Fig. 10.17). The interior of the lymph node is populated by a multitude of cells, but some regions of the node have higher concentrations of cells than others (Fig. 10.18). The connective tissue stroma of the lymph node's interior contains many reticular fibers together with the cells that formed these fibers, the reticular cells, which are derived from mesenchyme. Thus, reticular connective tissue constitutes the connective tissue stroma of a node. Blood vessels and nerves supply all areas of the lymph node interior.

The lymph node is divided into an outer *cortex* and an inner *medulla* (Plate 19C). Many closely packed cells are organized into spherical aggregations called *lymphatic nodules*, which are located in the cortex (Fig. 10.17). The lymphatic nodules stain dark blue with hematoxylin because of the large number of closely packed, nucleated cells with heterochromatin (Plate 19C). Cords of cells extend from the cortical lymphatic nodules into the central region or medulla of the lymph node; these are called *medullary cords* (Plate 19C; Fig. 10.17). They also stain dark blue with hematoxylin because of the many closely packed, nucleated cells. Surrounding the cortically placed lymphatic nodules, which are continuous with the medullary cords, are a number of lighter stained regions called *sinuses* (Plate 19C). These sinuses have different names, depending upon their location within the lymph node. Immediately internal to the capsule is a *subcapsular sinus*, which completely invests the convex surface beneath the capsule (Figs. 10.17, 10.18). Lymph that comes to the lymph

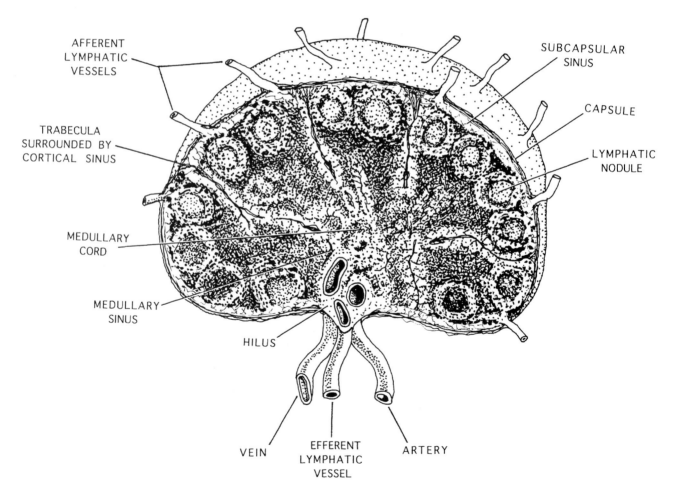

AFFERENT LYMPHATIC VESSELS

SUBCAPSULAR SINUS

CAPSULE

TRABECULA SURROUNDED BY CORTICAL SINUS

LYMPHATIC NODULE

MEDULLARY CORD

MEDULLARY SINUS

HILUS

VEIN

EFFERENT LYMPHATIC VESSEL

ARTERY

Figure 10.17. Diagram illustrates a section of a lymph node. Afferent lymphatic vessels that contain valves pierce the capsule and communicate with the subcapsular sinus, cortical sinus, and medullary sinus and exit the node as an efferent lymphatic vessel that also contains valves. The more cellular regions of the node include the lymphatic nodules with germinal centers, internodular cortex, and medullary cords. Arteries enter the node at the hilus and branch many times to supply the node and nodules. Veins also exit the node at the hilus.

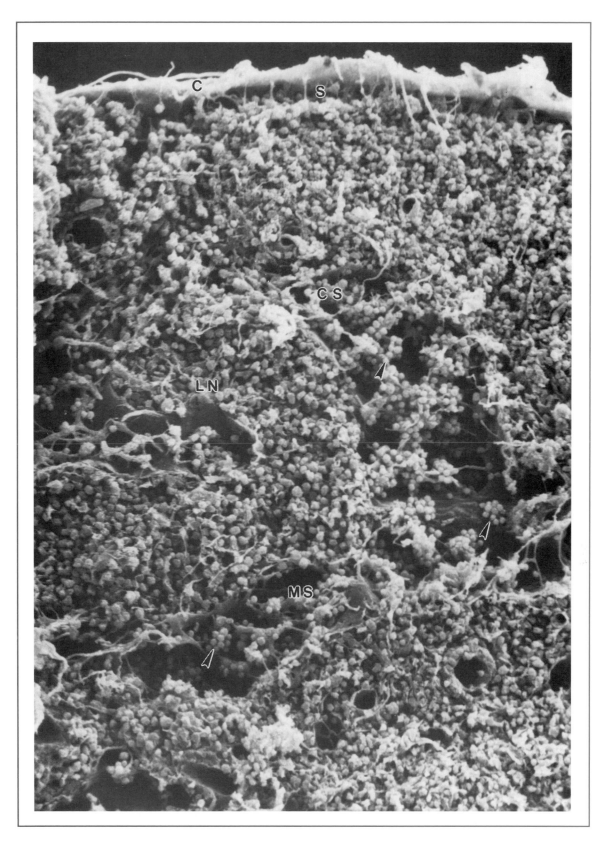

Figure 10.18. SEM of lymph node, cut section. Capsule (C), subcapsular sinus (S), lymphatic nodule (LN), cortical sinus (CS), and medullary sinus (MS) are identified. Note the clusters of small cells (arrowheads) in the sinuses. These represent a macrophage covered by lymphocytes. ×550. (From R. Kessel and R. Kardon, *Tissues and Organs: A Text-Atlas of Scanning Electron Microscopy.* W.H. Freeman, New York, 1979)

node in the afferent lymphatic vessels immediately enters the subcapsular sinus to which these vessels are connected. The subcapsular sinus is continuous with a system of channels between the lymphatic nodules that are called *cortical sinuses* because of their position (Plate 20A,B). The cortical sinuses, in turn, are continuous with a system of channels in the medulla of the node called *medullary sinuses* (Fig. 10.18). As indicated, the medullary sinuses converge into an efferent lymphatic vessel that exits the node at the hilus, the point at which blood vessels enter and leave the lymph node. The efferent lymphatic vessel also has one-way valves to direct the flow of lymph. The circulation of lymph throughout the lymphatic system is largely dependent upon body activity and muscle contractions. Thus, lymph nodes are encapsulated aggregations of lymphatic tissue that are placed in the path of afferent lymphatic vessels and serve to filter and modify the lymph as it drains away in efferent vessels. Further, the cellular concentration inside the node is much greater in the primary lymphatic nodules and medullary cords than in the system of sinuses through which the lymph percolates on its way through the node and out the efferent lymphatic vessel.

Lymph

Lymph originates as excess tissue fluid that forms from capillaries. Tissue fluid is drained, in part, from the intercellular spaces by entering blind-end lymphatic capillaries that permeate the tissues and organs. It is then called *lymph*. The lymphatic capillaries and small vessels join together, ultimately converging into two large trunks, the thoracic duct and the right lymphatic duct, which connect to the venous circulatory system. The thoracic duct enters the venous system at the junction of the left subclavian and left internal jugular veins. The right lymphatic ducts enters the venous system at the junction of the right subclavian and right internal jugular veins. Both lymphatic vessels continuously empty their contents into the venous side of the circulatory system, so that all tissue fluid formed is ultimately returned to the blood.

Cellular diversity

Early in their development, lymph nodes are seeded or colonized by T lymphocytes from the thymus and by B lymphocytes from the bone marrow. Lymphocytes can exit the lymph node by either blood vessels or lymphatic vessels and circulate throughout the body. T lymphocytes (thymus-dependent regions of lymph nodes) are located near the junction of the cortex and medulla.

After birth, the central region of each *primary lymphatic nodule* is lighter stained and is known as the *secondary lymphatic nodule* or *germinal center* region (Plate 20A,B). The central region of a nodule is more lightly stained because of a number of relatively large cells with large nuclei containing considerable amounts of euchromatin. In sectioned and stained lymphatic tissue, the cytoplasm of many cell types is not apparent; thus, cells must be distinguished largely on the basis of nuclear characteristics. The cell types that are especially numerous in the germinal center of a secondary lymphatic nodule are the macrophages, reticular cells, B lymphoblasts, and B lymphocytes. The macrophages have rounded, euchromatic-staining nuclei, and the cytoplasm may contain granules representing digestive vacuoles or other forms of lysosomal heterophagy. The reticular cell nuclei tend to be elongated and lightly stained with hematoxylin because of the presence of considerable euchromatin. A prominent nucleolus may also be evident in these nuclei. The B lymphoblasts have rounded nuclei with considerable euchromatin and have a distinct rim of stained cytoplasm. In contrast, the surrounding B lymphocytes are smaller cells with small nuclei that exhibit more heterochromatin. The cytoplasm is often difficult to discern in LM preparations. The darker-stained periphery of a lymphatic nodule consists principally of B lymphocytes that have resulted from the division of activated B lymphoblasts in the germinal center region. The lymphatic nodule is a site where activated B lymphocytes enlarge into mitotic B lymphoblasts that produce many programmed progeny. These progeny move into the medullary cords, where they differentiate into plasma cells and initiate the synthesis and release of specific humoral antibody as a defense against the specific foreign protein that elicited their formation (Plate 20D; Plate 21C,D). Plasma cell formation is common in medullary cords. Additional types of cells present in the medullary cords include macrophages (Plate 21A,B), reticular cells and reticular fibers (Plate 20C), and other blood cells such as eosinophils and mast cells. Plasma cells can move from the nodes through the blood vascular system or through the lymph drainage. T lymphocytes from the thymus populate a region near the cortical-medullary junction in the lymph node.

The various sinuses in the lymph node are less concentrated with cells. Perhaps the most numerous cell is a highly branched one called the reticular cells; the nature of this branching is usefully displayed by SEM (Figs. 10.19–10.21). The network of many branched reticular cells in the sinuses creates a cytoreticulum that serves as a baffle, creating turbulence in the flow of lymph through the sinuses. In addition, the macrophages are positioned and supported in the forks of the branched reticular cells, as is evident in SEM (Figs. 10.19–10.23). The ability of reticular cells to form a coarse cytoreticulum in the lymph node sinuses reflects an interesting association between the reticular cells and the reticular fibers that they form. Once the reticular cells have synthesized the fibers, they are exported from the cell, but the fiber bundles remain ensheathed or wrapped by the

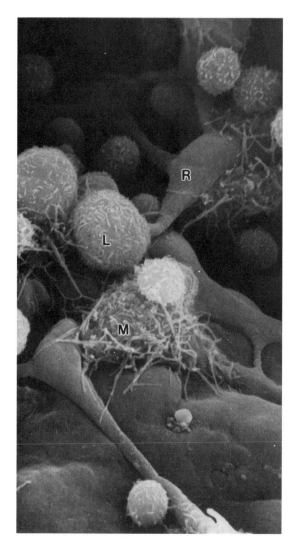

Figure 10.19. SEM of lymph node sinus. Highly branched smooth reticular cells (R) and macrophages (M) with tendrils are identified. Leukocyte (L) ×3325. (From R. Kessel and R. Kardon, *Tissues and Organs: A Text-Atlas of Scanning Electron Microscopy.* W.H. Freeman, New York, 1979)

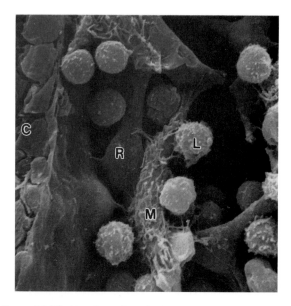

Figure 10.20. Portion of medullary cord (C) and sinus (S) in lymph node. Highly branched reticular cells (R), macrophages (M) and leukocytes (L) are identified. ×1345. (From R. Kessel and R. Kardon, *Tissues and Organs: A Text-Atlas of Scanning Electron Microscopy.* W.H. Freeman, New York, 1979)

to antigen recognition, processing, and presentation. The wide distribution of macrophages throughout the sinus system is thus functionally very important.

Functions

General functions of the lymph node include (1) straining and filtering of lymph, (2) phagocytosis of material by macrophages as the lymph percolates through the

branched reticular cell processes (Figs. 10.24–10.26). This relationship is best illustrated in TEM and SEM images in which a reticular cell branch is fractured, revealing the enclosed reticular fibers (Fig. 10.21). Therefore, the reticular fibers cannot actually be seen during passage through the lymphatic sinuses since the fibers are completely surrounded or ensheathed by the reticular cells. This relationship does not exist in the lymphatic nodules and medullary cords, where, once the reticular fibers are exported from the reticular cell, they do not remain ensheathed but are freely exposed. In addition to fluid lymph, lymphocytes and other blood cell types are distributed through the circulating fluid. Because many antigen-presenting macrophages are present in the sinuses, and because of the possible circulation of antigen in the lymph, this setting is conducive

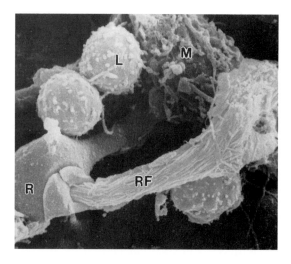

Figure 10.21. A process or extension of a reticular cell (R) was fractured away, revealing a group of reticular fibers (RF). Macrophage (M). Leukocytes (L). ×5170. (From R. Kessel and R. Kardon, *Tissues and Organs: A Text-Atlas of Scanning Electron Microscopy.* W.H. Freeman, New York, 1979)

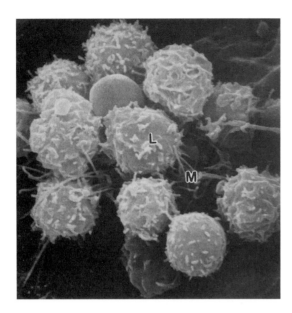

Figure 10.22. Macrophage (M) in a lymph node sinus is covered by so many lymphocytes (L) that it is barely visible. ×6145. (From R. Kessel and R. Kardon, *Tissues and Organs: A Text-Atlas of Scanning Electron Microscopy*. W.H. Freeman, New York, 1979)

node, (3) storage for T lymphocytes, (4) a place for the antigenic stimulation of B lymphocytes, with participating macrophages and T lymphocytes in some cases, and (5) the production of humoral antibody-producing plasma cells. As a result, the lymph nodes produce B lymphocytes (memory) and plasma cells, which can enter either the blood circulation or the lymphatic circulation. Blood-borne and lymph-borne antigens flow freely through lymph nodes.

SPLEEN

General organization

The spleen is an encapsulated lymphatic tissue designed to filter blood and respond to blood-borne antigens. It is about the size of a clenched fist and resides in the shelter of ribs 9, 10, and 11. It is soft in consistency and reddish purple in color due to the large amount of stored blood. The connective tissue *capsule* that surrounds the spleen contains some smooth muscle; thus the organ is somewhat compressible. An external layer of simple squamous cells, called *mesothelial cells*, and connective tissue comprise the serosa or *mesentery*. Elements of the capsule called *trabeculae* extend into the substance of the spleen and carry branches of the splenic artery. In addition to the capsule and trabeculae, many irregularly shaped *reticular cells* (Fig. 10.27) that produce *reticular fibers* are distributed throughout the spleen. In the parenchyma macrophages (Fig. 10.28) abound, and there are numerous B lymphoblasts, B lymphocytes, T

lymphoblasts, and *T lymphocytes*. Extensive numbers of erythrocytes, leukocytes, and platelets are present in the spleen since one function of this organ is to store blood.

White pulp

The principal cellular mass of the spleen is known as the *splenic parenchyma* or *pulp* and is organized into *white pulp* and *red pulp* (Plate 22A,B; Fig. 10.29). The white pulp contains a high concentration of B lymphoblasts and B lymphocytes, as well as CDC4+ and CDC8+ T lymphocytes that were sent from the thymus to colonize the spleen. Plasma cells, reticular cells, fibers, and macrophages (Plate 22D) also are widely distributed in the white pulp. White pulp consists of periarterial lymphatic sheaths and splenic nodules (Figs. 10.29, 10.30). The *periarterial lymphatic sheaths* (*PALS*) surround the arteries that leave the trabeculae to enter the parenchyma. The PALS of lymphocytes are continuous with those comprising the *splenic nodules* (Malpighian nodules) and the central artery branches to become the follicular arteriole in the splenic nodules (Plate 22B,C). The PALS and splenic nodules can be distinguished after birth by the presence (PALS) or absence (splenic nodule) of the central artery. The germinal centers in splenic nodules contain B lymphoblasts, B lymphocytes, macrophages, and reticular cells. The thymus-dependent region of the spleen containing T lymphocytes is in the central region of the PALS, while the periphery of the PALS contains principally B lymphocytes. Many lymphocytes, lymphoblasts, and other lymphatic tissue cells that surround the central artery are collectively called the *periarterial lymphatic sheaths* (*PALS*) (Fig. 10.29). Germinal centers

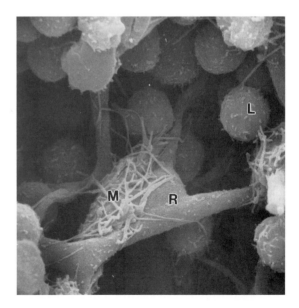

Figure 10.23. Lymph node sinus. Reticular cell (R), macrophage (M), and lymphocytes (L). ×3760. (From R. Kessel and R. Kardon, *Tissues and Organs: A Text-Atlas of Scanning Electron Microscopy*. W.H. Freeman, New York, 1979)

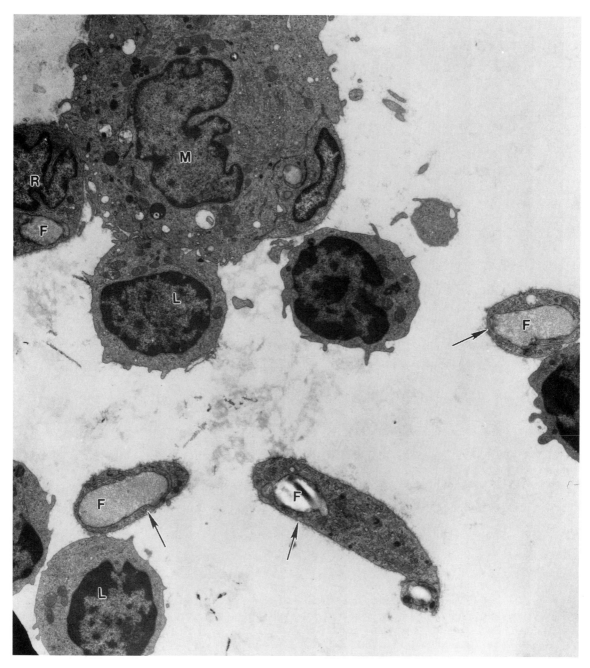

Figure 10.24. TEM of lymph node sinus. Reticular cells (R) and processes (arrows) ensheath groups of reticular fibers (F). Macrophage (M), lymphocytes (L). ×6875. (From R. Kessel and R. Kardon, *Tissues and Organs: A Text-Atlas of Scanning Electron Microscopy.* W.H. Freeman, New York, 1979)

are due to a reaction with antigen and hence do not appear until after birth. While transverse sections of the PALS appear spherical, very much like the splenic nodules, they contain the central artery in section. Depending upon the plane of section, lymphatic nodules may appear as localized expansions of the PALS, in which case the central artery may be displaced or eccentric and not central in position (Plate 22A,B). The proliferation of B lymphoblasts is largely restricted to the germinal center of splenic nodules (Fig. 10.30). The subsequent differentiation into plasma cells occurs at

the periphery of the splenic nodule, in a region called the *marginal zone*, and in the neighboring red pulp (Fig. 10.31).

Red pulp

The white pulp is surrounded by *red pulp*, which is named from the fact that in the fresh or living, this region appears red because of the presence of large amounts of blood (Fig. 10.31). The red pulp has two major constituents: highly cellular (*Billroth cords*), *red*

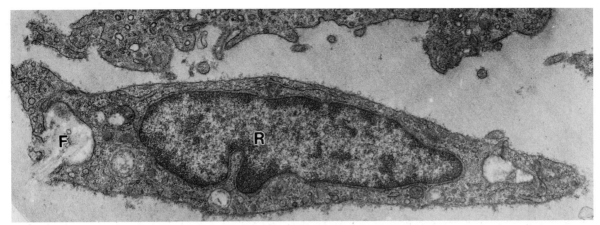

10.25

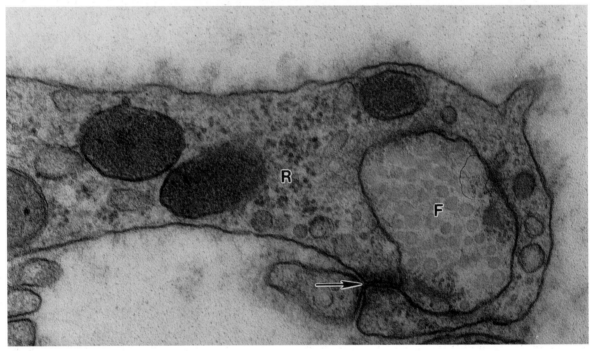

10.26

Figures 10.25, 10.26. TEM of reticular cells (R) and reticular fibers (F). Note how the reticular cell process closely surrounds the reticular fibers in Figure 10.30, but the fibers are in fact extracellular (arrow). ×12,800; ×67,230. (From R. Kessel and R. Kardon, *Tissues and Organs: A Text-Atlas of Scanning Electron Microscopy.* W.H. Freeman, New York, 1979)

pulp cords, which are riddled with many vascular channels called *splenic sinusoids* (Fig. 10.31). The splenic sinusoids are characterized by a large lumen, thin walls, incomplete basal laminae, and an endothelium with rather wide intercellular spaces—all features that facilitate easy, rapid movement of cells between the sinusoids and surrounding red pulp cords (Plate 23A–C). Reticular fibers in the red pulp cords are invested by branched reticular cells. The red pulp cord meshwork contains macrophages, plasma cells, and large numbers of erythrocytes and platelets. In some organisms, megakaryocytes and monocytes are located in the red pulp cords. The red pulp contains considerable amounts of stored blood, and macrophages ingest and digest worn-out erythrocytes and platelets here. In a number of mammals, as well as in human embryos, there are islands of hemopoietic tissue in the red pulp that contains erythroblasts, myeloblasts, and megakaryocytes.

Circulation

Branches of the splenic artery traverse the splenic capsule and are conveyed into the interior within trabeculae as trabecular arterteries. The trabecular blood vessels leave the trabeculae and are designated *central arteries* (either small, muscular arteries or arterioles) as they extend through the PALS and splenic lymphatic nodules. In the Malpighian nodules, the arterioles may be displaced to one side of the germinal center. Small

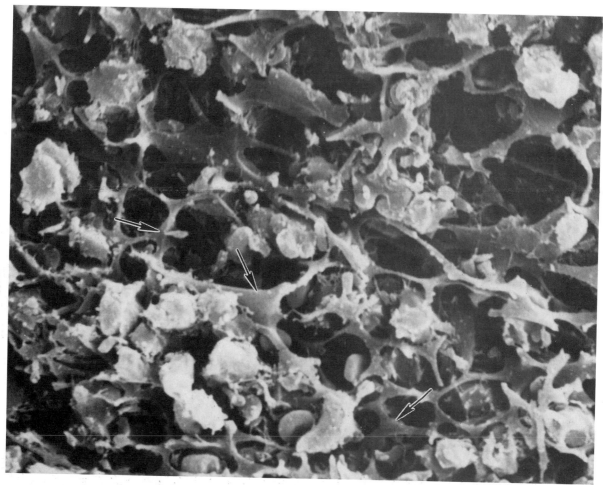

Figure 10.27. SEM of red pulp illustrates many highly branched reticular cells (arrows) with blood cells in the interstices of the branched reticular cells. ×950 (From R. Kessel and R. Kardon, *Tissues and Organs: A Text-Atlas of Scanning Electron Microscopy*. W.H. Freeman, New York, 1979)

Figure 10.28. TEM of a splenic macrophage (M) with many digestive vacuoles (V). Macrophages abound in the spleen, especially in the red pulp, where worn-out erythrocytes are ingested and digested. Macrophages are also involved in antigen presentation to T and B lymphocytes in the spleen. ×7595. (From R. Kessel and R. Kardon, *Tissues and Organs: A Text-Atlas of Scanning Electron Microscopy*. W.H. Freeman, New York, 1979)

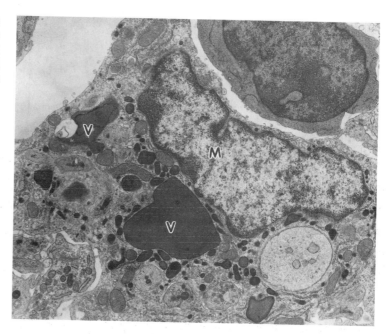

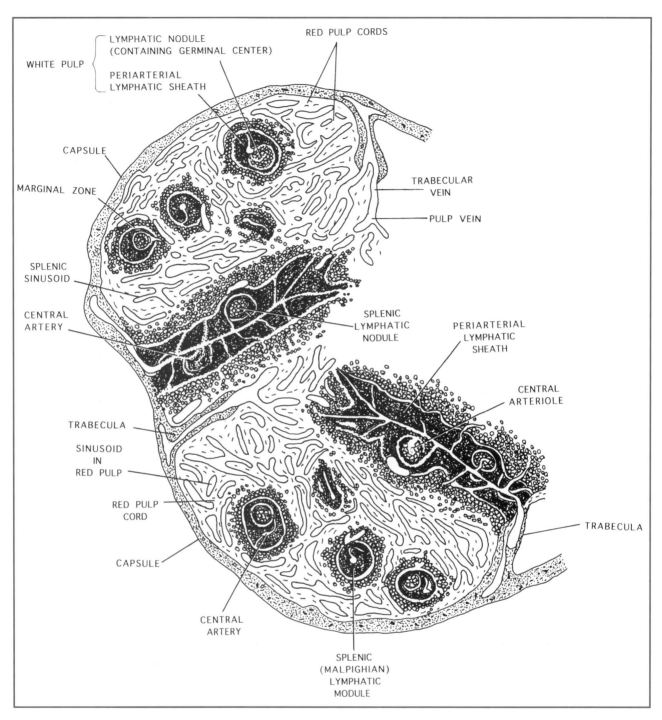

Figure 10.29. Diagram illustrates part of the spleen and depicts its organization. The white pulp consists of periarterial lymphatic sheaths and lymphatic (splenic) nodules, which are illustrated in different section planes. The white pulp consists of the surrounding venous sinuses and intervening red pulp cords (of Billroth). The connective tissue capsule extends into the parenchyma and conveys branches of the splenic artery and vein called the *trabecular artery* and *trabecular vein*. As the trabecular artery leaves the trabecula, it is surrounded by periarterial sheaths of lymphocytes as a central artery. Branches of this central artery supply the ger-minal center of the splenic (Malpighian) nodules as follicular arterioles. The follicular arterioles communicate with the marginal sinuses. Vessels that emerge from the white pulp enter the red pulp, where most of them terminate in the red pulp cords, while some terminate close to or with the venous sinuses. The many sinuses drain into pulp veins, which then drain into trabecular veins. (Redrawn and modified from L. Weiss, and M. Tavossoli, 1970, Anatomical hazards to the passage of erythrocytes through the spleen. *Semin. Hematol.* 7, 372, with permission)

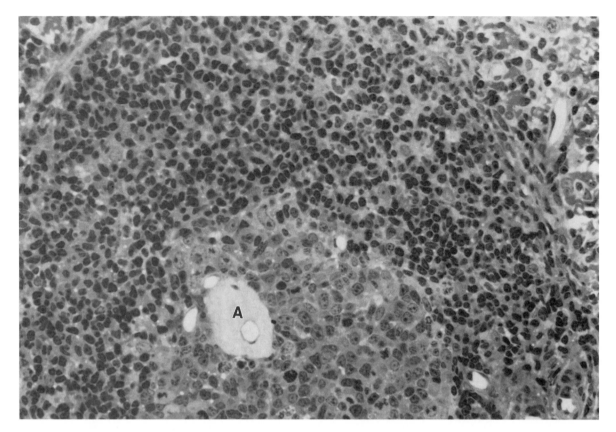

Figure 10.30. LM section of splenic (Malgiphian) nodule with a lighter-staining germinal center that contains a central arteriole (A). The red pulp is at the upper extreme right. ×500. (From R. Kessel and R. Kardon, *Tissues and Organs: A Text-Atlas of Scanning Electron Microscopy*. W.H. Freeman, New York, 1979)

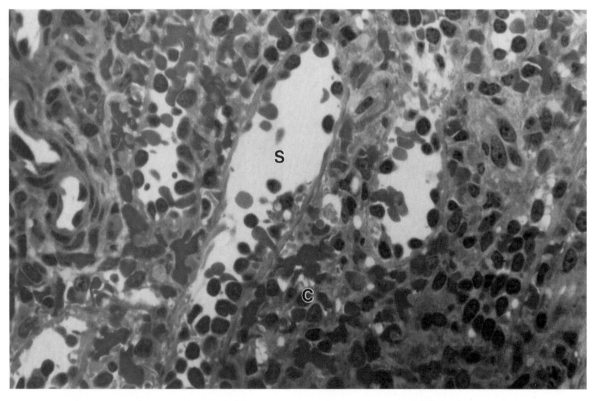

Figure 10.31. LM photomicrograph of red pulp, which consists of sinusoids (S) and red pulp cords (C) of Billroth. The red pulp cord is a site of blood storage; thus all types of blood cells may be present, as well as macrophages, reticular cells, and fibers. ×800. (From R. Kessel and R. Kardon, *Tissues and Organs: A Text-Atlas of Scanning Electron Microscopy*. W.H. Freeman, New York, 1979)

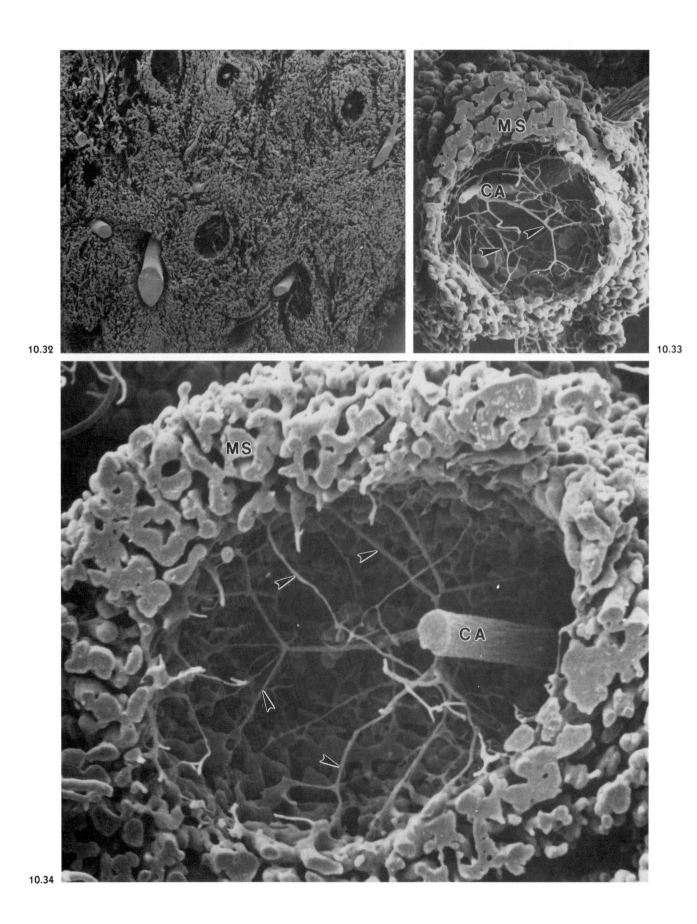

10.32

10.33

MS

CA

MS

CA

10.34

Table 10.5 Comparative Structural Features

Feature	Lymph Node	Spleen
Cortex/medulla	Yes	No
Lymphatic nodules	Yes (in cortex)	Yes (splenic nodules)
Central artery in lymphatic tissue	No	Yes (in PALS)
Smooth muscle in capsule, trabeculae	No	Yes
Afferent lymphatic supply	Yes	No
Efferent lymphatic drainage	Yes	Yes
Lymph sinuses	Yes	No
Blood sinuses or sinusoids	No	Yes
Fat associated with periphery	Yes	No
Filters lymph or blood	Lymph	Blood

branches called *follicular arterioles* radiate from the central arteriole in the Malpighian nodule toward the marginal zone near the adjacent red pulp, where they may be continuous with a marginal zone of sinuses (Figs. 10.32–10.34). Some of the vessels become continuous with penicillar arterioles in the red pulp and then either terminate in the red pulp cords or communicate with the many splenic sinusoids that riddle the red pulp. The numerous venous sinuses in the red pulp drain into pulp veins that are continuous with trabecular veins that ultimately join to form the splenic vein.

Structural comparison: lymph node and spleen

Comparative structural features of the lymph node and spleen are denoted in Table 10.5.

Functions

The spleen plays a major role in producing *humoral antibodies* to counteract blood-borne antigens. Associated with this function, a large number of B lymphocytes typically populate the spleen. Thus considerable amounts of Ig are produced in the spleen by the plasma cells located there and that resulted from the stimulation of B lymphocytes by blood-borne antigens. The spleen also plays a major role in the elimination or *disposal* of de-

fective or worn-out *blood cells*. To perform this role, a large number of resident macrophages are located in the spleen. These macrophages are extremely active in phagocytosis of senescent or damaged platelets, erythrocytes, and leukocytes, as well as any debris or particulate material that may be circulating in the blood. Another function of the spleen is to *recycle iron*. Hemoglobin is injested by macrophages and degraded into heme and globin. Iron is freed from heme and stored in the macrophage as ferritin or hemosiderin. Heme is degraded to bilirubin by the macrophages and released into the blood, where it binds to albumin. It is then transported to the liver, where hepatocytes conjugate the bilirubin to glucuronic acid and excrete this into the bile. In addition, the spleen serves as a *storage depot* for blood, from which it can be released into the bloodstream under conditions of increased need (Figs. 10.35, 10.36). The spleen is not essential to life, however; other hematopoietic tissues can assume its functions if the spleen is removed. In the fetus, the spleen plays a role in the formation of leukocytes. However, it does not normally participate in active myeloid hematopoiesis in adult life.

DIFFUSE LYMPHATIC TISSUE

It is common to find aggregations of lymphatic nodules widely distributed under moist epithelial membranes in

---

Figures 10.32–10.34. SEMs illustrating the microvasculature of the spleen; all cellular elements have been digested away. The marginal zone of sinuses and many red pulp sinusoids are replicated in Figure 10.32. Figures 10.33 and 10.34 illustrate centrial arterioles (CA) and follicular arteri-

oles (arrowheads) that communicate with the marginal zone of sinuses (MS). Figure 10.32, ×25; Figure 10.33, ×120; Figure 10.34, ×280 (From R. Kessel and R. Kardon, *Tissues and Organs: A Text-Atlas of Scanning Electron Microscopy.* W.H. Freeman, New York, 1979)

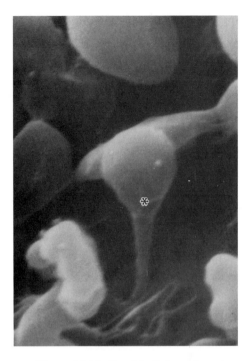

Figure 10.36. Dumbbell-shaped erythrocyte (*) undergoing diapedesis or movement through the splenic sinusoidal wall. ×14,438.

ithelial lining of this tube are particularly abundant in parts of the ileum where the lymphatic nodules comprise *Peyer's patches.* Lymphatic nodules are present at the esophageal-gastric junction, in the appendix, and in the recto-anal region. Collectively, the lymphatic nodules present in the digestive tract comprise the *gut-associated lymphatic tissue (GALT).* Lymphatic nodules are sometimes present under the moist epithelium of the inner eyelid and under the epithelium in bronchi as well. The rationale for their presence under moist epithelia is that the epithelia are imperfect barriers to foreign substances or antigen. Therefore, the lymphatic nodules are strategically positioned to respond early to the entry of antigen into the body. This accounts for the frequent presence of plasma cells in these lymphatic nodules. The plasma cells have been induced to form so as to produce humoral Ig to counteract the antigen.

Tonsils represent an amplification of this protective function. Tonsils consist of many *lymphatic nodules* under the moist epithelium of the oral cavity and pharynx. The *pharyngeal tonsils* or adenoids are located in the roof of the pharynx. The *palatine tonsils* are paired and located at the posterior part of the oral cavity between the faucial pillars. The *lingual tonsils* are located under the epithelium covering the posterior portion of the tongue. There are many lymphatic nodules comprising the lingual tonsils. Because the epithelium covering the tonsils is folded into crypts, these areas can be obstructed with bacteria and other debris, becoming inflammed or infected, hence the necessity to remove these lymphatic tissues. Most of the lymphatic nodules within tonsils, as well as those in diffuse lymphatic tissue, contain germinal centers after birth.

the body. These lymphatic nodules consist of a closely packed cellular population that includes many B lymphocytes and B lymphoblasts, as well as plasma cells and perhaps T cells. In addition, macrophages and reticular cells are present. The solitary lymphatic nodules that are present in the alimentary canal under the moist ep-

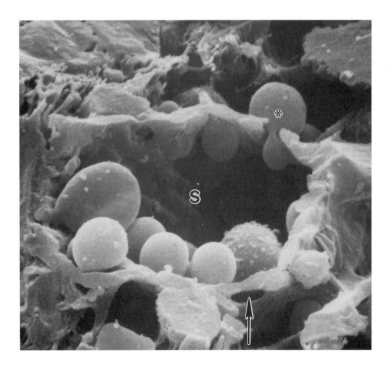

Figure 10.35. SEM of a transverse section through a splenic sinusoid (S). Note the pores between the sinusoid lining cells (arrows) and one erythrocyte that appears to be in the process of moving through the sinusoid (*). ×5750.

SELECTED BIBLIOGRAPHY

Alberts, B., Bray, D., Lewis, J., Raff, M., Roberts, K., and Watson, J. (1994). The immune system. In *Molecular Biology of the Cell*, 3rd ed., Garland, New York.

Albright, J., and Oppenheim, J. (1991). Contributions of basic immunology to human health. *FASEB J.*, 5, 265–270.

Berek, C. (1992). The development of B cells and the B-cell repertoire in the microenvironment of the germinal center. *Immunol. Rev.* **126**, 5–19.

Brodsky, F.M., and Guagliardi, L.E. (1991). The cell biology of antigen processing and presentation. *Annu. Rev. Immunol.* **9**, 707–716.

Claman, H. N. (1992). The biology of the immune response. *JAMA.* **268**, 2790–2796.

Groom, A.C., Schmidt, E.E., and MacDonald, I.C. (1991). Microcirculatory pathways and blood flow in spleen: new insights from washout kinetics, corrosion casts, and quantitative intravital videomicroscopy. *Scanning Microsc.* **5**, 159–174.

Klausner, R., Lippincott-Schwartz, J., and Bonifacino, J. (1990). The T cell receptor: insights into organelle biology. *Annu. Rev. Cell Biol.* **6**, 403–432.

Kopp, W.C. (1990). The immune functions of the spleen. In *The Spleen: Structure, Function and Clinical Significance*, A.J. Bowdler, ed. Chapman and Hall, London.

Lewis, C.E., and McGee, J., eds. (1992). *The Natural Immune System. The Natural Killer Cell.* IRL Press and Oxford University Press, Oxford.

O'Garra, A. (1989). Interleukins and the immune system. *Lancet* **1**, 943–954.

Oilier, W., and Symmons, D. P. (1992). *Autoimmunity.* BIOS Scientific, Oxford.

Pardoll, D., and Carrera, A. (1992). Thymic selection. *Curr. Opin. Immun.* **4**, 162–165.

Roitt, I.M., Brostoff, J., and Male, D.K. (1993). *Immunology*, 3rd ed. Mosby, St. Louis.

Savill, J., Fadak, V., Henson, P., and Haslett, C. (1993). Phagocyte recognition of cells undergoing apoptosis. *Immunol. Today* **14**, 131–136.

Smith, K. (1990). Interleukin-2. *Sci. Am.* **262**, 48–57.

Suzuki, T. (1991). Signal transduction mechanisms through Fc_r receptors on mouse macrophage surface. *FASEB J.* **5**, 187–193.

vonGaudecker, B. (1991). Functional histology of the human thymus. *Anat. Embryol.* **183**, 1–26.

CHAPTER 11

Muscle Tissue

M uscle is one of four basic tissues, the one most highly specialized for contractility. The contractility is due to the presence, large quantity, and precise organization of several *contractile* and regulatory *proteins*.

TYPES OF MUSCLE

There are two major types of muscle. One type is called *striated* because of repeating cross-bands or striations. There are two subtypes of striated muscle: *skeletal muscle* and *cardiac muscle*. Skeletal muscle is associated with the bony skeleton and consists of cylindrical *fibers* that are *multinucleate*. The skeletal muscle fiber is a *syncytium* resulting when originally separate cells, called *myoblasts*, fuse to form the muscle fiber in the embryo. The term *muscle fiber* is used to refer to a muscle cell; its meaning is thus unlike that of fiber described in connective tissues (Chapter 5). Skeletal muscle fibers are innervated by cerebrospinal nerves; hence, contraction is under voluntary control. The second subtype of striated muscle is *cardiac muscle* that comprises the heart. Cardiac muscle consists of separate cellular units and is uninucleate. Furthermore, cardiac muscle is characterized by rhythmic, involuntary contractions controlled by autonomic innervation.

The second type of muscle is called *smooth muscle.* Smooth muscle consists of spindle-shaped, fusiform, uninucleate cells that do not exhibit striations. Smooth muscle is involuntary and is innervated by the autonomic nervous system. Smooth muscle is widely distributed throughout the digestive tube and in the tubular portions of many organs; it is also present in the walls of many blood vessels.

SKELETAL MUSCLE

ORGANIZATION

A named muscle such as the deltoid consists of many *muscle bundles* or *fascicles* (Fig. 11.1). Each muscle bundle is surrounded or delineated by connective tissue that is continuous with an external connective tissue sheath surrounding the entire muscle. Each muscle bundle or fascicle consists of a variable number of *muscle fibers;* the muscle fiber is the basic structural unit of skeletal muscle. The muscle fiber is a long, cylindrical structure that is multinucleate (Plate 24A,B).

The connective tissue that surrounds the entire anatomically named muscle is called *epimysium.* Connective tissue elements extend inward, surrounding the muscle bundles or fascicles comprising the muscle; this connective tissue is called *perimysium* (Fig. 11.2) Smaller amounts of connective tissue extend inward, surrounding individual muscle fibers; this connective tissue is called *endomysium* (Fig. 11.2). All connective tissue elements are continuous and decrease in amount into the interior of the muscle around individual fibers. The connective tissue conducts blood vessels, lymphatic vessels, and nerves into the interior of the muscle, bringing them close to the individual muscle fibers.

MUSCLE FIBER AND MYOFIBRILS

The muscle fiber is a long, multinucleate cylinder. While an individual fiber is isodiametric, different fibers can vary in both length and width. Most fibers are 1–40 mm long, but some may be several centime-

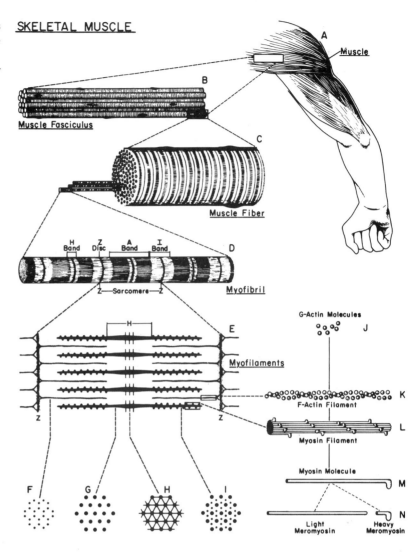

Figure 11.1. Diagram illustrates the organization of skeletal muscle tissue. (From D. Fawcett, *A Textbook of Histology*, Chapman & Hall, New York 1994, with permission)

ters in length. The width of muscle fibers ranges from about 10 to 100 μm. The plasma membrane of the muscle fiber is called the *sarcolemma*. The nuclei in a muscle fiber are all located at the periphery of the muscle fiber in contact with the sarcolemma (Plate 24B,D). The sarcolemma is supported by a basal lamina similar to that associated with epithelia. Myofibrils are linked to each other by desmin IFs that are also anchored to the sarcolemma by proteins, one of which is dystrophin. The interior of the muscle fiber contains a variable number of longitudinally oriented structural units called *myofibrils*, which are all in register. Myofibrils usually range from 1 to 2 μm in diameter (Plate 24C,D; Fig. 11.2). Each of the many myofibrils in a single muscle fiber consists of many (perhaps well over 100) *myofilaments* (Figs. 11.3, 11.4). These myofilaments, which are oriented longitudinally within the individual myofibrils, are of two types: *thick* and *thin* (Figs. 11.5, 11.6).

BANDING PATTERN

In the LM, H&E-stained striated skeletal muscle illustrates alternate light and dark transverse banding along the fibers (Plate 24A,B). The hematoxylin-stained dark bands are the *A bands*, while the alternate bands that do not stain with hematoxylin are the *I bands*. However, the bands were initially named as they appeared in the polarizing microscope. With polarized light, the hematoxylin-stained dark bands, as viewed by LM, were found to be anisotrophic (birefringent) or double refractile. Thus, the *A* is derived from the term *anisotrophic*. Actually, with polarized light, the A bands appear bright. With polarized light, the light-staining I bands are isotropic or singly refractile. Hence, the I band designation comes from the term *isotropic*. The I bands appear dark with polarized light. In a relaxed muscle, the A band is approximately 1.5 μm in length, while the I band is approximately 1 μm in length (Figs. 11.3, 11.5).

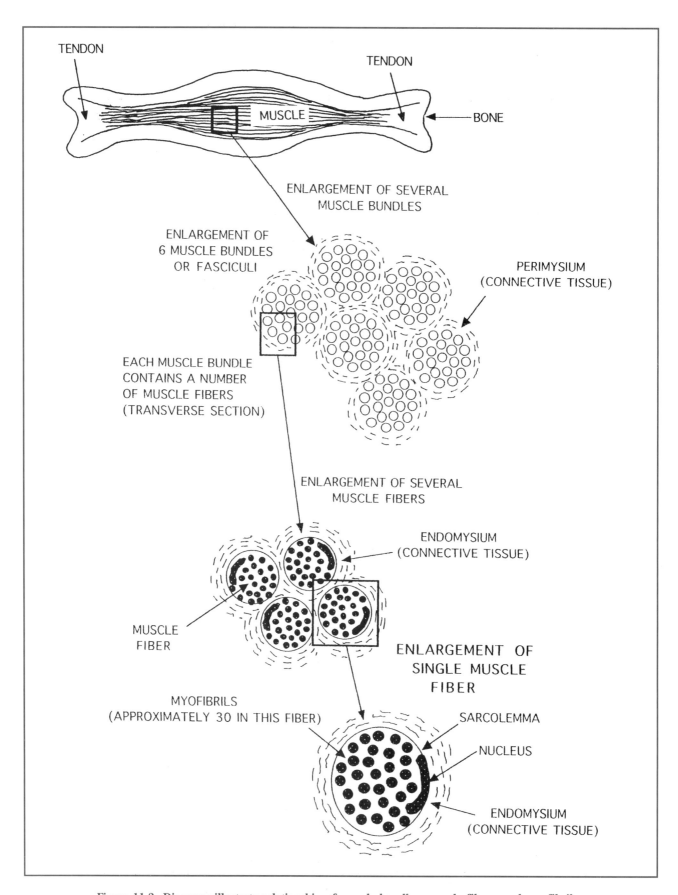

TENDON

TENDON

MUSCLE

BONE

ENLARGEMENT OF SEVERAL
MUSCLE BUNDLES

ENLARGEMENT OF
6 MUSCLE BUNDLES
OR FASCICULI

PERIMYSIUM
(CONNECTIVE TISSUE)

EACH MUSCLE BUNDLE
CONTAINS A NUMBER
OF MUSCLE FIBERS
(TRANSVERSE SECTION)

ENLARGEMENT OF SEVERAL
MUSCLE FIBERS

ENDOMYSIUM
(CONNECTIVE TISSUE)

MUSCLE
FIBER

ENLARGEMENT OF
SINGLE MUSCLE
FIBER

MYOFIBRILS
(APPROXIMATELY 30 IN THIS FIBER)

SARCOLEMMA

NUCLEUS

ENDOMYSIUM
(CONNECTIVE TISSUE)

Figure 11.2. Diagrams illustrate relationship of muscle bundles, muscle fibers, and myofibrils.

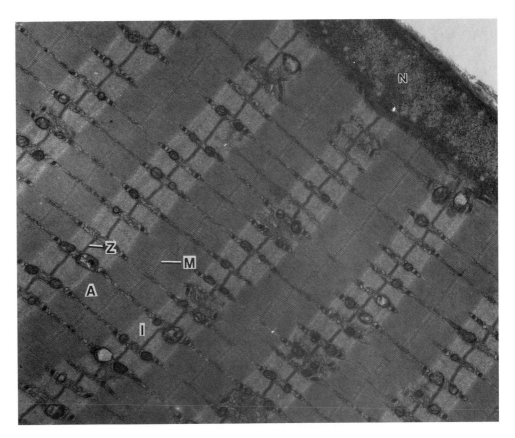

Figure 11.3. Low-magnification TEM of muscle fiber. The nucleus (N) is present under the sarcolemma at the top. The boundary of the fiber is at the lower left. Although individual myofibrils are aligned in register, approximately 15 myofibrils can be counted in this longitudinal section of a fiber. A, I, M, Z = A, I, M, Z lines. ×15,500.

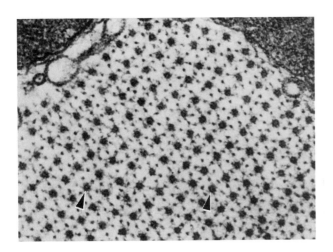

Figure 11.4. TEM, transverse section of a portion of one myofibril, illustrating both myosin thick filaments (arrowhead) and smaller actin thin filaments in register. Note also the thin cross-bridges between the thick and thin myofilaments. Portions of two mitochondria are present at the top of the figure. ×97,900. (From R. Kessel and R. Kardon, *Tissues and Organs: A Text-Atlas of Scanning Electron Microscopy.* W. H. Freeman, New York, 1979, with permission)

A thin *Z line* bisects the I band; this can sometimes be seen by oil immersion LM observation. The *H band*, which bisects the A band, can also sometimes be observed in suitable LM preparations. Finally, an *M band* bisects the H band but is apparent only in TEM. The M band or M line traverses the center of the A band and consists of fine cross-filaments that appear to connect thick filaments to each other (Figs. 11.5, 11.6).

The term *sarcomere* refers to the unit of distance between adjacent Z lines and is the fundamental unit of contraction. The length of the sarcomere is approximately *2.5 μm* for *mammalian skeletal muscle*, but the length varies with the degree of contraction (Fig. 11.5). The sarcomere consists of one A band and one-half of two contiguous I bands. Both the *H bands* and *I bands* decrease in length (shorten) during contraction, but the length of the A band does not change. The longitudinal striations apparent in muscle fibers are due to the presence of myofibrils. Furthermore, the myofibrils are all aligned within a single fiber. As a result, the I, A, H, and Z bands all appear in register.

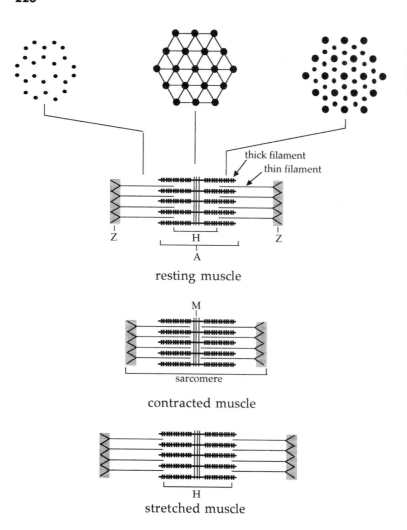

thick filament
thin filament

Z   H   Z
A

resting muscle

M

sarcomere

contracted muscle

H

stretched muscle

SARCOPLASM

The protoplasm of the muscle fiber, called *sarcoplasm,* surrounds the many myofibrils that are present in each fiber. The sarcoplasm includes a Golgi complex, small amounts of rER, glycogen, and lipid. In addition, numerous, often large mitochondria are distributed around the myofibrils. Further, a prominent system of sER, called the *sarcoplasmic reticulum* is present around the myofibrils and plays an important role in Ca^{2+} ion regulation during muscle contraction. The sarcoplasm of skeletal muscle fibers also contains the protein *myoglobin,* which has some similarities to hemoglobin in that the pigment can take up and release oxygen. It is present in relatively low concentration in humans. Myoglobin is reddish brown, and muscle fibers that contain rather substantial amounts of myoglobin are called *red fibers.* Red fibers are also called *slow twitch fibers* and have a smaller diameter than white fibers. They have a red color due to the amount of myoglobin present, as well as a rich vascular supply. These fibers also have many large mitochondria and lipid droplets. The fibers generally contract more slowly and are quite resistant to fa-

tigue; thus, they are used in maintaining posture. *White fibers,* also called *fast twitch fibers,* are larger in diameter than red fibers and have fewer mitochondria. The fibers contract rapidly with considerable force. Since they fatigue more rapidly, white fibers are more suited to short, intense bursts of activity. Other muscle fibers have different amounts of myoglobin; thus fibers can be distinguished as red, white, or intermediate fibers. Most human muscle contains all three types of fiber.

THICK MYOFILAMENTS (MYOSIN)

The myosin-containing thick filaments are approximately *1.5 μm long* and *12 to 15 nm in diameter.* The myosin thick filament is slightly wider in the middle than at either end. Each thick myofilament contains approximately 400 individual myosin molecules. The myosin molecule has the shape of a golf club with two "heads" (Figs. 11.7–11.10). If treated with proteolytic enzymes, the myosin molecule is cleaved into two portions: a *light meromyosin (LMM)* fragment and a *heavy meromyosin (HMM)* fraction (Fig. 11.11).

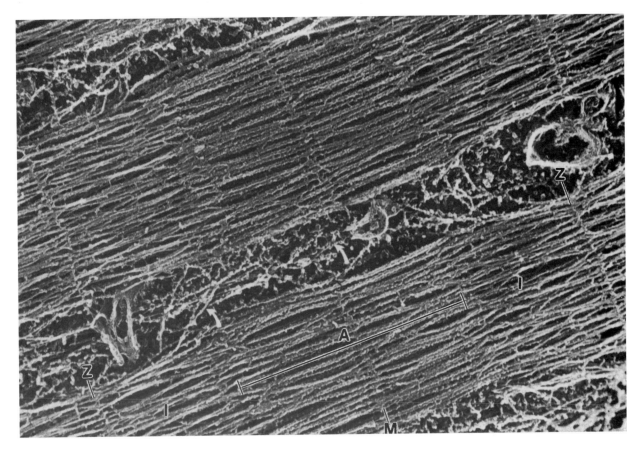

Figure 11.6. Quick free-deep etch preparation of amphibian skeletal muscle. Parts of two myofibrils are present. Thick myofilaments of the A band (A), thin myofilaments of the I band (I), Z disc (Z), and M line (M) are identified. Intermediate filaments in the sarcoplasm between the myofibrils are identified at white arrows. ×40,000. (Micrograph courtesy of Dr. Wallace Ip)

The ~400 myosin molecules in a thick filament are bundled together such that one-half of the molecules have their heads pointing toward one end of the thick filament, while the remaining half of the molecules have their heads pointing toward the opposite end (Fig. 11.9). This arrangement results in a bare zone in the center of the A band where there are no myosin heads. This molecular organization explains in part why two sets of thin filaments in a sarcomere are pulled toward each other, that is, toward the center of the A band. It is also important to note that the myosin molecules have a staggered position in the thick filament because the heads have a helical arrangement along the thick filament. In this configuration, two pairs of myosin heads or cross-bridges are arranged opposite each other at a given level. Then the next pair of cross-bridges are displaced 14.3 nm along the length of the filament and rotated 120° relative to the adjacent pair, as illustrated in Figure 11.10.

It is possible to disrupt the HMM fragment to obtain two subfragments called SF_1 and SF_2. The SF_1 subfragment consists of two globular heads. It has been shown that three important biochemical features are localized in this region of the molecule. The SF_1 subfragment possesses ATPase activity, has actin-binding affinity, and has affinity for ATP. If myosin is treated with urea, the myosin dissociates into six polypeptide chains. There are two H chains (the molecular weight of each is about 200,000) and four very small L chains associated with the myosin heads in a manner indicated by the diagram. The myosin molecule has a "hinge" or is flexible in two different regions: one is at the junction of the LMM and HMM, and the other is at the neck region near the two globular heads (Figs. 11.11–11.13).

THIN (ACTIN) MYOFILAMENT

The principal protein in the thin filament is actin, but in vertebrates there are two major regulatory proteins closely associated with the actin. The filamentous or *fibrous (F) actin* of the thin filament is formed by the polymerization of many *globular (G) actin* monomers (Fig. 11.14). *G actin* is a globular protein shaped like a marble that is about 55 Å in diameter. Each thin filament consists of a twisted double strand of G actin molecules

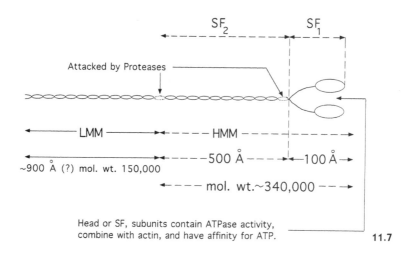

Attacked by Proteases

SF₂ · · · SF₁

LMM ──── HMM

~900 Å (?) mol. wt. 150,000 · 500 Å · 100 Å

mol. wt.~340,000

Head or SF, subunits contain ATPase activity,
combine with actin, and have affinity for ATP.

11.7

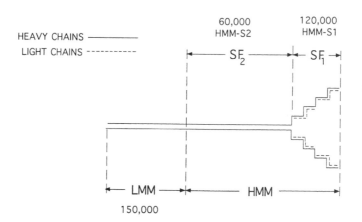

HEAVY CHAINS ────
LIGHT CHAINS --------

60,000
HMM-S2 · 120,000
HMM-S1

SF₂ · SF₁

LMM ──── HMM

150,000

SIX POLYPEPTIDE CHAINS OF MYOSIN 11.8

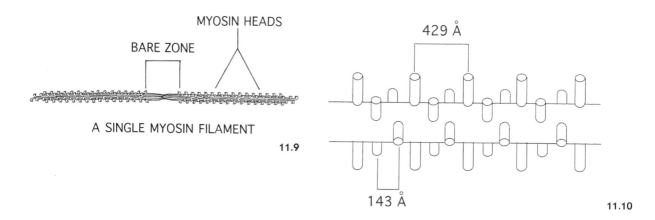

MYOSIN HEADS

BARE ZONE

A SINGLE MYOSIN FILAMENT

11.9

429 Å

143 Å

11.10

Figures 11.7–11.10. All figures illustrate details of the myosin molecule. The globular heads, L and H chains, and the six polypeptide chains of myosin are illustrated. An assembled thick myosin myofilament is also shown; the central bare zone is due to the opposite orientation of myosin molecules in each half of the thick filament. Adjacent pairs of globular myosin heads are located at a distance of 143 Å along the thick filament and rotated 120°, resulting in a complete circle around the thick filament every 429 Å.

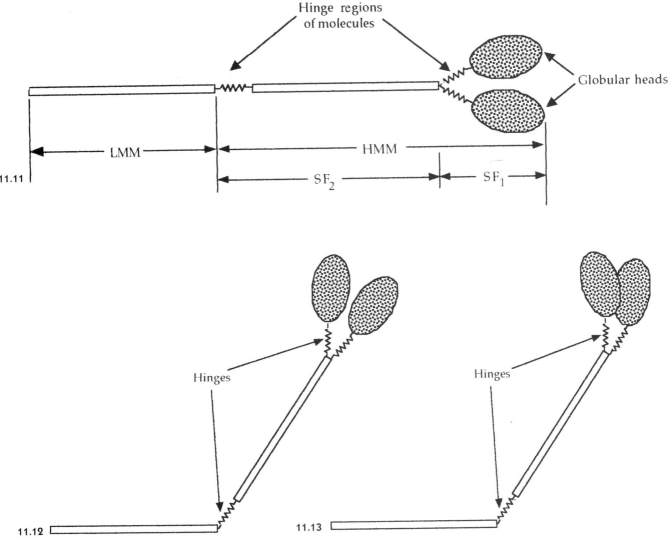

Figures 11.11–11.13. Diagrams of myosin molecules showing conformational changes at the "hinge" regions during contractions.

that gives a beads-on-a-string appearance (Fig. 11.14). The G actin molecule has a polarity that is different on either side of the Z line. G actin thus behaves as if it has a functional "front and back," which can be emphasized by applying different colors to each half of the "marble" (Fig. 11.15). The thin filaments comprise the I band of muscle. Each thin filament is about 1 μm long and 6–7 nm in diameter. Each thin filament in mammalian skeletal muscle contains *300–400* G actin molecules. In the region of the Z line (band or disk), the TEM shows a zigzag arrangement of Z filaments to which the thin filaments are attached. The electron density of the Z disc is due to alpha actinin, a 100-kD actin-binding protein; *zeugmatin*, a 200-kD protein; and *filamin*, another actin-binding protein. When actin filaments that have been "decorated" with HMM are examined by TEM, they exhibit arrowheads that indicate the polarity of the actin filament. The pointed end of the barb is called

the *minus end*, and the barbed end is called the *plus end*. The myosin heads "walk" in a single direction along an adjacent actin filament, and movement is toward the actin filament's plus end. It has been estimated that a myosin head attaches and dissociates from actin about five times per second during rapid contraction.

ACTIN-ASSOCIATED REGULATORY PROTEINS

Tropomyosin

Tropomyosin is a long, thin molecule about 40 nm long (Fig. 11.14). It is a needle-shaped, coiled-coil dimer that binds along the groove of the F actin helix in a head-to-tail arrangement (Fig. 11.15). One tropomyosin molecule is closely associated with 7 G actin molecules. Furthermore, tropomyosin molecules are associated with both strands of the actin thin filament. Therefore, since

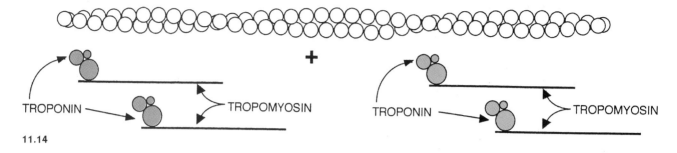

11.14

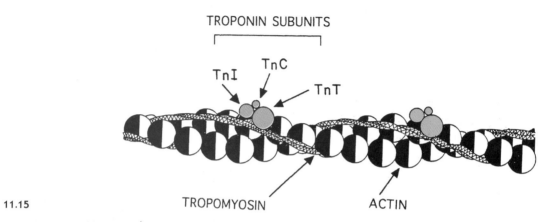

11.15

Figures 11.14, 11.15. Diagrams illustrate G actin molecules (that have a functional front and back), which are assembled into a thin filament as a twisted (helical) double strand of globular molecules, resulting in F (fibrous) actin. Tropomyosin is a long, thread-like molecule extending over seven actins; tropomyosins oriented end to end are associated with each of the two actin strands. Troponin consists of three subunits that are associated with each tropomyosin near the end of the molecule. The assembled thin filament is illustrated below. The double strand of actin molecules with functional polarity (which is reversed on either side of the Z band), the tropomyosin filaments, and troponin subunits are illustrated. The TnT subunit has affinity for tropomyosin; the TnC subunit has affinity for calcium; the TnI subunit has affinity for actin.

there are 300–400 G actin molecules in one thin filament, there are 40–60 tropomyosin molecules in this same actin myofilament. In the relaxed state, the tropomyosin molecules cover those sites on the G actin molecules that are capable of reacting with myosin heads.

Troponin

Troponin is a globular regulatory protein molecule present in the thin filament. One globular troponin molecule resides near the end of a single tropomyosin molecule. Therefore, one troponin molecule is present at a regular interval of about 40 nm, which is the length of the tropomyosin molecule. Troponin is composed of three subunits (Figs. 11.15, 11.16). One of the subunits has a high affinity for calcium and is called *troponin C*. A second troponin subunit (*troponin T*) has a high affinity for tropomyosin, and a third troponin subunit (*troponin I*) has a high affinity for actin. When calcium ions bind to the troponin C subunit, this has the effect of sending a message to the tropomyosin molecule indicating that it should move slightly to uncover the active

site on the actin molecules, which it covers so that myosin heads can bind to this specific site. When calcium is released from the sarcoplasmic reticulum, it binds to the troponin subunit C. This event causes tropomyosin to move slightly so that the reactive sides on the actin molecules are uncovered for interaction with the myosin heads (Fig. 11.16). The characteristics of sarcomere proteins are summarized in Table 11.1.

Other muslce proteins

Three M band proteins have been identified: *M protein* (a single polypeptide chain of 165,000 molecular weight), *M band protein* (an isozyme of creatinine kinase), and *myomesin*, which has a molecular weight of 185,000. Phosphocreatinine in the M band is the source of high-energy phosphate groups and, upon activation, phosphorylcreatinine is transphosphorylated by creatinine kinase to yield ATP for contraction when additional energy is required. Several other proteins are present in the myofibril, and are thought to maintain the precise architecture of the myofibril and to provide elasticity to the myofibril. *Alpha-actinin* is an actin bundling

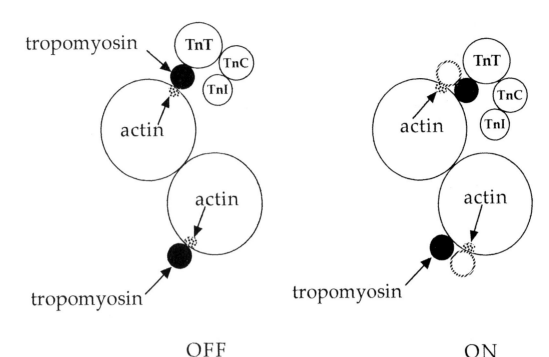

OFF   ON

Figure 11.16. End-on model of thin filaments in resting (left) and active (right) states. At rest, tropomyosin covers myosin reactive sites on actin molecules. When calcium
is released from the SR, it binds to TnC, which causes
tropomyosin to move slightly to uncover the myosin reactive
sites on the G actin molecules (stippled regions at arrows).

protein that links actin filaments together in the Z disc
(Fig. 11.17). *Myomesin* is a myosin-binding protein present in the M line in the middle of the A band. *C protein* is also a myosin-binding protein that is located in
stripes on either side of the M line. The nature, distribution, and function of still other proteins in the sarcomere have recently received attention. One of these,
called *titin*, is a fibrous protein whose molecules span
half a sarcomere from the M line to the Z line and are
closely associated with the myosin thick filaments (Fig.
11.18). The carboxy-terminal end of each titin is anchored to the M line apparently by two M-line proteins,

Table 11.1 Characteristics of Sarcomere Proteins

	Myosin Thick Filament	Actin Thin Filament	Tropomyosin	Troponin
Length	1.5 μm	1 μm		
Diameter	15 nm	6–7 nm		
Spacing	45 nm			
Number of molecules	~350–400	300–400	40–60 per thin filament	40–60 per thin filament
Length of molecule	300 nm	5.5-nm dia.	~40 nm	Globular molecule; one molecule per tropomyosin molecule
Width of molecule	2–3 nm	Extremely thin: <5 Å		Three subunits to molecule—affinity for calcium, troponin, actin
Distance between heads	14 nm			
Rotation between heads	120°			

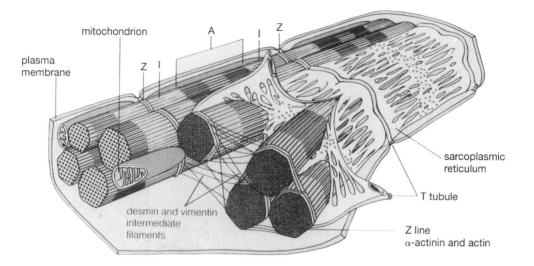

plasma
membrane

mitochondrion

A   Z

Z I

sarcoplasmic
reticulum

T tubule

desmin and vimentin
intermediate
filaments

Z line
α-actinin and actin

Figure 11.17. Diagram illustrates how the sarcoplasmic reticulum is distributed around the individual myofibrils in a muscle fiber. The distribution of desmin and vimentin in- termediate filaments is also illustrated. (From E. Lazarides. Reprinted with permission from *Nature*, 283, 249–256, © 1980, Macmillan Magazines Limited)

myomesin and M-protein. The amino-terminal end of titin is anchored to the Z line, perhaps through interaction with *α-actinin*. Titin filaments appear to play a role in centering the thick filaments during contraction and in generating elastic tension when sarcomeres are stretched. Another protein, *nebulin*, is attached to Z discs and is oriented parallel to actin filaments in vertebrate skeletal muscle (Fig. 11.18). Nebulin may be involved in the regulation of thin filament length, but details are still incomplete. It has been estimated that striated muscle contains perhaps an additional 20 proteins of unknown functional significance.

CYTOSKELETON

A cytoskeletal system is present in the muscle fiber. Each myofibril is surrounded by a sleeve of 10-nm intermediate filaments. The Z lines or disks and the thick and thin myofilaments in each myofibril appear to be held in place by cytoskeletal filaments. In particular, IFs containing the proteins *desmin* (skeletin), *vimentin*, and *synemin* have been described to be concentrated in the Z lines (Fig. 11.17). An actin-binding protein called *filamin* has been identified at the periphery of the Z line as well. *Costameres* are small densities at places where Z

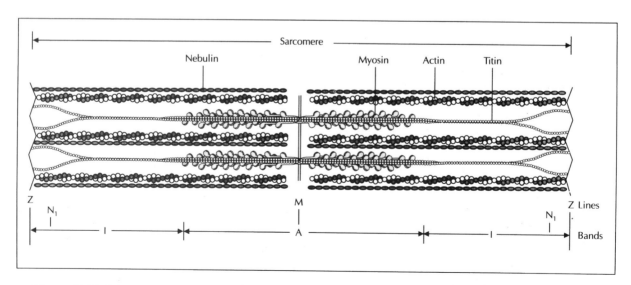

Figure 11.18. Diagram illustrates the distribution of two proteins, titin and nebulin, in the sarcomere. (From T. Keller, Structure and function of titin and nebulin. *Current* *Opinion in Cell Biology*, 7, 32–38, © 1995 Cell Biology Ltd., with permission)

lines of peripheral myofibrils attach to the sarcolemma by IFs and filaments of the cytoskeleton. *Vinculin* is an anchoring protein in costameres.

INITIATION OF CONTRACTION

MYONEURAL JUNCTION

The number of skeletal muscle fibers innervated by a single motor neuron varies from about 100 to more than 1700, based to some extent on muscle size. Large muscles in the arms and legs have hundreds to over 1000 fibers innervated by a single motor neuron. At a motor end plate (Fig. 11.19) or myoneural junction, the arrival of a nerve impulse results in the release of a neurotransmitter (acetylcholine), which causes a depolarization of the sarcolemma that is conducted into the interior of the muscle fiber by transverse (*T*) tubules (Fig. 11.20). The transverse tubules are long, finger-like invaginations of the sarcolemma at the level of all the A/I band junctions in the muscle fiber. The interior of the T tubule is thus continuous with the extracellular space. While the transverse tubules of mammalian skeletal muscle are present at the level of the junction of the *A and I* bands, the transverse tubules are positioned at the level of the *Z bands* in frog skeletal muscle and in cardiac striated muscle. The transverse tubules conduct the wave of depolarization initiated at the sarcolemma of the motor end plate into the interior of the muscle fiber.

The T tubule and two adjacent parallel terminal cisternae of the SR comprise a *triad* or *T system*. The triads are all in register across the entire width of a muscle fiber.

SARCOPLASMIC RETICULUM

The sarcoplasmic reticulum (SR) is an extensive system of smooth-surfaced membranes in the form of interconnected cisternae and tubules surrounding all myofibrils present in a muscle fiber (Fig. 11.20). *Terminal cisternae* of the SR are positioned close to the T tubules so that, in section, three membranous elements are visible with the TEM (Fig. 11.20). These three elements, the T tubule and the two terminal cisternae, comprise the *triad* of muscle fibers. The triad is positioned at the level of the A/I band junction in mammalian skeletal muscle (Fig. 11.21); thus there are two T tubules, four terminal cisternae, and two T systems per sarcomere. In frog skeletal muscle and human cardiac muscle, however, the T systems are positioned at the level of the Z band (Fig. 11.20); therefore, there is only a single T

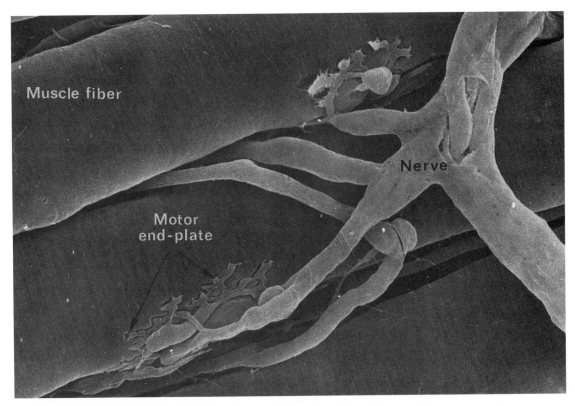

Figure 11.19. SEM of a nerve ending as motor end plates on the surface of muscle fibers. (From J. Desaki and Y. Uehara, The overall morphology of neuromuscular junc- tions as revealed by scanning electron microscopy. *Journal of Neurocytology* 10, 101–110, 1981, with permission)

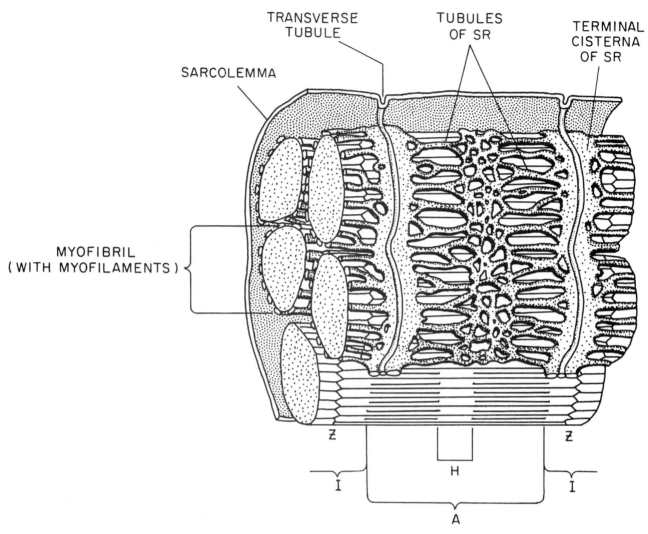

Figure 11.20. Diagram of several muscle myofibrils in a muscle fiber illustrates the relationship of the transverse tubule and terminal cisternae of the sarcoplasmic reticulum in the formation of the triad or T system of skeletal muscle.

tubule per sarcomere, two terminal cisternae per sarcomere, and one T system per sarcomere in this muscle.

Interaction between actin and myosin myofilaments occurs only when a signal is delivered to muscle by a motor nerve. The nervous signal causes a depolarization of the plasma membrane of the muscle fiber (sarcolemma) that is conducted into the interior of the fiber along many T tubules. The T tubules are positioned close to the terminal cisternae of the SR, separated by a distance of only 10–20 nm. When electrically excited, by means not yet clear, a signal is conveyed from the T tubule to the adjacent terminal cisternae. This signal causes large *calcium release channels* in the terminal cisternae of the SR to open, permitting the bound calcium to flow into the cytosol around the many myofilaments where the calcium can bind to troponin C, initiating contraction. The signal resulting in calcium release from the SR requires only milliseconds. The main integral membrane protein in the SR is an enzyme called $Ca^{2+} + Mg^{2+}$*-dependent adenosine triphosphatase* (*ATPase*). From the energy of ATP, the enzyme rapidly pumps calcium ions from around the myofilaments of the myofibrils into the lumen of the SR for storage.

Figure 11.21. TEM illustrates two transverse tubules (arrowheads) and adjacent terminal cisternae (TC) of the sarcoplasmic reticulum (SR). Note the abundance of particulate glycogen surrounding the SR. ×120,000 (From R. Roberts, R. Kessel, and H. Tung, *Freeze Fracture Images of Cells and Tissues.* Oxford University Press, New York, 1991, with permission)

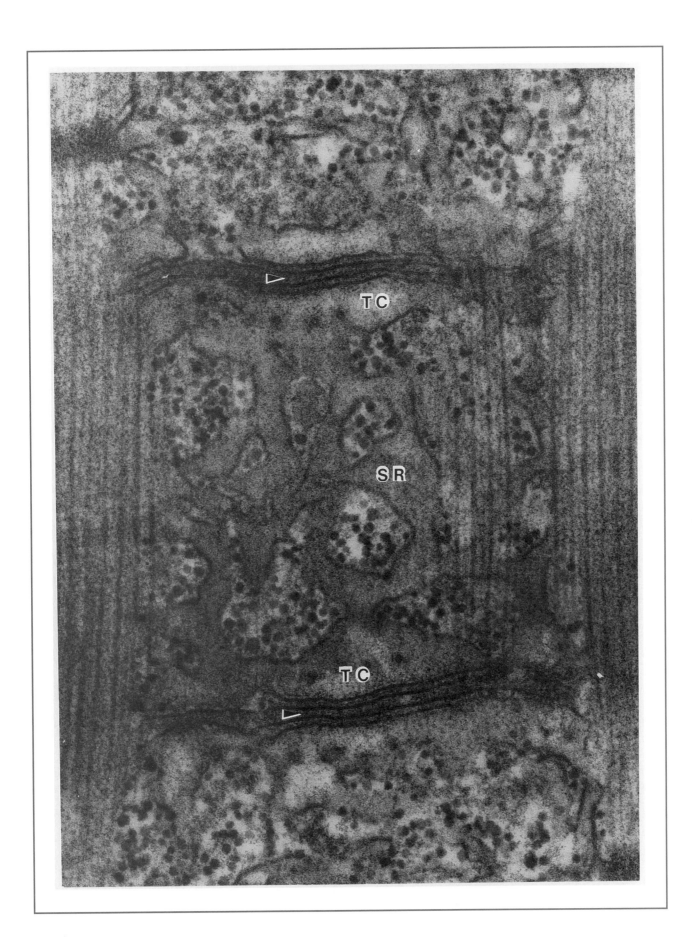

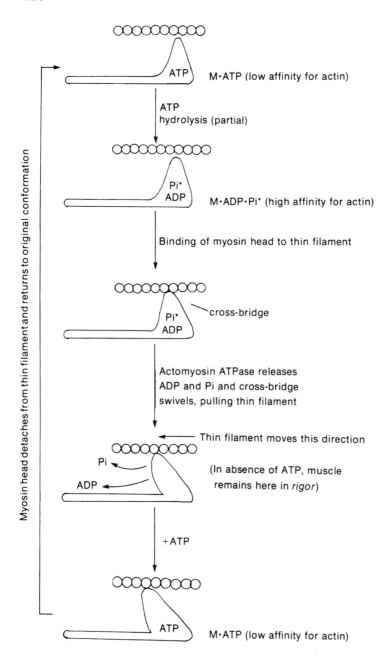

Figure 11.22. Diagrams illustrate sequences during muscle contraction. In the relaxed condition, myosin binds ATP and has low affinity for actin. ATP is split, and the resulting myosin-ADP-P_i complex has strong affinity for actin; thus the myosin heads attach to the binding site on the actin molecules. Dissociation of the myosin-ADP-P_i complex results in a tilting (swivel) of myosin heads and contraction. The myosin head again binds ATP, and myosin heads detach (relaxation). (From C.J. Flickinger, *Medical Cell Biology*, W.B. Saunders, Philadelphia, 1979, with permission)

A calcium-binding protein called *calsequestrin* is a peripheral membrane protein inside the SR that plays an important role in calcium storage. When Ca^{2+} and ATP are added to an isolated myofibril in culture, the myofibril instantly shortens or contracts, thus demonstrating their importance to the contraction process. In summary, the SR plays an important role in the storage and release of calcium ions to the myofilaments in the myofibrils surrounded by the SR.

CONTRACTION

The arrangement and polarity of actin and myosin myofilaments, the presence or absence of calcium ions, and the hydrolysis of ATP are important for muscle contraction. Contraction is an energized process of rapid make-and-break cyclic connections between the myosin heads and adjacent localized sites on actin molecules. Figure 11.22 summarizes the major events in the contraction process.

It should be stressed that myosin, when bound to ATP, has a low affinity for actin; thus cross-bridges are released from their connections to actin. However, with the partial hydrolysis of ATP, a *myosin-ADP-Pi complex* is formed that has a high affinity *for* actin. This complex is "split" but not dissociated. As a consequence of the high affinity of myosin-ADP-Pi for actin, the myosin heads bind to reactive sites on actin. The ATPase then releases the ADP-Pi complex in a dissociation process such that the cross-bridges now swivel and pull on the thin filament. After dissociation of the *ADP-Pi complex*, ATP once again binds to the myosin head, and since the myosin (M-ATP) now has a low affinity for actin, the cross-bridges detach from the actin molecules. In the absence of ATP, as in death, myosin heads remain bound to actin in a state of rigor mortis for several hours.

ATP hydrolysis results from the interaction between myosin and actin. Myosin initially binds to ATP, followed by ATP hydrolysis. While the hydrolysis of ATP to a myosin-ADP-iP complex is rapid, the dissociation or release of the products is much slower. This rate-limiting step reflects the fact that ADP and iP remain noncovalently bound to the myosin molecule. The binding of actin to the myosin-ADP-iP complex accelerates the release of the ADP and iP. The weak binding of myosin-ADP-iP to actin triggers the release of inorganic phosphate, which causes myosin heads to bind actin more tightly and to undergo the conformational change ("swivel") in structure that results in the power stroke to move the thin filament. This is possible since the myosin molecule has two "hinge" regions, one at the junction of the SF1 and SF2 units and the other at the LMM and SF2 region (Figs. 11.12, 11.13). The ADP is released and another ATP binds to the myosin head, which causes detachment from the actin filament and the return of the myosin head to its original position in preparation for a second cycle. Mg^{2+} ions are required for the reactions.

ENERGY (ATP)

ATP is necessary for both contraction and relaxation of muscle. ATP is necessary for the cyclic events associated with the myosin heads during contraction and for pumping calcium ions into the SR, a necessary preliminary for muscle relaxation. The energy required for resynthesis can be derived from oxidative phosphorylation in the metabolism of glucose, glycogen, and free fatty acids. ATP can also be resynthesized during contraction by combining it with phosphate groups from creatine phosphate. Creatine phosphokinase appears to be localized to the M band of muscle based on immunocytochemical studies.

DEVELOPMENT

Myoblasts are uninucleate cells that form skeletal muscle fibers in the embryo. Myoblasts divide repeatedly, and many fuse to form long, multinucleated structures called *myotubes*. Over a period of time the myotubes form many myofibrils. Most of the skeletal muscle fibers develop before birth in humans; nearly all are formed by the end of the first year after birth. However, some

uninuculeate cells, called *satellite cells*, are closely apposed to the fibers and are enclosed in the same basal lamina. Satellite cells are distributed at intervals in surface depressions of muscle fibers; the cells appear to be a relatively undifferentiated type of myoblast capable of some muscle repair. During postnatal growth, skeletal muscles can increase in length and width. After the first year of life, the growth of muscle is believed to occur by hypertrophy of existing muscle fibers, not to an increase in the number of fibers (hyperplasia). Skeletal muscle is capable of only limited repair in adults.

CARDIAC MUSCLE

STRUCTURE

Cardiac muscle consists of separate uninucleate cells. Occasionally, binucleate cells are present. Cardiac muscle fibers branch and anastomose (Plate 25A). The individual cells making up the fibers are joined end to end by specialized junctions. As a result of the branching, small spaces are present between fibers that contain connective tissue *endomysium* with blood vessels, lymphatic vessels, and nerves. Cardiac muscle fibers display the same banding pattern as skeletal muscle (Fig. 11.23). With LM and iron hematoxylin staining, it is possible to observe additional thin, dense lines that traverse cardiac muscle fibers. These lines are called *intercalated disks* and represent the *boundaries* between individual cardiac muscle cells. Their ultrastructure will be described subsequently. Cardiac muscle is striated but involuntary; thus, it will contract without a nerve supply. However, in life, specialized *pacemaker cells* that are innervated by the autonomic nervous system are responsible for the rate of depolarization. The heartbeat is a function of special cardiac muscle (pacemaker) cells, but the rate of contraction is regulated by the autonomic nervous system. Cardiac muscle cells are surrounded by a basement membrane. The myofibrils in cardiac muscle anastomose and vary in diameter, unlike those in skeletal muscle. In skeletal muscle, the myofibrils are more discrete and uniformly cylindrical. The mitochondria are larger and more numerous in cardiac muscle fibers than in skeletal muscle fibers. Glycogen granules, lipid droplets, and Golgi complexes are found principally at the poles of the centrally located nucleus. Thus, the central location of the nucleus in cardiac muscle is unlike the situation in skeletal muscle, where the nuclei are in contact with the sarcolemma. Modified cardiac muscle cells called *Purkinje fibers* comprise the bundle of His in the heart, a part of the impulse-conducting system. Purkinje fibers differ from regular cardiac muscle cells in being wider, having fewer myofibrils, and containing abundant glycogen (Fig. 11.24).

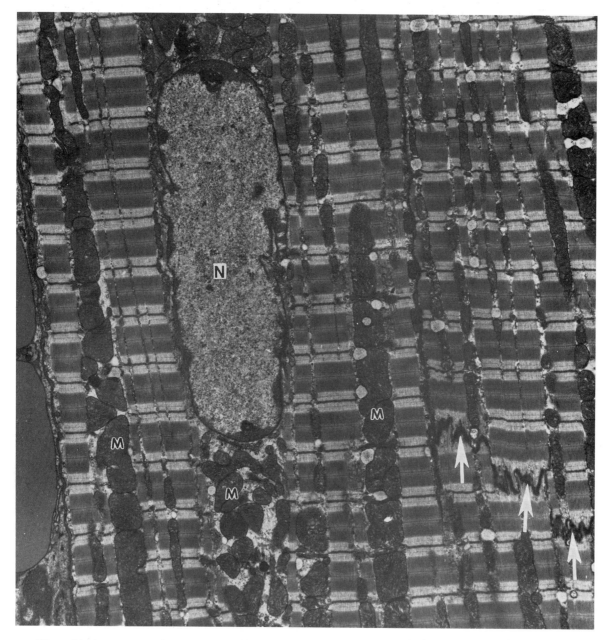

Figure 11.23. TEM of cardiac striated muscle. Note the nucleus (N) and the banding pattern. The intercalated disks are denoted by the arrows. Mitochondria (M). ×5000. (From R. Roberts, R. Kessel, and H. Tung, *Freeze Fracture Images of Cells and Tissues.* **Oxford University Press, New York, 1991, with permission)**

INTERCALATED DISK

Intercalated disks cover the ends of adjacent and contiguous cardiac muscle cells at the level of the *Z line*. This specialized attachment is called a *fascia adherens* and is somewhat similar to a zonula adherens of an epithelial cell. However, the fascia adherens is plate-like and has many more actin filaments associated with the membrane in this region. In addition, the transverse portion of the disk contains desmosomes or maculae adherentes (Figs. 11.25, 11.26). Vimentin and desmin IFs are closely associated with the desmosomes. The lon-

gitudinal portion of the intercalated disk contains large gap or communicating junctions (Fig. 11.27). Small gap junctions can also be located along the transverse portion of the disk. The gap junctions provide direct electrical communication between adjacent muscle cells, and this is maximal in the large gap junctions in the longitudinal portion of the intercalated disk. Intercalated disks thus function in (1) providing strong attachment between adjacent cells, (2) transmitting the pull generated by contraction, and (3) permitting electrical communication so that impulses for contraction can spread from cell to cell over the heart.

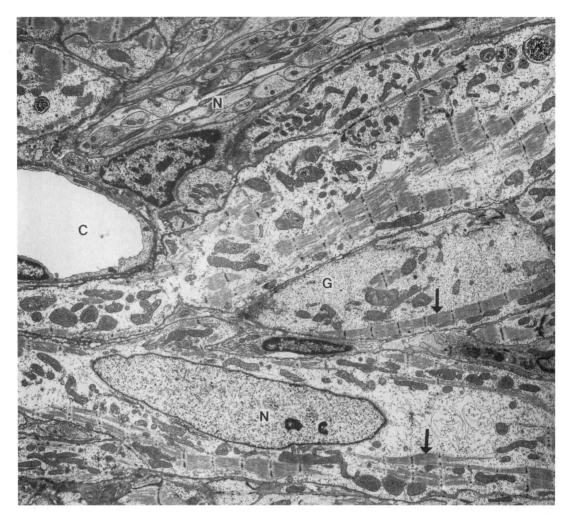

Figure 11.24. TEM of Purkinje fibers in the heart. These conductive fibers are modified cardiac muscle cells that have fewer myofibrils (arrows) and larger amounts of glycogen (G) than normal cardiac muscle cells. Unmyelinated nerve fibers (N) and capillaries (C) are present. ×5500.

T-TUBULES AND SARCOPLASMIC RETICULUM

The *SR* in cardiac muscle is less well developed than in skeletal muscle. The *terminal cisternae* are greatly reduced in cardiac muscle. In mammalian cardiac muscle, the T-tubules enter at the level of the Z lines; thus, there is only one T tubule per sarcomere. The T tubules in cardiac muscle are much wider than those in skeletal muscle.

ATRIAL NATRIURETIC FACTOR

The heart is an endocrine gland since it secretes a potent peptide hormone called *atrial natriuretic factor* (*ANF*). *Natriuresis* refers to excretion of sodium, and the concomitant *diuresis* refers to excretion of water. ANF is present in dense granules located in cardiac muscle cells in the atria and is released in response to atrial dis-

tention. ANF plays an important role in blood pressure, blood volume, and excretion of sodium, water, and potassium. In a manner that is unclear, ANF inhibits secretion of renin and directly inhibits secretion of aldosterone by the adrenal cortex. ANF also acts directly on various sites in the kidney to regulate water and sodium excretion, and causes relaxation of smooth muscle in the vascular system.

SMOOTH MUSCLE

DISTRIBUTION

Smooth muscle is found in the ducts of glands (e.g., gallbladder, bile duct), the urinary and genital ducts, arrector pili muscle of hair follicles, areola of mammary gland (erection of nipple), subcutaneous tissue of scrotum (wrinkling of the skin of the scrotum), and the iris

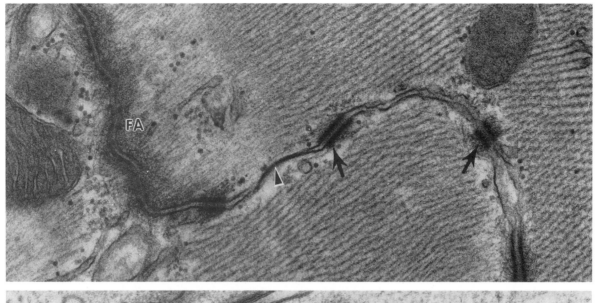

11.25

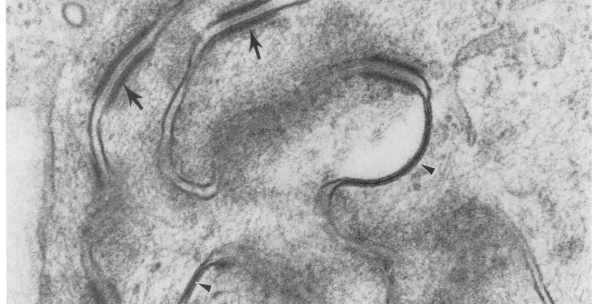

11.26

Figures 11.25, 11.26. TEMs of a portion of intercalated disks. The fascia adherens (FA), macula adherens (arrows), and gap junctions (arrowheads) are identified. Figure 11.25, ×62,250; Figure 11.26, ×93,000. (From R. Roberts, R. Kessel, and H. Tung, *Freeze Fracture Images of Cells and Tissues.* **Oxford University Press, New York, 1991, with permission)**

and ciliary body (constricting and dilating the pupil and in accommodation). Smooth muscle is widespread in the walls of tubular organs of the viscera and in many blood vessels. Smooth muscle is innervated by the autonomic nervous system and is involuntary. It plays an important role in regulating the diameter of organs, ducts, and vessels and in maintaining tonus.

STRUCTURE

Smooth muscle consists of separate cellular units called *smooth muscle cells* or *fibers* that have no cross-striations.

Each smooth muscle cell is a long, spindle-shaped or fusiform structure with a centrally located nucleus (Plate 25B–D). Individual smooth muscle cells in sheets of muscle are separated by about 50 nm. A PAS+ basal lamina or glycocalyx material is present in the intercellular spaces. When smooth muscle is arranged into sheets, the wide parts of the fusiform cells are positioned adjacent to the slender parts of adjacent cells. As a consequence, the thick portion of the cells containing the nucleus is juxtaposed to the thin end of adjacent cells. Thus, in section, many rounded or polygonal units of different size are apparent, only a few of which contain a nucleus (Plate 25B–D). Smooth muscle cells vary in

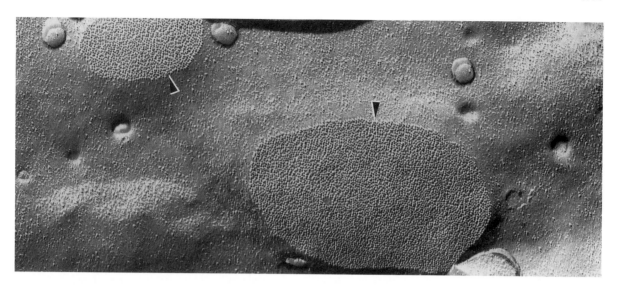

Figure 11.27. Freeze fracture replica of cardiac muscle illustrates two gap junctions (arrows), which consist of closely packed intramembranous particles. ×55,000. (From R. Roberts, R. Kessel, and H. Tung, *Freeze Fracture Images of Cells and Tissues.* Oxford University Press, New York, 1991, with permission)

length from about 20 μm in some arterioles to almost 1 mm in some visceral muscles. The cells are usually 5–8 μm wide. Smooth muscle cells in the walls of certain blood vessels can produce elastin and other intercellular substances. In the digestive tube, oviducts, and ureters, smooth muscle is arranged in circular and longitudinal layers (Fig. 11.28). Rhythmic contractions of these layers produce *peristaltic waves.* Smooth muscle constriction in the iris of the eye in bright light narrows the diameter of the pupil, so less light enters the eye.

Among the organelles confined to the cytoplasm at the poles of the nucleus are mitochondria, Golgi bodies, glycogen, and small amounts of rER. There is no T system in smooth muscle comparable to that in striated

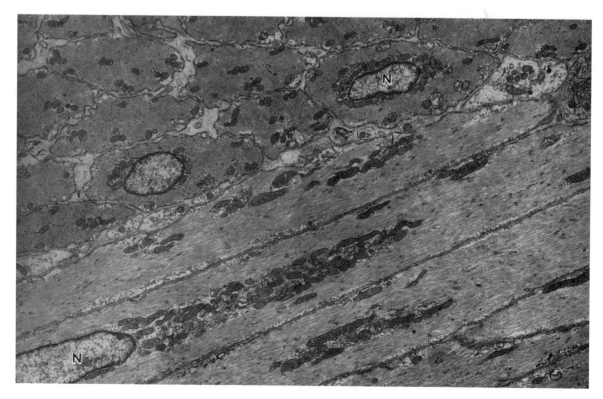

Figure 11.28. TEM, low-magnification view of smooth muscle sectioned transversely (at top) and longitudinally at the bottom of the illustration. Nuclei are present in some cells only because of the various section planes. ×5600.

muscles. The plasma membrane has numerous depressions called *caveolae*, which are flask-shaped and roughly uniform in size (Figs. 11.29, 11.30). When the necks of the caveolae are not included in the section, the caveolae appear as vesicles. The caveolae are usually grouped in rows that parallel the long axis of the cell; this is evident in freeze fracture replicas. They may occupy approximately 50% or more of the smooth muscle cell surface in the pulmonary artery. It has been estimated that the caveolae increase the surface area of the smooth muscle cell by up to 70%. They appear to be permanent structures, but their significance is unclear. It has been suggested that caveolae may represent sites of calcium transport across the cell membrane or sites for the control of cell volume. The caveolae are regarded by some as the possible counterparts of the T tubules. Single short, smooth, membranous lamellae are sometimes present between the caveolae in the smooth muscle cell when viewed with the TEM. It is unclear if these lamellae are related to SR membranes of other muscle types.

The sarcoplasm of smooth muscle contains both thick myosin and thin actin myofilaments, as well as a system of IFs. The demonstration of these filaments, especially myosin, in smooth muscle cells is difficult and requires especially good preservation in transmission electron micrographs. Electron-dense regions or plaques are present in both the cytoplasm and the inner surface of the plasma membrane of the smooth muscle cell. Smooth muscle thick filaments contain *myosin II* molecules that differ from striated muscle myosin molecules in the amino acid sequences of both the H and L chains. Smooth muscle thin filaments are anchored in *cytoplasmic dense bodies* that appear to be the functional equivalent of Z lines in striated muscle (Figs. 11.31–11.33). The cytoplasmic dense bodies contain α-actinin. The thin filaments between two adjacent cytoplasmic dense bodies together with associated thick filaments resemble an unorganized sarcomere. The proportion of thick filaments to thin filaments is 1:6 in striated muscle. In smooth muscle, however, there is 1 thick filament for approximately 12–18 thin filaments. IFs extend from the plasma membrane dense plaques to cytoplasmic electron densities. The regulatory protein tropomyosin is present in smooth muscle. Troponin is absent in smooth muscle cells, but the protein caldesmon seems to play a comparable role in smooth muscle contraction. *Caldesmon* is an important protein in smooth muscle that interacts with actin, myosin, tropomyosin, and calcium-calmodulin. Caldesmon appears to have a regulatory role in smooth muscle contraction and an organizational role in maintaining the proper orientation of myosin filaments. The system of 10-nm-wide IFs serves as a supporting framework for the

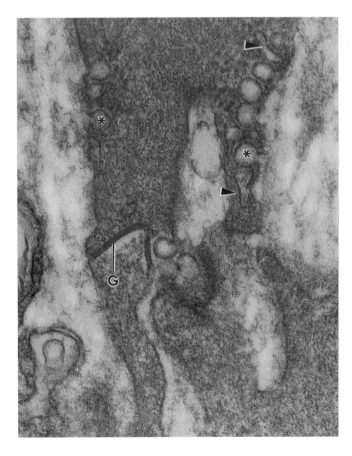

Figure 11.29. TEM of a portion of two smooth muscle cells in the region of the gap junction (G) (arrow). Note also the caveolae (*) and membranous elements (arrowheads) between the caveolae. ×75,000.

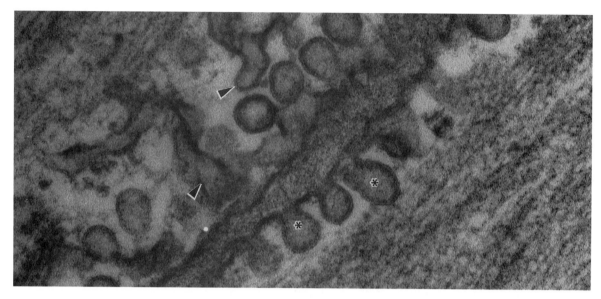

Figure 11.30. TEM of a small portion of the plasma membrane of two adjacent smooth muscle cells. Note the caveolae (*) attached to the plasma membrane and membranous elements (arrowheads). ×125,000.

smooth muscle cell. These IFs extend between the plasma membrane and numerous electron-dense bodies present in the interior of the smooth muscle cells (Fig. 11.34). Desmin is the principal IF protein in smooth muscle, although vimentin is present in vascular smooth muscle. The desmin IFs are organized into bundles that attach to electron-dense plaques along the inner surface of the plasma membrane. Based on fluorescent antibody staining, both vinculin and talin are also present in the electron-dense plaques associated with the plasma membrane

MECHANISM OF CONTRACTION

In smooth muscle, contraction is triggered by a rise in cytosolic Ca^{2+} but does not involve a troponin-tropomyosin complex, as in skeletal muscle. Rather, contraction is initiated as a result of the phosphorylation of one of the two myosin L chains. When the L chain is phosphorylated, myosin heads interact with adjacent actin filaments in contraction. When the L chain is dephosphorylated, the myosin heads dissociate from the actin and relaxation occurs. The enzyme *myosin light-*

Figures 11.31, 11.32. Sections of smooth muscle cells from arterioles. Note the electron-dense regions in the cell and associated with the cell membrane (arrows). Figure 11.31, ×7875; Figure 11.32, ×15,500.

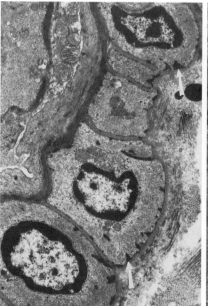

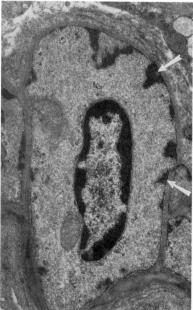

11.31

11.32

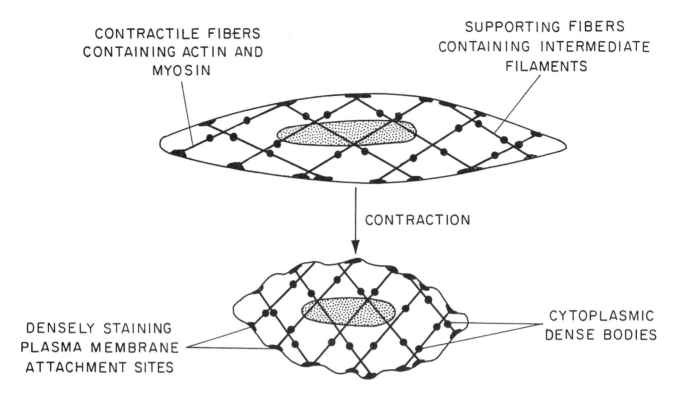

CONTRACTILE FIBERS
CONTAINING ACTIN AND
MYOSIN

SUPPORTING FIBERS
CONTAINING INTERMEDIATE
FILAMENTS

CONTRACTION

DENSELY STAINING
PLASMA MEMBRANE
ATTACHMENT SITES

CYTOPLASMIC
DENSE BODIES

Figure 11.33. Diagrams illustrate the distribution of contractile filaments and intermediate filaments in the smooth muscle cell and their attachment to cytoplasmic dense bodies and plasma membrane attachment plaques. The lower diagram illustrates the shape change that occurs in the smooth muscle cell during contraction.

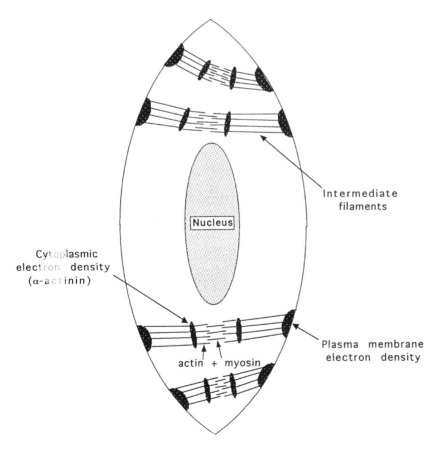

Figure 11.34. Alternative view of contractile and intermediate filament localization in smooth muscle cells. In this view, actin and myosin myofilaments are located between electron-dense cytoplasmic structures. Intermediate filaments predominate between cytoplasmic and plasma membrane densities.

Intermediate
filaments

Nucleus

Cytoplasmic
electron density
(α-actinin)

Plasma membrane
electron density

actin + myosin

chain kinase causes the *phosphorylation* of the *myosin head*. The action of this enzyme, in turn, requires its binding of a *calcium-calmodulin complex*. Therefore, calcium also controls contraction in smooth muscle, as in other muscle types. Because phosphorylation is a relatively slow process, contraction of smooth muscle is also slow relative to that of other muscle types. In addition, myosin hydrolyzes ATP much more slowly in smooth muscle than in skeletal muscle. Although smooth muscle contracts slowly, it is able to sustain contraction over comparatively longer time periods while utilizing less energy than does striated muscle.

As an example, when a hormone such as norepinephrine circulates in smooth muscle, it binds to receptors in the smooth muscle plasma membrane and causes the opening of calcium channels in the ER or plasma membrane. The opening of calcium channels often occurs through the inositol triphosphate/diacylglycerol second-messenger pathway. During smooth muscle contraction, calcium activates *calmodulin*, which then activates *myosin light chain kinase*, which, in turn, causes phosphorylation of regulatory light chains and the consequent attach-pull-release cycle of myosin and actin. In addition, there is an actin-linked pathway that involves *caldesmon*. The calcium-calmodulin complex induces a conformational change in caldesmon such that caldesmon is released from actin so as to uncover the myosin-binding sites on the actin filaments.

Smooth muscle cells in some organs have *gap junctions* that permit direct ion flow from one cell to the neighboring cell (Figs. 11.29, 11.35). These gap junctions provide a low-resistance connection between these electrically coupled cells. Contraction rates of smooth muscle are variable but are usually 10 to 1000 times slower than those of skeletal muscle. Smooth muscle cells in blood vessels have receptors for norepinephrine, angiotensin, and vasopressin, all of which stimulate contraction (vasoconstriction). Bradykinin and prostaglandins may cause loss of smooth muscle tone and *vasodilatation*. Smooth muscle cells in the wall of the uterus during pregnancy increase not only in size (hypertrophy) but also in number (hyperplasia). Mitotic figures can be observed among the smooth muscle cells in this case. New smooth muscle cells can also arise from pericytes that are distributed along the surface of small blood vessels. A comparison of skeletal, cardiac, and smooth muscle is summarized in Table 11.2.

CLINICAL CORRELATIONS

Satellite cells present in skeletal muscle fibers are a potential source of new myoblasts that can fuse with one another to form new skeletal muscle fibers. In postnatal life, myoblast cells can fuse with skeletal muscle fibers to lengthen them. Because of limited capability for re-

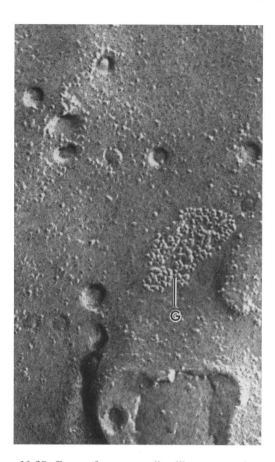

Figure 11.35. Freeze fracture replica illustrates a cluster of intramembranous particles characteristic of a gap junction (G) between two smooth muscle cells. ×64,000.

generation in postnatal life, damaged muscle is replaced by disorganized skeletal muscle and scar tissue. Although skeletal muscle regeneration is limited, these muscles can grow larger in mass and strength in response to frequent exercise. This is due to hypertrophy of existing muscles, not to the addition of new muscle fibers. A decrease in muscle mass may occur as individuals age. Changes in the nervous and circulatory systems of muscle with age may also adversely affect muscle function.

The inner surface of the sarcolemma has a 400-kD protein called *dystrophin*, which coats the cytoplasmic side of the sarcolemma and appears to provide support for the membrane. Dystrophin is structurally similar to spectrin and is thought to couple sarcolemma membrane proteins to actin myofilaments. In the disease Duchenne muscular dystrophy, dystrophin is lacking and a weakening of the sarcolemma results in damaged muscle fibers that are progressively replaced by connective tissue and adipocytes.

Myasthenia gravis involves a deficiency of acetylcholine receptors in the motor end plate. As a result, motor nerve impulses cannot elicit contraction of a sufficient number of muscle fibers for effective contrac-

Table 11.2 Comparison of Muscle Types

Muscle Characteristic	Skeletal	Cardiac	Smooth
Distribution	Skeletal muscles; sheets of abdominal muscle; middle ear ossicles	Heart	Alimentary canal; urogenital, respiratory tubes; blood vessels, large ducts of glands; eye ciliary muscle; arrector pili, hair follicle
Pseudonyms	Voluntary, striped, red and white fibers, skeletal	Heart	Involuntary, nonstriated
Cell shape	Cylindrical (isodiametric)	Branched cylinders; rectangular cell units	Fusiform, spindle-shaped
Branching of fiber	No	Yes	No
Length of fiber	~1–40 mm	<0.08 mm	~0.02–0.5 mm
Diameter of fiber	10–40 μm	~15 μm	8–10 μm at widest part
Sarcolemma	Plasma membrane, basal lamina, and reticular fibers	Consists of plasma membrane, basal lamina, and reticular fibers	Plasma membrane of cells and basal lamina
Control of contraction	Neurogenic; contracts in response to impulse in motor end plates; voluntary	Myogenic; rate controlled by autonomic nervous system; involuntary	Impulses from sympathetic and parasympathetic nervous systems; involuntary
Innervation	Cerebrospinal nerves	Autonomic nervous system (sympathetic, parasympathetic)	Autonomic nervous system
Nature of contraction	Rapid, powerful	Moderately rapid; short intervals between contractions	Slow, rhythmic, and sustained
Number of nuclei	Multinucleate (syncytium)	Uninucleate (occasionally binucleate)	Uninucleate
Position of nuclei	All peripheral (adjacent to sarcolemma)	Center of cell	Center of cell
Cross-striations	Present	Present	Absent
Intercalated discs	Absent	Present	Absent
Myofibrils	Myofibrils prominent and in register	Myofibrils moderately apparent	Poorly defined myofibrils, terminate in cytoplasmic dense plaques
Sarcomeres	Present (~2.5 μm long)	Present	Absent
Actin and myosin myofilaments	Myosin—1.5 μm long, 15 nm in diameter Actin—1 μm long; 7 nm in diameter	Similar to that of skeletal muscle	Myosin—1.5 to 2.2 μm long, 15 nm in diameter Actin—~4.5 μm long, 4–8 nm in diameter
Ratio of actin to myosin	2:1 to 4:1	Similar to that of skeletal muscle	12:1 to 14:1
Tropomyosin	Present	Present	Present
Troponin complex	Present	Present	Absent

Table 11.2 Comparison of Muscle Types *continued*

Muscle Characteristic	Skeletal	Cardiac	Smooth
Ca^{2+} role in contraction	Ca^{2+} binds troponin subunit; permits myosin heads to interact with actin (contraction)	Similar to that of skeletal muscle	Ca^{2+} binds calmodulin, activating myosin light chain kinase, which phosphorylates myosin (contraction)
T tubule	T tubules present at A-1 band junction (human)	T tubules wider, present at level of Z lines (human)	Surface pits (caveolae) may be a primitive T-tubule system
Sarcoplasmic reticulum	Well-developed system; terminal cisternae (triads)	Terminal cisternae less well developed (diads—1 T tubule and 1 terminal cisternae)	Sparse; located among surface caveolae
Cytoplasmic dense bodies	Absent	Absent	Present; contain α-actinin and desmin IFs
Intermediate filaments	Desmin	Desmin	Desmin (vimentin in vascular smooth muscle)
Mitochondria	Moderate size; numerous	Long (~2.5 μm long); numerous	Small
Junctional complexes	None	Desmosomes, gap junctions (ionic coupling), fascia adherens	Gap junctions
Glycogen	Abundant (0.5–1% muscle weight)	Moderate	Sparse
Lipid	Sparse	Abundant	Sparse
Basal lamina	Present	Present	Present

tion. The condition can result when patients develop antibodies to their acetylcholine receptors or, to a lesser extent, antibodies against titin.

Cardiac muscle does not divide, and few or no satellite cells are present. Thus, cardiac muscle has no capacity for muscular regeneration. If a part of the myocardium dies, it is replaced by scar tissue. Increased demands on the heart result in enlargement (hypertrophy) of existing muscle cells.

SELECTED BIBLIOGRAPHY

Amos, L.A. (1985). Structure of muscle filaments studied by electron microscopy. *Annu. Rev. Biophys. Chem.* **14**, 291–313.

Cooke, R. (1986). The mechanism of muscle contraction. *CRC Crit. Rev. Biochem.* **21**, 53–118.

Draeger, A., Amos, W.B., Ikebe, M., and Small, J.V. (1990). The cytoskeleton and contractile apparatus of smooth muscle. *J. Cell Biol.* **111**, 2463–2473.

Grounds, M.D. (1991). Towards understanding skeletal muscle regeneration. *Pathol. Res. Pract.* **187**, 1–22.

Hall, Z.W., and Sanes, J.R. (1993). Synaptic structure and development: the neuromuscular junction. *Cell* **72** (suppl), 99–121.

Holmes, K.C., Poss, D., Gebhard, W., and Kabsch, W. (1990). Atomic model of the actin filament. *Nature* **347**, 44–49.

Irving, M. (1987). Muscle mechanics and probes of the cross-bridge cycle. In *Fibrous Protein Structure*, J.M. Squire and P.J. Vibert, eds. Academic Press, Orlando, FL.

Katz, B. (1988). *Nerve, Muscle and Synapse*. McGraw-Hill, New York.

Keller, T. (1995). Structural and function of titin and nebulin. *Current Opin. Cell Biol.* **7**, 32–38.

Korn, E.D., and Hammer, J.A. (1990). Myosin I. *Curr. Opin. Cell Biol.* **2**, 57–61.

Morgan, J.P., Perreault, D.L., and Morgan, K.G. (1991). The cellular basis of contraction and relaxation in cardiac and vascular smooth muscle. *Am. Heart J.* **121**, 961–968.

Moss, R.L., and Hofmann, P.A. (1991). Cellular and molecular basis of muscle contraction. In *Fundamentals of Medical Cell Biology*, Vol. 5B, E. Bittar, ed. JAI Press, Greenwich, CT.

Payne, M.R., and Rudnick, S.E. (1989). Regulation of vertebrate-striated muscle contraction. *Trends Biochem. Sci.* **14**, 357–360.

Saito, A., Inui, M., Radermacher, M., Frank, J., and Fleischer, S. (1988). Ultrastructure of the calcium-release channel of sarcoplasmic reticulum. *J. Cell Biol.* **107**, 211–219.

Sever, N.J. (1990). The cardiac gap junction and intercalated disc. *Int. J. Cardiol.* **26**, 137–173.

Squire, J.M. (1986). *Muscle: Design, Diversity and Disease.* Benjaimin Cummings, Menlo Park, CA.

Squire, J.M., ed. (1989). Molecular mechanisms in muscular contraction. In *Topics in Molecular and Structural Biology*, Vol. 3, Academic Press, New York.

Titus, M.A. (1993). Myosin. *Curr. Opin. Cell Biol.* **5**, 77–81.

Trybus, K.M. (1991). Regulation of smooth muscle myosin. *Cell Motil. Cytoskeleton* **18**, 81–85.

Nervous Tissue

Nervous tissue is that type of tissue in which protoplasm is most highly adapted for excitability and conductivity, that is, the ability to respond to appropriate stimulation and to react by transmitting a nervous impulse. The fundamental unit of nervous tissue is the *neuron,* and the basic unit of information that is transmitted throughout the nervous system is an action potential. Nervous tissue is organized into the *central nervous system* (*CNS*), consisting of the brain and spinal cord, and the *peripheral nervous system* (*PNS*), which includes the cranial and spinal nerves and their receptor and effector endings. The *autonomic nervous system* (*ANS*) is a specialized portion of the PNS that is concerned with involuntary innervation of the organ systems.

Since nervous tissue and the organ systems into which it is organized are subjects of entire courses, as in neurobiology and neuroanatomy, the treatment of this topic will be limited. However, an objective of this chapter is to provide an overview of the neuron and its function, as well as the interrelations of nervous tissue to other tissue types that form the foundation for the construction of organ systems.

The principal cellular constituent of the CNS and PNS is a nerve cell or neuron that is both electrically and chemically excitable. Neurons are arranged into complex, integrated circuits over which nerve impulses travel. Neurons are unique in their ability to propagate action potentials. Nonnervous cells in the nervous system have a supportive and nutritive function and are called *neuroglia.* Phagocytic scavengers of the nervous system, called *microglia,* are widely distributed. The brain is extensively vascularized, but this circulatory system is separated from the neurons by a blood-brain barrier.

The nervous system is a derivative of the surface epithelium, the dorsal neuroectoderm of the embryo. Among its epithelial characteristics, the nervous system has relatively little intercellular space; it resides on a continuous basal lamina; and internally it has a free surface lined by ependyma cells with microvilli and cilia. There are also junctional complexes in the nervous system such as zonulae occludentes in the endothelium of blood vessels in the brain and gap junctions. However, no maculae adherentes are present in the CNS. Tight junctions are present between endothelial cells of brain capillaries and between epithelial cells of the choroid plexus. The gap junction is a high-speed, low-resistance pathway of limited distribution in the nervous system and may be utilized in coordinating and synchronizing certain nerve cells.

THE NEURON

The nervous system originates from neural ectoderm in the early embryo. Following gastrulation early in development, a thickening of the ectoderm on the dorsal embryo surface results in a neural plate. The margins of the neural plate fold (neural folds), then touch and fuse to form the neural tube. Cells differentiating from the neural tube include *neuroblasts, spongioblasts,* and *ependymal spongioblasts.* The neuroblasts develop into neurons of the CNS, while the spongioblasts develop into nonnervous *neuroglia cells* in the CNS. The human brain is thought to contain about 10^{11} neurons, or approximately the same number as the number of stars in our galaxy! As the neural folds fuse to form a neural tube, *neural crest* cells are released that migrate into diverse regions of the embryo and give rise to a variety of cell types including *dorsal root ganglion cells* and *sympathetic ganglion* cells, both of which are types of neurons outside the CNS. Neural crest cells also differentiate into melanocytes, smooth muscle of blood vessels, adrenal medullary cells, Schwann cells, dentin-producing cells in teeth, fibroblasts in the iris, and much of the cartilage and bone in the head.

The neuron is a highly branched cell that contains a *cell body* or *perikaryon* and cytoplasmic branches that include *dendrites* and *axons* (Fig. 12.1). *Dendrite* is a term derived from the Greek word meaning "tree" and indicates the tree-like branching that commonly characterizes dendrites. When dendrites are stimulated, they conduct impulses to the neuronal cell body. Frequently, a number of dendrites are associated with the neuronal perikaryon. A single axon merges from the cell body at a region called an *axon hillock*. At some point distally, the axon may branch at right angles to form collaterals. When stimulated, axons conduct impulses away from the cell body.

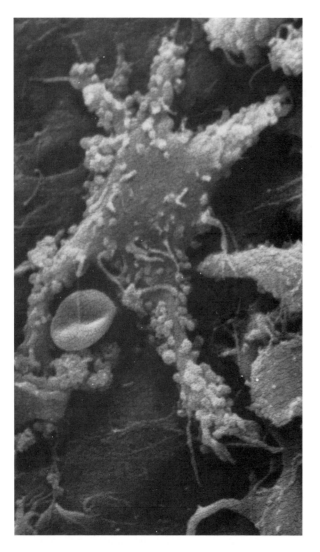

Figure 12.1. SEM of a neuronal perikaryon with several processes leading away from the cell body. Note the thread-like structures with expanded endings (synaptic boutons) associated with the cell body. ×3680.

Structurally, neurons may be classed as *unipolar, bipolar, pseudounipolar,* or *multipolar.* A unipolar neuron contains only one process that is functionally an axon. This type of neuron is found only in lower invertebrates. The bipolar neuron possesses two processes; while they both look like axons, one is functionally an axon and the other is a dendrite. Bipolar neurons can be found in the retina, ear, and olfactory mucosa. Pseudounipolar neurons have only one process that emerges from the cell body but shortly divides into two branches; one branch conducts impulses to the cell body, while the other conducts impulses away from the cell body. Dorsal root ganglion cells and many cranial ganglion cells are pseudounipolar. Multipolar neurons, as the name implies, have many processes extending from the cell body or perikaryon. Typically, many branching dendrites but only a single axon extend from the cell body. Most neurons in the CNS are multipolar.

The dendrites vastly amplify the surface area of the neuron and therefore increase the receptor area of the cell. By means of many specific contacts with other neuronal processes, dendrites permit the acquisition of a vast array of information. The dendritic tree of various neurons is remarkably variable and reflects functional diversity among neurons. Dendrites that emerge from the cell body of motor neurons extend for several millimeters in the spinal cord and have hundreds or thousands of inhibitory and excitatory synapses with other neurons. The axon distributes the information received by this neuron. The information may be modified and relayed by the axon and its terminal branching (arborization) to many effector neurons and structures. The axon provides the route by which information is transmitted to other neurons. Axons may be myelinated or unmyelinated, but dendrites are rarely myelinated and then only with a thin layer of myelin. While dendrites may contain polyribosomes and rER, the axon rarely, if ever, contains polyribosomes. Neurofilaments predominate in the axon, while microtubules are especially numerous in dendrites.

Neurons may also be classed functionally as *motor neurons, sensory neurons,* or *interneurons.* Motor neurons innervate and control effector cells including *muscle, gland cells, epithelium,* and other *neurons.* Motor neurons are *efferent* because they conduct impulses away from the CNS. Sensory neurons are *afferent* because they conduct impulses toward the CNS. Sensory neurons are concerned with receiving exteroceptive (from the immediate external environment), interoceptive (from viscera) and proprioceptive (from tendons and muscles) stimuli. Interneurons are concerned with connecting other neurons. *Sensory* neurons are *pseudounipolar,* while *motor* neurons and *interneurons* are *multipolar.*

The perikaryon is the part of the neuron that contains the nucleus and organelles but does not include the cell processes (axons and dendrites). Most neurons have a large, pale-staining nucleus with a single promi-

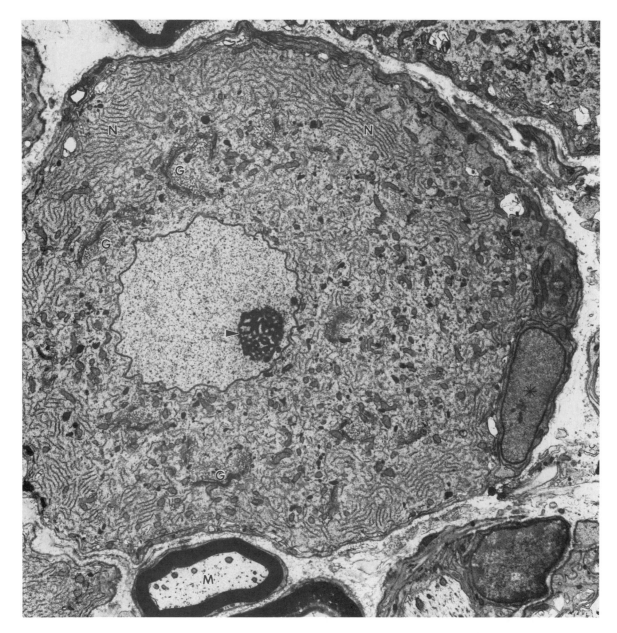

Figure 12.2. TEM of a neuronal perikaryon. Golgi complexes (G) and Nissl substance (N) are denoted. Perineu- **ronal satellite (*). Myelinated (M) nerve. Note the nucleolus (arrowhead) in nucleus. ×5000.**

nent nucleolus (Fig. 12.2). The nucleus is usually in the center of the perikaryon. The rER consists of well-developed stacks of parallel membranes with polyribosomes coating the membranes and polyribosomes are also present between the membranes in a stack (Fig. 12.2). With the LM and basophilic stains, the rER stains as basophilic clumps to which the name *Nissl substance* was earlier applied (Plate 26D). The Nissl substance is absent from the axon hillock and axon but may be present in dendrites. Free polyribosomes are also present and widely distributed in the perikaryon cytoplasm, where they are involved in the synthesis of structural proteins and proteins for export to the nerve endings. When a neuron is injured or under conditions of pro-

longed stimulation, a decrease in Nissl substance occurs in a process called *chromatolysis*. The Golgi apparatus of neurons consists of scattered groups of parallel, smooth-surfaced, membranous saccules and vesicles that are present in the perinuclear cytoplasm. Mitochondria are widely distributed in the neurons; they are present in the perikaryon, in dendrites and axons, and they are especially numerous in the axonal terminations (synaptic boutons).

Neurons contain cytoskeletal elements including filaments and tubules. Neurofilaments are IFs about 10 nm in diameter and of considerable length that are present in the perikaryon and in the neuronal processes. Neurofilaments aggregate in response to some fixatives.

When stained with silver and examined in the LM, they were initially called *neurofibrillae*. Microtubules, called *neurotubules* in the neuron, tend to be long, straight, and about 25 nm in diameter, as in other cell types. They are present in the perikaryon and in all neuronal processes. Both neurofilaments and neurotubules appear to be involved with the maintenance of the highly asymmetric neuronal cell shape. The microtubules also appear to play a role in guiding the movement of small components in the neuronal processes. The microtubule-organizing center (MTOC) of a neuron is associated with juxtanuclear centrioles at the beginning of axonogenesis. The centrioles appear to be embedded in a diffuse, amorphous substance that is thought to contain tubulin subunits. The positive (+) end of the polarized microtubule is toward the end of the axon outgrowth, while the minus (−) end of the microtubule is at the proximal or centriolar end of the microtubules. The thin cross-bridges commonly observed by TEM between microtubules and microfilaments in the neuron probably represent microtubule-associated proteins.

Some neuronal perikarya contain pigment granules such as melanin, but their significance is unknown. Lipofuscin (aging) pigment may also accumulate with age in the perikarya of some neurons (Plate 26F). Lysosomes, centrioles, and elements of the sER are present in neuronal perikarya. In addition, elements of the sER can be found in the neuronal processes.

The common constituents present in the axon include mitochondria, neurofilaments, neurotubules, vesicular and short lamellar elements of the sER, and some smooth vesicles (Fig. 12.3). The axonal ending terminates as a terminal arborization or branching called *telodendria*. The telodendria typically have small, localized swellings that have been called *bouton terminaux* (terminal swellings). The axon of one neuron may end in close synaptic relationship with a number of possible structures, including a *muscle fiber* (in a region called the *motor end plate* or *myoneural junction*), a *gland cell*, an *epithelial cell*, or another *neuron*. Furthermore, the axon termination may end on the *perikaryon* (axosomatic synapse) of another neuron, the *dendrite* (axodendritic synapse) of another neuron, or the *axon* (axoaxonic synapse) of another neuron.

AXONAL TRANSPORT

Axonal or axoplasmic transport is necessary in neurons because there is virtually no protein synthesis (polyribosomes) in the axon. Certain proteins and glycoproteins, as well as mitochondria and membranous vesicles,

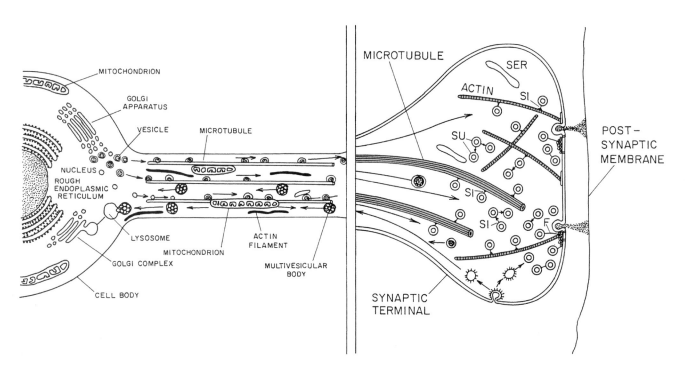

Figure 12.3. Diagram of an axon and an enlarged terminal region. Golgi vesicles and mitochondria may travel along the axon in association with microtubules (neurotubules) in anterograde movement. Multivesicular bodies, mitochondria, and other vesicles may also move retrograde. At the synaptic ending, synaptic vesicles are connected to each other, to microtubules, and to actin microfilaments by thin filaments of a protein called *synapsin I*. When a nerve impulse reaches the axon terminal, calcium enters the nerve and synapsin dissociates (through a phosphorylation process) from some of the synaptic vesicles, permitting them to move to the presynaptic membrane, dock with receptors located there, and then release neurotransmitter by exocytosis.

are continuously transported from the cell body toward the distal region of the axon, and this movement occurs at different rates. A *slow stream* of flow moves at a rate of only about 1–4 mm/day and involves cytosolic enzymes (e.g.: tyrosine hydroxylase, which is involved in the synthesis of the neurotransmitter norepinephrine), actin, myosin, and clathrin. A *fast-flowing stream* moves anterograde at a speed of about 50–400 mm/day. Movement at this rate includes vesicles filled with neurotransmitter. Mitochondria travel along the axoplasm at a rate that is *intermediate* between the slow and fast streams. The mechanism of movement involves membranous organelles and vesicles becoming attached to neurotubules (microtubules) by thin, cross-linking structures that possess ATPase activity (Fig. 12.3). Thus, energy from ATP is used to move the structures along microtubule tracks that serve to direct the flow. Some constituents may be transported from the axon to the cell body in what is called *retrograde* transport (Fig. 12.3). In retrograde transport, movement of material occurs from the synaptic endings to the perikaryon and is powered by cytoplasmic dynein, which is also an ATPase. Dynein plays an important role in movement of vesicles back to the cell body to regenerate new synaptic vesicles. It appears that surplus membrane at the synaptic terminal is packaged into multivesicular bodies that are transported retrograde to the cell body, where they are degraded by lysosomes. Mitochondria can be transported both anterograde and retrograde on an intermittent basis. However, transport of vesicles appears to be a continuous process. Anterograde transport toward the plus (+) end of the neurotubules involves the ATPase *kinesin*.

MYELINATED AND UNMYELINATED NERVES

Within the CNS, cell bodies or perikarya of neurons are found only in the gray matter, which also contains unmyelinated nerves. The white matter contains only myelinated neuronal processes, but nuclei of nonnervous neuroglia cells are present in both gray and white matter. In the PNS, neuronal perikarya are located in *ganglia* (*cranial, spinal, autonomic*), as well as in such sensory receptors as the eye and olfactory area (Plate 26D–F). A ganglion is a region of concentration of nerve cell bodies. In higher vertebrates, the substance of the brain and spinal cord is divided into gray and white matter. In humans, approximately 40% of a section of the brain is occupied by a glistening white substance called *myelin*, which coats nerves. The proportion of white to gray matter increases with progression up the evolutionary scale. In addition, most of the nerves that ramify throughout the body are coated with myelin, which provides insulation and increases the velocity of impulse transmission. Myelin was first named by Virchow; the term means "marrow." This reflects the fact that myelin is especially abundant in the marrow or core of the brain.

Nerve processes may be either *myelinated* or *unmyelinated*. The velocity of a nerve impulse in an unmyelinated nerve fiber increases with the square root of the fiber diameter. In contrast, the velocity of a nerve impulse in a myelinated fiber or process essentially varies with the diameter of the process.

Myelin in the PNS is a differentiation of the *Schwann cell* plasma membrane. Schwann cells are formed early in embryonic development from *neural crest* cells that migrate throughout the body to take up a position on the surface of many nerve processes and over a period of time slowly form a myelin sheath around the nerve process. During myelin formation, the Schwann cell (neurilemma sheath) surrounds the fiber like a hand grasping a wrist (Fig. 12.4). The Schwann cell then moves around and around the fiber so as to build up successive layers of plasma membrane (Figs. 12.5–12.7). The thickness of the myelin or the number of layers of Schwann cell plasma membrane is somewhat variable in different nerve fibers. Junctions between successive segments of myelin are called *nodes of Ranvier* (Plate 27A). Nodes are functionally important regions of the nerve process, for in this region the axon plasma membrane, or axolemma, is bare and the membrane in this region contains a high concentration of Na^+ and K^+ channels that are important in conducting a nerve action potential. The myelinated portion of an axon between successive nodes is called an *internode* or *internodal segment*. At the node of Ranvier, the axolemma is exposed to tissue fluid. A basement membrane surrounds the Schwann cell and extends over the nodes of Ranvier (Figs. 12.4, 12.8). Since exchange of ions between the inside of the axon and the extracellular space occurs at the node of Ranvier, excitation of the membrane jumps from node to node. Conduction of an impulse is therefore faster in a myelinated nerve than in an unmyelinated nerve. The jumping of the nerve impulse from one node of Ranvier to another along the length of the axon is called *saltatory conduction* (Latin: *saltare*, "to leap").

Oligodendroglia cells that form myelin in the CNS have several short branches (Plate 28C,D). The oligodendroglia processes, and thus their complete form, are very difficult to display in routine histologic preparations (Plate 28D). A single oligodendroglia cell can myelinate several nerve processes in the CNS. This is unlike the situation in the PNS, where a Schwann cell can myelinate only a portion of a single nerve process. Further, entire oligodendroglia cells cannot rotate around the nerve processes during myelin formation; only a tongue-shaped extension of the cell's cytoplasm produces the myelin. Thus, the method by which myelination occurs by oligodendroglia and Schwann cells is different. As the oligodendrocyte process raps around an axon, apposing cytoplasmic faces of the layers be-

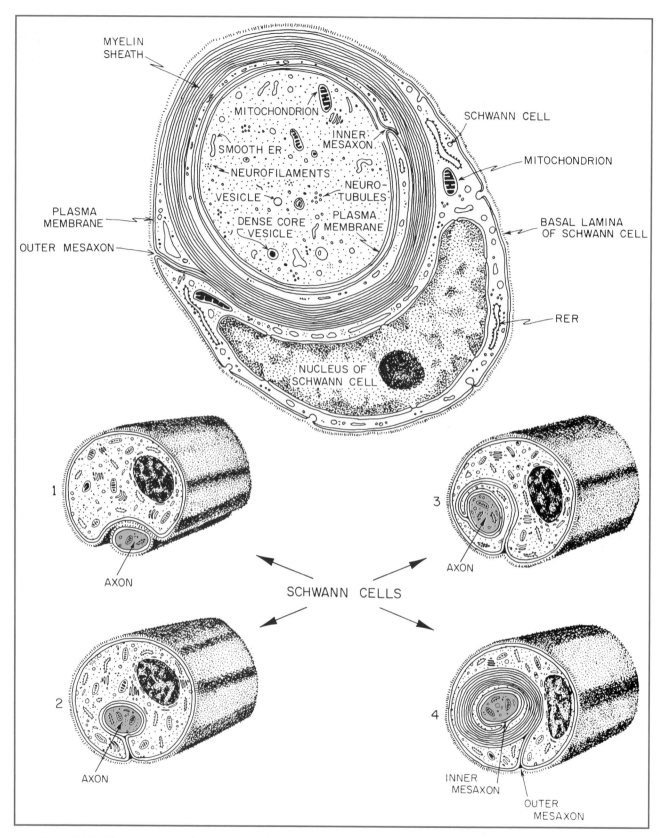

Figure 12.4. Diagram of a myelinated axon, with all major constituents labeled. Lower diagrams illustrate how the Schwann cell rotates around the axon and forms a myelin sheath.

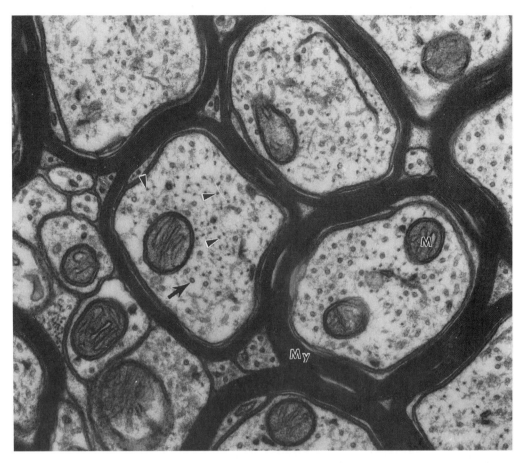

Figure 12.5. TEM of myelinated nerves. Myelin sheath (My). Neurotubules (arrows), neurofilaments (arrowheads), and mitochondria (M) in nerve processes are identified. ×69,000.

come bonded with adhesion molecules. This region of close apposition of cytoplasmic leaflets in TEM takes the form of an electron-dense line usually called the major dense line. The major dense lines (only ~30 Å thick) alternate with interperiod lines that contain an electron-lucent region (~90 Å thick) and a thin line formed by the close apposition of the extraplasmic or outer faces of the plasma membrane of the successive layers of oligodendrocyte plasma membrane. The thickness of myelin in the CNS corresponds directly to the diameter of the axon. While myelination of the PNS is largely complete before birth, myelination of the brain and spinal cord is not. In the PNS, Schwann cells can divide; therefore, some remyelination can occur if a nerve is damaged. Myelin for nerve processes in the white matter of the CNS is formed by *oligodendroglia* cells. These cells cannot divide and do not regenerate after an injury. Therefore, loss of myelin in the brain and spinal cord, as occurs in multiple sclerosis, is extremely serious.

Some afferent and autonomic nerve fibers have no myelin sheath. These *unmyelinated nerve fibers* nevertheless are partially surrounded and supported by Schwann cells (Figs. 12.9–12.11). Furthermore, a number of nerve processes are associated with a single Schwann cell. The nerve processes reside in surface concavities of the Schwann cell, sometimes in deep recesses. While the nerve processes superficially appear to reside within the Schwann cell cytoplasm, they are in fact extracellular.

STAINING OF NERVE PROCESSES

In routine histologic preparations examined by LM, the lipid of the myelin sheath surrounding nerve fibers dissolves during dehydration and clearing (Plate 27A–C). The nerve fibers are pale-staining, and the nuclei of Schwann cells and a thin rim of their cytoplasm are apparent. Osmic acid treatment of myelinated nerves retains the myelin sheath but does not stain the nerve process or the Schwann cell cytoplasm. Heavy metal impregnation (e.g., silver, gold) is used to display the nerve process itself, but this shows little detail in other components of the myelinated nerve fiber. Camillo Golgi was especially concerned with the development of the

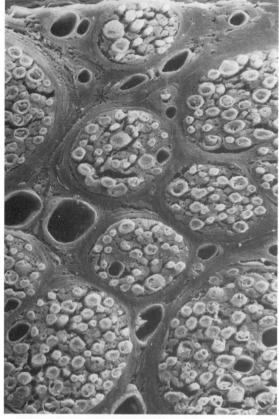

12.6

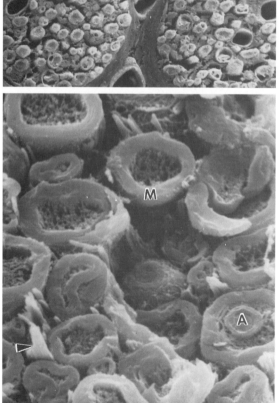

12.7

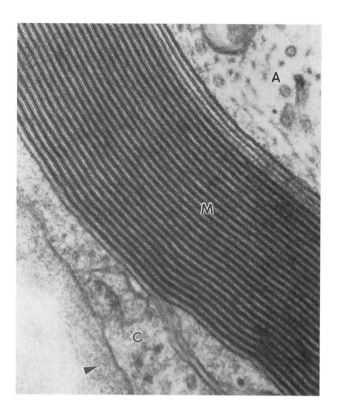

Figure 12.8. TEM of a myelin sheath (M). Axon (A), Schwann cell cytoplasm (C), basal lamina (arrowhead). ×128,000.

Figures 12.6, 12.7. SEMs of myelinated nerves in transverse section. Perimysium (*) around nerve bundles contains many empty blood vessels. Blood vessels are also present within fascicles in endomysium. A variable number of nerves comprise each fascicle. One fascicle is enlarged in Figure 12.7. An axon (A), a myelin sheath (M), and connective tissue fibers of the endoneurium (arrowheads) are denoted. Figure 12.6, ×585; Figure 12.7, ×3,120. (From R. Kessel and R. Kardon, *Tissues and Organs: A Text-Atlas of Scanning Electron Microscopy*. W.H. Freeman, New York, 1979, with permission)

Figure 12.9. Transverse section of spinal nerve. TEM. Both myelinated (M) and unmyelinated nerves (U) are present, Schwann cell nucleus (N). Collagen (C). ×13,230.

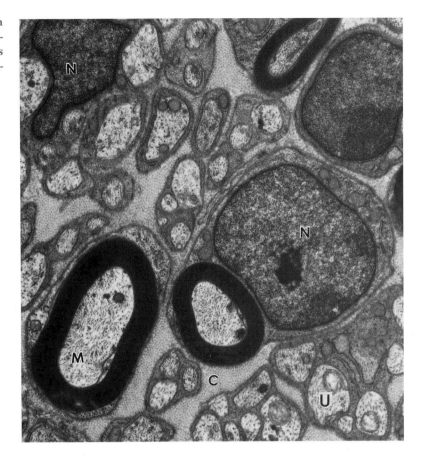

silver impregnation technique, which was used initially to display the Golgi complexes in the perikaryon of barn owl spinal ganglia. Golgi, an Italian neurologist who set up a histologic laboratory in his kitchen, was a physician and surgeon at the University of Pavia. He soaked brain tissue in potassium bichromate for a time and then soaked the same tissue in silver nitrate. The silver was deposited on many of the nerve cell processes, outlining the nerve tracts. Santiago Ramon y Cajal was an outstanding Spanish neurohistologist working at the same time as Golgi. He made some improvements in Golgi's technique and also introduced gold impregnation methods. By using their staining methods, Cajal and one of his students, Pio del Rio-Hortega, were able to distinguish different types of neuroglia cells in nervous tissue. In addition, del Rio-Hortega developed a weak silver carbonate method that was useful for staining microglia in the CNS. Golgi and Cajal shared the Nobel Prize in Biology and Medicine in 1906.

NERVE IMPULSE

The ability of a neuron to transmit an impulse resides in the properties of the axolemma, or the neuron plasma membrane. The underlying mechanism of the nerve impulse involves permeability changes in the ax-

olemma and a "flow" of ions. It was previously noted that the plasma membrane is a bimolecular layer of lipid in which there are protein "icebergs" of different kinds that can float in the plane of the membrane under appropriate conditions such as temperature.

Like other cells, the neuron can maintain a fluid whose composition is markedly different from the extracellular fluid on the outside of the neuron. This difference is especially striking in connection with sodium and potassium ions. Thus, in the "resting" axolemma, the extracellular medium is about 10× richer in Na^+ ions than the cytoplasm (axoplasm) (Fig. 12.12). Conversely, the axoplasm is about 10× richer in K^+ ions than the extracellular fluid outside the axolemma. In the resting condition, the permeability of the axolemma to sodium ions is low so that there is almost no counter flow of sodium ions from the exterior to the interior of the neuron despite the concentration difference in sodium ions. However, K^+ *ions* (which are about 30% larger than a Na^+ ion) can leak through the membrane to the outside more freely. This potassium flow gives rise to a net deficit of positive charges on the inside surface of the axolemma. As a result of this and the sodium pump to be described, the inside of the axolemma is *electronegative* with respect to the outside. This voltage difference has been found to be about −*70 mV.*

A pump in the axolemma maintains this differen-

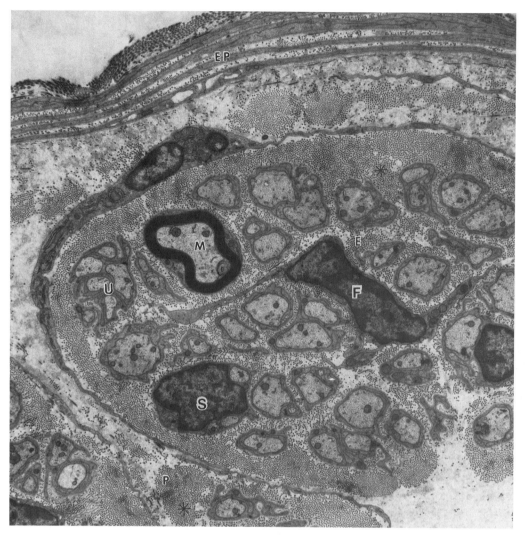

Figure 12.10. TEM of vagus nerve showing myelinated (M) and unmyelinated (U) nerves. The epimysium layer (EP) surrounds the nerve bundles. Many collagenic fibrils (*) are present in the endomysium (E) and perimysium (P). Schwann (S) cell nucleus, fibroblast (F). ×8920.

tial distribution of sodium and potassium ions. The pumping of ions is accomplished by an integral membrane protein called the *sodium-potassium adenosine-triphosphatase pump* (or *sodium pump*). The protein is about *275,000 daltons* and measures about *6 × 8* nm. Each integral membrane protein pump (these pumps can vary in different parts of the axolemma) can harness the energy stored in the phosphate bond of ATP to exchange three sodium ions on the inside of the cell for two potassium ions on the outside of the cell (Fig. 12.12). During the maximum rate of pumping, each pump can move ~200 Na^+ ions and ~130 K^+ ions per second.

The propagation of the nerve impulse coincides with the sudden change in permeability of the *axon* membrane to sodium and potassium ions. This involves a localized lowering in voltage difference across the axon membrane. Immediately ahead of the electrically altered region in the direction in which the nerve impulse is to be propagated, *sodium channels* in the membrane open and sodium ions pour into the axon locally. This process is self-reinforcing; that is, the flow of sodium ions through the membrane opens more channels and makes it easier for additional sodium ions to follow. The sodium ions that pour into the axon change the internal potential of the membrane locally from negative to positive. But soon after a sodium channel opens, it closes. Then *potassium channels* open to let K^+ ions flow out of the axon so that the resting voltage inside the axon locally returns to its resting value of −70 mV. This sharp positive and then negative localized change shows up as a "spike" on an oscilloscope and is called the *action potential*. It is the electrical manifestation of the nerve impulse. Eventually, the original distribution of sodium ions outside and potassium ions inside the axon is restored by the *sodium pump*. The wave of voltage sweeps along the axon until it reaches the end of an axon, much

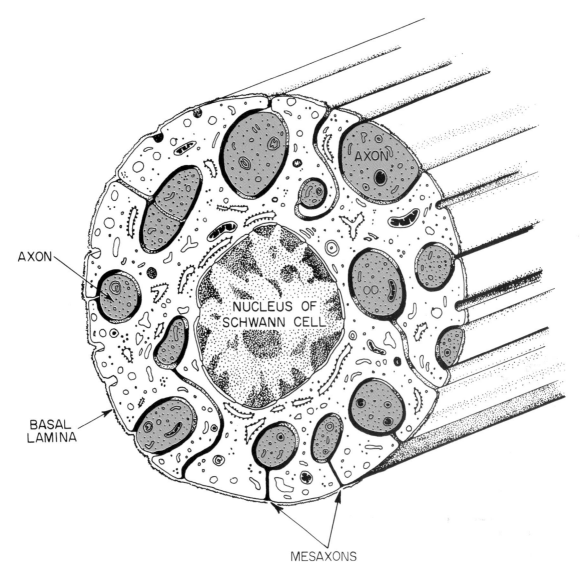

Figure 12.11. Diagram of the transverse section of unmyelinated nerve. Schwann cell with a number of axons of different sizes located in surface concavities (i.e., they are extracellular). (Modified from T.L. Lenz, *Cell Fine Structure.* W.B. Saunders Company, Philadelphia, 1971, with permission)

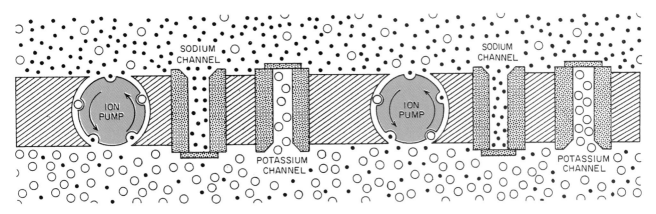

Figure 12.12. Diagram illustrates the sodium-potassium ATPase pump (Na$^+$, pump) in the neuron plasma membrane, as well as sodium channels and potassium channels. Larger circles represent potassium ions and smaller dots represent sodium ions. Through the operation of the Na$^+$ pump, which requires energy, approximately 10× more sodium ions are located outside the axolemma than inside, and approximately 10× more potassium ions are located inside the axolemma than outside. Each Na$^+$ pump transfers three sodium and two potassium ions.

like the flame that travels along the fuse of a fire-cracker.

The gating mechanism that regulates the opening and closing of the membrane channels may be (1) *voltage gated* when the channel protein opens and closes in response to voltage differences across the membrane, as in the propagation of an action potential, or (2) *chemically gated* when the channel protein opens when a transmitter molecule binds to a specific receptor or channel protein, as occurs in the postsynaptic membrane at a synapse. The chemically gated channels are found at the synapse and are concerned with translating the chemical signals produced by the axon terminals into permeability changes during synaptic transmission. Conformational changes in the channel proteins that are composed of subunits form the basis for gating, as they open and close the channel by slight movement.

THE SYNAPSE

STRUCTURE

The principal means of communication in the nervous system occurs through the regulated exocytosis of neurotransmitter, which occurs at the synapse. Since an axon terminal can form a synapse with any part of the surface of another neuron, *axodendritic, axosomatic,* and *axoaxonal* synapses can be found. Synapses between two dendrites (*dendrodendritic*), between the perikaryon or soma of two neurons (*somatosomatic*), and between soma and dendrites (*somatodendritic* and *dendrosomatic*) are also possible. At the synapse, an impulse is transmitted in one direction.

The synaptic region involves a presynaptic portion or terminal and a postsynaptic portion or terminal. The end of an axon terminal of a presynaptic neuron is typically enlarged slightly into an end bulb or end foot (bouton terminaux), and the axolemma in this region is called the *presynaptic membrane* (Fig. 12.13). At a distance of only 20–30 nm is the axolemma of the postsynaptic neuron, called the *postsynaptic membrane*. The intervening region is called a *synaptic cleft* (*20–30 nm wide*). The presynaptic portion of the synapse is characterized by the presence of many mitochondria and an abundance of synaptic vesicles that are about 40–50 nm in diameter.

THE NEUROMUSCULAR SYNAPSE (NEUROMUSCULAR JUNCTION, MOTOR END PLATE)

The motor end plate is the specialized termination of a nerve on a muscle fiber and is a principal effector structure (Plate 30A,B). Where the axon of a motor

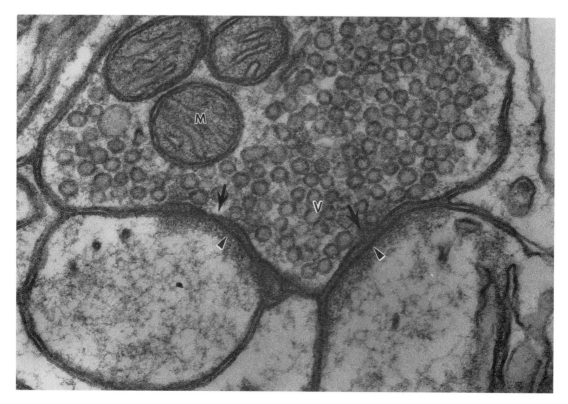

Figure 12.13. TEM of a synapse. The presynaptic membrane (arrow) and postsynaptic membrane (arrowheads) contain a diffuse, electron-dense material adjacent to the axolemma. Note that numerous synaptic vesicles (V) and mitochondria (M) are present in the axon terminal. ×100,000. (From R. Roberts, R. Kessel, and H. Tung. *Freeze Fracture Images of Cells and Tissues.* Oxford University Press, New York, 1991, with permission)

nerve terminates on a muscle fiber, the myelin sheath is lost and the nerve terminal is somewhat enlarged and occupies a depression or gutter in the sarcolemma of the muscle fiber (Figs. 12.14, 12.15). The expanded synaptic ending of the nerve terminal contains mitochondria, many synaptic vesicles 40–50 nm in diameter, and tubular elements of the sER, as well as filaments and neurotubules. The sarcolemma opposite the nerve terminal is typically thrown into junctional folds (or subneural folds). The intercellular space between the synaptic nerve terminal and the sarcolemma, called the *synaptic* (or *subneural*) *trough* or *cleft*, is about 60–100 nm wide (Fig. 12.14). A basal lamina is located in the cleft and follows the contour of the folded sarcolemma. A number of electron densities may be associated with the presynaptic membrane. A thin, electron-dense layer is usually associated with the inner surface of the postsynaptic membrane as well.

During neuromuscular transmission, the neurotransmitter acetylcholine, (ACh), which is released from the stimulated nerve terminal, diffuses across the synaptic cleft and attaches to postsynaptic acetylcholine receptors (AChR) (Fig. 12.14). The binding of two or more ACh molecules to a single AChR causes AChR to undergo a conformation change that results in opening of ion channels, permitting the influx of Na^+ ions and efflux of K^+ ions across the muscle postsynaptic membrane. This wave of depolarization is conducted over the sarcolemma and along the transverse tubules into the interior of the muscle fiber. Ultimately, it causes release of Ca^{2+} ions from the terminal cisternae of the SR at the myofibril level.

SYNAPTIC TRANSMISSION

During synaptic transmission, as the action potential arrives at the nerve terminal, there is an *opening* of voltage-gated *calcium channels* and an *influx* of *calcium* ions into the nerve terminal, followed by *exocytosis* of

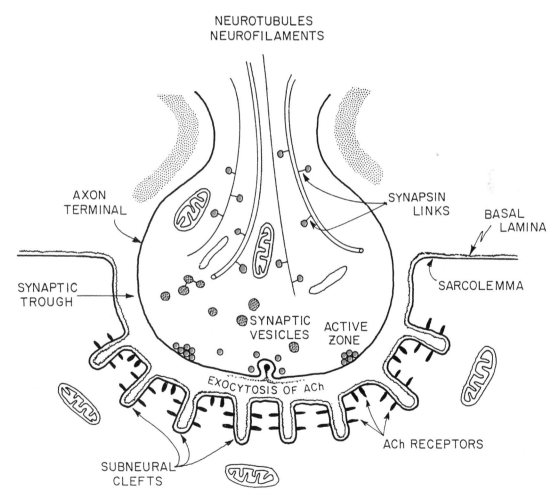

Figure 12.14. Diagram illustrates nerve ending on muscle (motor end plate). Impulse causes calcium entry into the nerve terminal, resulting in exocytosis of acetylcholine (ACh) into the synaptic trough. ACh receptors are present in folded sarcolemma of muscle fiber. (Modified from T.L. Lentz, *Cell Fine Structure.* W.B. Saunders Company, Philadelphia, 1971, with permission)

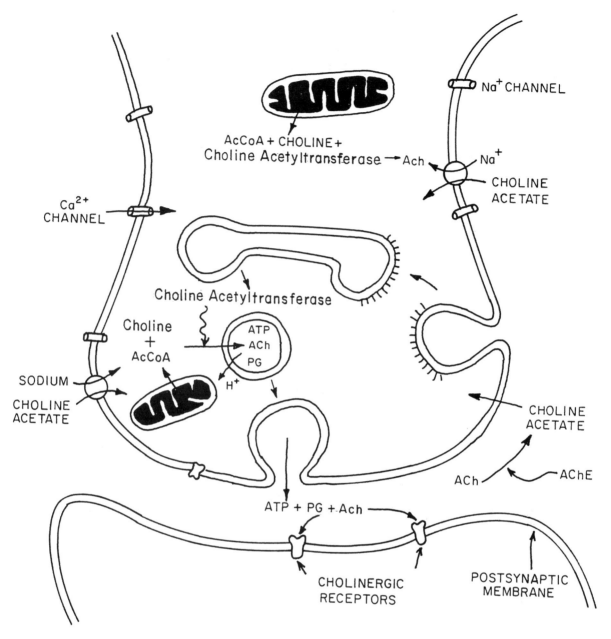

Figure 12.15. Diagram illustrates recycling of ACh and refilling of synaptic vesicles at the synapse, as described in text.

neurotransmitter-filled synaptic vesicles and binding of neurotransmitter to receptors in the postsynaptic membrane, resulting in its depolarization. Calcium ions are pumped to the exterior of the nerve ending by *calcium pumps* in the plasma membrane. The neurotransmitter molecules that are released into the synaptic cleft interact with neurotransmitter receptors in the postsynaptic membrane and produce an electrical response in the postsynaptic membrane (Fig. 12.14). In many synapses, the neurotransmitter depolarizes the postsynaptic membrane. These are excitatory synapses, which result in the generation of impulses in the postsynaptic

neuron. Some synapses, however, produce a neurotransmitter that *hyperpolarizes* the *postsynaptic membrane*. These synapses are inhibitory, since they reduce the likelihood that impulses will be produced in the postsynaptic neuron. *Excitatory neurotransmitters* such as *ACh* increase the permeability of the postsynaptic membrane to ions, particularly opening sodium channels that permit entry of sodium ions into the postsynaptic neuron. *Inhibitory transmitters* such as γ-aminobutyric acid (*GABA*) open anion channels such as *chloride channels*, which increase the electronegativity of the postsynaptic membrane and reduce the probability of neuronal firing.

SYNAPTIC VESICLE TURNOVER OR FILLING

Neurotransmitter is released from 50-nm vesicles that can undergo many rounds of fusion and recycling at the presynaptic membrane. Some of the neurotransmitter-loaded vesicles are concentrated near the presynaptic membrane in regions called *active zones*, and fusion of these docked vesicles with the presynaptic membrane occurs when the intracellular calcium level rises upon arrival of an action potential. Other loaded synaptic vesicles comprise a reserve pool and are organized by cytoskeletal elements to be described subsequently.

Prolonged fusion of synaptic vesicles with the presynaptic membrane could contribute significant amounts of membrane to the presynaptic terminal. However, following exocytosis of synaptic vesicles, they can be reinternalized by endocytosis and refilled with neurotransmitter, as in the case of ACh. After exocytosis of synaptic vesicle and neurotransmitter discharge, the membrane is internalized by *endocytosis* as *coated vesicles*. The clathrin coats are lost and the vesicles filled with ACh and ATP. The internalized vesicles may also fuse with elements of the sER in the nerve terminal, and new synaptic vesicles are then released form the sER containing newly formed neurotransmitter (Fig. 12.15). ACh is a transmitter that can be synthesized locally in presynaptic membranous cisternae from precursors, and from enzymes synthesized in the perikaryon, and transported along the axon to the synaptic bouton. Once ACh is discharged, it is hydrolyzed to choline and acetate by *acetylcholinesterase* (*AChE*) in the synaptic cleft area. Both choline and acetate can be transported into the nerve terminal to be reutilized in neurotransmitter recycling. Synaptic vesicle membranes contain a *proton pump* that is able to drive the uptake of neurotransmitters by an electrochemical gradient across the synaptic vesicle membrane, permitting refilling of empty synaptic vesicles with neurotransmitter at the nerve terminal (Fig. 12.15).

An action potential can result in the release of 100–300 synaptic vesicles, each of which may contain as many as 10,000 molecules of ACh. Further, two ACh molecules are necesary to activate one AChR. At the motor end plate, ACh is inactivated almost instantaneously by the acetylcholinesterase (AChE) located in the synaptic cleft. AChE thus limits the duration of the response. ACh is hydrolyzed into choline and acetate, which can be reutilized in the nerve terminal to form new ACh.

In addition to the synaptic vesicles with clear centers, vesicles 40–60 nm in diameter containing a dense granule (dense-cored vesicles) are found in regions of adrenergic nerve fiber endings. These synaptic vesicles contain catecholamines such as noradrenaline (norepinephrine), adrenalin (epinephrine), and dopamine.

POSITIONING OF SYNAPTIC VESICLES IN THE TERMINAL

Synapsins are phosphoproteins that coat synaptic vesicles and connect them to each other, to microtubules, or to actin filaments at the axon terminal. Synapsin I is not an integral membrane protein of the vesicle, for it can be dissociated from the vesicle by increasing the ionic strength of the medium or by lowering the pH. The synapsins appear to be involved in positioning the synaptic vesicles in the nerve terminal and to play a role in determining which, and how many, synaptic vesicles can move to the plasma membrane and discharge. *Ca²⁺ influx* through the presynaptic Ca^{2+} channels *activates Ca^{2+}/calmodulin-dependent kinase*, which *phosphorylates synapsin*. The *phosphorylated synapsin* detaches from synaptic vesicles, which are then able to move to the presynaptic membrane for exocytosis.

NEUROTRANSMITTERS

A neuron typically can produce only a single kind of transmitter. The transmitter molecules are prepared by the modification of a precursor molecule, often an amino acid, by enzymatic reactions. For ACh, only one enzymatic step is required, but for norepinephrine, three enzymatic steps are required. *ACh* is an excitatory neurotransmitter because it causes positively charged *sodium* ions to move into the postsynaptic cell, which depolarizes it. *GABA* has a receptor whose pore is permeable only to negatively charged chloride ions. When chloride ions enter a postsynaptic cell, they increase the voltage across the membrane and inhibit transmission of the impulse. Dopamine and norepinephrine utilize a second messenger, cAMP, in producing their effects.

In addition to *ACh*, which is a major neurotransmitter, there are a group of monoamines that include the catecholamines dopamine, epinephrine (adrenalin), norepinephrine (noradrenalin), serotonin (5′-hydroxytryptamine), and histamine. Several amino acids including glutamate, aspartate, GABA, and glycine can also serve as neurotransmitters, especially at high concentration. While GABA and glycine are inhibitory neurotransmitters, glutamate and aspartate are excitatory neurotransmitters.

Glutamic acid and aspartic acid have excitatory effects on most neurons. The simplest of all amino acids, *glycine*, is an inhibitory transmitter in the spinal cord. The most common inhibitory transmitter in the brain is *GABA*. This amino acid is not incorporated into proteins. Perhaps one-third of the synapses in the brain have GABA as a neurotransmitter.

Neurotransmitters

Chemical	Class of Neurotransmitter	Principal Feature
Glutamate	Glutamatergic	Main excitatory neurotransmitter—brain
γ-Aminobutyric acid	GABA ergic	Main inhibitory neurotransmitter—brain; role in pain perception
Glycine	Glycinergic	Main inhibitory neurotransmitter—spinal cord
Acetylcholine	Cholinergic stimulating; in CNS, PNS, ANS	Degenerate in Huntington's chorea
Dopamine	Monoaminergic	Depleted in parkinsonism, schizophrenia
Epinephrine	Catecholaminergic	Sympathetic nervous system
Norepinephrine	Catecholaminergic, usually stimulatory	Regulates mood (brain)
Serotonin	Monoaminergic— indolaminergic, usually inhibitory	Low level: depression, insomnia; elevated level: mania (may play a role in sleep)
Endorphins	Peptidergic—opioid	Pain suppression, morphine-like properties
Enkephalins	Peptidergic—opioid	Pain suppression (inhibits substance P)
Dynorphins	Peptidergic—opioid	Pain suppression (?)
Substance P	Peptidergic—nonopioid	Pain transmission—receptors to CNS (excitatory)
Somatostatin	Peptidergic—nonopioid	Reduced level in brain of patients with Alzheimer's disease

CONNECTIONS BETWEEN CNS AND PERIPHERY

The peripheral regions of the body are connected to the brain and spinal cord via two types peripheral nerves: *cranial* and *spinal*. These are paired structures that usually contain both sensory and motor nerve processes. Sensory receptors in the periphery are connected by way of *afferent nerves* that conduct *impulses to the CNS. Motor neurons* in the CNS also use the peripheral nerves to extend *efferent nerves* to the *periphery*. The spinal cord is connected to paired *dorsal* and *ventral roots* (nerves) that are segmentally arranged along the length of the spinal cord. The dorsal and ventral roots fuse just adjacent to the spinal cord to form the *spinal nerve*, which then extends to the sensory and motor structures. The dorsal roots have small swellings containing nerve cell bodies or ganglia called *spinal, posterior root*, or *dorsal root ganglia*. The neurons in the dorsal root ganglia are *sensory* neurons, *pseudounipolar* in type. One of the processes extends into the gray matter of the spinal cord, while the longer branch extends to innervate the sensory structure at the periphery.

The gray matter of the spinal cord resembles an H in transverse section. Neuronal cell bodies are restricted to the gray matter, which contains principally unmyelinated nerves. The gray matter is organized into dorsal,

lateral, and ventral horns. Cell bodies of motor neurons are located in the ventral horn of gray matter in the spinal cord. The axon of these neurons leaves the spinal cord by the ventral root and extends through the spinal nerves to the motor end plates

The white matter surrounds the gray matter of the spinal cord and is so named because of the appearance of the nerve fibers, which are sheathed by meylin (produced by oligodendroglia). Neuronal cell bodies are not present in the white matter, but cell bodies of astrocytes, oligodendroglia, and microglia are located there. Motor neurons that innervate facial and extraocular muscles are present in nuclei located within the gray matter of the brain stem.

PERIPHERAL NERVES

Most peripheral nerves are mixed, containing both afferent and efferent fibers and containing both myelinated and unmyelinated nerve fibers (Figs. 12.6, 12.7). A large peripheral nerve contains many bundles or *fascicles* of nerve fibers. The entire peripheral nerve is surrounded by a connective tissue sheath called the *epineurium*. Some connective tissue from the epineurium extends inward into the nerve, subdividing the nerve into fascicles of nerve fibers; this connective tissue is called the *perineurium*. Some connective tissue also extends into the fascicles to surround individual nerve fibers present; this connective tissue is called the *endoneurium*. Blood vessels, lympatic vessels, and nerves are distributed in the connective tissue elements of the peripheral nerve.

RECEPTORS

Receptors are involved in receiving specific sensations and in transmitting them to the CNS. The sensations of touch, pressure, heat, cold, pain, smell, sight, and hearing, as well as the recognition of position of various parts of the body, cause the discharge of afferent nerve endings. The impulses produced by these stimuli are conducted along afferent neurons to ascending fiber tracts in the white matter of the spinal cord to sensory areas of the cerebral cortex.

Sensory receptors are those that are affected by stimuli such as touch, pressure, pain, temperature, smell, sight, and hearing and are called *exteroceptors*. *Proprioceptors* are affected by stimuli arising within the body wall, such as nerve endings in muscle, tendons, and joints. *Interoceptors* are affected by stimuli arising from visceral organs such as the digestive, excretory, and circulatory systems.

Afferent sensory receptors in muscles (*neuromuscular spindle*), tendons (*neurotendinous spindles*), and joints (*joint receptors*) provide input to the CNS that makes possible an awareness of the kind and speed of movements in different parts of the body.

Stretch receptors called *muscle spindles* or *neuromuscular spindles* are associated with most muscles of the body (Plate 30C,D). The muscle spindle registers muscle length and provides information about the degree of stretch in skeletal muscle. The muscle spindle consists of several muscle fibers that are invested with a connective tissue capsule in the midportion of the fibers. Those fibers that are invested with a connective tissue capsule are called *intrafusal muscle fibers* (intrafusal, "inside a spindle") to distinguish them from ordinary muscle fibers (extrafusal, "outside a spindle"). The detailed innervation of the neuromuscular spindle is outside the scope of this chapter.

Golgi tendon organs, or *neurotendinous organs*, are encapsulated receptors present on *tendons* near their junction with muscles (Plate 30E,F). The myelinated afferent nerve fiber that supplies a tendon organ loses its myelin sheath, and the terminals ramify between the collagen bundles of the tendon. The tendon organ is stimulated as the nerve terminals are twisted or compressed when the tendon is subjected to tension. There is no efferent innervation of tendon organs. When the Golgi tendon organ is stimulated, it reflexively inhibits firing of the motor neurons that supply the adjacent muscle so as to terminate the contraction reflex caused by stretching.

FREE NERVE ENDINGS

A number of sensory receptors are located in different regions of the integument. Free nerve endings terminate among the epithelial cells in the basal layers of the epidermis and are thought to be *thermoreceptors* and *nociceptors* (pain). Free nerve endings are also associated with the hair follicles and represent a type of mechanoreceptor since they respond to displacement of the hairs. Free nerve endings are also attached to specialized cells, called *Merkel cells*, in the stratum germinativum of the skin, as well as on the surface of the hands and feet. *Merkel endings* are thought to be *mechanoreceptors*.

ENCAPSULATED NERVE ENDINGS

Pacinian corpuscles are ovoid structures about 1–2 mm long. They are encapsulated and are scattered throughout the dermis and subcutaneous tissue (Plate 29C,D). The myelinated nerve that supplies the corpuscle loses the myelin inside the receptor and is encapsulated by many layers of flattened cells. Pacinian corpuscles detect *deep pressure* and *vibrations*. *Meissner's corpuscles* are mechanoreceptors that respond to *touch* or *tactile stimuli* (Plate 29A,B). They are often present in thick skin in the connective tissue papillae of the dermis. They are also associated with the feet, lips, eyelids, external genitalia, and nipples. The nerve ending is surrounded by flattened cells that are probably modified Schwann cells. *Ruffini corpuscles* are located in the dermis and subcutaneous tissue, where they are closely asssociated with collagen bundles. These endings are structurally quite similar to Golgi tendon organs. They were once considered to be heat receptors, but they are now thought to be *mechanoreceptors* that respond to tension in collagen fibers, very much like the Golgi tendon endings. *Krause's end bulbs* are lightly encapsulated receptors located in connective tissue such as that in the dermis. They were once considered to be cold receptors, but they are now thought to be *mechanoreceptors*.

WALLERIAN DEGENERATION

Cutting or crushing a peripheral nerve results in a number of changes collectively called *Wallerian degeneration*. The nerve fiber totally degenerates distal to the cut. A slight degeneration may or may not occur proximal to the cut. Shortly after the cut or injury, the neuronal perikaryon swells, the nucleus becomes displaced, and the Nissl substance disappears (chromatolysis). Macrophages migrate into the area of the degenerating fiber and phagocytose the debris remaining from the degeneration process. Several days after injury, there is total degeneration of the nerve fiber and macrophages remove the resulting debris. In approximately 1 week following injury and degeneration, the Schwann cells begin to proliferate and form a tube into the region of degeneration, which guides the regenerating nerve process. Nerve process (axon) regeneration occurs at a rate of about 1–4 mm/day. It is after nerve fiber regeneration that the myelin sheath begins to reform. A considerable period of time is required for the myelin to regain its former thickness.

CENTRAL NERVOUS SYSTEM

NEUROGLIA

The most numerous type of cell in the CNS is the neuroglia, which is estimated to outnumber neurons in the brain by a ratio of 9:1 and to occupy more than half of the brain volume. These nonnervous cells have long been considered to have a supportive role in the CNS. The neuroglia can be subdivided into *macroglia* (including the *astrocytes* and *oligodendrocytes*), the *ependymal cells*, and *microglia* (Fig. 12.16). The ependyma cells are epithelial cells that line the fluid-filled central canal system of the brain and spinal cord. The functions of oligodendroglia, astrocytes and microglia are summarized in Table 12.1.

OLIGODENDROGLIA

Oligodendrocytes are smaller than astrocytes and have fewer and shorter processes (Fig. 12.16). They are clas-

sified as *perineuronal satellite* cells when they are located in close proximity to nerve cell bodies in the gray matter. Another class of oligodendrocyte, called the *interfascicular oligodendrocyte*, is located between myelinated nerve processes in the white matter. Both perineuronal satellite cells and interfascicular oligodendrocytes can form myelin. Recent in vitro evidence suggests that perineuronal satellite cells may express a nerve growth factor. The cell bodies of oligodendrocytes are concentrated in the white matter, and they are usually aligned in rows between myelinated nerve fibers (Plate 28A). The cells have several short cytoplasmic branches, and the ends of the branches are often expanded into a flap-like structure, each of which can wrap around and around adjacent nerve processes to build up concentric layers during the myelination process (Fig. 12.16). Therefore, a single oligodendrocyte may form a number of internodal segments on several different nerve processes. Oligodendroglia are of different sizes but generally have a cell body containing a large nucleus and a prominent nucleolus, such that they sometimes appear as miniature editions of neuronal perikarya. Once oligodendrocytes begin to form myelin, they do not divide. The cell body of an oligodendrocyte contains mitochondria, rER, free polyribosomes, an extensive Golgi complex, and many microtubules and glial filaments.

ASTROCYTES

Astrocytes are macroglial cells of neuroectodermal origin that provide support for neurons and other cells in

Table 12.1 Functional Roles of Oligodendrocytes, Astrocytes, and Microglia

Cell Type	Functions
Oligodendroglia	
Interfascicular oligodendrocytes	Form myelin; are located between myelinated nerve processes in white matter
Perineuronal satellite cells	May express neurotrophic factors in vitro; thus may play a role in providing a suitable metabolic environment for the neuron; can also form myelin
Astrocytes	May provide a potassium sink when neurons are subject to prolonged depolarization
	Remove (take up) neurotransmitters (serotonin, GABA) from synapse
	Produce neurotrophic factors (in explants)
	Produce cytokines, inflammatory proteins in vitro
	Wall off damaged brain tissue
Microglia	Can retract process and migrate to inflammatory or degenerating regions of CNS—become phagocytic
	Role as antigen-presenting cells—express class II MHC proteins (transformed monocytes)
	Produce IL-1

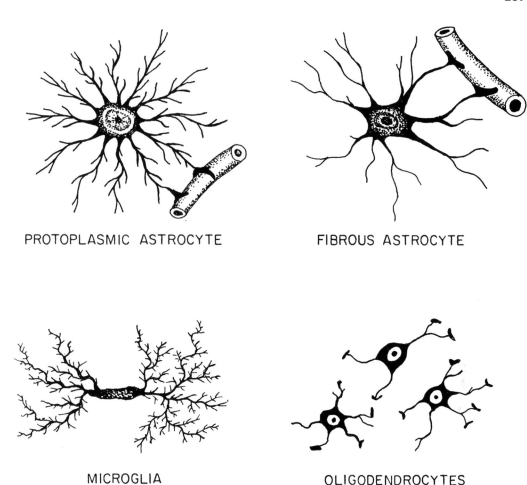

PROTOPLASMIC ASTROCYTE   FIBROUS ASTROCYTE

MICROGLIA   OLIGODENDROCYTES

Figure 12.16. Diagram of protoplasmic astrocytes, fibrous astrocytes, microglia, and oligodendrocytes, showing their usual morphology.

the CNS (Fig. 12.17). Astrocytes were named from the fact that they appeared to be star-shaped with special staining methods (silver carbonate, gold sublimate). The cells are highly branched, and the ends of many of the branches have expanded tips called *astrocyte (end) feet.* The endings of astrocytes terminate on a variety of structures, including nerve cell bodies, dendrites, synapses, walls of blood vessels, and the inner surface of the pia mater. Some of the feet that end on capillaries are called *perivascular feet* (Plate 27E; Fig. 12.17).

Astrocytes contain small amounts of rER and free polyribosomes. A Golgi complex, lysosomes, glycogen granules, and glial filament bundles are present in the cell bodies. Glial filaments also occur in bundles in most of the processes. The highly attenuated astrocyte processes have numerous microtubules and 10-nm intermediate (glial) filaments oriented parallel to the long axis of the processes. The intermediate filaments in astrocytes contain a protein, *glial fibrillary acidic protein,* and some vimentin as well. Gap junctions are associated with the astrocyte plasma membrane. Astrocytes are classified as either *fibrous* or *protoplasmic.* Fibrous astrocytes are located primarily in the white matter and have sev-

eral long, slender, and usually unbranched processes (Plate 27E). Protoplasmic astrocytes, in contrast, are located predominantly in the gray matter and have shorter, broader, and more highly branched processes (Plate 27D).

Protoplasmic astrocytes are sensitive to the extracellular potassium concentration, and it has been suggested that the cells serve a buffering role by taking up excess K^+ when adjacent neurons are stimulated for prolonged periods. Thus, protoplasmic astrocytes appear to serve as a potassium sink under appropriate conditions so that active neurons can be protected from depolarization due to localized elevations in extracellular potassium ion concentration. Protoplasmic astrocyte processes end in close proximity to synaptic areas and have the ability to remove and take up such neurotransmitters as serotonin and GABA from synaptic clefts.

Astrocytes have long been thought to provide some degree of support to the delicate, soft tissue of the brain, which has no connective tissue. Astrocytes appear able to produce factors influencing neurons since they secrete nerve growth factor, brain-derived growth factor, and glial-derived growth factor, which promote growth

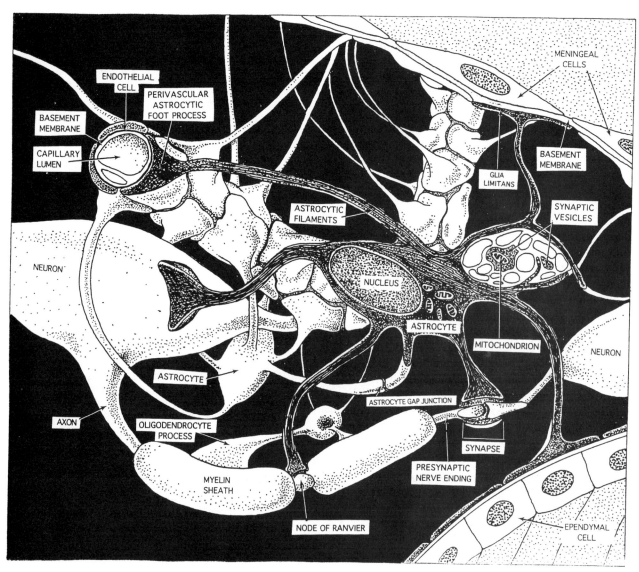

Figure 12.17. Diagram shows how astrocyte end feet terminate in relation to various structures in brain. (Adapted from H. Kimelberg and M. Norenberg, *Astrocytes.* **Copyright**

and survival of neurons in explant culture. They also appear to play a role in the elimination of neurotoxins, and they respond to various neural insults that result in damaged tissue. Astrocytes can express transforming growth factor (TGF-β1), a cytokine with a regulatory role in many immmune and inflammatory responses. Under some experimental conditions involving destruction of nervous tissue, astrocytes tend to wall off the damaged brain tissue. They may play some role in removal of neuronal debris as well.

MICROGLIA

Microglia can be specifically stained by the weak silver carbonate method of del Rio-Hortega, which stains the cell body and the long, angular processes (Plate 28E,F).

However, the cytoplasm is difficult to demonstrate in routine cytologic preparations. Based on silver impregnation methods, processes extend from either end of the small oval cell body, and the processes branch after extending from the cell body (Fig. 12.16). Microglia are about evenly distributed in gray and white matter. The cells are *migratory* and somewhat *phagocytic.* The cells are thought to be derived from mesenchyme, and represent transformed monocytes that leave the blood capillaries and invade the CNS. In response to inflammatory or degenerative processes in the CNS, the microglia proliferate. Some of them retract their cytoplasmic processes and migrate to the site of injury, where they become phagocytic and remove the debris, which is transported to the region of blood vessels. The microglia are antigen-presenting cells that express class II MHC molecules. They have relatively low phagocytic activity to particulate materials. Microglia reportedly are able to produce IL-1. They are observed at the interface between the CNS and blood, as well as within parenchyma of the CNS.

The functional roles of oligodendrocytes, astrocytes, and microglia are summarized in Table 12.1.

BLOOD–BRAIN-BARRIER

The interstitial fluid that surrounds the neurons in most areas of the brain is highly regulated by a blood-brain barrier. The barrier is achieved by the presence of *continuous tight junctions* between *endothelial* cells in capillaries of the brain. Thus, the intercellular spaces between capillary endothelial cells in the brain are sealed off, and substances that enter or leave the capillaries in the brain must do so by passing through, not between, the endothelium. Those capillaries participating in the blood-brain barrier carry out very little transendothelial transport by micropinocytosis. As an additional structural feature, the *basal lamina* or basement membrane is relatively thick, and the outer surface of the capillaries is rather densely covered with processes and *end feet* of glial cells, principally *astrocytes* (Fig. 12.18). The blood-brain barrier shields the neurons from contents of the blood that might act as neurotransmitters. The

barrier also protects the neurons from various harmful substances such as bacterial toxins and drugs.

EPENDYMA, CHOROID PLEXUS (CP), AND CEREBROSPINAL FLUID (CSF)

ORGANIZATION OF CP AND CSF CIRCULATION

Glia cells that line the ventricles of the brain and the central canal of the spinal cord (Plate 26B) are called *ependymal cells*, and the lining itself is called *ependyma*. The cells are simple cuboidal or low columnar in shape, and cilia and microvilli are associated with the apical ends of the cells. The ependyma covers the CP, and here the layer is called the *choroid plexus epithelium* (Figs. 12.19, 12.20). Ependyma cells are unusual in that they do not have a basement membrane. A CP is present in the roof of the third and fourth brain ventricles and in the medial wall of each lateral ventricle. The CP is highly folded into the ventricle. The epithelium is underlain by a connective tissue stroma that is richly vascularized. The endothelial cells of the vessels in the CP contain fenestrations that permit rapid production of tissue fluid, facilitating the production of a watery *cerebrospinal fluid* (*CSF*) by the epithelial cells. The CPs continually secrete CSF. The CSF flows through the brain ventri-

Figure 12.18. Diagram illustrates the basis of the blood-brain barrier. See text for futher details.

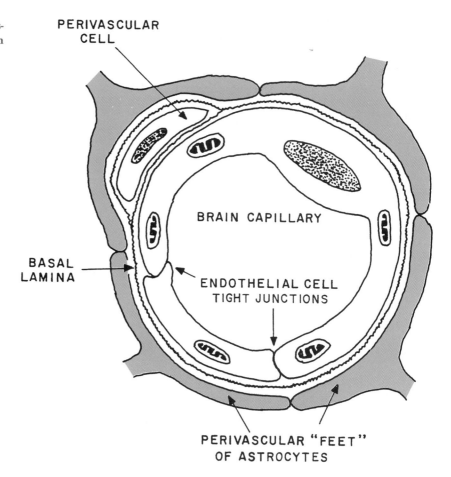

PERIVASCULAR CELL

BRAIN CAPILLARY

BASAL LAMINA

ENDOTHELIAL CELL TIGHT JUNCTIONS

PERIVASCULAR "FEET" OF ASTROCYTES

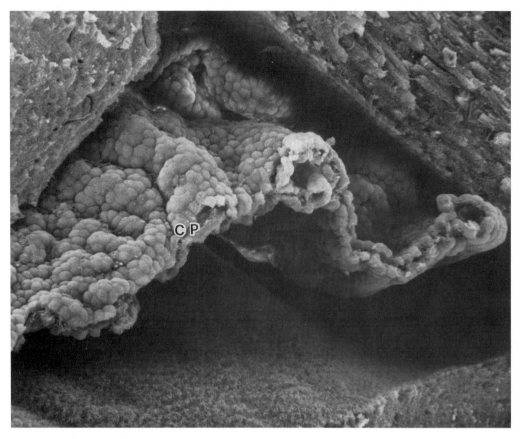

Figure 12.19. SEM of choroid plexus (CP) projecting into brain ventricle. The plexus has been cut. ×340. (From R. Kessel and R. Kardon, *Tissues and Organs: A Text-Atlas* *of Scanning Electron Microscopy.* **W. H. Freeman, New York, 1979, with permission)**

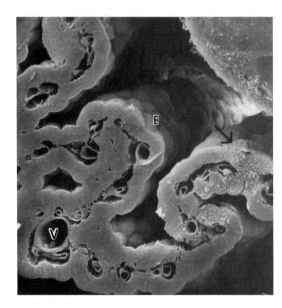

Figure 12.20. SEM of section of choroid plexus shows epithelium (E), blood vessels (V), and an apparent macrophage (arrow) on the surface of epithelium. ×675. (From R. Kessel and R. Kardon, *Tissues and Organs: A Text-Atlas of Scanning Electron Microscopy.* W. H. Freeman, New York, 1979, with permission)

cles, in the spinal cord central canal as well as around the spinal cord, and into the subarachnoid space surrounding the brain. The CSF drains into the blood of the superior sagittal sinus through structural specializations called the *arachnoid granulations*. The CP and the arachnoid membrane comprise a blood-CSF barrier.

FORMATION OF CSF

The cytoplasm of the CP epithelial cells contains many mitochondria that provide the energy necessary for active transport of CSF. There are also vesicles, lysosomes, rER, sER, and microfilaments. The plasma membrane at the basal surface of the cells is highly folded. At the apical end of the cells, the lateral plasma membranes have circumferential tight junctions (zonulae occludentes) that seal off the intercellular space and prevent leakage of CSF between the epithelial cells. Zonulae adherentes and gap junctions are also present between epithelial cells. The microvilli of the epithelial cells contain Na^+,K^+-ATPase. With the use of a strong sodium pump in the microvilli membranes, sodium ions are pumped into the ventricle lumen (Figs. 12.21, 12.22). Water pas-

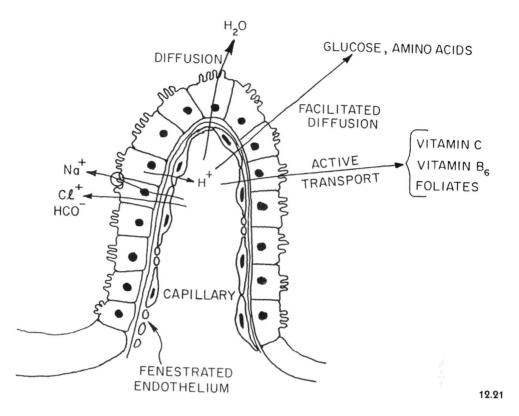

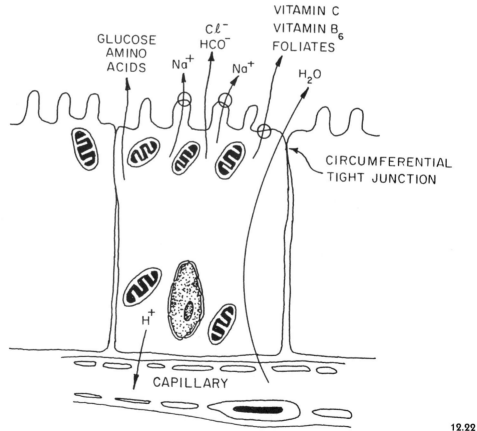

Figures 12.21, 12.22. Diagrams of choroid plexus epithelium indicating the principal functions of these cells in the formation of CSF for the ventricles. Additional details are presented in text.

sively follows the transported sodium ions and passes through the paracellular pathway. CSF circulates between the four ventricles of the brain, and the cilia facilitate this circulation. The fourth ventricle is continuous with the central canal of the spinal cord. The CSF provides buoyancy and diminishes the weight of the brain some 30-fold. The CSF facilitates the distribution of hormones and growth factors throughout the CNS. The CP secretes about 90% of the CSF and provides the fluid with nutrients extracted from blood. The ependymal cells that line the ventricles are linked by gap junctions. The CSF is replaced about every 3–4 hours, and the CSF drains into venous blood through the arachnoid granulations that act as one-way valve. The CSF is 99% water and contains Na^+, Cl^-, K^+, HCO^{3-}, Ca^{2+}, ascorbic acid, folates, and vitamin B_6, which are transported into the CSF by epithelial cells. There are no lymph vessels in the brain.

Macrophages are present within the stroma of the CP and on the epithelial surface of the CP, where they are called *Kolmer* or *epiplexus cells* (Fig. 12.23). It has been suggested that the Kolmer cells located on the apical surface of the CP epithelium may have an important role in the removal of debris from the ventricles.

MENINGES

The brain and spinal cord are located in the cranium and vertebral column and are protected by these bony constituents. In addition, the brain and spinal cord are covered by three connective tissue investments, the *meninges*. The innermost meninge is called the *pia mater* and is very delicate. It consists of a few collagen and elastic fibers plus a continuous layer of simple squamous epithelial cells. In these respects, the pia resembles a

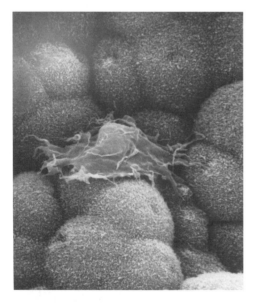

Figure 12.23. SEM of a macrophage (microglia) on the surface of choroid plexus epithelium. ×2170.

mesothelium. The pia mater also contains fibroblasts, macrophages, and blood vessels. Blood vessels that extend into the brain are covered by an extremely thin layer of connective tissue (a perivascular sheath), as well as by pia. Between the pia and connective tissue is sometimes an extremely thin perivascular space that is actually a continuation of the *subarachnoid space* (also filled with *CSF*).

The *arachnoid* is the middle meninge and is connected to the pia mater by fine connective tissue trabeculae. The arachnoid is constructed of collagen fibers, elastic fibers, and a continuous layer of epithelium much like that associated with the pia mater. The space between the arachnoid and pia is called the *subarachnoid space* and contains CSF.

The *dura mater* is the outermost meninge. It is constructed of dense connective tissue, primarily collagen fibers. The potential space between the inner surface of the dura and the outer surface of the arachnoid is called the *subdural* space.

CEREBRUM

The cerebral cortex has a highly organized cellular organization. The cerebral cortex is extremely important and complex, for it is here that sensory information is integrated and motor responses are initiated and coordinated. Such useful activities as memorization, language, and learning occur in the cerebral hemispheres.

The surface of the cerebral hemispheres consists of a series of folds, called *gyri* (sing., *gyrus*) separated by grooves called *sulci* (sing., *sulcus*). The layers of the cerebral cortex include (1) an *outer molecular layer* consisting mainly of nerve processes of cells that are located deeper in the cortex; (2) an *outer granular layer* that contains cell bodies of small neurons; (3) the *pyramidal cell layer*, so called because the cell bodies of neurons located here have the shape of a pyramid; (4) an *inner granular layer* that also contains cell bodies of many small neurons; (5) an *internal pyramidal layer*, again so called because of the presence of pyramid-shaped cell bodies of neurons located here (in one area of the motor cortex, the pyramidal cells are so large that they are called the *cells of Betz* to distinguish them); and (6) a layer of *polymorphic cells* because, as the name implies, the cells in this layer have many shapes. The dominant cerebral hemisphere is usually the left. The interpretive and speech centers are located in this hemisphere.

Unlike the components of the brain stem, the positions of gray and white matter are reversed in the cerebral hemispheres and the cerebellum. Thus the cerebral hemispheres and cerebellum have a covering of gray matter.

CEREBELLUM

The cerebellum is concerned with processing and integrating proprioceptive information from the periphery, visual information from the eyes, and equilibrium sensations from the inner ears. The cerebellum thus regulates the muscles of the body that are necessary to maintain balance and equilibrium. The cerebellum is also concerned with coordinating movements involving groups of muscles.

The gray matter in the cortex of the cerebellum is arranged in three layers (Plate 26C). The superficial layer is (1) the *outer molecular layer*, since it consists of many unmyelinated nerve processes but only a few small neurons; (2) the middle layer consists of very large neurons called *Purkinje cells*; and the (3) *inner granular layer* contains many small neurons. The dendritic tree of the Purkinje cells is huge, and extends into and fills much of the outer molecular layer.

AUTONOMIC NERVOUS SYSTEM (ANS)

Although skeletal muscle contraction is voluntary and can occur at will, many other responses in the body are not under the control of the will. The *efferent innervation* of the *exocrine glands, heart muscle*, and *smooth muscle* (including that of the viscera and circulatory system) is achieved by the ANS. The ANS is actually a specific functional subset of the PNS. The remainder of the PNS is called the *somatic nervous system*. Furthermore, most smooth muscle and exocrine glands, as well as the heart, are innervated by both divisions of the ANS.

The ANS has two divisions, *sympathetic* and *parasympathetic*, and these divisions are functionally antagonistic. Another feature of the ANS is that both sympathetic and parasympathetic divisions have their *origin* in the *CNS*, but in *different* regions which will be described. Still another important feature of the ANS is that *two efferent neurons* are always required to connect the CNS with the *heart muscle, smooth muscle*, or *glands* innervated. Moreover, while the cell body of the first efferent neuron of both divisions is located in different regions of the CNS, the second efferent neuron in both divisions is usually located in a *ganglion outside the CNS*. Finally, the two efferent neurons are called the *preganglionic neuron* (the one located in the CNS) and the *postganglionic neuron* (the one located outside the CNS—in a ganglion).

Autonomic ganglia have a connective tissue covering and framework, and contain *ganglion cells and capsule cells*. Nerve cells in autonomic ganglia are *multipolar*, unlike those in spinal ganglia. Nerve cell bodies of autonomic ganglia tend to be smaller than those of spinal ganglia and have fewer capsule cells. In addition, the nucleus of an autonomic ganglion cell tends to be eccentrically located in autonomic ganglion cells, while those in spinal ganglia tend to be more centrally located.

SYMPATHETIC DIVISION

The cell bodies of the first efferent neurons of the sympathetic division reside in the lateral column of gray matter in the thoracic and upper lumbar portions of the spinal cord (Fig. 12.24). The lightly myelinated axons (*preganglionic fibers*) of these preganglionic neurons exit the spinal cord by way of the *anterior (ventral) nerve root*. These processes then leave the spinal nerve by a small trunk, called a *white ramus communicans* (pl. *rami communicantes*), since the contained nerve processes have some whitish myelin. A series of paired *paravertebral ganglia* are located along the spinal cord, and they are connected to the spinal nerves by both *white* and *gray rami communicantes* on both sides of the cord. The gray rami are so named because the nerves within them lack myelin. All of the paired segmental paravertebral ganglia are connected, and the resulting structures comprise the *sympathetic trunks*. The paravertebral ganglia may contain the cell body of the second efferent neuron (called the *postganglionic neuron*). The preganglionic fibers of the preganglionic neuron enter the white ramus and may then synapse with the second efferent neuron (postganglionic neuron), whose cell body may be located there. Then the *postganglionic fiber* of the postganglionic neuron may either (1) exit the gray ramus to enter a spinal nerve for distribution, or, more commonly, (2) extend through a connection (called a *sympathetic nerve*) between the paravertebral ganglion and one of three *prevertebral ganglia* (these are named the *coeliac ganglion, superior mesenteric ganglion*, and *inferior mesenteric ganglion*) located close to organs of the viscera. If the preganglionic nerve extends to a prevertebral ganglion, it then synapses with several postganglionic neurons. The postganglionic fibers of these postganglionic neurons then extend to the smooth muscle of the digestive tract or another organ part to be innervated.

PARASYMPATHETIC DIVISION

The parasympathetic division innervates most structures innervated by the sympathetic division, and generally it is antagonistic in action (Fig. 12.24). The cell bodies of the *first efferent neurons* are located either in the nuclei of the gray matter in the midbrain and medulla or in the lateral horn of the gray matter in the sacral portion of the spinal cord. Thus, the parasympathetic division has widely divergent origins (from head and tail: cranial-sacral outflow). The preganglionic fibers of these neurons exit the brain by way of the 3rd, 7th, 9th, and 10th cranial nerves or exit the spinal cord by way of the *2nd, 3rd*, and *4th sacral nerves*. The preganglionic fibers are much longer than those of the sympathetic ganglion and generally extend to the organ being innervated. The *second efferent neuron (postganglionic neuron)* of the parasympathetic division may be located in a small cranial ganglion next to the organ innervated or the second efferent neuron cell body may be located in the organ itself. Thus, the neuronal cell bodies located between the circular and longitudinal smooth muscles

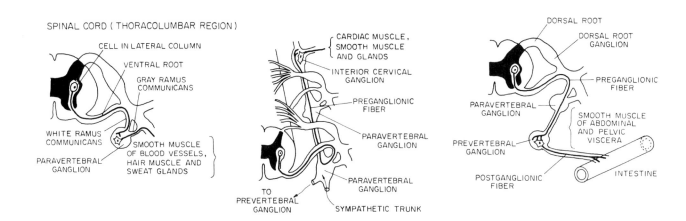

PARASYMPATHETIC DIVISION

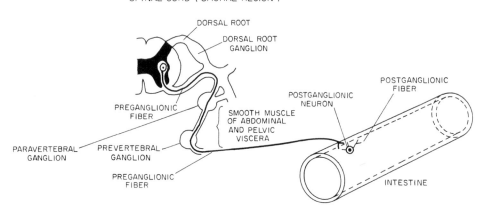

Figure 12.24. Diagrams illustrate possible routes taken by presynaptic and postsynaptic neurons of the sympathetic and parasympathetic nervous systems. See text for additional details about the actions of these antagonistic systems.

Comparison of ANS Divisions

	Sympathetic Division	Parasympathetic Division
Location of preganglionic neuron (first efferent neuron cell body)	Lateral horn, gray matter, spinal cord (thoracic, lumbar)	Gray matter of midbrain and medulla + lateral horn gray matter, sacral region of spinal cord
Location of postganglionic neuron (second efferent neuron cell body)	In ganglia outside CNS— in paravertebral or prevertebral ganglia	In cranial ganglia (head) or in wall of organ innervated (posterior portion)
Structures innervated	Heart, smooth muscle, glands	Heart, smooth muscle, glands
Action	Often inhibitory (e.g., peristalsis) (but stimulates heart, sweat glands)	Often stimulatory (e.g., peristalsis) (but inhibits heart, sweat glands)
Neurotransmitter released at presynaptic nerve terminal	Cholinergic (ACh)	Adrenergic (NE) (except sweat glands)
Neurotransmitter released at postsynaptic nerve terminal	Cholinergic (ACh)	Cholinergic (ACh)

of the intestine (Auerbach's plexus) represent the second efferent neuron cell bodies of the parasympathtic division. Therefore, the postganglionic fibers of the postganglionic neuron are usually quite short in the parasympathetic division.

SYNAPSES IN THE ANS

The *preganglionic fibers* of both the *sympathetic* and *parasympathetic* divisions of the ANS are *cholinergic*. That is, the chemical transmitter released at the synapse between the pre- and postganglionic neuron is *ACh*. The neurotransmitter released from the *postganglionic fibers* of the sympathetic nervous system (except for sweat glands) is *norepinephrine or noradrenalin*. These endings are therefore *adrenergic* (an exception: postganglionic sympathetic endings on sweat glands are cholinergic). *Sympathetic nervous innervation* is frequently *inhibitory* with respect to function. Thus, sympathetic innervation of the smooth muscle of the digestive tract has the effect of slowing peristalsis. Furthermore, sympathetic stimulation of the heart tends to speed up the heart rate.

The neurotransmitter released at the *postganglionic nerve endings* of the *parasympathetic* division is *ACh*. Thus, both preganglionic and postganglionic fibers of the parasympathetic division are *cholinergic*. The parasympathetic division's cholinergic fibers generally stimulate peristalsis, for example, or secretion in the case of glands. The sympathetic division activates or inhibits organs as needed for stressful situations ("flight or fight"), while the parasympathetic division activates or inhibits activities to bring about a "rest" or "repose" response.

SELECTED BIBLIOGRAPHY

Bamburg, J.R. (1988). The axonal cytoskeleton: stationary or moving matrix? *Trends Neuroscience* **11**, 248–249.

Barres, B.A. (1991). New roles for glia. *Neuroscience* **11**, 3685–3694.

Benfenati, F., and Valtorta, F. (1993). Synapsins and synaptic transmission. *NIPS* **8**, 18–23.

Bradbury, M.W.B. (1985). The blood-brain barrier. Transport across the cerebral endothelium. *Circ. Res.* **57**, 213.

Brown, D.A. (1986). Synaptic mechanisms. *Trends Neurosci.* **9**, 468–470.

Brown, M.C., Hopkins, W.G., and Keynes, R.J. (1991). *Essentials of Neural Development*. Cambridge University Press, Cambridge.

Deber, C.M., and Reynolds, S.J. (1991). Central nervous system myelin: structure, function, and pathology. *Clin. Biochem.* **24**, 113–134.

DeCamilli, P., Benferati, F., Valtorta, F., and Greengard, P. (1990). The synapsins. *Annu. Rev. Cell Biol.* **6**, 403–432.

de Waegh, S.M., Lee, V.M., and Brady, S.T. (1992). Local modulation of neurofilament phosphorylation, axonal caliber, and slow axonal transport by myelinating Schwann cells. *Cell* **68**, 451–463.

Goldstein, G.W., and Betz, A.L. (1986). The blood-brain barrier. *Sci. Am.* **253**(3), 74–83.

Greengard, P., Valtorta, F., Czernik, A.J., and Benfenati, F. (1993) Synaptic vesicle phosphoproteins and regulation of synaptic function. *Science* **259**, 780–785.

Hall, Z.W. (1992). *An Introduction to Moleuclar Neurobiology*. Sinauer, Sunderland, MA.

Heuser, J.E., Reese, T.S., Dennis, M.J., Yan, Y., Jam, L., and Evans, L. (1979). Synaptic vesicle exocytosis captured by quick freezing and correlated with quantal transmitter release. *J. Cell Biol.* **81**, 275.

Hubbard, J.I., ed. (1974). *The Peripheral Nervous System*. Plenum, New York.

Jessell, T.M., and Kandel, E.R. (1993). Synaptic transmission: a bidirectional and self-modifiable form of cell-cell communication. *Cell* **72**(10), 1–30.

Kandel, E.R., Schwartz, J.H., and Jessel, T.M. (1992). *Principles of Neural Science*, 3rd ed. Appleton & Lange, Norwalk, CT.

Keynes, R.D., and Aidley, D.J. (1991). *Nerve and Muscle*, 2nd ed. Cambridge University Press, Cambridge.

Martenson, R.E. (1992). *Myelin: Biology and Chemistry*. CRC Press, Boca Raton, FL.

Marx, J. (1979). New information about the development of the autonomic nervous system. *Science* **206**, 413–437.

Murphy, S., ed. (1993). *Astrocytes: Pharmacology and Function*. Academic Press, San Diego, CA.

Sargent, P.B. (1989). What distinguishes axons from dendrites? Neurons know more than we do. *Trends Neurosci.* **12**, 203–205.

Smith, S.J. (1992). Do astrocytes process neural information? *Prog. Brain Res.* **94**, 119–136.

Stevens, C.F. (1993). Quantal release of neurotransmitter and long-term potentiation. *Cell* **72**(10), 55–64.

Stewart, P.A., and Coomber, B.L. (1986). Astrocytes and the blood-brain barrier. In *Astrocytes*, S. Fedoroff and A. Vernadakis, eds. Academic Press, New York.

Travis, J. (1994). Glia: the brain's other cells. *Science* **266**, 970–972.

Trimble, W.S., Linial, M., and Scheller, R.H. (1991). Cellular and molecular biology of the presynaptic nerve terminal. *Annu. Rev. Neurosci.* **14**, 93.

Tuomanen, E. (1993). Breaching the blood-brain barrier. *Sci. Am.* **268**, 80–85.

Vallee, R.B., and Bloom, G.S. (1991). Mechanism of fast and slow axonal transport. *Annu. Rev. Neurosci.* **14**, 59.

Nervous Tissue: The Eye

ORGANIZATION

The human eye is roughly spherical, with a diameter of ~2.5 cm. It focuses an image of an individual's environment on a photosensitive layer called the *retina*, which generates impulses conveyed via the optic nerve to the brain. The eye is located in a bony orbit that contains extraocular muscles, fat, blood vessels, nerves, and a lacrimal gland. Adipose tissue in the orbits protects the eyeballs by absorbing shock. Three pairs of extraocular muscles are attached to each eyeball and permit a wide range of movement. Two different blood vascular systems supply the eye. One system supplies the optic nerve and the inner surface of the retina. The other system supplies the outer surface of the eye and the vascular layer of the choroid. The photoreceptors and outer pigment layer of the retina receive blood from the choriocapillaris of the choroid.

The eye is invested with three coats or tunics (Fig. 13.1). The external tunic is called the *sclera* and continues anteriorly as the transparent *cornea*. The junction of the cornea and sclera is called the *limbus*. The middle layer of the eye, called the *uvea*, consists of pigmented connective tissue, smooth muscles, and epithelium. The uvea consists of the *choroid layer*, which continues anteriorly as the *ciliary body* and the *iris*. The inner tunic or layer is the photosensitive *retina*, which ends anteriorly at the *ora serrata*.

EYELIDS

The eyelids and associated hairs protect the anterior portion of the eye. The eyelid contains a number of glands (Fig. 13.2). The *Meibomian glands* are sebaceous glands in the upper and lower eyelids. They produce an oily substance that coats the tears, thereby reducing evaporation. *Glands of Zeis* are modified sebaceous glands associated with the hair follicles of the eyelashes. *Glands of Moll* are sweat glands. Tears are produced by *lacrimal glands* located below the conjunctiva in the upper lateral portion of the eye. *Accessory tear glands* (*tarsal glands*) are located in the inner surface of both the upper and lower eyelids. The eyelids have two muscles, the *levator palpebrae* and the *orbicularis oculi*, for opening and closing the eyelids.

ORIGIN

The retina and optic nerve develop as an outgrowth of the embryonic brain and are thus derived from neural ectoderm. The neural ectoderm gives rise to the optic nerve, vitreous body (a portion originates from mesenchyme), neuroepithelium of the retina, pigmented epithelium of the retina, iris, and ciliary body, as well as the iris muscle (pupillary dilator and sphincter). As this outgrowth (optic cup) approaches the superficial ectoderm (epidermis), the epidermal cells thicken, detach, and become associated with the optic cup to form the lens and anterior epithelium of the cornea. The lens, anterior epithelium of the cornea, conjunctiva, and lacrimal gland have their origin from surface ectoderm. The mesoderm gives rise to the sclera, stroma of the ciliary body, cornea, iris, and choroid. The extraocular muscles, hyaloid system, sheath of the optic nerve, and a portion of the vitreous are also formed from mesoderm.

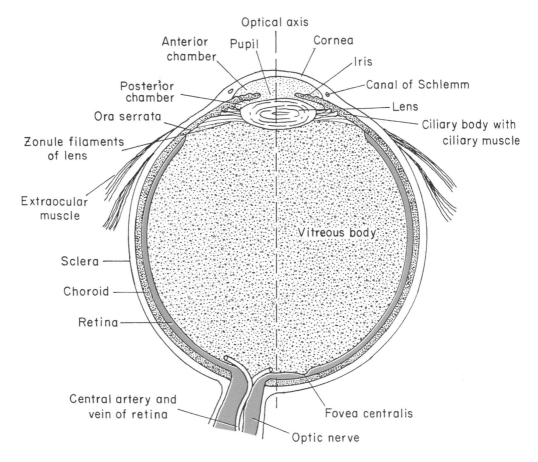

Figure 13.1. A median sagittal section of the eye at the level of the optic nerve, with basic structures and layers identified.

SCLERA

The sclera is about 0.5 mm wide and consists of collagen fibers, fibroblasts, and intercellular substance (Fig. 13.1). The extraocular muscles attach on the sclera. Where the optic nerve exits the eye, the sclera consists of fenestrated layers of collagen fibers, called the *lamina cribrosa*, through which the optic nerve fibers pass into the optic nerve (Fig. 13.1). The sclera not only protects the eye but plays an important role in maintaining its normal size and shape. Its importance is illustrated by the fact that if the axial length of the eye is increased by only 1 mm, a condition of severe *myopia* (nearsightedness) results. If the axial length of the eye is decreased by only 1 mm, a refractive deviation called *hyperopia* (or farsightedness) results.

CORNEA

The sclera is continuous anteriorly with a transparent cornea that comprises the "white" of the eye (Fig. 13.3). The junction of the cornea and sclera is called the *limbus*. While the cornea is innervated, it has no blood supply. The cornea is the primary refractive portion of the

eye (refractive index = 1.376; air = 1.0), but the lens also plays an important role in light refraction. Nourishment of the cornea is from the aqueous humor, which is present in the anterior eye chamber. The five layers of the cornea, from outside to inside the eye, are illustrated in Plate 31A and are described in the following sections.

ANTERIOR CORNEAL EPITHELIUM

This is a layer of stratified squamous, nonkeratinizing epithelium about five cells thick with a very smooth anterior surface. The anterior corneal epithelium is continuous laterally with the bulbar conjunctiva (Figs. 13.2, 13.3). The *bulbar conjunctiva* is folded to form the *palpebral conjunctiva*, which lines the inner surface of the eyelid (Fig. 13.2). Mucus-producing goblet cells may be distributed in both the bulbar and palpebral conjunctivae.

BOWMAN'S MEMBRANE

Bowman's membrane is a homogeneous, noncellular layer ~30 μm thick (Plate 31A). The layer consists of a

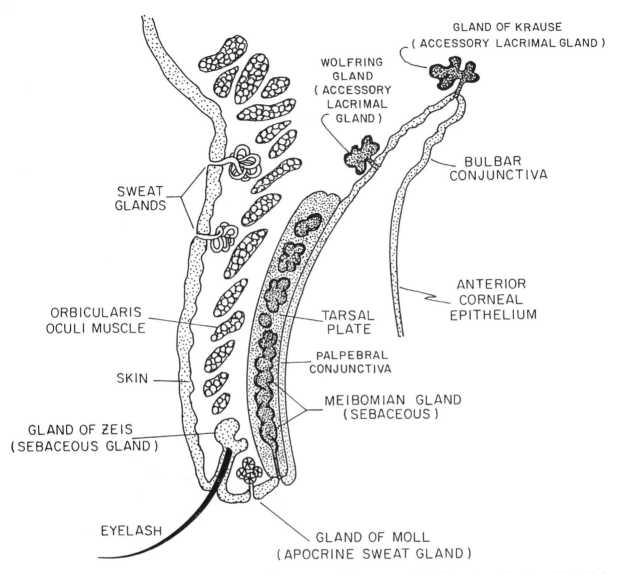

Figure 13.2. Diagram illustrates the microscopic anatomy of the upper eyelid. The various glands are identified.

feltwork arrangement of short collagen fibrils embedded in intercellular substance. This layer is resistant to bacterial invasion and, once destroyed, does not regenerate.

SUBSTANTIA PROPRIA OR CORNEAL STROMA

This layer comprises most of the cornea (Plate 31A). The substantia propria contains many layers of collagen fibrils that have different orientations in successive layers (Fig. 13.4). Keratocytes form the collagen and are present between the layers of fibers. A ground substance containing chondroitin and keratan sulfates surrounds the collagen fibrils. During inflammation, neutrophils and lymphocytes are able to migrate between the layers of the corneal stroma. The fibroblast-like cells (keratocytes) that form collagen are derived from the neural crest.

DESCEMET'S MEMBRANE

This is a layer 5–10 μm thick that represents the basement membrane of Descemet's endothelium (Fig. 13.4). Descemet's membrane can regenerate after an injury. It extends peripherally beneath the sclera as a meshwork called the *pectinate ligament*, which terminates in the ciliary muscle and sclera.

DESCEMET'S ENDOTHELIUM

A layer of simple squamous epithelium covers the posterior surface of the cornea (Fig. 13.4), and at the periphery of the cornea, the endothelium covers the trabeculae of the trabecular meshwork (Fig. 13.5). The corneal endothelium (Descemet's endothelium) appears to play a role in the transport of water out of the cornea and the diffusion of nutrients into the avascular

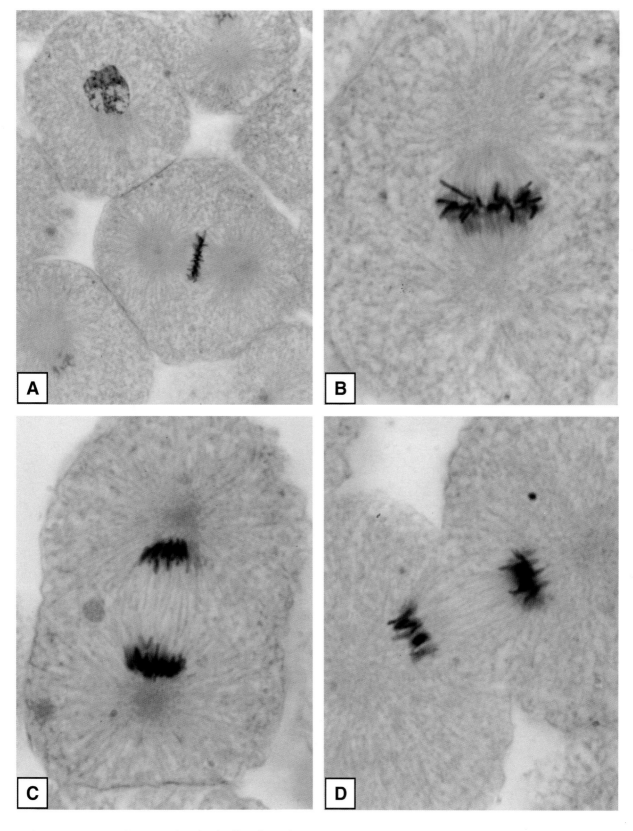

PLATE 1 *A* Whitefish blastula mitosis. Prophase (upper) and metaphase (lower) stages are illustrated. ×740. *B*

Metaphase. ×1850. *C* Anaphase. ×1850. *D* Telophase. ×1850.

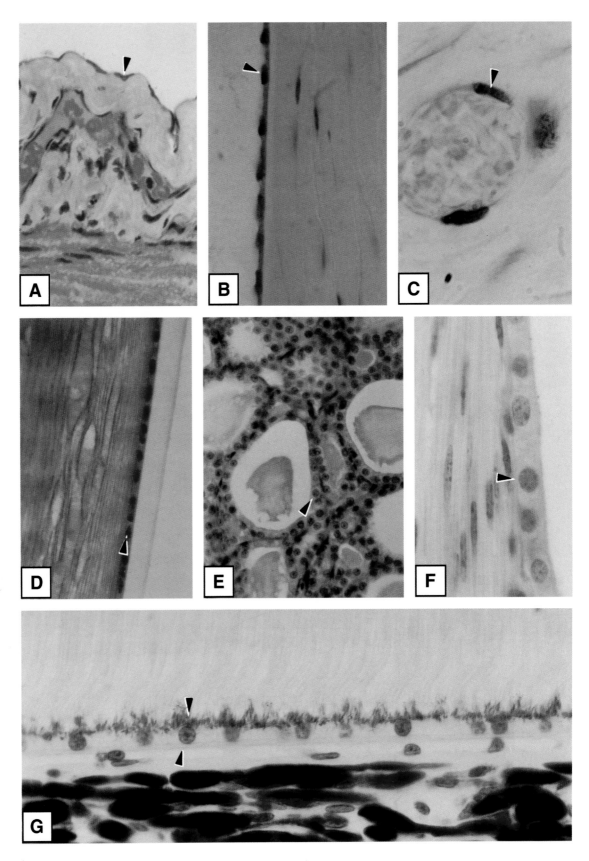

PLATE 2 *A* Mesothelial cells (arrowhead) (simple squamous epithelium) of serosa (1.5 μm, H&E). ×400. *B* Simple squamous epithelium (arrowhead) of inner epithelium
of cornea. H&E. ×740. *C* Capillary (simple squamous epithelium) endothelium (arrowhead), X-section H&E. ×1600.
D Simple cuboidal epithelium (arrowhead), anterior lens epithelium. H&E. ×400. *E* Simple cuboidal epithelium (arrowhead), glandular epithelium (thyroid). H&E. ×320.
F Simple cuboidal epithelium (arrowhead). H&E. ×740.
G Simple cuboidal epithelium, pigmented epithelium of
retina (arrowhead), contains melanin (brown). H&E. ×740.

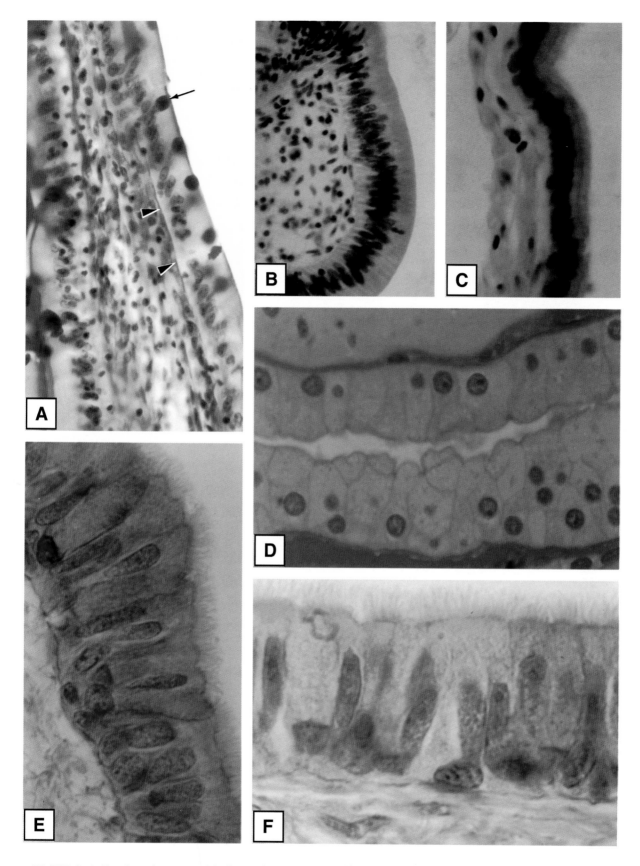

PLATE 3 *A* Simple columnar epithelium with goblet cells (arrow). PAS reaction stains basement membrane (arrowheads), mucigen granules in goblet cell, and striated border a magenta color. ×465. *B* Simple columnar epithelium, gastric pits of stomach. H&E. ×320. *C* Simple columnar, ciliated epithelium, bronchiole in lung. H&E. ×510. *D* Simple columnar epithelium in collecting duct of kidney. 1.5-μm section, H&E. ×1600. *E* Pseudostratified, ciliated columnar epithelium with goblet cells (blue). Trachea, Masson's stain. ×1660. *F* Pseudostratified, ciliated columnar epithelium with goblet cells (blue). Trachea, Masson's stain. ×1850.

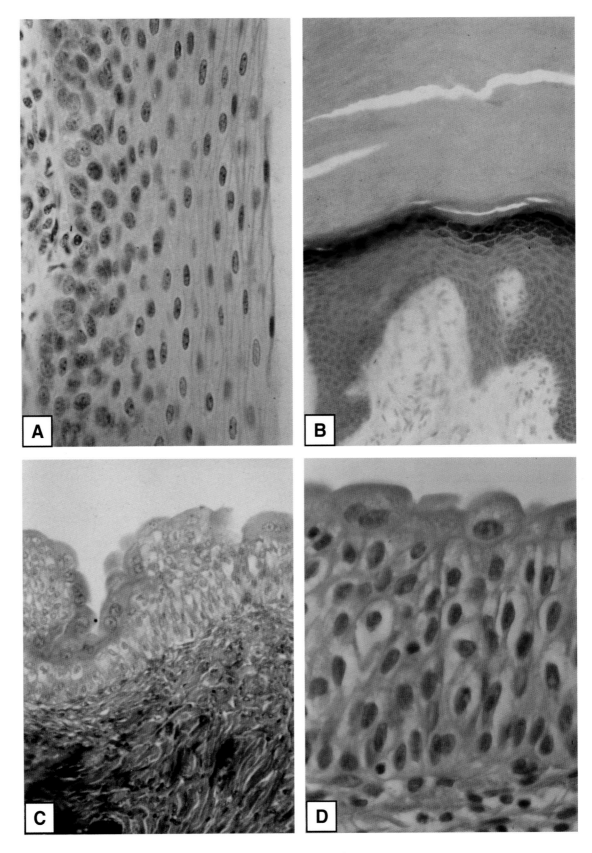

PLATE 4 *A* Stratified squamous, nonkeratinized epithelium, esophagus. H&E. ×320. *B* Stratified squamous, keratinized epithelium (thick skin). H&E. ×160. *C* Transitional epithelium, urinary bladder, relaxed. Masson's stain. ×330. *D* Transitional epithelium, urinary bladder, relaxed, H&E. ×740.

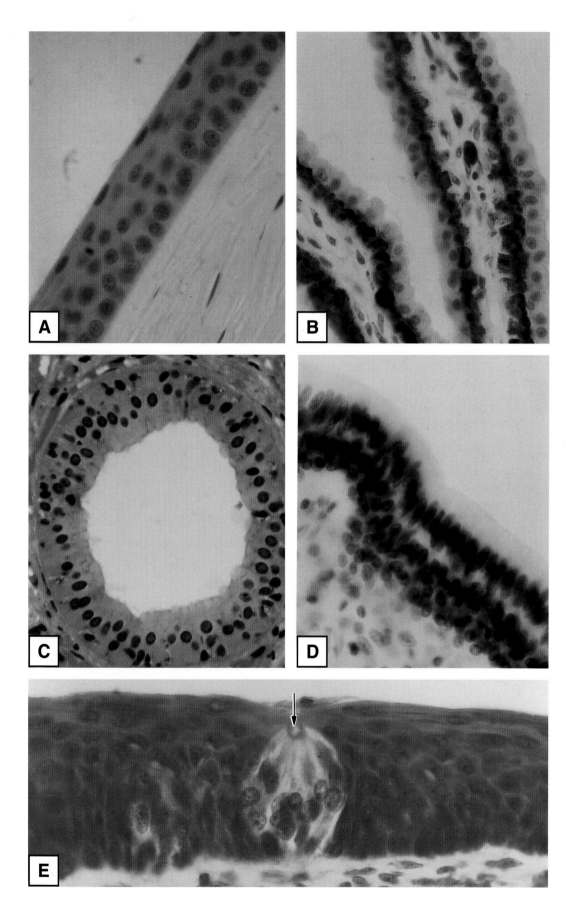

PLATE 5 *A* Stratified squamous, nonkeratinized epithelium; anterior epithelium of cornea, H&E. ×640. *B* Stratified cuboidal epithelium, ciliary processes of eye. One layer of the epithelium contains melanin pigment. H&E. ×460. *C* Thin, stratified columnar epithelium, interlobular duct of gland. H&E. ×400. *D* Thick, stratified columnar epithelium, male penile urethra. H&E. ×700. *E* Stratified squamous epithelium of tongue contains a taste bud, an example of neuroepithelium. Taste pore denoted by arrow. H&E. ×740.

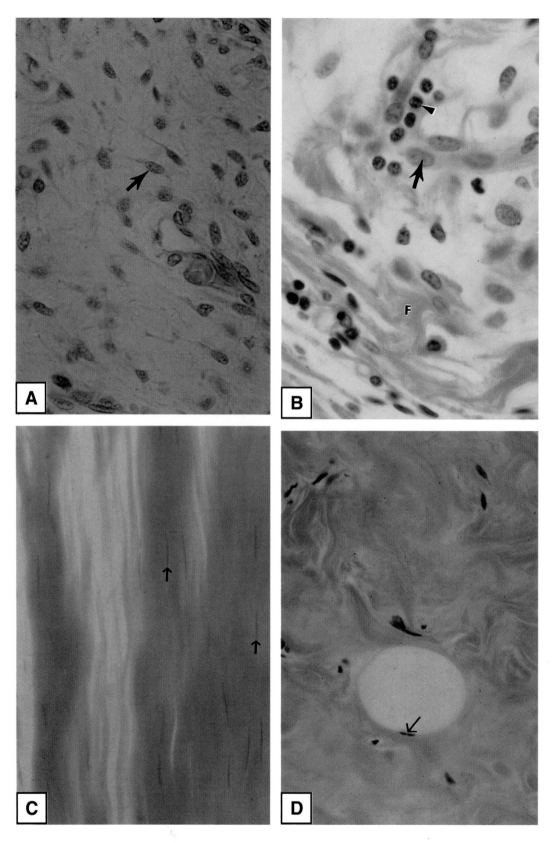

PLATE 6. *A* Section of mesenchyme from mammalian embryo. Mesenchyme cells are undifferentiated, spindle-shaped (arrow), and form a loose packing. Blood vessel with erthrocyte is located in lower right. H&E. ×510. *B* Section of loose connective tissue illustrates acidophilic (pink) collagen fibers (F), fibrocyte nuclei (arrow), and macrophage (arrowhead) nuclei. Spaces in living tissue contain amor-

phous intercellular substances. H&E. ×740. *C* Dense, regularly arranged white fibrous connective tissue. Section of tendon with flattened nuclei (arrows) of fibroblast compressed between collagen fibers. H&E. ×320. *D* Dense collagenic fibers are pink, with fibroblast nuclei between fibers. A single fat cell (adipocyte) contains nucleus (arrow) compressed at cell periphery. H&E. ×320.

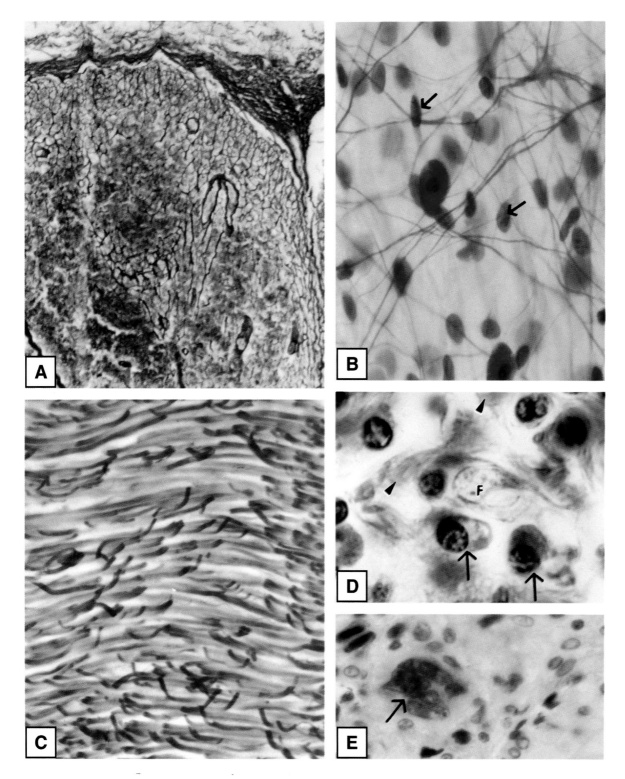

PLATE 7. *A* Section of lymph node stained with silver to show argyrophilic reticular fibers that form a meshwork for the node. Silver stain. ×185. *B* Whole mount of mesentery. Large, faintly stained nuclei are of mesothelial cells comprising mesothelium to which loose connective tissue adheres. Fibroblasts (arrows) are smaller, oval, and more darkly stained. Large cells are mast cells whose cytoplasm contains granules. Pink (acidophilic) fibers are collagen, while the many thin purple-stained fibers are elastic fibers.

Amorphous intercellular substances are dissolved from the preparation. ×740. *C* Section of elastic fiber ligament stained with resorcin orcein, which (like resorcin fuchsin) is used to stain elastic fibers. This is an example of dense, regularly arranged, elastic connective tissue. ×465. *D* Loose connective tissue in mammary gland shows plasma cells (arrows) and collagen (arrowheads). Masson's stain. ×1600. *E* Section of pregnant uterus with two large, multinucleate cells (arrow) that are foreign body giant cells. H&E. ×640.

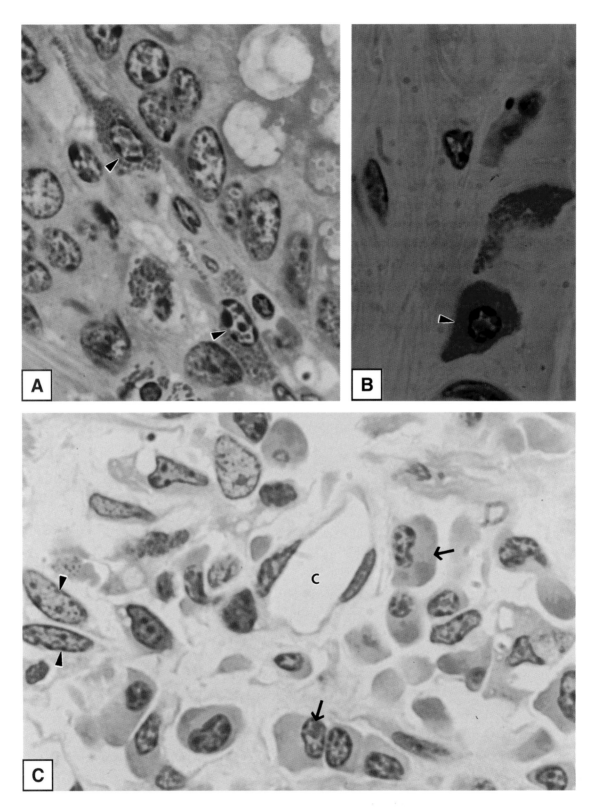

PLATE 8. *A, B* Section of connective tissue in intestine illustrates mast cells (arrowheads) with distinct cytoplasmic granules. H&E. ×1850. *C* Section of monkey cardiac stom-ach. 1.5-μm section, H&E. Plasma cells (arrows), fibroblasts (arrowheads), and capillary (C) are identified. ×1850.

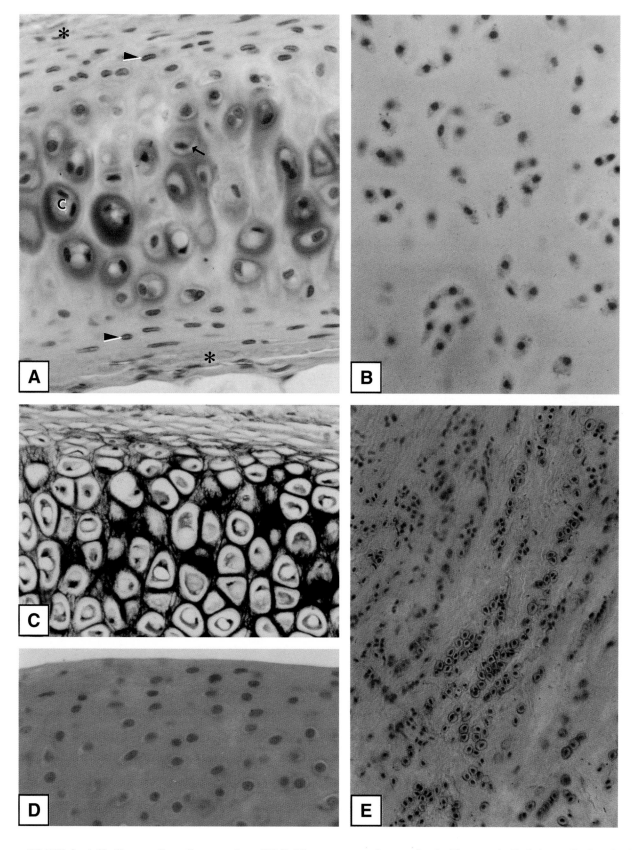

PLATE 9. *A* Hyaline cartilage from trachea. H&E. Fibrous layer of perichondrium (*), chondrogenic layer of perichondrium (arrowheads), vacuolated chondrocytes (C), and lacuna (arrow). Note additional basophilic capsular matrix immediately surrounding chondrocytes. ×465. *B* Embryonic cartilage. H&E. Note large numbers of small chondrocytes in isogenous cell nests. ×465. *C* Elastic cartilage, external ear stained with resorcin fuchsin to display elastic fibers (blue). ×450. *D* Articular cartilage. Note absence of perichondrium and smooth, articulating surface of cartilage at top of figure. ×465. *E* Fibrocartilage. The large number of collagen fibers in matrix causes chondrocytes to be organized in linear arrays and matrix to stain acidophilic. ×310.

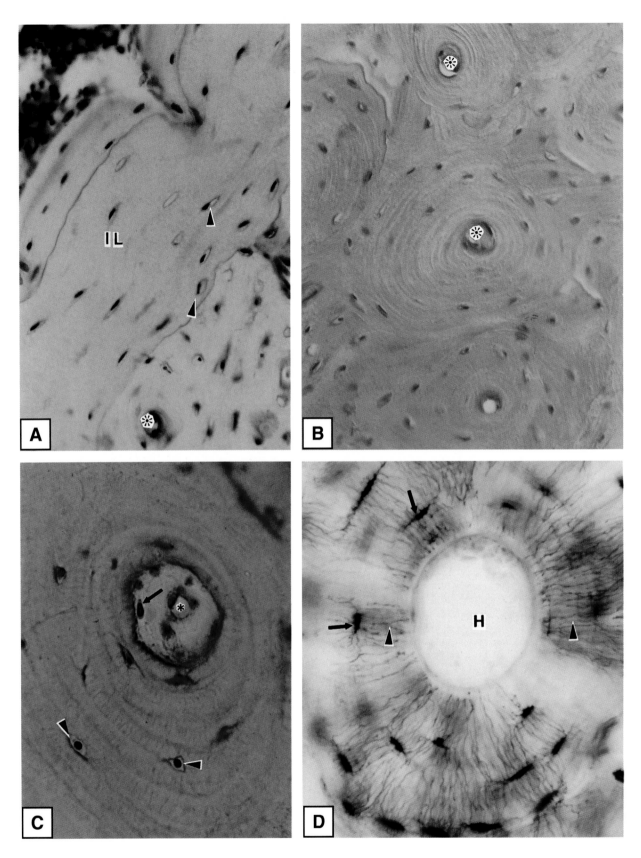

PLATE 10. *A, B* Decalcified sections of compact bone. H&E. Haversian canal (*), inner circumferential lamellae (IL), and nuclei (arrowheads) of osteocytes are identified. ×400. *C* Enlarged portion of decalcified bone illustrates a blood vessel (*) and endosteum (arrow) in a Haversian canal and osteocyte nuclei (arrowheads) in lacunae surrounded by bone matrix. H&E. ×1200. *D* Ground bone, x-section. Haversian (H) canal, lacunae (arrows), and thin, radiating canaliculi (arrowheads) are identified. ×1700.

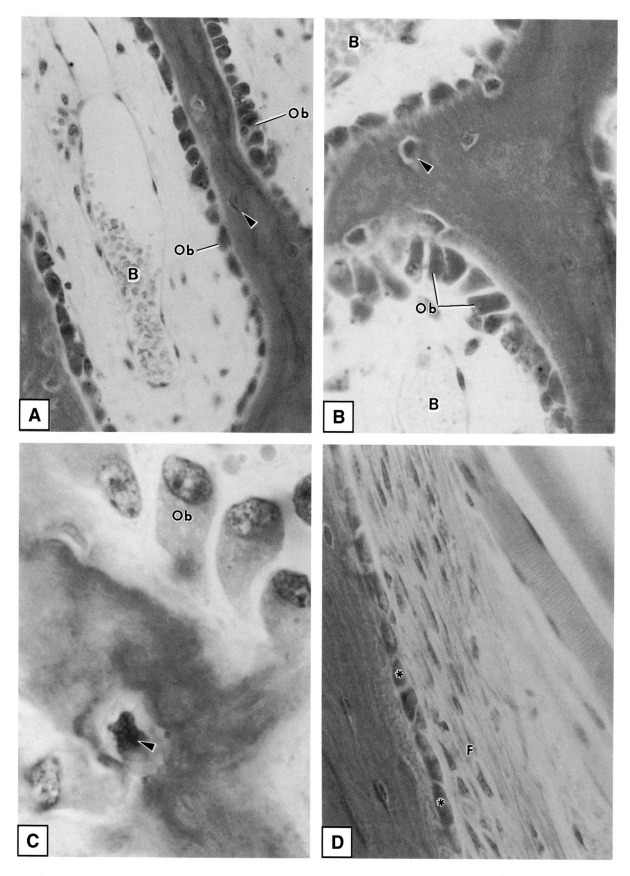

PLATE 11. *A, B, C, D* Cancellous bone, decalcified, H&E. Osteoblasts (Ob), osteocytes (arrowheads), and blood (B) vessels. Fibrous (F) and osteogenic (*) layer of periosteum. *A*, ×465; *B*, ×750; *C*, ×1850; *D*, ×740.

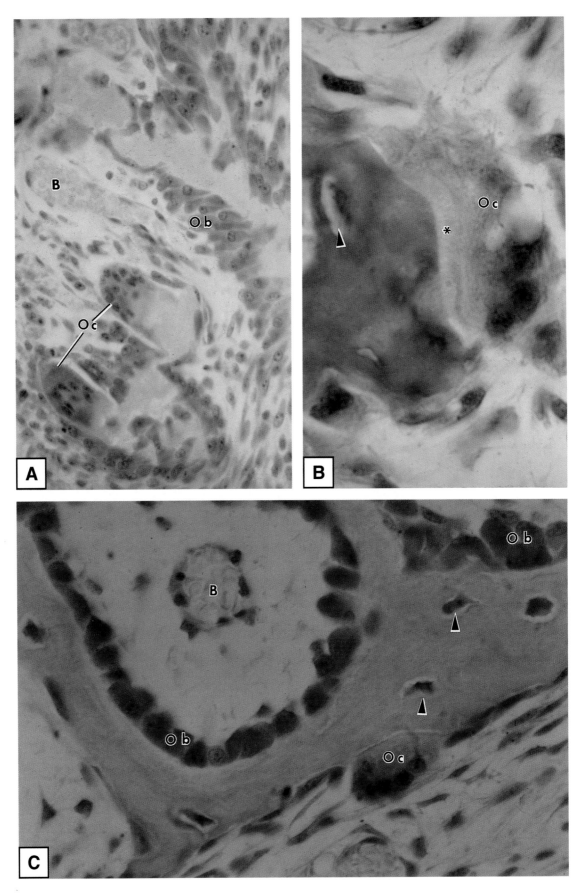

PLATE 12. *A, B, C* Intramembranous ossification. H&E. Osteoblasts (Ob) on surface of spicules of bone matrix. A few osteocytes (arrowheads) have become trapped in bone matrix. Osteoclasts (Oc) with ruffled border (* in *B*). Blood (B) vessels in mesenchyme. *A,* ×400; *B,* ×1600; *C,* 740.

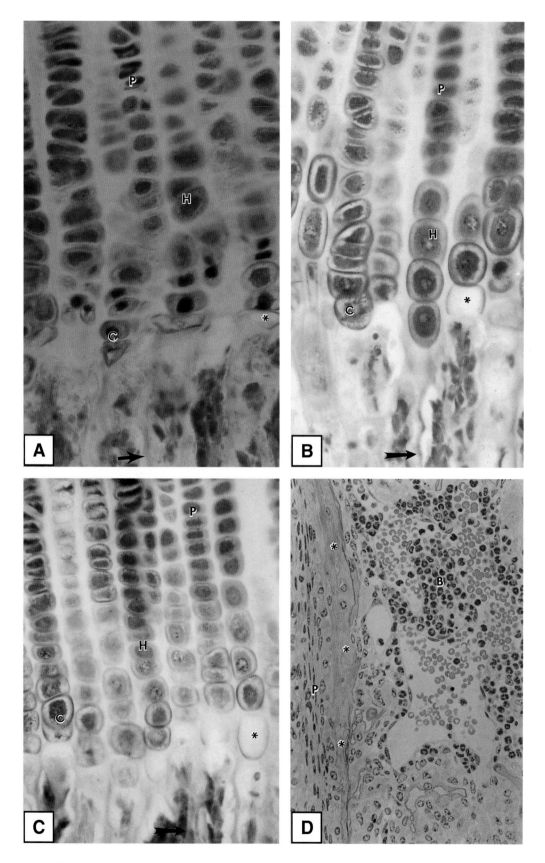

PLATE 13. *A* The figures illustrate endochondral (or intracartilagenous) ossification. Marrow cavity and active bone deposition are located toward the bottom of the figures. Zone of proliferating cartilage (P), zone of hypertrophic (H) or maturing cartilage, and zone of calcified (C) cartilage are identified. In region of calcified cartilage, some

chondrocytes have pyknotic nuclei and are degenerate, while in other areas empty lacunae (*) remain. H&E. *A, B,* ×460; *C,* ×385. *D* Section of daphyseal region of developing long bone. H&E. Periosteum (P), bone matrix (*) of the diaphysis, and blood (B) cells of the marrow are identified. ×225.

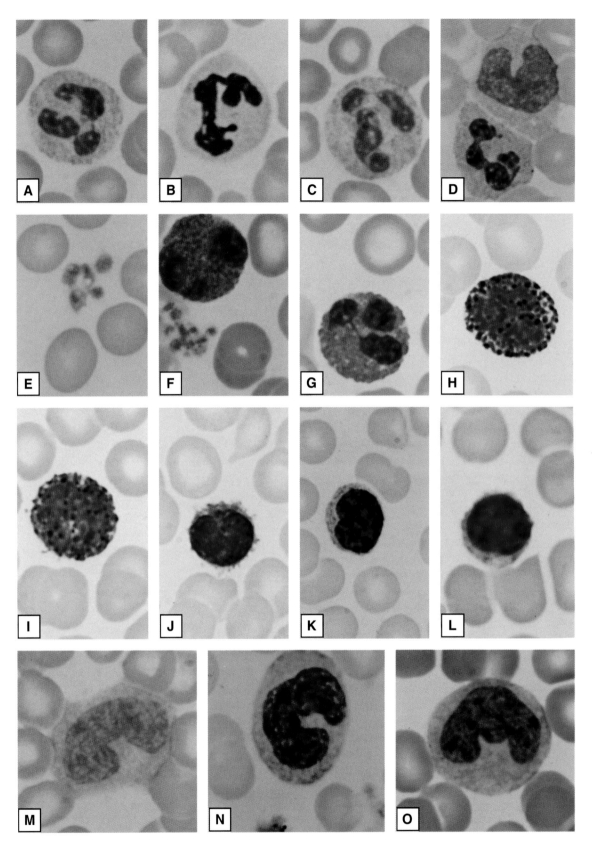

PLATE 14. All color illustrations are magnified approximately 1600×. Giemsa stain. *A,B,C,D* illustrate neutrophils with lobated nucleus and neutrophilic granules *A*. Barr body apparent in *B*. A monocyte is also present at the top in *D*. Platelets are shown in *E* and have a central pink granulomere and a light blue-staining outer hyalomere. Eosinophils are shown in *F,G*; note lobated nucleus and numerous eosinophilic-staining cytoplasmic granules. Ba-

sophils are illustrated in *H,I*; note large basophilic-staining granules. Lymphocytes are illustrated in *J,K,L*; note some difference in size, the heterochromatic-staining nucleus, and a few azurophilic granules (*K,L*) in some cells. Monocytes are illustrated in *M,N,O*; note large size of cells, kidney-shaped nucleus, and presence of azurophilic granules in some cells.

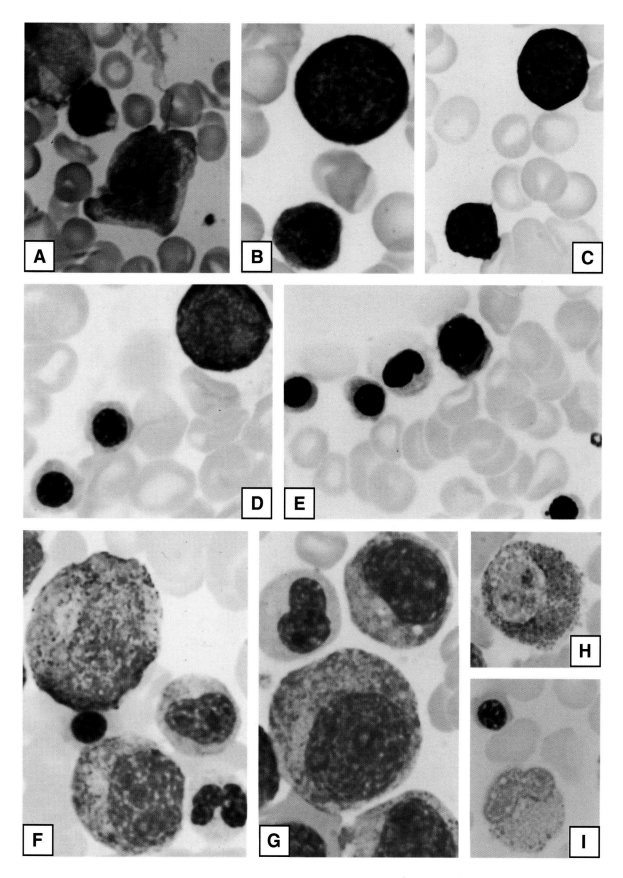

PLATE 15. *A* Large proerythroblast. ×1280. *B* Large basophilic erythroblast at top. Note heterochromatic-staining nucleus and intensely basophilic cytoplasm. ×1850. *C* Small basophilic erythroblast (top). ×1600. *D* Basophilic erythroblast at top; two polychromatophilic erythroblasts. ×1850. *E* Several polychromatophilic erythroblasts. ×1600. *F* Marrow showing large and smaller promyelocytes (left) with azurophilic-staining granules. Neutrophilic myleocyte is located at center, right. ×1850. *G* Promyelocyte is located in center of field, while neutrophilic myelocytes are located above and below the promyelocyte. ×1850. *H* Eosinophilic myelocyte; spherical nucleus, eosinophilic cytoplasmic granules. ×1600. *I* Eosinophilic metamyelocyte (nucleus indented). Both figures ×1600.

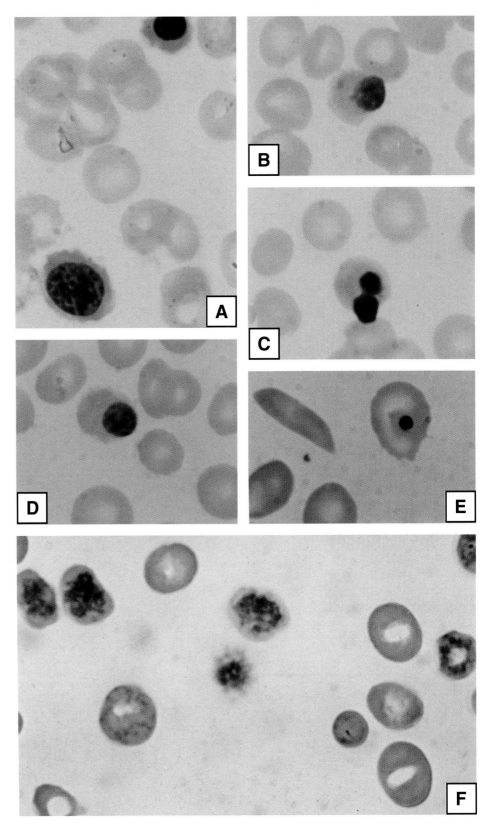

PLATE 16. *A* Polychromatophilic erythroblasts. ×1850. *B,C,D,E* All illustrate terminal differentiation of erythrocytes and the process of nuclear extrusion. A piece of chromatin (Howell-Jolly body) remains in the erythrocyte in E. ×1850.

F Reticulocytes lack a nucleus but contain polyribosomes, which, when stained with new methylene blue, form a blue-staining "reticulum." ×1850.

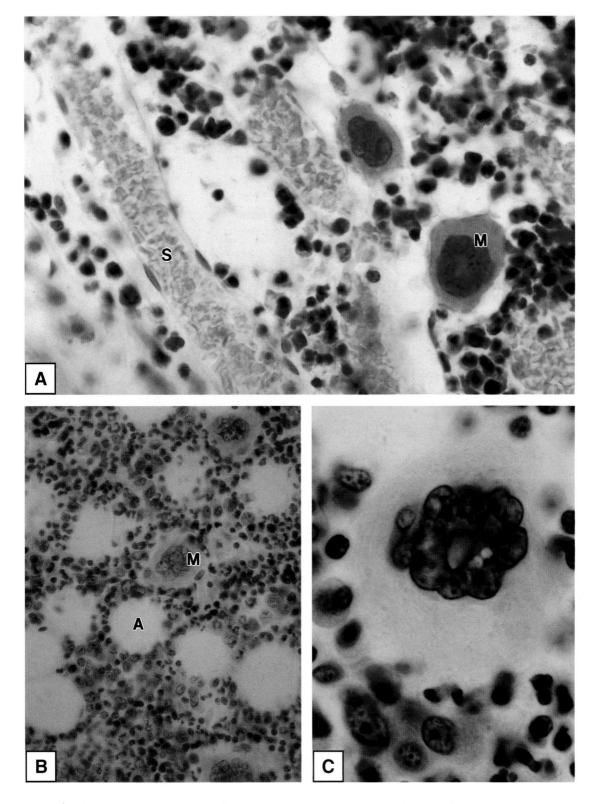

PLATE 17. *A* Bone marrow. H&E. Sinusoid (S) with erythrocytes and megakaryocytes (M) are identified. ×640. *B* Section of bone marrow with megakaryocytes (M) and adipocytes (A) are identified. ×400. *C* Megakaryocyte. Note lobated nucleus and extensive cytoplasm. ×1280.

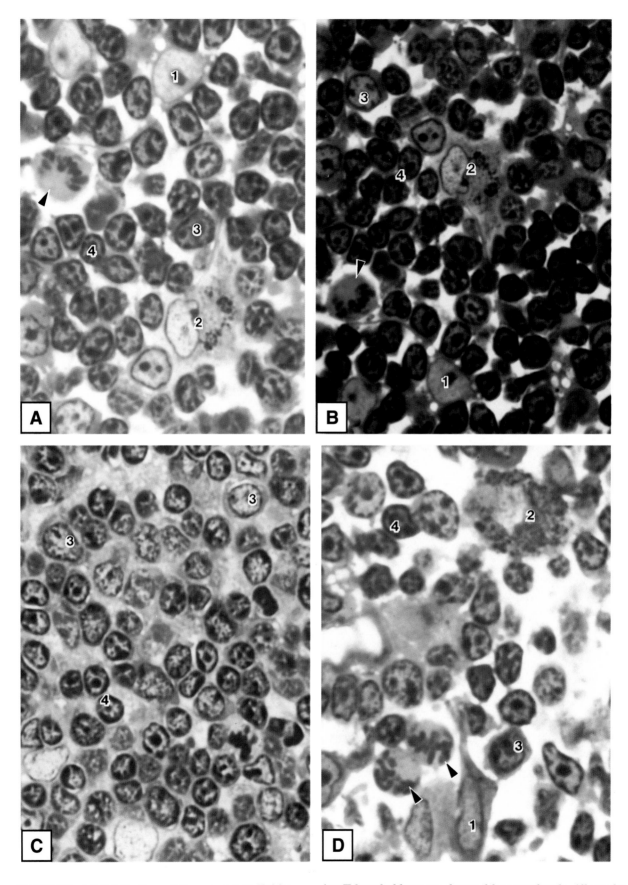

PLATE 18. *A,B,C,D* Section of thymus cortex. Epithelial reticular cells (or nuclei) (1), macrophages (2), T lymphoblasts (3), and T lymphocytes (4) are identified. Dividing T lymphoblasts are denoted by arrowheads. All rat thymus. 1.5-μm sections. ×465.

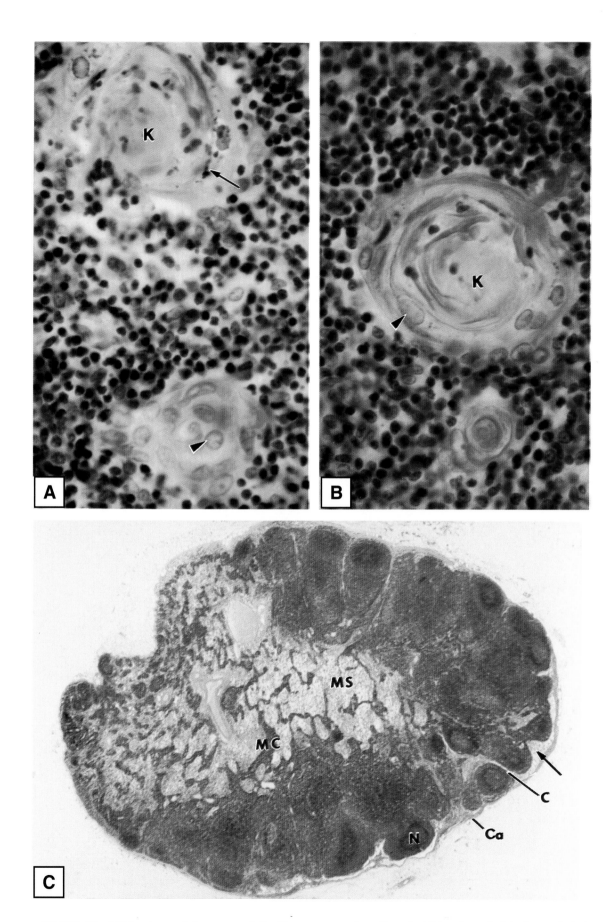

PLATE 19. *A,B* Sections of thymus medulla illustrate Hassall's corpuscles, consisting of keratin (K), keratohyalin (arrow), and epithelial reticular cells (arrowheads). Human infant. ×640. *C* Low-magnification view of lymph node section. Capsule (Ca), subcortical (subcapsular) sinus (arrow), lymphatic nodules (N), cortical sinus (C), medullary sinus (MS), (lightly stained) and medullary cords (MC) (darker stained). ×35.

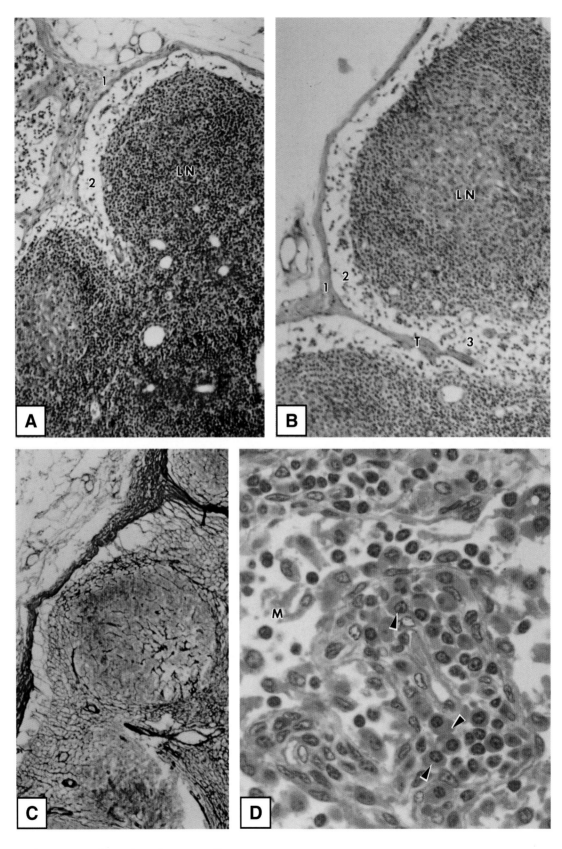

PLATE 20. *A,B* Sections of lymph node cortex. Capsule (1), subcapsular sinus (2), cortical sinus (3), and lymphatic nodules (LN). Trabecula (T). *A,* ×160; *B,* ×185. *C* Section of lymph node cortex stained with silver to show distribution of argyrophilic reticular fibers (black). ×130. *D* Section of lymph node medulla. Medullary cord has several plasma cells (arrowheads) and medullary sinus (M). 1.5 μm, H&E. ×465.

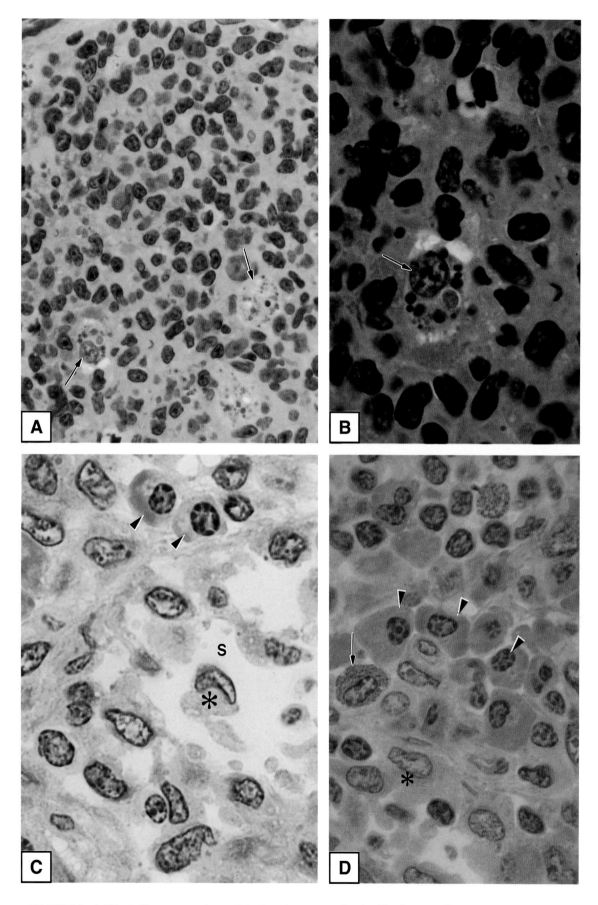

PLATE 21. *A,B* Both illustrate sections of the lymphatic nodules with germinal centers. Macrophages (arrows) contain cytoplasmic granules, some of which are digestive vacuoles. Numerous B lymphocytes are located in the lymphatic nodules. *A,* ×850; *B,* ×1600. *C* Lymph node medullary cord (top) with plasma cells (arrowheads) and a medullary sinus (S). Reticular cell (*). ×740. *D* Medullary cord of lymph node. Mast cell (arrow) and many plasma cells (arrowheads) are present, as well as reticular cell (*). 1.5 μm, H&E. ×1600.

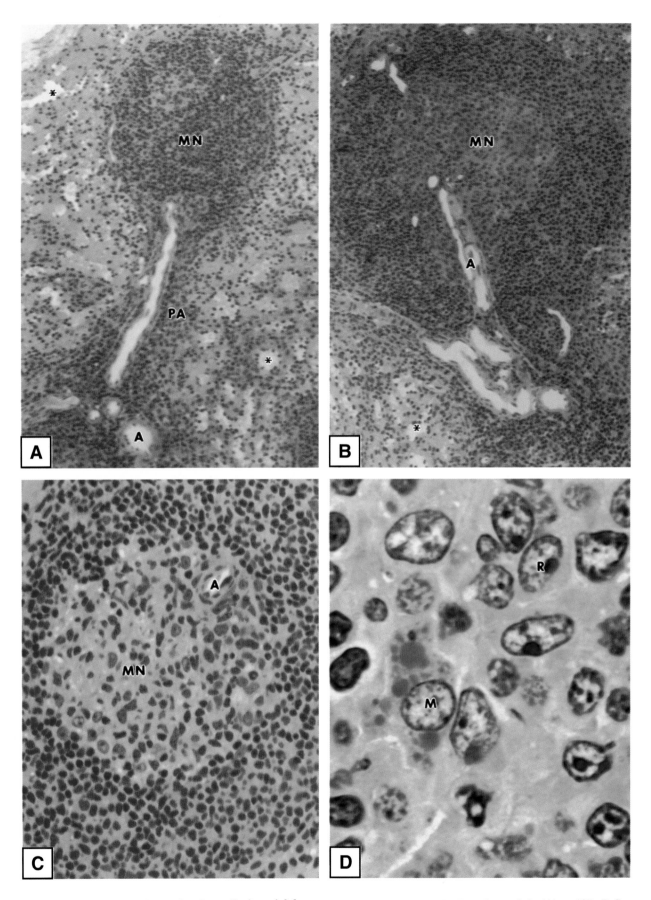

PLATE 22. *A,B* Sections of spleen. Periarterial lymphatic sheaths (PA) and splenic (Malpighian) nodules (MN) comprise the white pulp. The red pulp consists of pulp cords riddled with many sinusoids (*). Central arteriole (A). ×180. *C* Section of Malpighian nodule with lighter-staining germinal center region (MN) and arteriole (A). ×465. *D* Center of Malpighian nodule of spleen shows a macrophage (M) (with digestive vacuoles in the cytoplasm) and a reticular cell nucleus (R). ×1850.

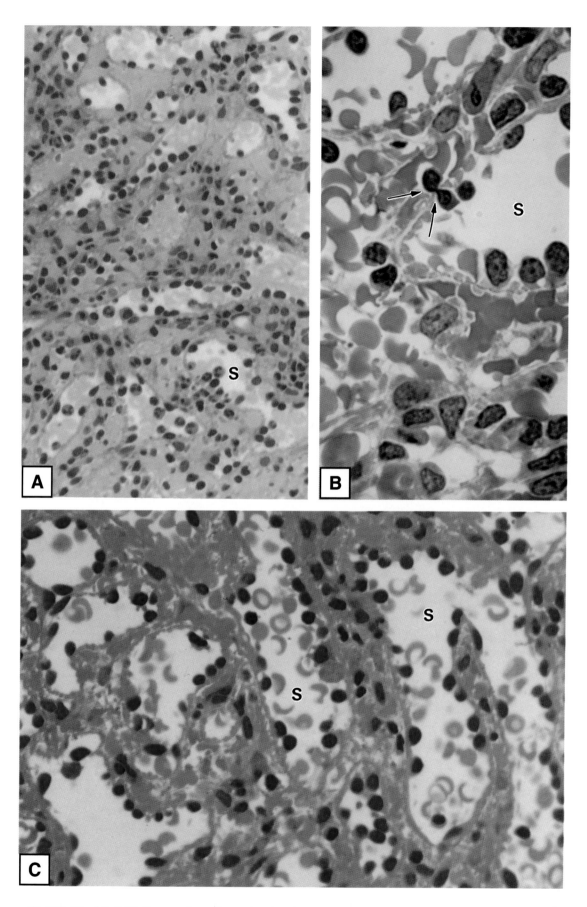

PLATE 23. *A,B,C* All figures show the red pulp with splenic sinusoids (S) and intervening red pulp cords of Billroth. The red pulp cords contain most of all possible types of blood cells, macrophages, and reticular cells. Blood cells can move easily across the sinusoidal wall (S), as illustrated at arrows in *B. A,B,C* 1.5 μm, H&E. *A,* ×465; *B,* ×640; *C,* ×740.

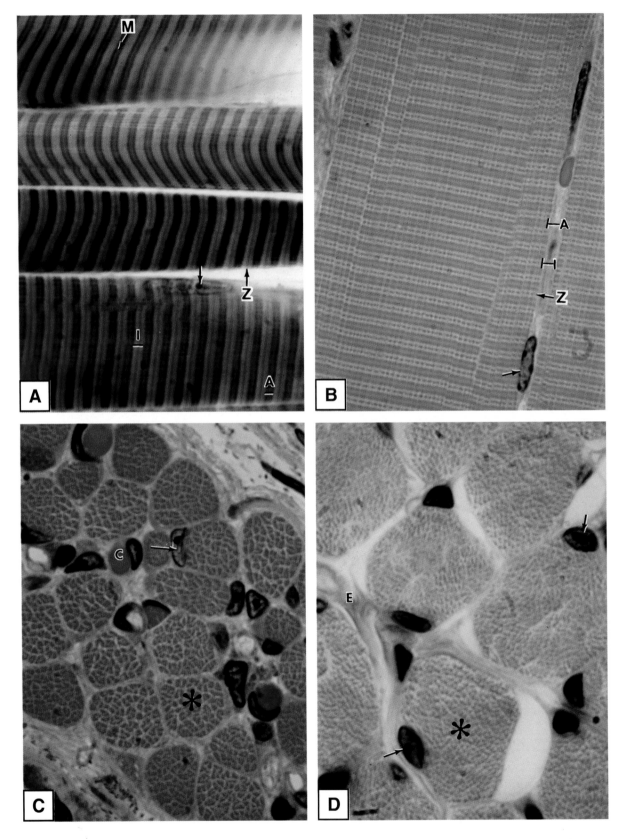

PLATE 24. *A* Longitudinal section of several muscle fibers. H&E. stain. The A, M, I, and Z bands can be identified. Nucleus of muscle fiber under sarcolemma at arrows. ×1600. *B* Longitudinal section of muscle fiber. 1.5. μm. H&E. A, I, and Z bands are evident. Nucleus of fiber at arrow. ×1600. *C,D* Both illustrate transverse sections of muscle fibers with internal myofibrils (*). Nuclei of muscle fibers are denoted at arrows; endomysium (E) and capillaries (C). ×1600.

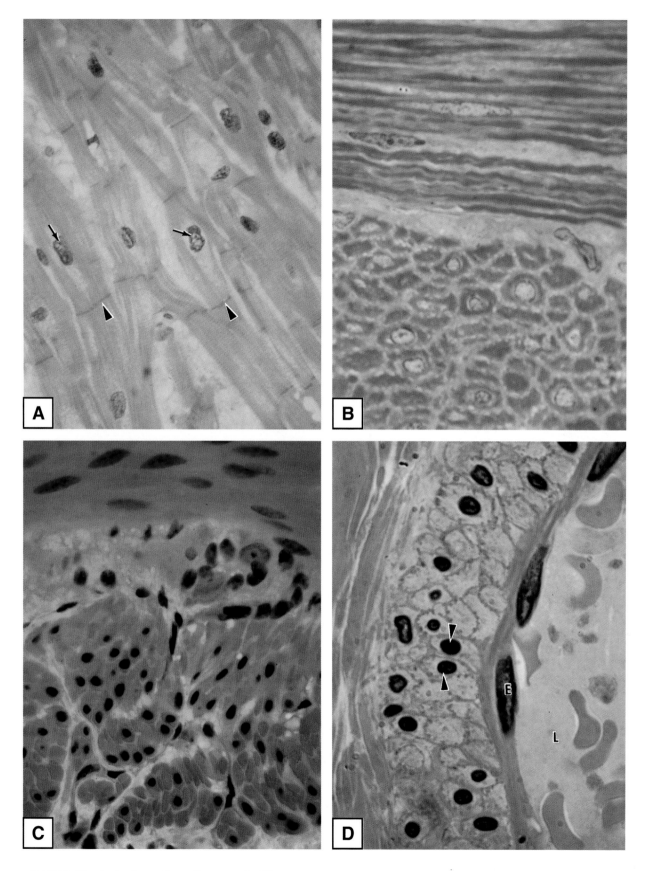

PLATE 25. *A* Section of cardiac muscle illustrates branching and anastomosis of fibers, central nuclei (arrows), and intercalated disks (arrowheads). ×840. *B* Longitudinal (top) and transverse (bottom) section of smooth muscle cells in the wall of the digestive tract. ×840. *C* Smooth muscle in transverse section (top) and longitudinal section (bottom) in the wall of the digestive tract. ×840. *D* Transverse section of smooth muscle in the wall of a large arteriole. Only some of the smooth muscle cells are sectioned to include the nucleus (arrowheads). The endothelium (E) and lumen (L) with red blood cells. ×1600.

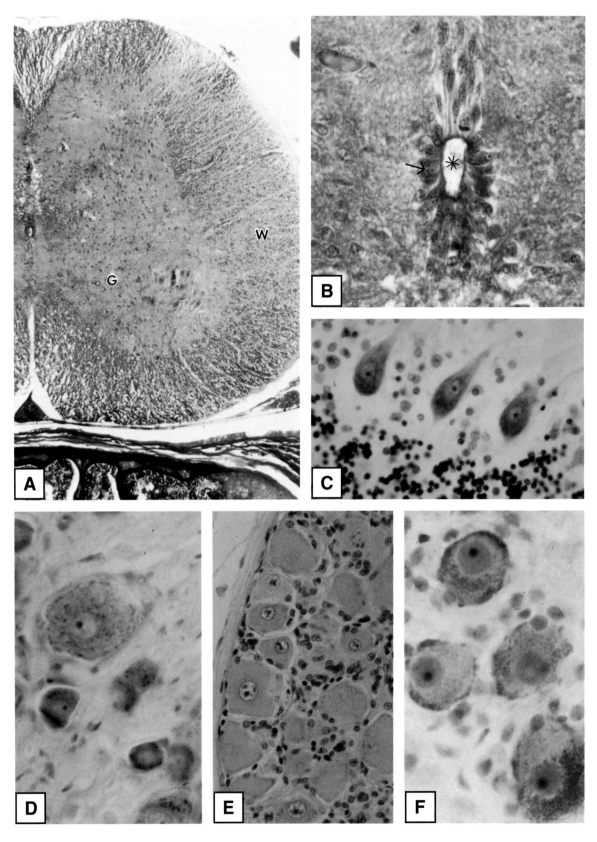

PLATE 26. *A* Cross section of spinal cord. Mallory's stain. Dorsal is toward top of figure. Gray matter (G), white matter (W). Motor neuron cell bodies are evident in the ventral horn of the gray matter. ×90. *B* Cross section of the spinal cord shows the central canal (*), which is surrounded by columnar ependyma cells (arrow). Mallory's stain. ×465. *C* Cerebellum includes part of the outer molecular layer, inner granular layer, and layer of Purkinje cells. Purkinje cells contain a nucleus, nucleolus, and basophilic-staining Nissl substance in cytoplasm. ×400. *D* Nerve cell bodies in the spinal ganglion. Blue-staining material in the neuronal perikarya is Nissl substance. ×740. *E,F* Nerve cell bodies in autonomic ganglia. H&E. Note the eccentric position of the nuclei in the cell bodies and lipofuschin pigment in the cytoplasm. ×740. Nerve processes do not stain well in H&E preparations.

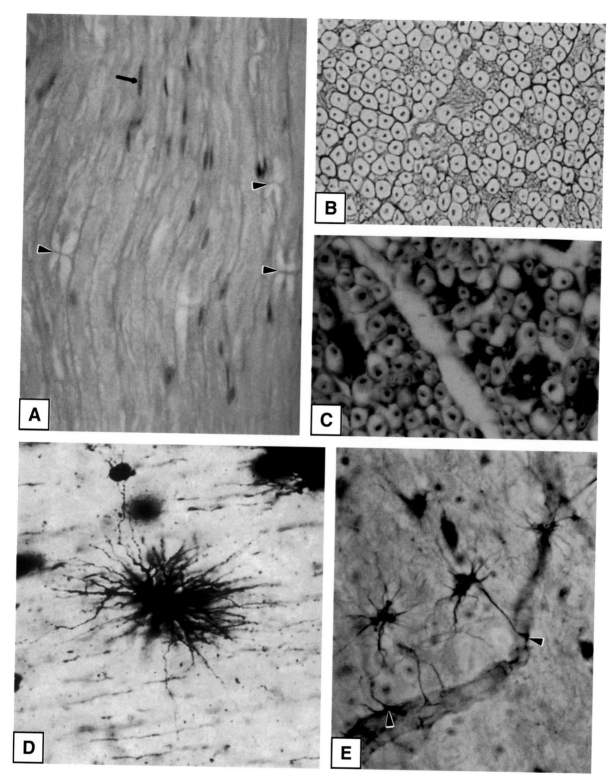

PLATE 27. *A* Longitudinal section of myelinated nerve. H&E. ×400. Nodes of Ranvier are denoted by arrowheads; Schwann cell nuclei are denoted by the arrow. *B* Cross section of myelinated nerve. Mallory's stain. Nerve processes stain as dark dots surrounded by a clear halo that represents dissolved myelin sheaths. Blue-staining material around the nerve processes is connective tissue endoneurium. ×285.

C Cross section of myelinated nerve. Silver stain. Nerve processes and connective tissue elements of the endomysium stain black. The clear region surrounding the nerve processes represents the dissolved myelin sheaths. ×285. *D* Protoplasmic astrocyte. ×740. *E* Fibrous astrocyte (arrowheads). ×640.

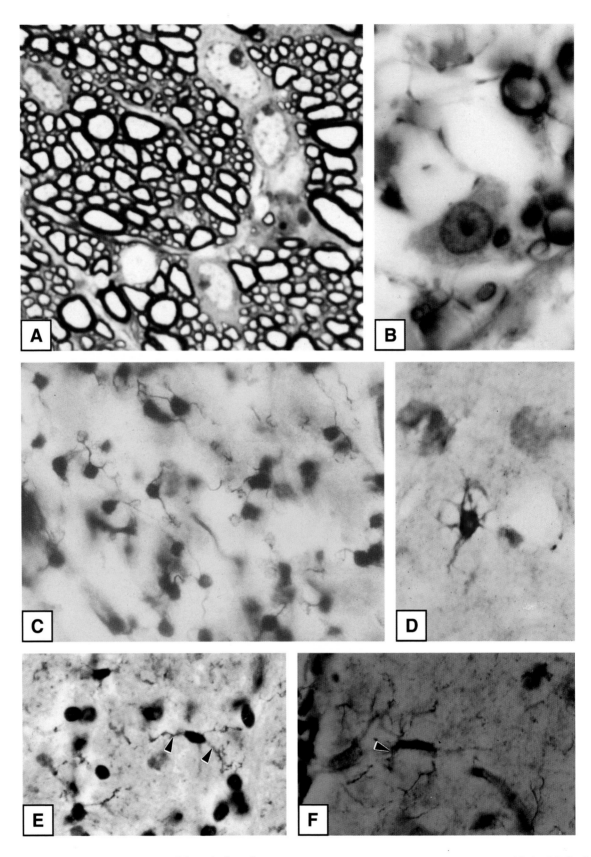

PLATE 28. *A* Section of white matter of the spinal cord. Methylene blue. Dark blue circles of different sizes are myelin sheaths. Cell bodies are those of oligodendrocytes. ×1850. *B* White matter of spinal cord. H&E. The cell body and nucleus of an oligodendrocyte are present and are sur-rounded by myelinated nerve processes. ×1850. *C,D* Both figures display oligodendroglia cells and some of their processes. *C*, ×465; *D*, ×740. *E,F* Both figures illustrate microglia and the fine cytoplasmic branches that emerge from the cell body (arrowheads). ×740.

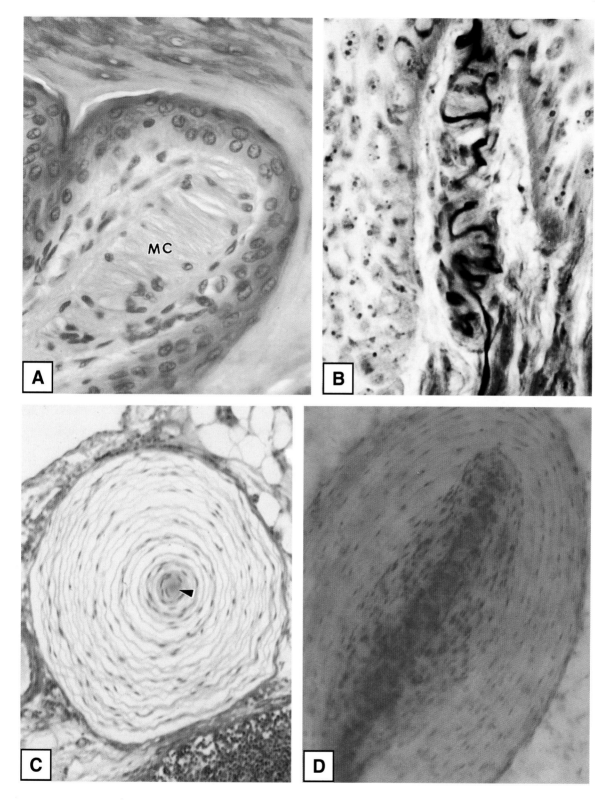

PLATE 29. *A* Longitudinal section of Meissner's corpuscle (MC) in connective tissue papilla of skin (fingertip). H&E. ×645. *B* Longitudinal section of Meissner's tactile corpuscle stained with silver to display the nerve (black) that traverses this sensory receptor. ×645. *C* Transverse section of Vater-Pacini corpuscle. The nerve is located in the center (arrowhead) and is surrounded by flattened supporting cells. ×185. *D* Whole mount preparation of entire Pacinian corpuscle in a mesentery. The nerve is located in the central region, and nuclei of encapsulating cells appear as small red dots. ×225.

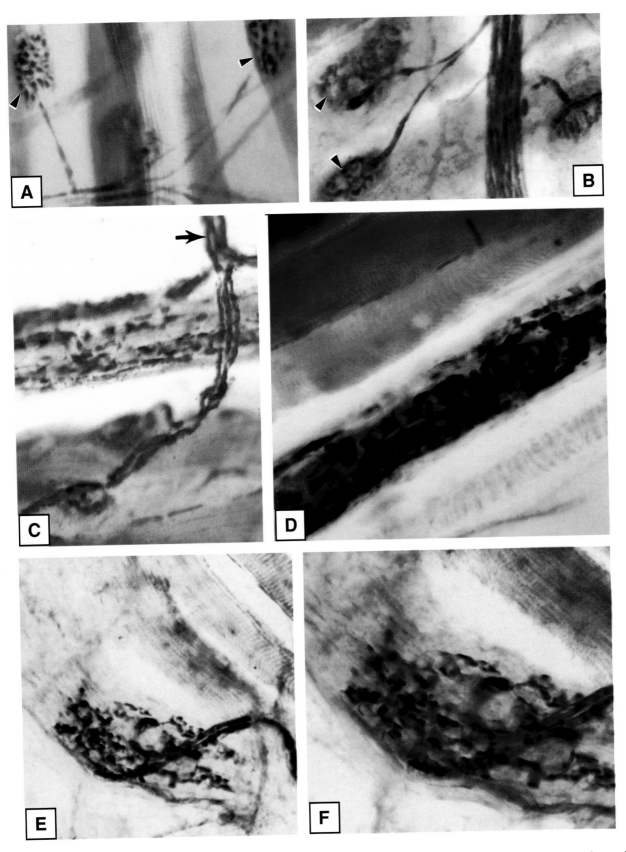

PLATE 30. *A,B* Whole mount preparations of muscle fibers and the motor end plates (arrowheads) (myoneural junctions) associated with these fibers. ×450. *C* Whole mount preparation of muscle fiber and nerve (arrow) supplying both a muscle spindle (top) and motor end plates (bottom). ×465. *D* Whole mount preparation of muscle showing a muscle spindle (darkly stained). ×640. *E,F* Both figures illustrate tendon spindles (darkly stained regions). The nerve endings are darker stained, and the tendon is lighter stained. *E,* ×465; *F,* ×740.

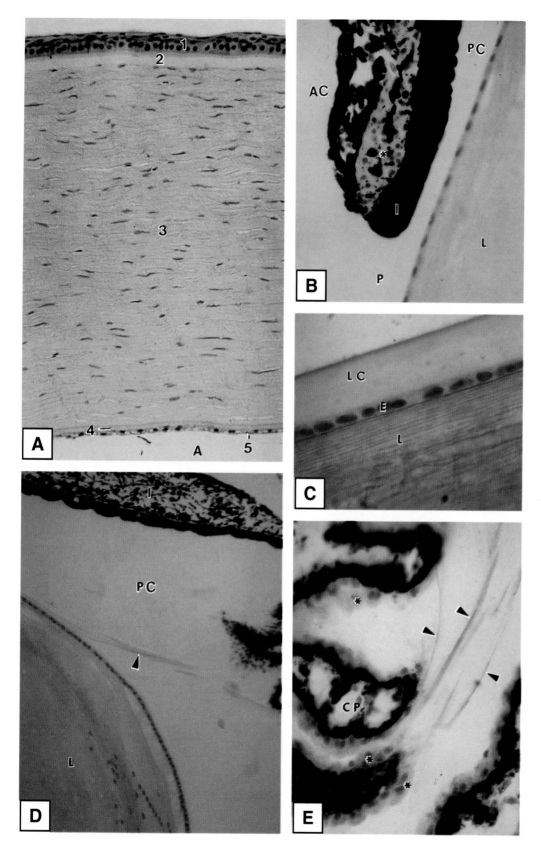

PLATE 31. *A* Section of cornea. From top to bottom; 1 = anterior corneal epithelium; 2 = Bowman's membrane; 3 = corneal stroma or substantia propria; 4 = Descemet's membrane; and 5 = Descemet's endothelium (simple squamous); A = anterior chamber. ×1300. *B* Section of eye. H&E, iris (I) and pupillary constrictor muscle (*), pupil (P), lens (L), anterior chamber (AC), posterior chamber (PC). ×400. *C* Section of lens. H&E. Lens capsule (LC), lens ep-ithelium (E), and lens fibers (L). ×640. *D* Section of anterior portion of eye. Iris (I), posterior chamber (PC), lens (L), and zonule filaments (arrowhead). ×160. *E* Ciliary processes (CP) illustrates both inner, nonpigmented epithelium (*) and outer, pigmented epithelium. Note that the zonule filaments (arrowheads) terminate in relation to the inner, nonpigmented epithelium. ×400.

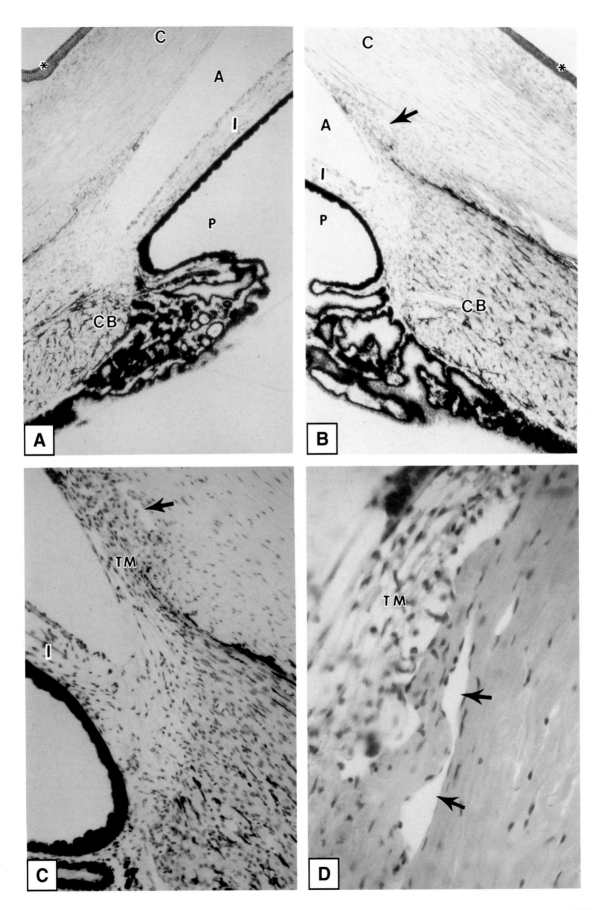

PLATE 32. *A,B* Sections of the anterior portion of the eye illustrate the cornea (C), bulbar conjunctiva (*), anterior chamber (A), posterior chamber (P), iris (I), ciliary body (CB), ciliary processes, and canal of Schlemm (arrow). *A,* ×160; *B,* ×185. *C,D* The iris (I), trabecular meshwork (TM), and canal of Schlemm (arrows) are illustrated. *C,* ×160; *D,* ×400.

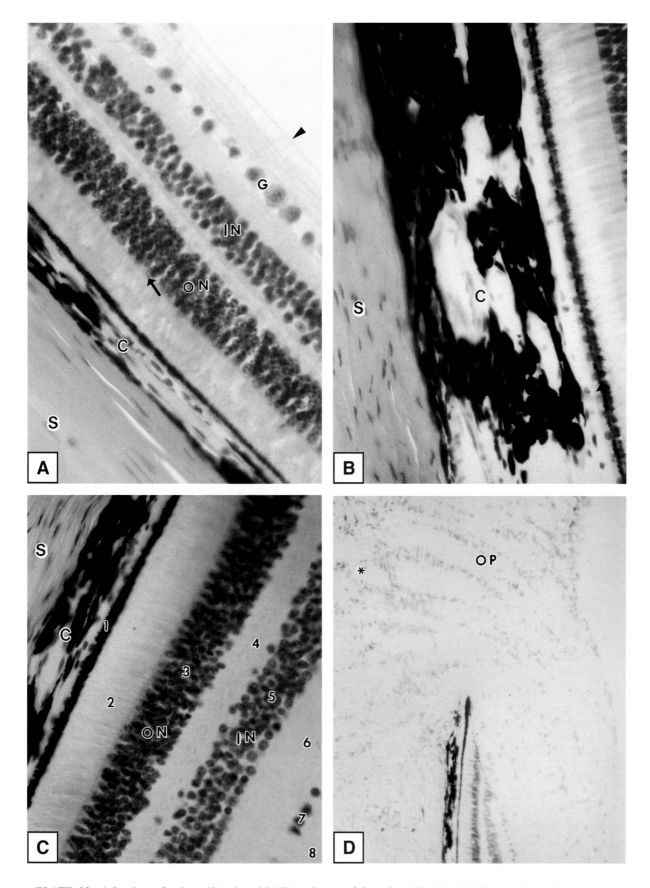

PLATE 33. *A* Section of sclera (S), choroid (C) and retina. The inner (arrowhead) and outer (arrow) limiting membranes, ganglion cell layer (G), inner nuclear layer (IN), and outer nuclear layers (ON) are identified. ×465. *B* Sections of the sclera (S), choroid (C), and pigmented epithelium of the retina (arrow) are identified. ×400. *C* Sections of the sclera (S), choroid (C), and layers 1 through 8 of the retina are denoted. 3 = outer nuclear layer (ON); 5 = inner nuclear layer (IN). ×400. *D* Optic papilla (OP) region of the eye, where axons of ganglion cells leave the eyeball in the optic nerve (*). ×160.

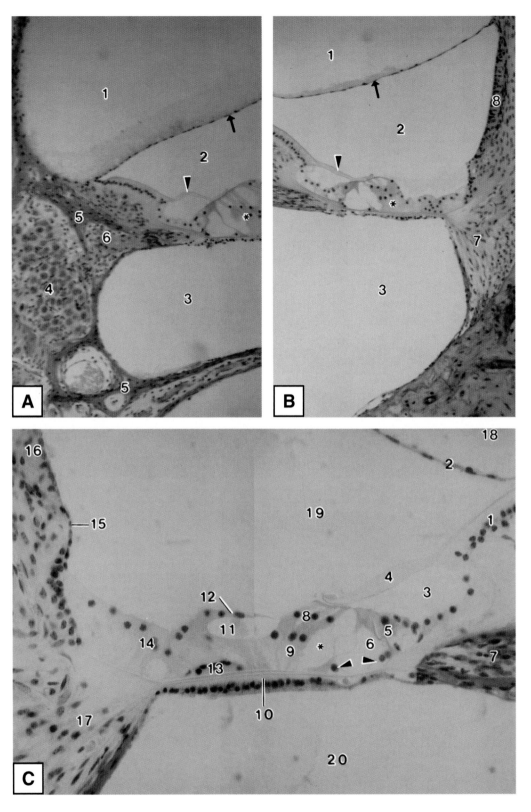

PLATE 34. *A,B* Light photomicrographs of the cochlea and organ of Corti. The following structures are identified: 1 = scala vestibuli; 2 = cochlear duct; 3 = scala tympani; 4 = spiral ganglion; 5 = osseous spiral lamina; 6 = membranous spiral lamina; 7 = spiral ligament; 8 = stria vascularis; arrow = Reissner's vestibular membrane; arrowhead = tectorial membrane; (*) = organ of Corti. H&E. ×160. *C* Organ of Corti. The following structures are identified from medial to lateral: 1 = interdental cells; 2 = Reissner's vestibular membrane; 3 = internal spiral sulcus; 4 = tector-ial membrane; 5 = inner hair cell; 6 = inner (Corti's) tunnel; 7 = tympanic lip of membranous spiral lamina; 8 = outer hair cells; 9 = outer phalangeal (Deiter's) cells; 10 = basilar membrane; 11 = outer tunnel; 12 = Hensen's cells; 13 = Boettcher cells; 14 = Claudius' cells; 15 = spiral prominence; 16 = stria vascularis; 17 = spiral ligament; 18 = scala vestibuli; 19 = cochlear duct; 20 = scala tympani; space of Nuel (*), inner pillar cells, and outer pillar cells are denoted by arrowheads. H&E. ×400.

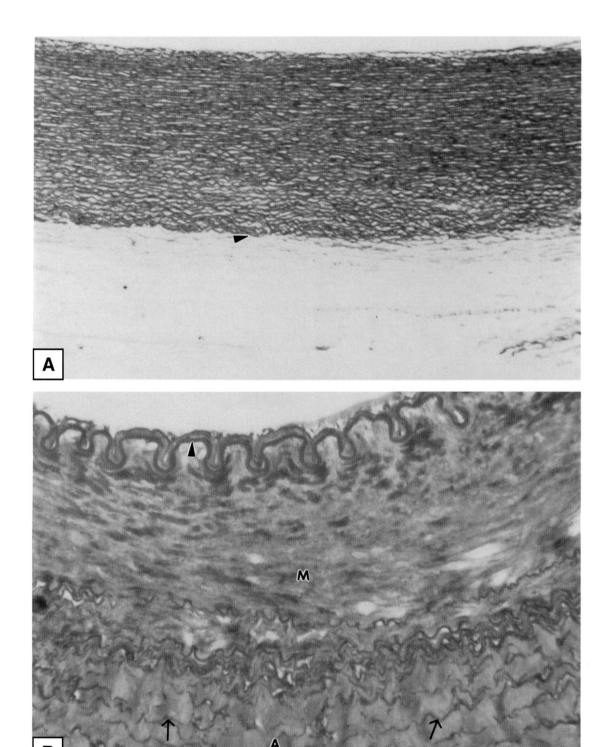

PLATE 35. *A* Low-magnification view of the aorta stained for elastic fibers, are abundant in the tunica intima and tunica media. Junction between the tunica media and tunica adventitia is denoted by an arrowhead. Weigert stain. ×185. *B* Section of a medium-sized or muscular artery. The tunica intima at the top is separated from the tunica media (M) by a thick, folded elastic fiber (arrowhead) called the *internal elastic lamina* (*of Henle*). The border tunica between the media and tunica adventitia contains a number of elastic fibers (arrows). Collagen (green) and elastic fibers (purple) are present in the tunica adventitia (A) at the bottom. Masson's stain. ×185.

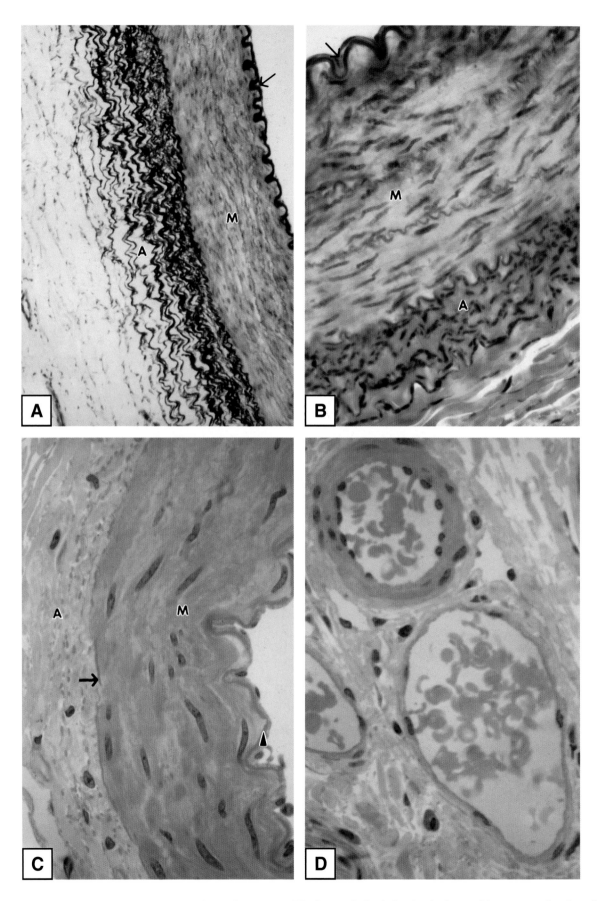

PLATE 36. *A,B* Both figures illustrate sections of muscular arteries stained with Weigert's stain to demonstrate elastic fibers (dark blue or purple). The tunica intima (arrows), tunica media (M), and tunica adventitia (A) are identified. *A,* ×160; *B,* ×400. *C* H&E section of muscular artery. The internal elastic lamina is denoted by an arrowhead, and the external elastic lamina is denoted by an arrow. Tunica media (M) and tunica adventitia (A) are identified. ×640. *D* Transverse section of an arteriole (top) and its companion venule (bottom); both contain erythrocytes. ×640.

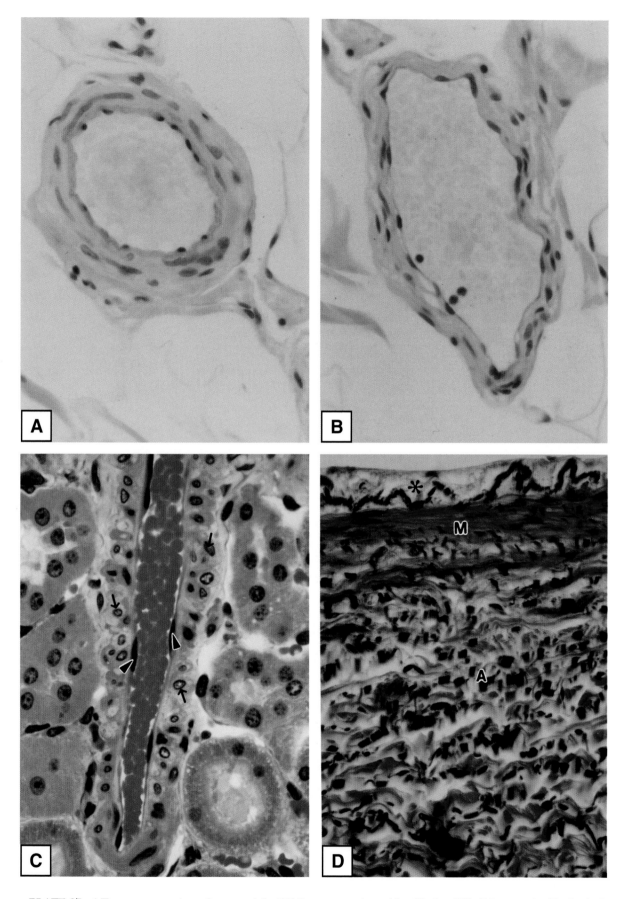

PLATE 37. *A* Transverse section of an arteriole. H&E. ×465. *B* Transverse section of a companion venule. H&E. ×465. *C* Longitudinal section of an arteriole in the kidney. Endothelial cells (arrowheads) and smooth muscle cells (ar-

rows) are identified. ×640. *D* Large vein. Tunica intima (*) at the top; the tunica media (M) contains circular smooth muscle, and the tunica adventitia (A) contains collagen and elastic fibers. ×400.

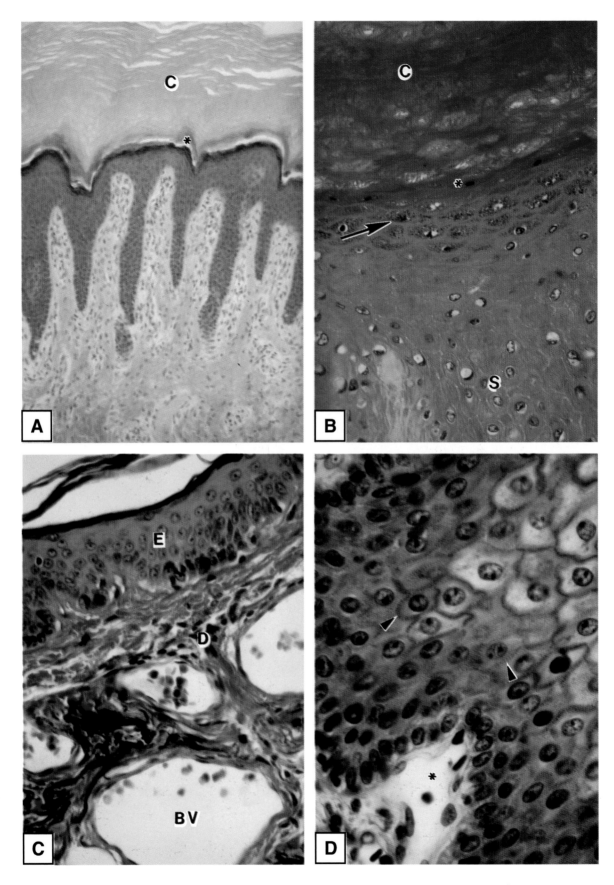

PLATE 38. *A* Thick skin, fingertip. H&E. Stratum corneum (C), and stratum lucidum (*) are identified. ×160. *B* Thick skin, fingertip, H&E. Stratum corneum (C), pyknotic nuclei in stratum lucidum (*), cells in stratum granulosum (arrow), stratum spinosum (S). ×400. *C* Thin skin. Wiegert's stain. Epidermis (E), dermis (D), blood vessels (BV). Collagen fibers are red; elastic fibers are dark. ×400. *D* Stratified squamous epithelium stained with Heidenhain's iron hematoxylin shows the stratum spinosum or spiny layer, which is due to many spot desmosomes (arrowheads) between these cells. Blood vessel (*). ×640.

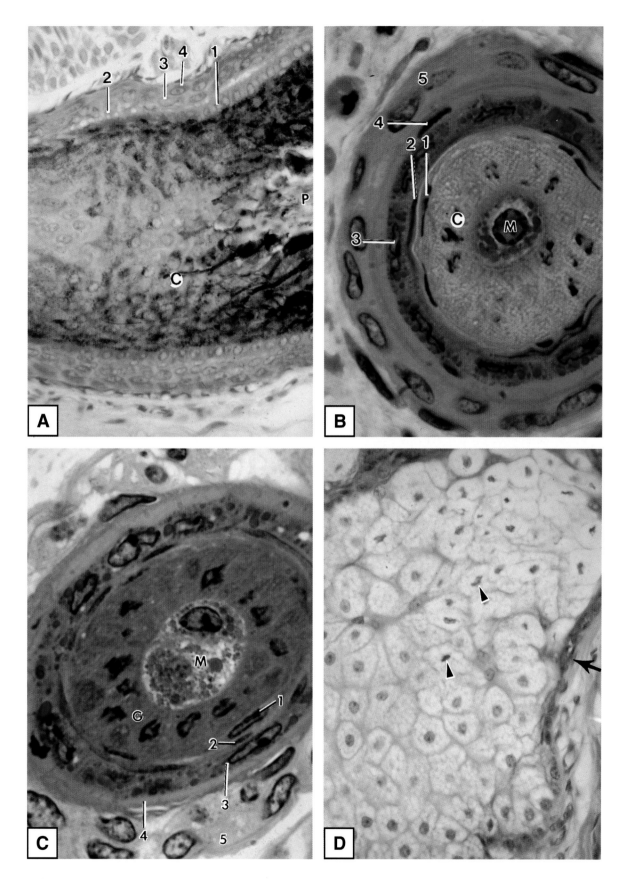

PLATE 39. *A* Oblique section of a hair follicle. The thick, pigmented hair cortex (C), connective tissue papilla (P), cuticle of hair (1), cuticle of inner root sheath (2), Huxley's layer (3), and Henle's layer (4) are identified. ×400. *B,C* Sections of an embryonic hair follicle. Medulla (M), hair cortex (C), cuticle of hair (1), cuticle of inner root sheath (2), Huxley's layer (3), Henle's layer (4), and external sheath (5) are identified. ×1600. *D* Sebaceous gland; cells are vacuolated due to dissolving of sebum; some pyknotic cell nuclei (arrowheads) and a region of myoepithelial cells (arrow) are denoted. ×400.

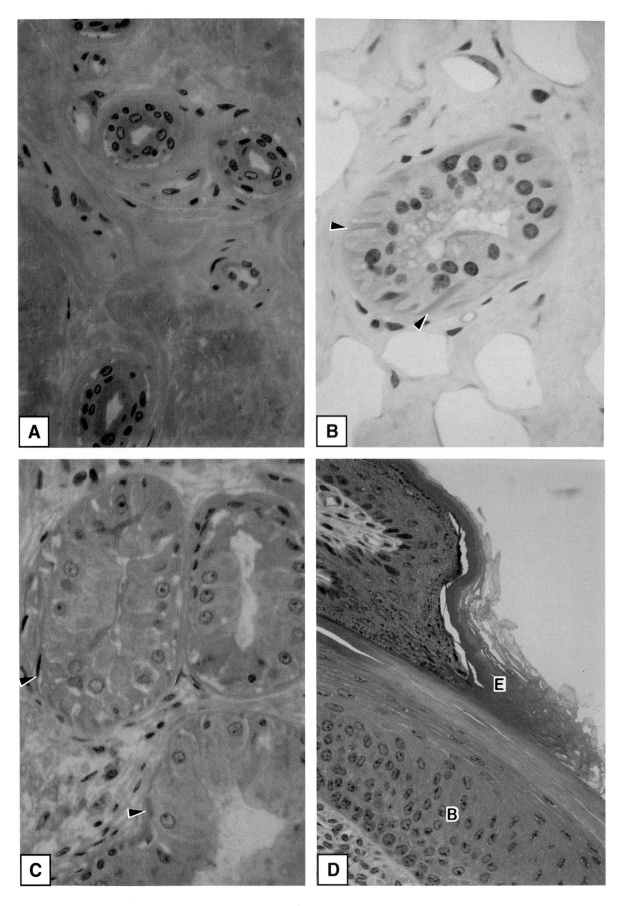

PLATE 40. *A,B,C* Sweat gland ducts *A* stratified cuboidal epithelium. Gland portion in *B,C.* Note the pink regions around the gland, which represent processes of my-oepithelial cells (arrowheads) in *B,C,* ×400; *B,* ×640. *D* Section of a nail. H&E. Nail bed (B) and cuticle or eponychium (E) are identified. ×400.

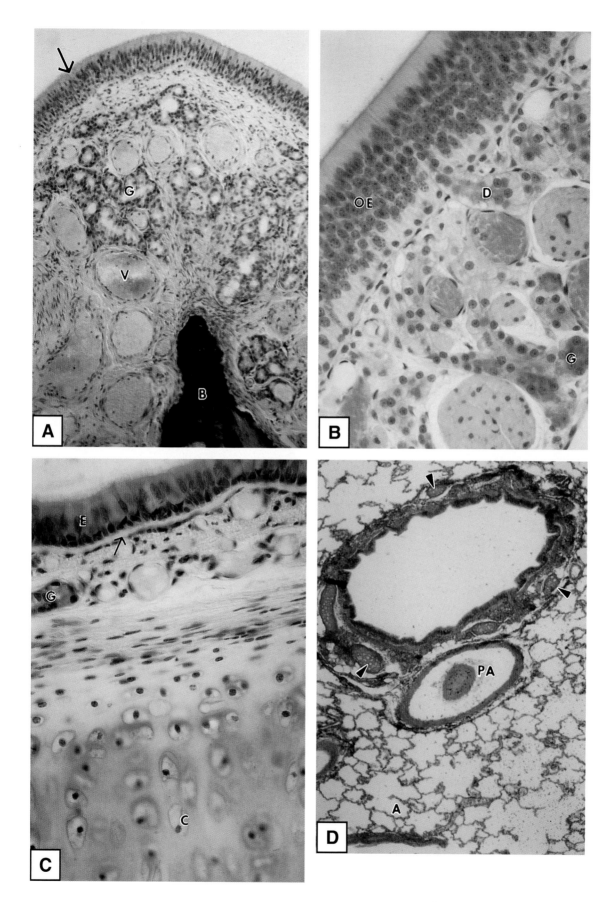

PLATE 41. *A* Section of a nasal cavity. Bone (B) of septum, venous sinuses (V), seromucous glands (G), and respiratory (pseudostratified ciliated columnar) epithelium (arrow). H&E. ×160. *B* Olfactory epithelium (OE). Bowman's glands (G) and ducts (D). H&E. ×400. *C* Trachea section. Epithelium (E), elastic lamina (arrow), gland (G), and hyaline cartilage (C). H&E. ×400. *D* Low-magnification view of lung shows a section of an intrapulmonary bronchus. Cartilages are denoted by arrowheads. Branch of the pulmonary artery (PA) and alveoli (A). Masson's stain. ×160.

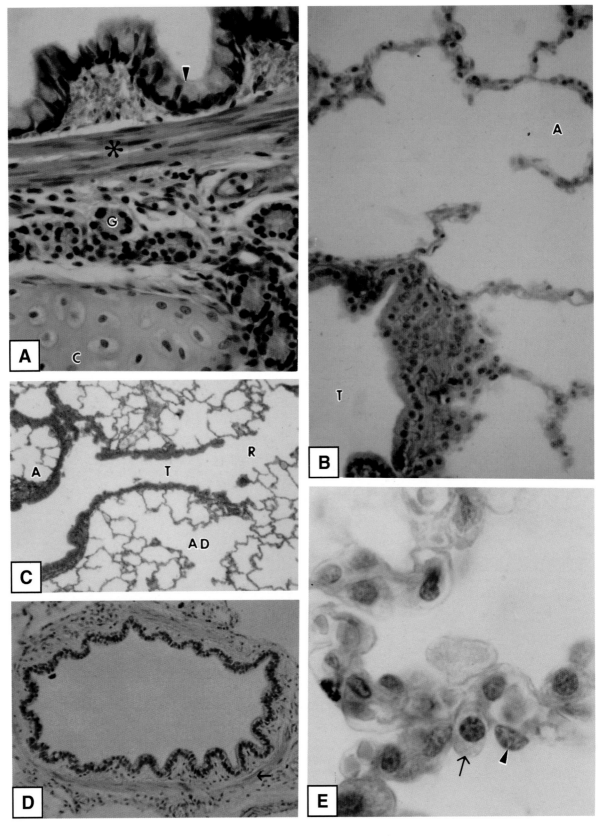

PLATE 42. *A* Section of an intrapulmonary bronchus; pseudostratified, ciliated columnar epithelium (arrowhead), smooth muscle (*), glands (G), and hyaline cartilage (C) are denoted. H&E. ×160. *B,C* Sections of lung with terminal bronchioles (T), respiratory bronchioles (R), alveolar ducts (AD), and alveoli (A). Masson's stain. *B,* ×400; *C,* ×160. *D* Transverse section of an intrapumonary bronchiole. Smooth muscle bands (arrow). ×160. *E* Interalveolar septa in lung. Masson's stain. Erythrocytes in capillaries stain yellow. Alveolar type II cells (arrow) and alveolar type I cell (arrowhead) are denoted. ×640.

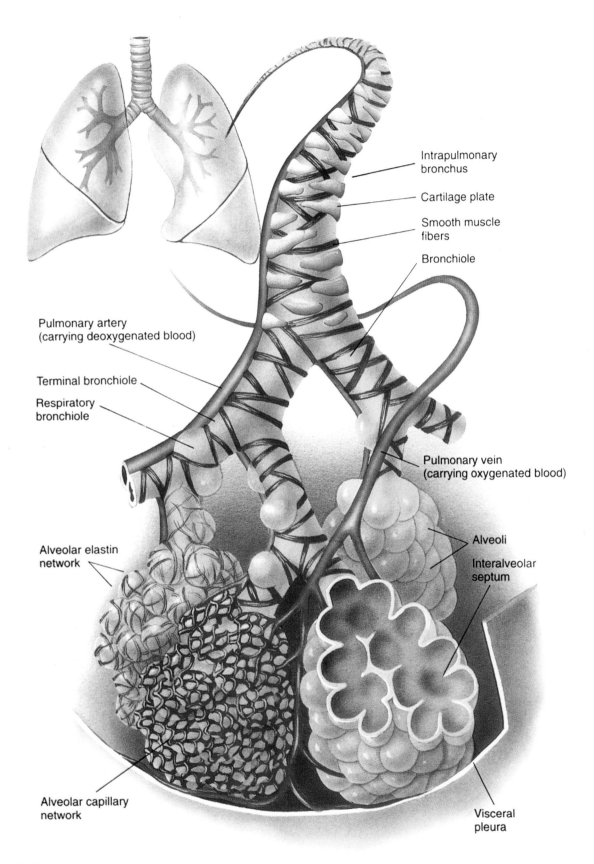

Intrapulmonary bronchus

Cartilage plate

Smooth muscle fibers

Bronchiole

Pulmonary artery (carrying deoxygenated blood)

Terminal bronchiole

Respiratory bronchiole

Pulmonary vein (carrying oxygenated blood)

Alveoli

Interalveolar septum

Alveolar elastin network

Alveolar capillary network

Visceral pleura

PLATE 43. Diagram illustrates the relationships of the intrapulmonary bronchus, terminal and respiratory bronchioles, and alveoli. (From L.P. Gartner and J.L. Hiatt, *Color Atlas of Histology*, 2nd ed., Williams & Wilkins, Baltimore, 1994, Reproduced with permission)

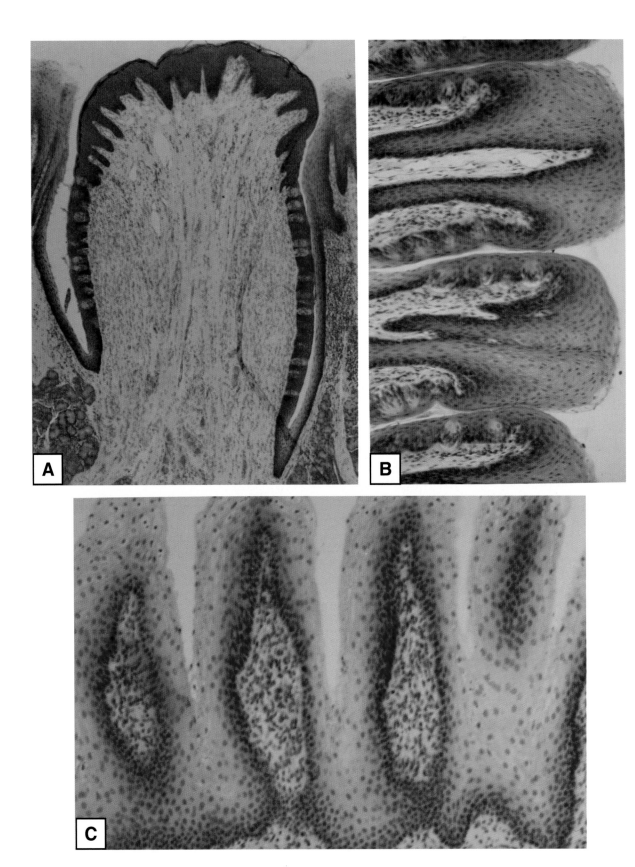

PLATE 44. *A* Circumvallate papilla, longitudinal section. H&E. Taste buds (lighter regions in the epithelium) are located along the sides of the papilla. Serous glands (of von Ebner) are located in the connective tissue lamina propria at the base of the papilla and open by ducts into the base of the vallum or rampart. ×185. *B* Foliate papillae. H&E. Note the deep extensions of epithelium into the lamina propria. Taste buds are located along the sides of the papillae. These papillae are rudimentary in humans and may be located along the sides of the tongue, but they are well developed in rabbits. ×160. *C* Filiform papillae, longitudinal section, H&E. In humans, these tapering papillae are covered with nonkeratinizing, stratified squamous epithelium and contain a central core of lamina propria (connective tissue). ×465.

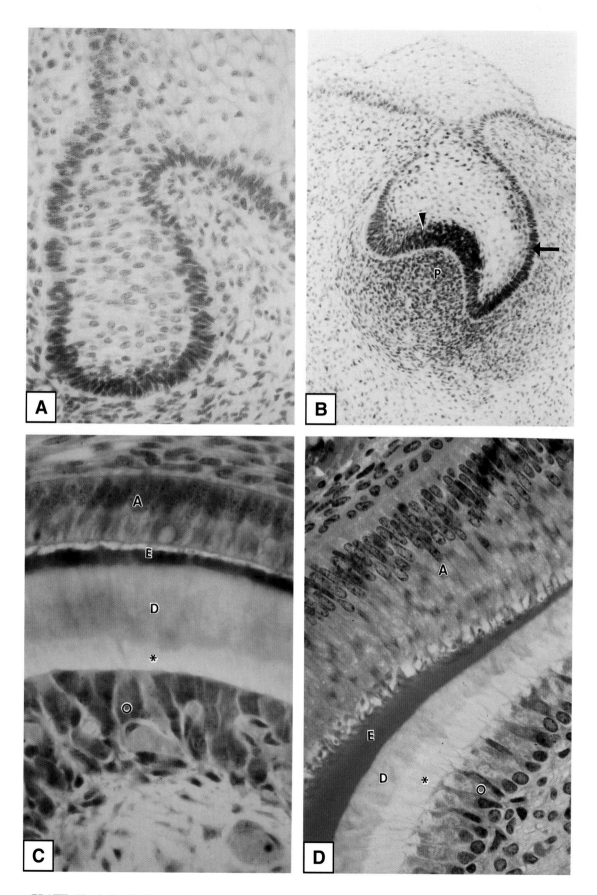

PLATE 45. *A–D* All figures illustrate tooth development. An early downgrowth of the oral epithelium (tooth bud) is illustrated in *A*, ×400. In *B*, the downgrowth has invaginated at its base so that the inner (arrowhead) and outer (arrow) enamel epithelia can be distinguished. ×185. A condensation of mesenchyme is present in the dental papilla (P). *C* illustrates the odontoblasts (O), predentin or uncalcified dentin (*), dentin (D), enamel (E), and ameloblasts (A). ×640. *D* also illustrates ondontoblasts (O), predentin (*), dentin (D), enamel (E), and tall ameloblasts (A). 1.5 μm, H&E. ×640.

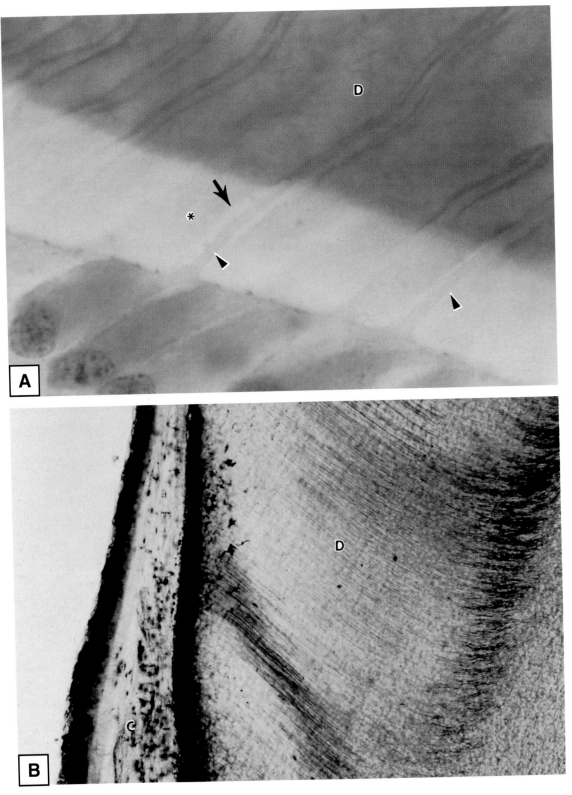

PLATE 46. *A* Enlargement of enamel organ showing apical ends of odontoblasts with slender extensions of these cells—odontoblastic processes (arrowheads) in the dentinal tubules (arrows), predentin (*), and dentin (D). ×1500. *B* Ground tooth includes dentin (D) and cellular cementum (C). Uncalcified regions of dentin (called the *granular layer of Toomes*) appear dark. ×150.

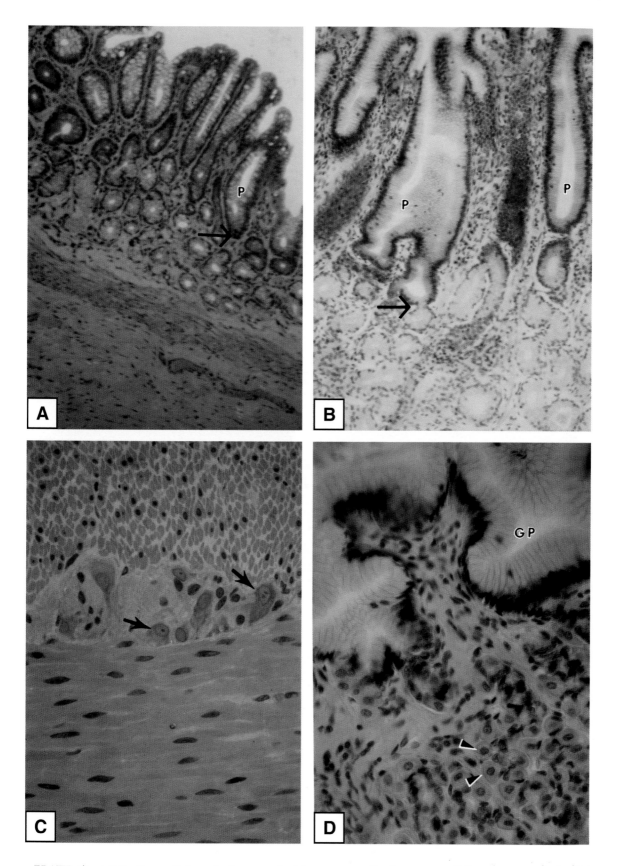

PLATE 47. *A,B* Sections of the pyloric stomach. The gastric pits or faveolae (P) are lined with columnar cells that produce mucus. The junction with the pyloric glands is denoted by the arrows. The pyloric glands contain numerous mucous gland cells and thus appear light. *A,* ×160; *B,* ×360. *C* Section of circular and longitudinal smooth muscle layers with neurons (arrows) of Auerbach's plexus (they are post-ganglionic neurons of the parasympathetic division of the ANS). 1.5 µm, H&E. ×400. *D* Portion of a gastric gland from the body of the stomach. The gastric pits are shorter (GP) and the glands are longer. The rounded, acidophilic cells (arrowheads) in the glands are parietal cells with surrounding mucous cells. ×400.

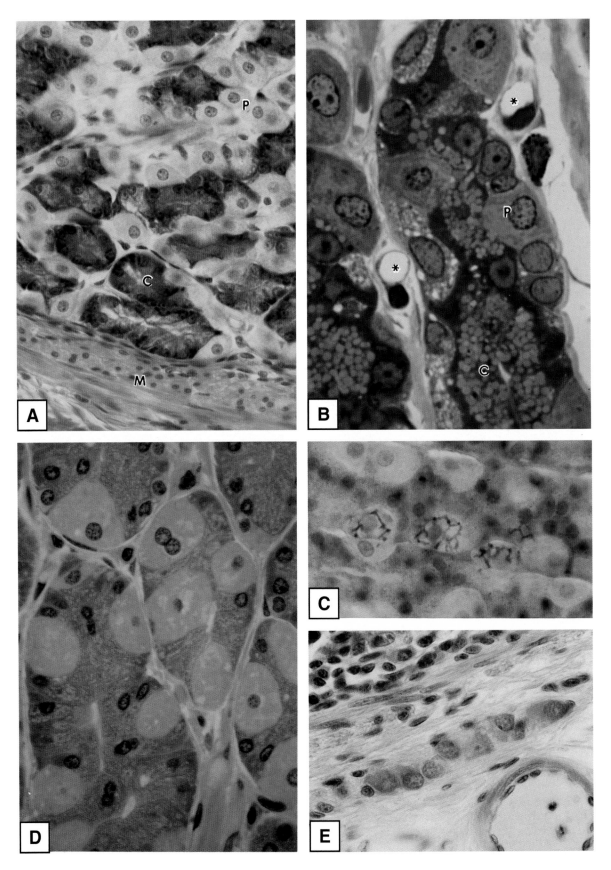

PLATE 48. *A,B* Both figures illustrate part of the gastric gland from the corpus of the stomach. Light acidophilic-staining cells and light blue-staining cells are parietal (P) cells. Chief or zymogenic cells (C), capillaries in the lamina propria (*), and muscularis mucosa (M) in *A,* ×465; *B,* ×640. *C* Several parietal cells have been stained with silver, which deposits in the intracellular canaliculus (dark network), which is apparent in these cells. ×500. *D* Section of a gastric gland in the corpus or fundus. Larger, pink cells are parietal cells and darker-staining cells are chief cells. ×640. *E* Section of stomach showing neurons (postganglionic parasympathetic) located in the submucosa and constituting part of Meissner's submucosal plexus. ×400.

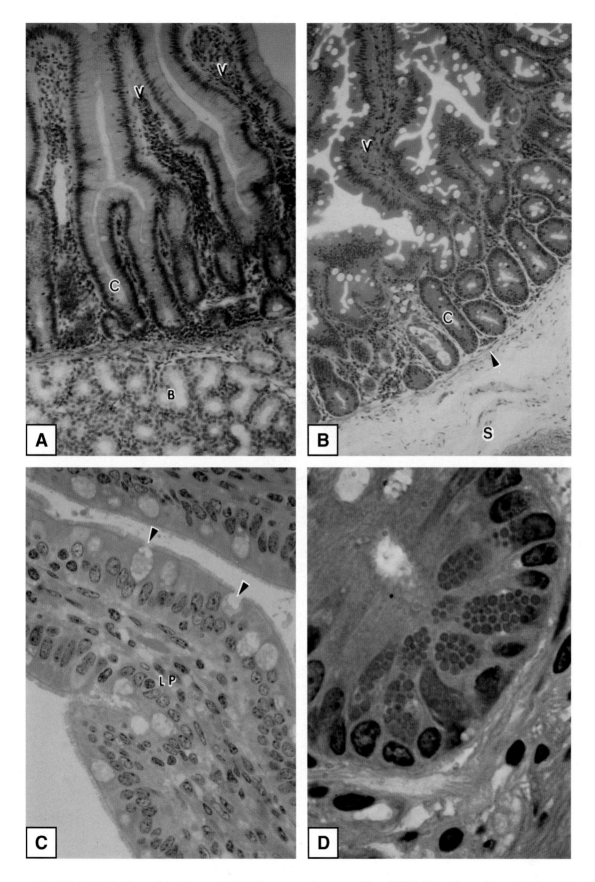

PLATE 49. *A* Section of duodenum. Villi (V), crypts of Lieberkuhn (C), Brunner's glands (B) in the submucosa are identified. H&E. ×160. *B* Section of jejunum showing villi (V) and crypts (C) of Lieberkuhn surrounded by lamina propria. The muscularis mucosa (arrowhead) and submucosa (S) are also denoted. H&E. ×160. *C* Longitudinal section of a villus. H&E. Note the goblet cells (arrowheads) and the connective tissue core of lamina propria (LP). ×640. *D* Section of the base of a crypt of Lieberkuhn (or intestinal gland). Paneth cells contain many acidophilic-staining granules. H&E. ×1600.

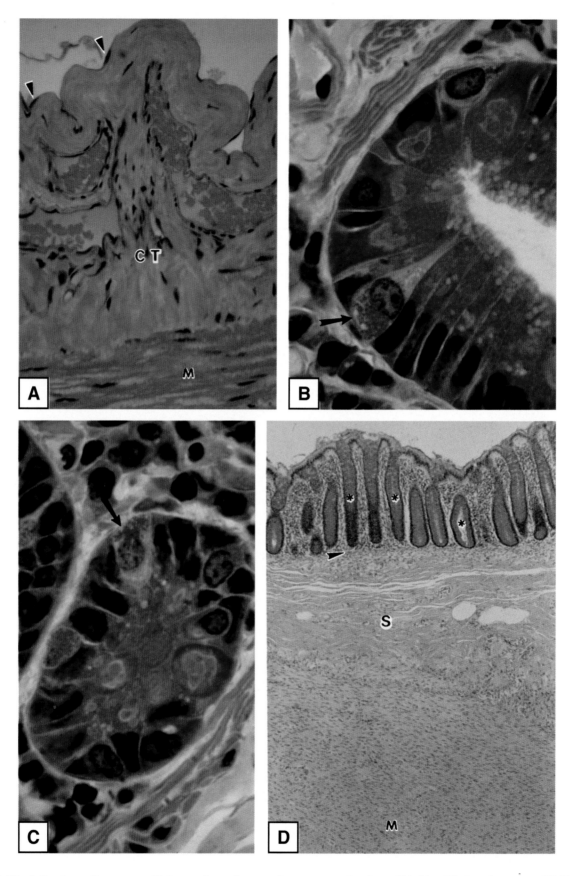

PLATE 50. *A* Section of serosa, which consists of mesothelial cells (arrowheads) and connective tissue (CT) surrounding a muscularis externa (M) layer. H&E. ×400. *B* Section of the base of a crypt of Lieberkuhn. An enteroendocrine cell is denoted at the arrow. 1.5 μm, H&E. ×1600. *C* Transverse section through a crypt of Lieberkuhn. An-other enteroendocrine cell is identified at the arrow. H&E. ×1600. *D* Section of colon. Crypts of Lieberkuhn (*) are surrounded by lamina propria. Submucosa (S) and muscularis externa (M) are also identified. Muscularis mucosa is located at the arrowhead. H&E. ×120.

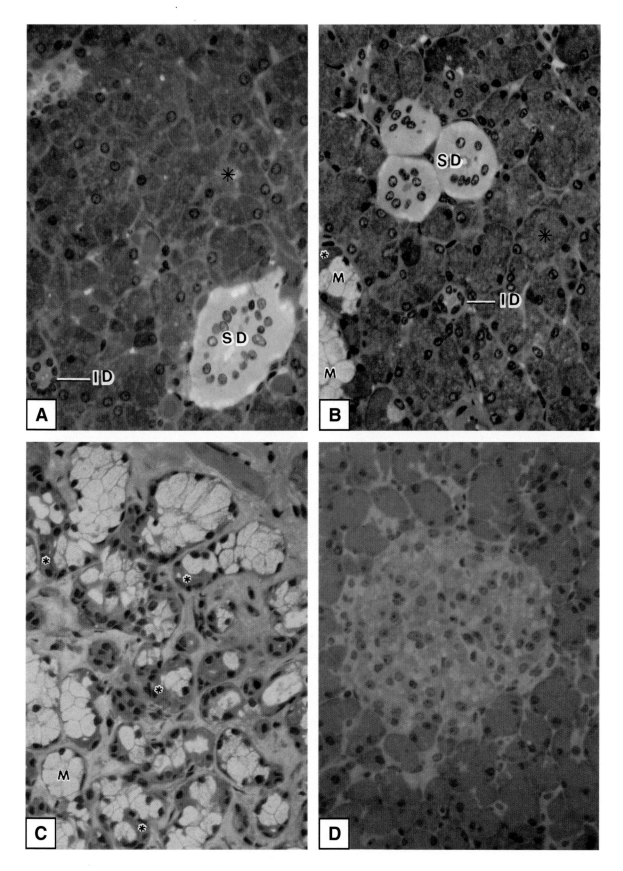

PLATE 51. Section of the parotid gland; serous secretory alveoli (*), intercalated (ID) intralobular ducts, and striated (SD) intralobular ducts are shown. 1.5 μm, H&E. ×400. B Submandibular gland; serous secretory alveoli (*), mucous alveoli (M) capped by serous demilunes (*), striated in-tralobular duct (SD), intercalated duct (ID). 1.5 μm, H&E. ×400. C Sublingual gland. Mucous (M) alveoli capped by serous demilunes (*). 1.5 μm, H&E, monkey. ×400. D Pancreas with an islet of Langerhans in the center of the field. 1.5 μm, H&E. ×400.

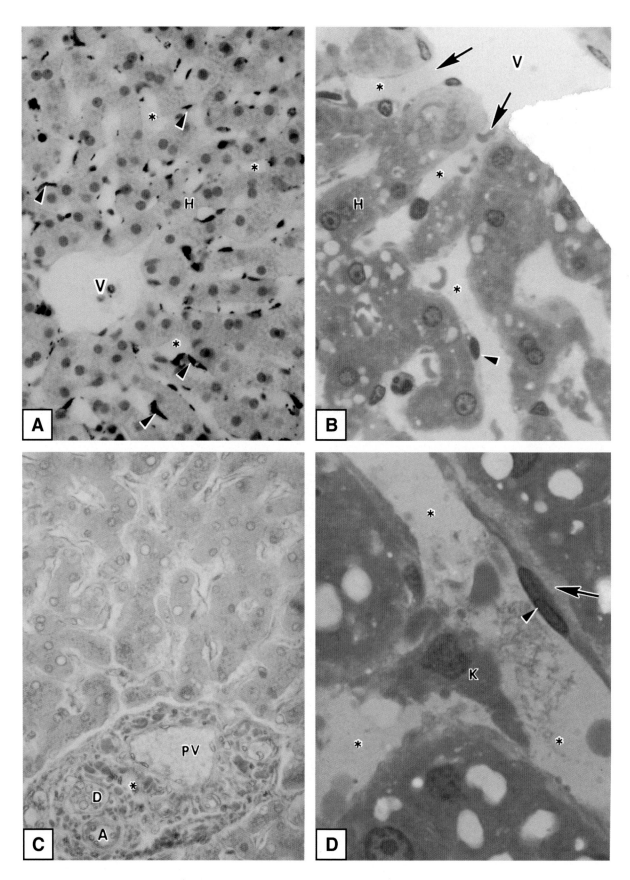

PLATE 52. *A* Section of a liver lobule; the central venule (V) and Kuppfer cells (arrowheads) have phagocytized black particulate material. Hepatocyte (H), sinusoids (*). H&E. ×400. *B* Hepatocytes (H) and sinusoids (*) draining (arrows) into a central venule (V). Endothelial cell nuclei (arrowhead). 1.5 μm, H&E, monkey. ×740. *C* Section of a portal tract (portal area or portal radicle) with branches of the hepatic portal vein (PV), hepatic artery (A), bile duct (D). The connective tissue (*) surrounding these components appears green. Hepatocytes and sinusoids surround the portal areas. Masson's stain. ×400. *D* Kuppfer (K) cells and endothelial cells (arrowhead) in the sinusoids (*). The space of Disse is denoted by the arrow. 1.5 μm, H&E, monkey. ×1850.

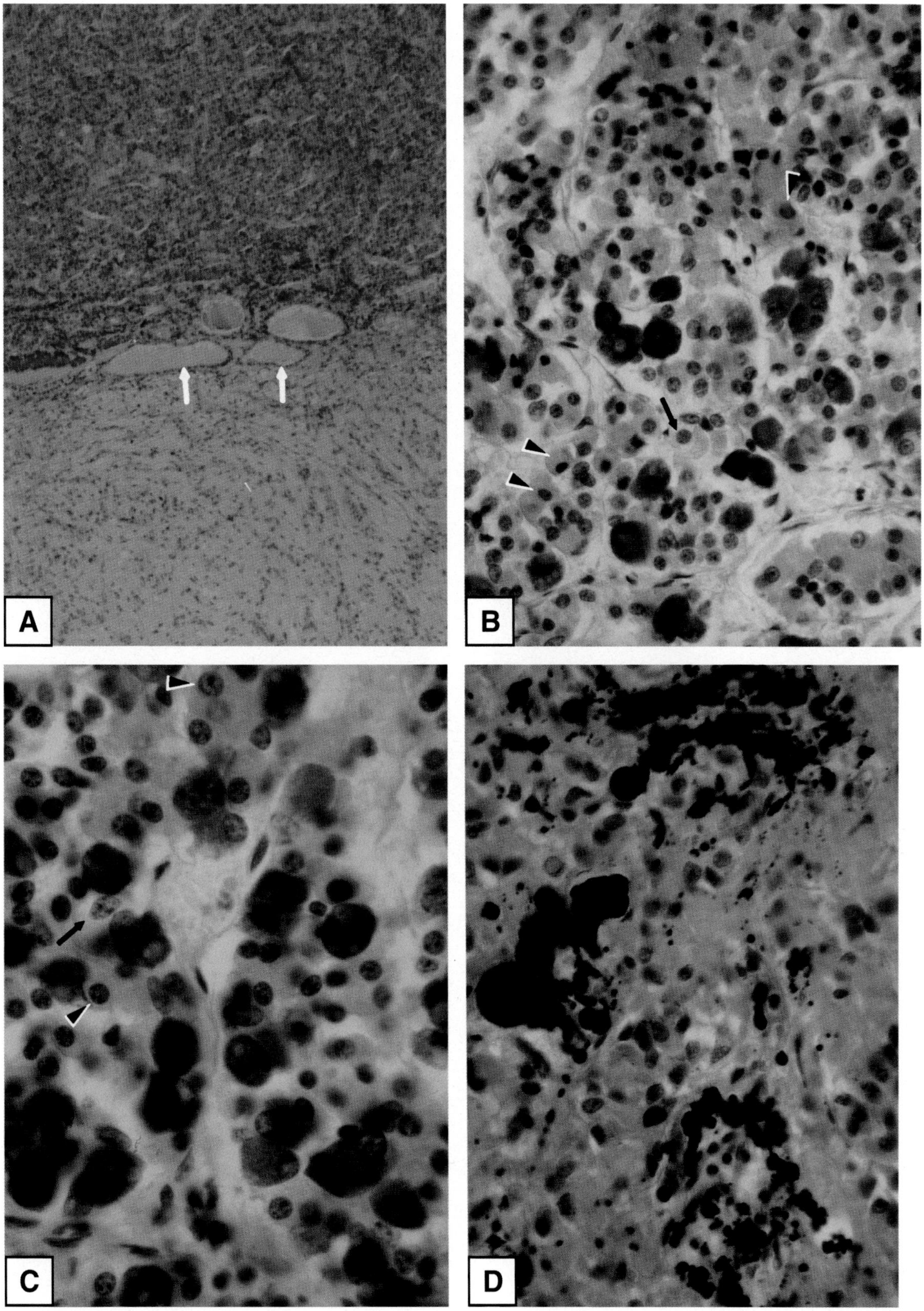

PLATE 53. *A* Section of the pituitary gland. The pars distalis is shown at the top; the thin pars intermedia contains several fluid-filled follicles (arrows), and the lighter-staining pars nervosa is toward the bottom. H&E. ×185. *B* Section of the pars distalis illustrates large, darkly staining basophils, acidophils (arrowheads), and several chromophobes (arrow). H&E. ×400. *C* Portion of the pars distalis with acidophils (arrowheads), chromophobe (arrow), and larger, more basophilic-staining basophils. H&E. ×640. *D* Section of the pineal gland (epiphysis cerebri). H&E. Note the darkly staining corpora arenacea ("brain sand granules"). The cells present include neuroglia and pinealocytes. H&E. ×400.

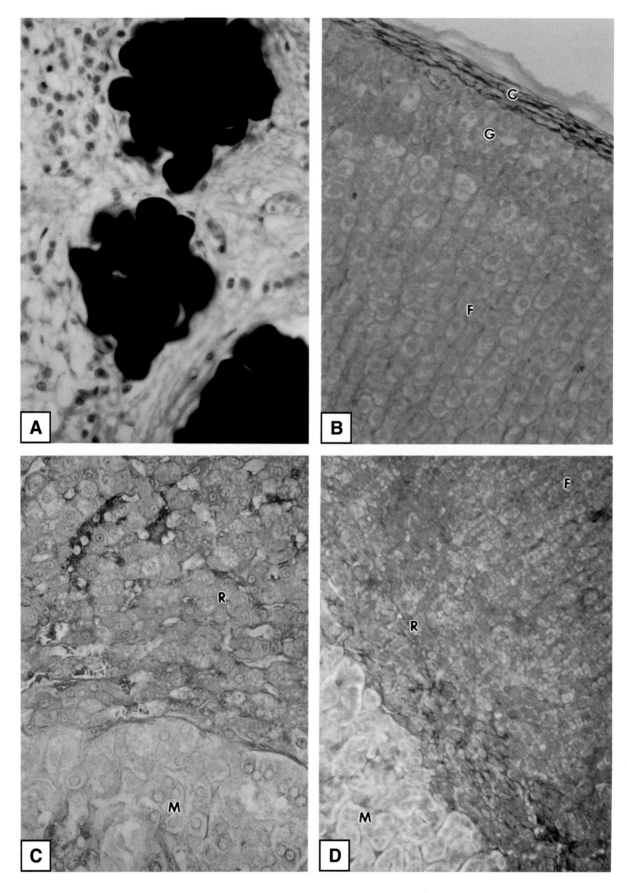

PLATE 54. *A* Section of the pineal gland illustrates several large corpora arenacea (or acervuli). ×400. *B–D* Sections of the adrenal gland illustrate the capsule (C), zona glomerulosa (G), zona fasciculata (F), zona reticularis (R) and medulla (M). Mallory's stain. *B*, ×370; *C,D*, ×400.

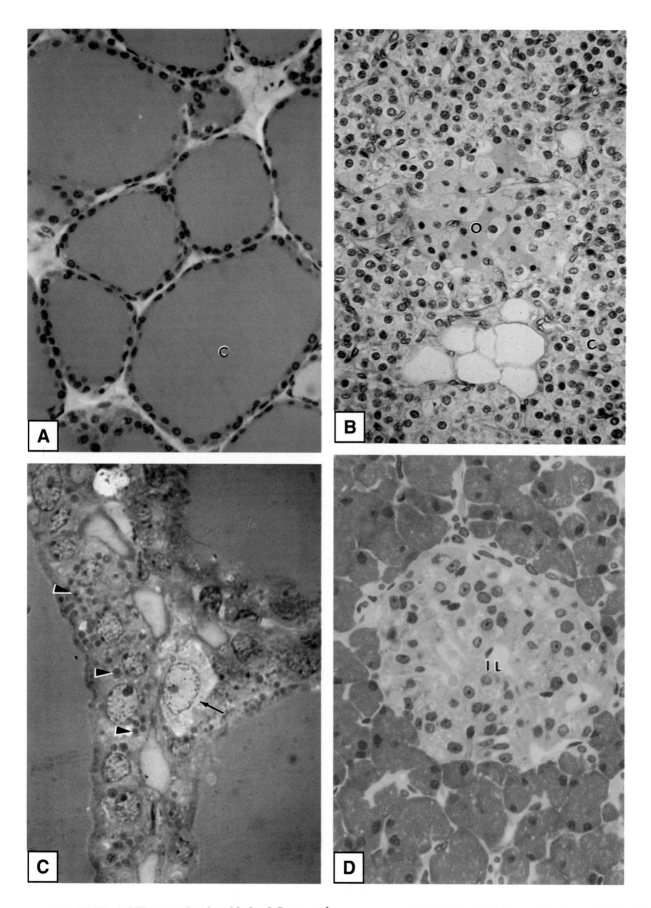

PLATE 55. *A,C* Illustrate the thyroid gland. Large, colloid (C)-filled follicles contain thryoglobulin. Follicle cells in *C* contain intracellular thyroglobulin (arrowheads) which has been incorporated into the cell for digestion. Parafollicular (C cell) cell which produces calcitonin is present (at arrow) in *C. A,* H&E. ×400; *C,* toluidine blue, ×1600. *B* Section of the parathyroid gland with clusters of oxyphils (O) and chief (C) cells. ×400. *D* Islet of Langerhans (IL) in monkey pancreas. ×740.

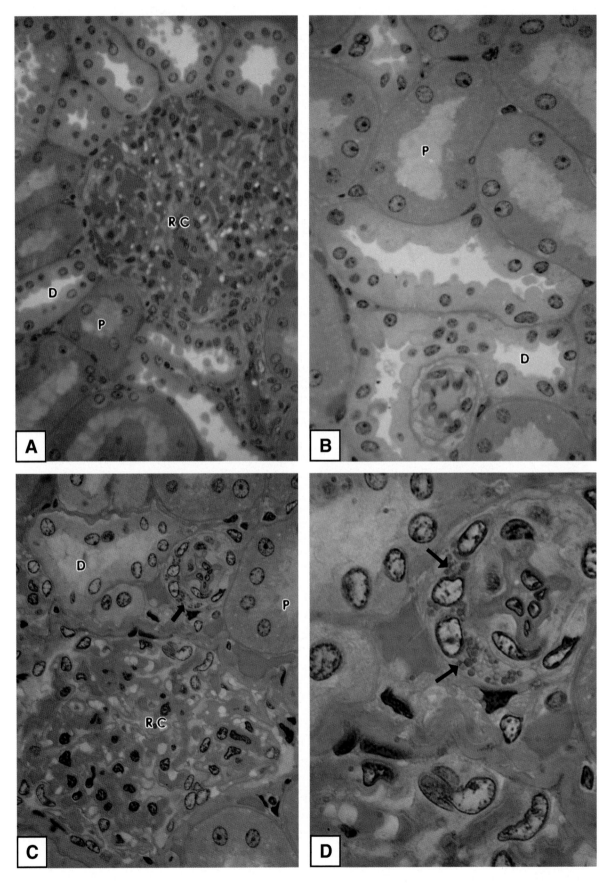

PLATE 56. *A* Portion of renal cortex showing the renal corpuscle (RC) and proximal (P) and distal (D) convoluted tubules. 1.5 μm, H&E. ×400. *B* Renal cortex with proximal (P) and distal (D) convoluted tubules. 1.5 μm, H&E. ×640. *C* Monkey kidney with renal corpuscle (RC) and proximal (P) and distal (D) convoluted tubules; afferent arteriole with JG cells and granules (arrow) 1.5 μm, H&E. ×640. *D* Monkey kidney showing acidophilic granules (arrows) in JG cells of the afferent arteriole. ×1600.

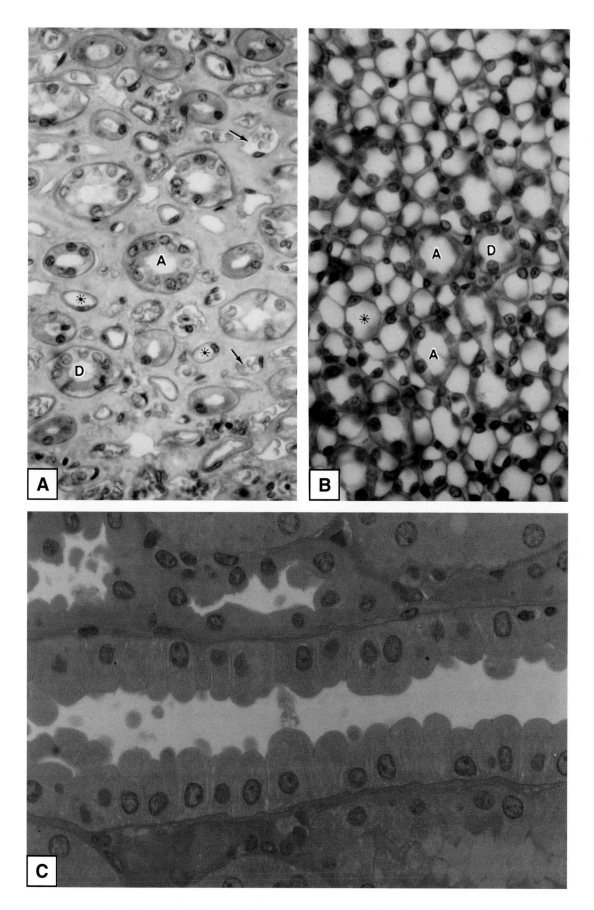

PLATE 57. *A* Medulla of the kidney showing vasa rectae and capillaries (arrows) containing erythrocytes, thin
limbs of the loop of Henle (*), and thick descending (D)
and thick ascending (A) limbs of the loop of Henle. Masson's stain. ×400. *B* Renal medulla of the rat with closely
packed portions of the uriniferous tubules; thin limbs of the
loop of Henle (*) and thick descending (D) and thick ascending (A) limbs of the loop of Henle are denoted. H&E.
×640. *C* Longitudinal section of a collecting duct contains
columnar epithelium. 1.5 μm, H&E. ×740.

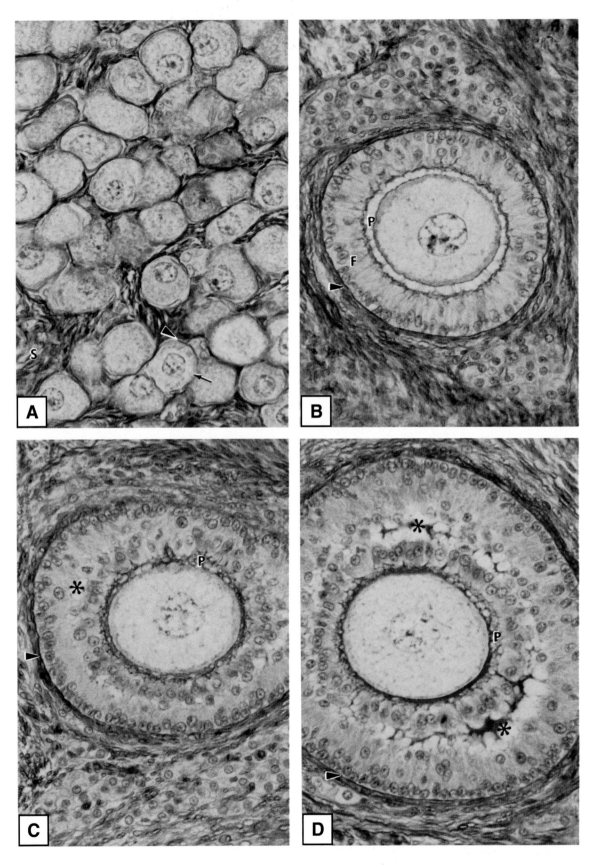

PLATE 58. Figures *A–D* illustrate Mallory-stained paraffin sections of monkey ovary. Numerous primordial follicles (arrow), surrounded by ovarian stromas, appear in the ovarian cortex *A;* an activated follicle in *B* is in transition to a multilaminar follicle. Zona pellucida (P), follicle cells (F). The arrowhead identifies basement membrane between granulosa follicle cells and surrounding theca folliculi (ovarian stroma). Slightly later stages of multilaminar follicles are also illustrated; the zona pellucida (P) surrounding the oocyte stains blue, as does the follicle liquor in the vacuoles of Call-Exner (*). Glassy (basement) membrane (arrowheads) separates granulosa follicle cells and theca folliculi. All figures ×370.

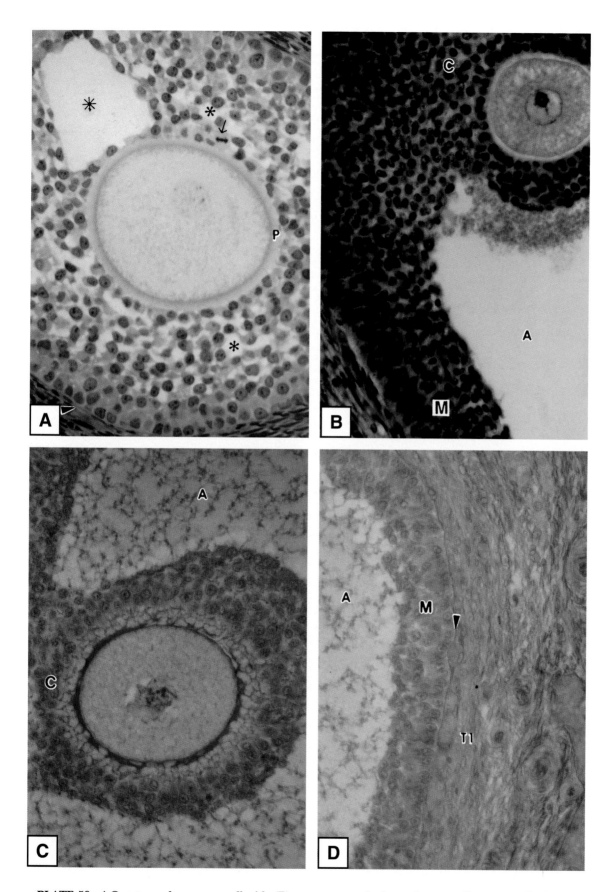

PLATE 59. *A* Oocyte nucleus, zona pellucida (P), vacuoles of Call-Exner (*) and forming antrum (*) are shown. The boundary between the follicle (granulosa) cells and theca folliculi is indicated by the arrowhead. A mitotic figure is denoted by the arrow. *A*, ×400. *B–D* illustrate parts of a nearly mature Graafian follicle. The oocyte, nucleus, nucleolus and surrounding zona pellucida (arrowheads) are present in *B,C*. The cells comprising the cumulus oophorus (C) and membrana granulosa (M) as well as the antrum (A) are denoted. In *D*, the glassy membrane (arrowhead) and theca interna (TI) are denoted. *B*, ×285; *C,D*, ×400.

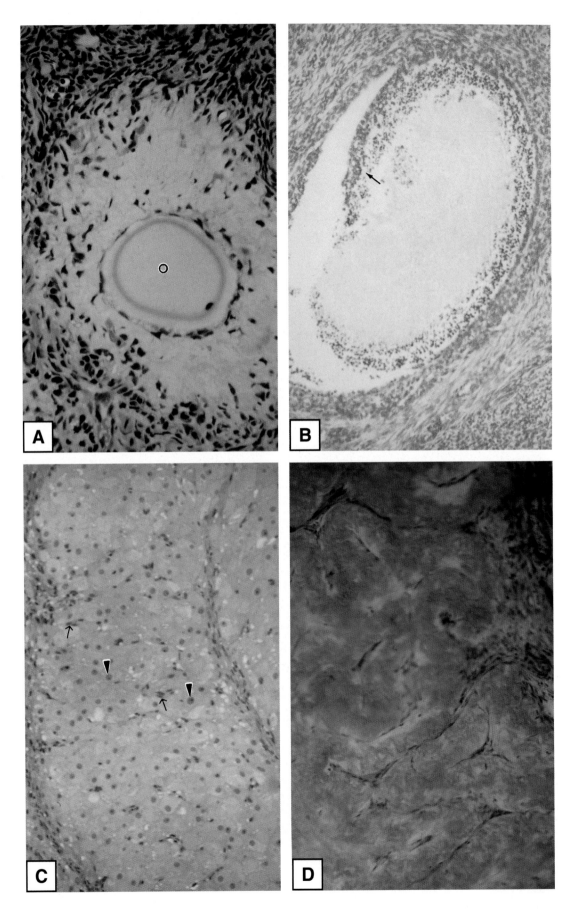

PLATE 60. *A,B* illustrate attretic follicles. In *A*, scar tissue is present around the oocyte (O) and zona pellucida. In *B*, the cells of the membrane granulosa have separated (arrow) and are dispersed in the antrum. *C*, illustrates part of a corpus luteum; larger granulosa lutein cells are denoted by arrowheads, small theca lutein cells by arrows. *D* is a section of a small part of a corpus albicans, which is largely scar tissue and noncellular. *A,C,D*, ×400; *B*, ×160.

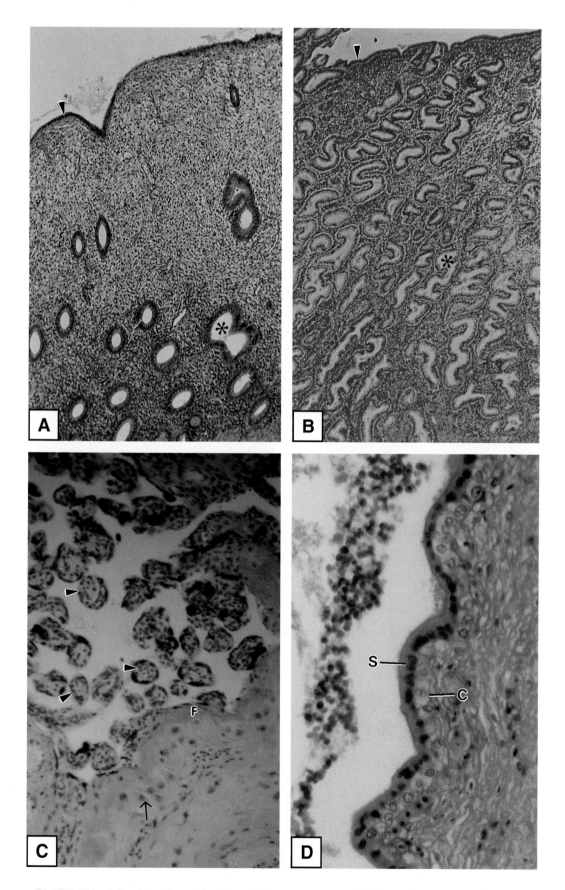

PLATE 61A. *A* Section of proliferative (follicular, estrogenic) uterus showing uterine glands (*) and surrounding endometrial stroma; surface epithelium is at the top (arrowhead). *B*, secretory or progestational endometrium with numerous coiled uterine glands (*). *C* (pregnant uterus) illustrates decidua basalis and decidua cells (arrows), fibrinoid (F), and sections of many chorionic villi at the arrowheads. *D* shows part of the fetal placenta (chorionic villi), in which both cytotrophoblast (C) and syncytiotrophoblast (S) cells are present; maternal blood cells appear at the left. *A,B,* ×160; *C,* ×160; *D,* ×400.

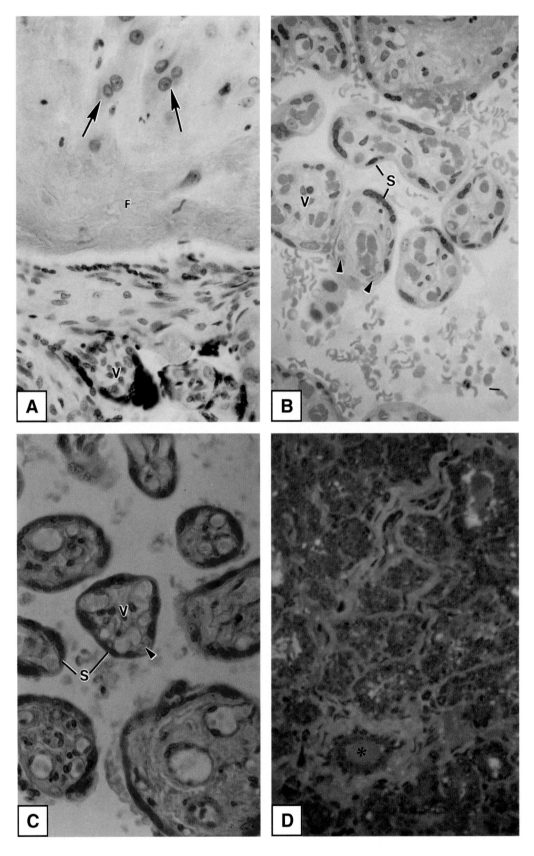

PLATE 62. *A* Section of decidua basalis with decidual cells (arrows), fibrinoid (F), and fetal chorionic villi (V) (H&E). *B* shows chorionic villi with syncytiotrophoblast (S) and scattered cytotrophoblast (arrowheads) cells. Fetal red blood cells are found in vessels in the villi, and maternal red blood cells are located around the villi (1.5 μm, H&E). *C* illustrates chorionic villi. The syncytiotrophoblast (S) stains red, while scattered cytotrophoblast cells (arrowhead) are lighter. The connective tissue cores of the villi (V) stain green (Masson's stain). Maternal blood surrounds the villi. *D*, lactating mammary gland (1.5 μm, H&E); note the secretion (*) in the lumens of secretory alveoli. *A*, ×640; *B,D*, ×400; *C*, ×465.

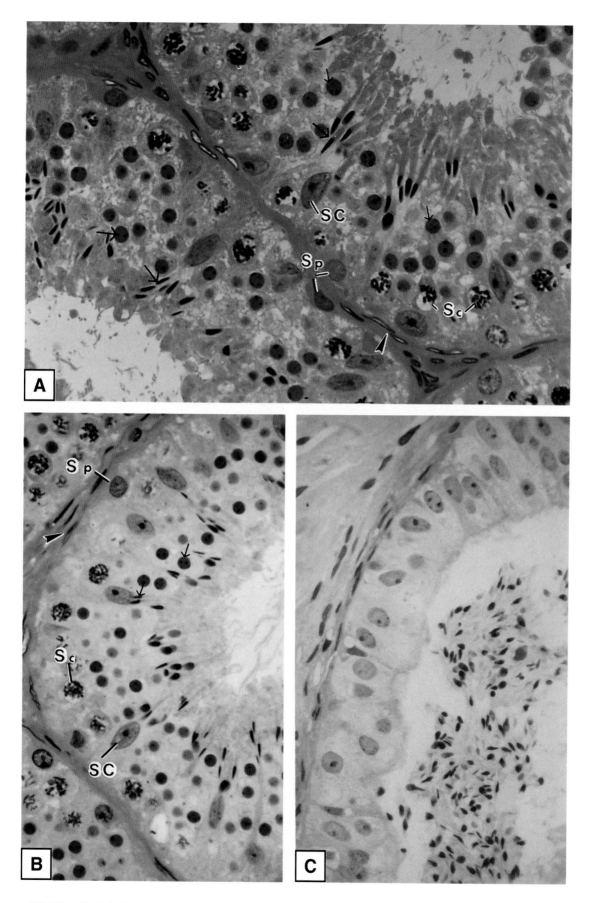

PLATE 63. *A,B* Sections of monkey seminiferous tubules. 1.5 μm, H&E. Cell types identified are spermatogonia (Sp), primary spermatocytes (Sc), early and late spermatids (arrows), and nuclei of Sertoli cells (SC). Myoid cells (arrowheads) are present in the connective tissue septuli testis. *A*, ×740; *B*, ×640. *C* Section of human ductuli efferentes. 1.5 μm, H&E. The epithelium has a festooned appearance, consisting of tall and short columnar cells, some of which are ciliated. Spermatozoa are present in the lumen. ×640.

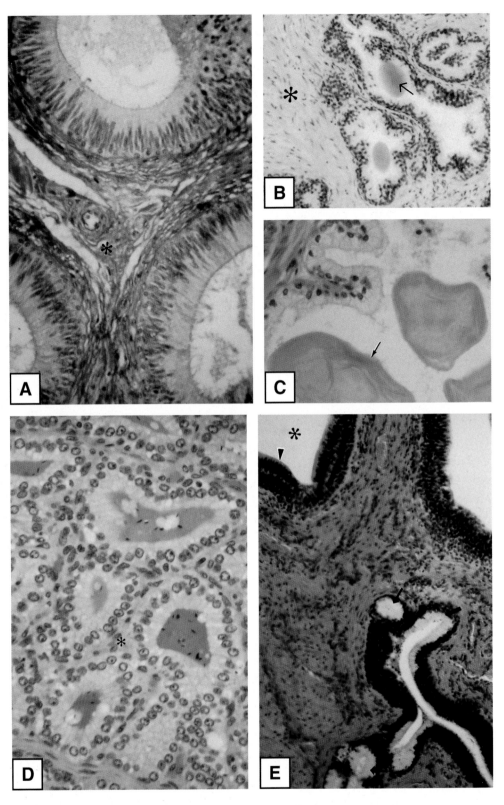

PLATE 64. *A* Section of the ductus epididymidis. Masson's stain. Pseudostratified epithelium with stereocilia. Connective tissue (*) is present between the tubule sections. ×550. *B,C* Section of the prostate gland (H&E); the glandular epithelium is usually tall columnar and highly folded. Connective tissue and smooth muscle (*) surround the epithelium. Calcified concretions (arrows) are sometimes present in the lumen, as shown here. *B,* ×160; *C,* ×400. *D* Sections of monkey seminal vesicle. 1.5 μm, H&E. The epithelium of the highly coiled tubes is simple columnar or pseudostratified. Secretory product is present in the cavities; connective tissue and smooth muscle (*) surround the epithelium (*). ×400. *E* Sections of the corpus spongiosum of the penis. The penile urethra (*) is lined by stratified columnar epithelium (arrowhead). The light-staining glands of Littré (arrows) in the epithelium produce mucus. Connective tissue, blood vessels, and nerves largely comprise the remainder of the corpus cavernosum urethrae (or corpus spongiosum). ×275.

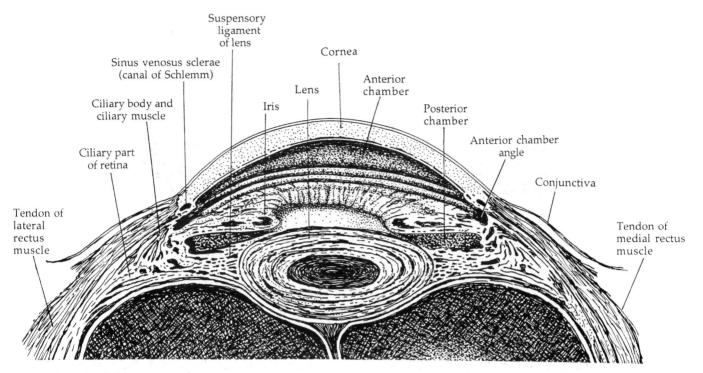

Figure 13.3. Microscopic anatomy of the anterior portion of the eye.

cornea. The cells contain numerous mitochondria involved in ion pumping. If water is not continuously removed from the cornea, it does not remain transparent. The endothelial cells have tight junctions and desmosomes.

CHAMBERS OF THE EYE

ANTERIOR CHAMBER

The anterior chamber is bounded anteriorly by the cornea and posteriorly by the lens and iris (Fig. 13.3). The volume of the anterior chamber is only about 0.2 ml. Aqueous humor fills the anterior chamber and contains most of the soluble constituents of the blood. Since the cornea and vitreous body are both avascular, the aqueous humor plays an important role in providing nutrients to these structures. Aqueous humor has been described to contain sodium, chloride, bicarbonate ions, free amino acids, ascorbic acid, and a low protein concentration. Fluid turnover rate is estimated at about 2 mm³/min.

In the region of the corneal-sclera junction called the *limbus*, near the *pectinate ligament*, there are a number of columns and spaces that comprise the *trabeculae* and *spaces of Fontana* (Figs. 13.3, 13.5, 13.6). The spaces of Fontana communicate medially with the anterior chamber of the eye and laterally with the *canal of Schlemm*. The trabecular meshwork includes the trabec-

ulae and spaces of Fontana, through which aqueous humor drains from the anterior chamber. Aqueous humor leaves the anterior chamber by way of spaces of Fontana, then through the canal of Schlemm (Plate 32D) and away from the eye in the anterior ciliary vein. Any obstruction that interferes with the normal drainage of aqueous humor through the spaces of Fontana can result in increased intraocular pressure. If the pressure is sufficiently high over a period of time, retina degeneration can result. Such a condition can occur in the eye disease called *glaucoma*.

POSTERIOR CHAMBER

The posterior chamber is bounded by the iris anteriorly, the lens and zonule filaments posteriorly, and the ciliary body laterally (Fig. 13.3). The lens forms the medial margin of this chamber (Plate 31D). The aqueous humor is produced by the inner, nonpigmented epithelium of the ciliary body. The aqueous humor then flows through the pupil into the anterior chamber. Both posterior and anterior chambers are filled with aqueous humor.

VITREOUS SPACE

The vitreous space is a large compartment surrounded by the lens, retina, and pars plana of the ciliary body.

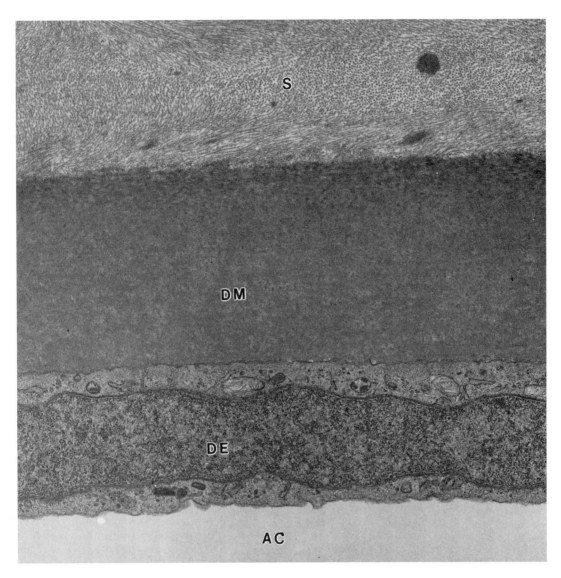

Figure 13.4. TEM of the posterior portion of the cornea. Collagenic fibrils of the substantial propria (S), De-scemet's membrane (DM), Descemet's endothelial cell (DE), and anterior chamber (AC). ×6265.

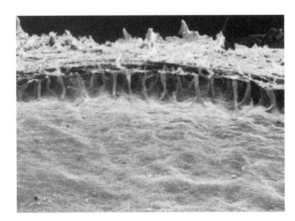

Figure 13.5. SEM of trabeculae and spaces of Fontana at higher magnification. The simple squamous Descemet's epithelium (endothelium of the cornea) is continuous with the simple squamous cells covering the trabeculae. ×85. (From R. Kessel and R. Kardon, *Tissues and Organs: A Text-Atlas of Scanning Electron Microscopy*, W. H. Freeman, New York, 1979, with permission)

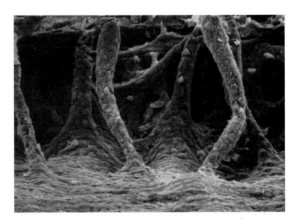

Figure 13.6. SEM illustrates a view from within the anterior chamber. The cornea has been removed, and the iris is located in the lower half of the image. The columns and spaces are the trabecular meshwork and spaces of Fontana. ×25. (From R. Kessel and R. Kardon, *Tissues and Organs: A Text-Atlas of Scanning Electron Microscopy*, W. H. Freeman, New York, 1979, with permission)

It contains a transparent, viscous, gelatinous material (volume ~4 ml) called the *vitreous body* (vitreous humor), which is ~99.9% water. It also contains collagenous fibrils and hydrophilic polysaccharides such as hyaluronic acid. A canal called the *canal of Cloquet* extends across the vitreous and represents the remains of the embryonic hyaloid vessels, including the hyaloid artery. These vessels are present during eye formation but disappear after the eye has differentiated.

UVEA

Uvea is the term used to collectively designate the choroid, ciliary body, and iris. This is a heavily pigmented portion of the eye that is richly vascularized.

CHOROID COAT

The choroid layer is composed of connective tissue, blood vessels, and melanophores; the choroid, which is dark brown, absorbs reflected light and minimizes glare (Plate 33B,C). An outer layer, called the *epichoroid*, consists mainly of elastic fibers. The remainder of the choroid consists of a *vessel layer* and *choroidal stroma* containing collagenous fibers, melanocytes, and numerous arteries and veins. Mast cells and lymphocytes are also present. An inner *choriocapillaris* (Fig. 13.7) contains fenestrated capillaries that facilitate rapid exchange between the blood and nearby pigmented epithelium of the retina. The inner layer of the choroid is called *Bruch's membrane*. This thin layer is located adjacent to the pigmented epithelium of the retina and includes the basal lamina of the pigmented epithelium among the thin components (Fig. 13.7). Bruch's membrane consists of the basal lamina of the choriocapillaris, fine collagenic fibrils and elastic fibers, and the basal lamina of the pigmented epithelium.

The central artery enters the eye in the optic nerve and branches at the junction of the vitreous and inner limiting membrane (Fig. 13.1). These vessels supply all of the retina except for rods and cones. The vessel endothelium has circumferential tight junctions that comprise part of the blood-retinal barrier. The rods and cones are supplied by the choriocapillaris of the choroid layer. These endothelial cells also have circumferential tight junctions, as do the pigmented epithelial cells of the retina.

CILIARY BODY

The ciliary body extends anteriorly from the choroid at a region marked by the most anterior extent of the retina called the *ora serrata* (Fig. 13.1). The inner and anterior portions of the ciliary body consist of many (about 70) highly folded processes called the *pars plicata* or *ciliary processes* (Figs. 13.8, 13.9). More posteriorly, the inner surface of the ciliary body is flattened and is called the *pars plana* of the ciliary body. In addition to two layers of cuboidal epithelium that cover the pars plica and pars plana, the ciliary body consists of connective tissue, blood vessels, and smooth muscle (Plate 31E). The ciliary zonule filaments (*zonule fibers, suspensory ligaments of the lens, ligaments of Zinn*) are attached at one end to the lens capsule and are inserted into the basal lamina of the inner layer of epithelial cells covering the pars plica and pars plana of the ciliary body (Fig. 13.9).

The interior of the ciliary body contains smooth muscles that are meridionally, radially, and circularly arranged (Plate 32A,B). The ciliary smooth muscle controls the focal power of the lens. By the contraction or relaxation of the smooth muscle, the shape of the lens is changed in accommodation. *Accommodation* refers to a process in which the shape of the lens is changed so that the eye can see at different distances. In positive accommodation for short distances, the ciliary muscle contracts. In negative accommodation of the eye for long distances, the ciliary muscle relaxes.

CILIARY EPITHELIUM

Bruch's membrane of the choroid continues anteriorly as a double lamina between the stroma and epithelium of the ciliary processes (Fig. 13.7). The inner layer of this lamina extends between epithelial cells of the ciliary processes and serves in part as attachment sites for the ciliary zonule filaments (Plate 31E). The two epithelial layers of the ciliary body originate from the inner and outer layers of the optic cup but adhere strongly to each other. The apical portions of the two cell layers are adjacent to each other, and the basal surfaces, covered by basal lamina, are directed away from each other. The basal lamina associated with the outer pigmented epithelium is continuous with the basal lamina of the pigmented epithelium of the retina. The ciliary zonule filaments have their attachment and origin in the basal lamina covering the inner, nonpigmented epithelial layer. This basal lamina is continuous with the inner limiting membrane of the retina.

The inner lining of the ciliary body thus consists of two layers of cuboidal cells, a stratified cuboidal epithelium, derived from neuroectoderm (Fig. 13.10). The inner, nonpigmented layer has a basement membrane that abuts upon the vitreous. The zonule fibers are apparently produced by the inner, nonpigmented ciliary epithelium. Well-developed tight junctions, circumferential zonulae occludentes, are present between the epithelial cells and constitute the basis of the *blood-aqueous humor barrier*. The inner, nonpigmented epithelial cells also secrete the aqueous humor by an active transport process. The basal region of the cells adjacent to the posterior chamber has a highly folded

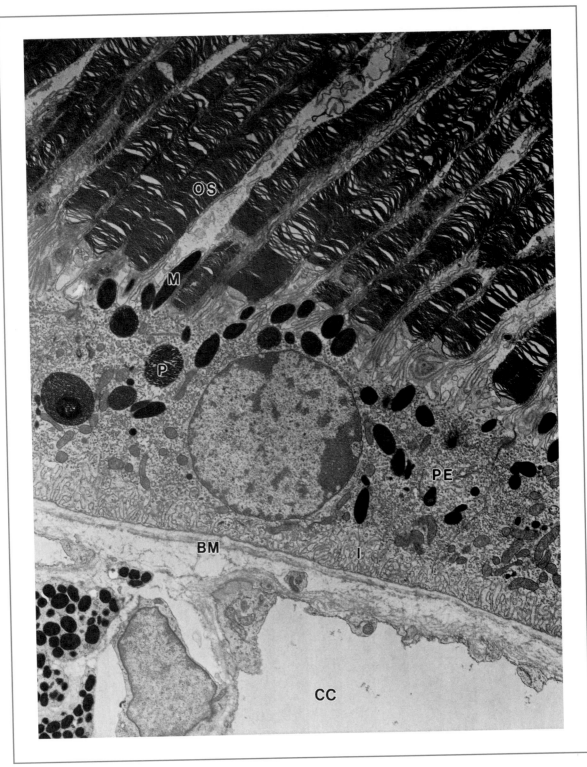

Figure 13.7. TEM of retinal pigmented epithelium (PE). Melanin (M), phagocytized (P) rod discs, rod outer segments (OS), plasma membrane infoldings (I), Bruch's membrane (BM), and choriocapillaris (CC) are identified. ×6900.

Figure 13.8. SEM view from within the eye toward the ciliary processes (CP) or pars plica and the iris (I), which is extremely dilated, resulting in a large circular hole, the pupil (P). The lens was removed. ×25. (From R. Kessel and R. Kardon, *Tissues and Organs: A Text-Atlas of Scanning Electron Microscopy*, W. H. Freeman, New York, 1979, with permission)

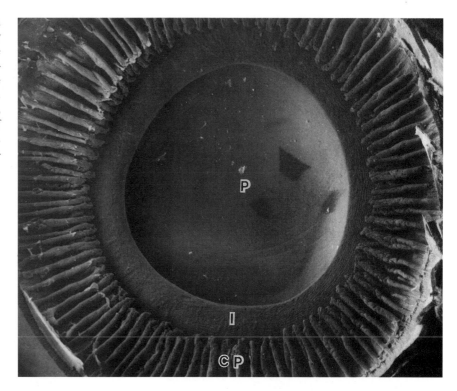

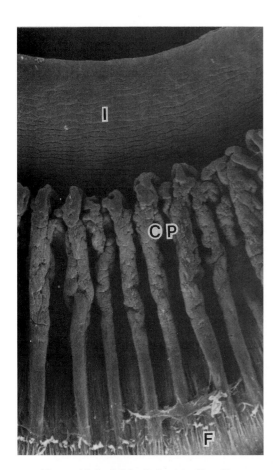

Figure 13.9. SEM of the iris (I), ciliary process (CP), and zonule filaments (F). ×45. (From R. Kessel and R. Kardon, *Tissues and Organs: A Text-Atlas of Scanning Electron Microscopy*, W. H. Freeman, New York, 1979, with permission)

plasma membrane, and many mitochondria are present in the cells (Fig. 13.10). The outer, pigmented epithelial cells have a basement membrane that abuts upon the connective tissue stroma of the ciliary body. These cells also have well-developed basal plasma membrane infoldings and melanin granules (Fig. 13.10).

IRIS

The iris is a flat, perforated sheet that extends medially from the ciliary body anterior to the lens (Figs. 13.1, 13.8, 13.9). The central opening in the iris is called the *pupil,* and its size can be varied by smooth muscles in the iris. The size of the pupil can be altered between 2 and 7 mm, which is comparable to varying the f stop of the eye from 12.0 to 3.5. The iris is thus comparable to the diaphragm of a camera and is important in controlling the amount of light that enters the eye and the depth of field.

The iris consists of connective tissue, blood vessels, epithelial cells, and smooth muscles. The anterior surface of the iris consists of an incomplete layer of fibroblasts and melanocytes. The interior of the iris contains connective tissue, blood vessels, smooth muscle, and melanocytes. The inner or posterior surface of the iris is continuous with the pigmented layer of the retina, and the cells are heavily pigmented (Plate 32A,B). The pigment in the cells of the iris is responsible for eye color. If only a few melanocytes are present in the iris stroma, eye color is determined by the reflection of light

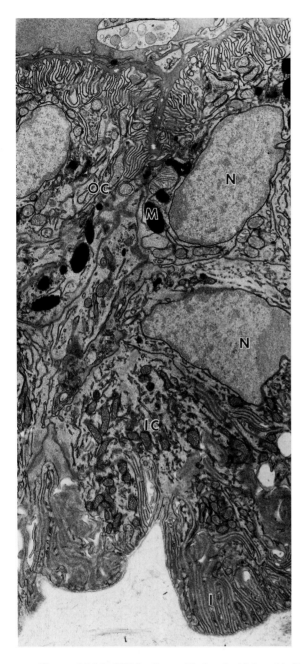

Figure 13.10. TEM of stratified cuboidal epithelium covering ciliary processes. Outer pigmented epithelium (OC) contains melanin (M) granules at the top. Inner, non-pigmented epithelium (IC) is located at the bottom. Both cells layers have infolded (I) plasma membranes. Nuclei (N). ×7500.

from the pigment in cells of the posterior iris epithelium and the color is blue. With increasing amounts of pigment in the stroma of the iris, eye color progresses from blue to shades of greenish-blue, gray, and finally brown. The pupillary sphincter is a circular band of smooth muscle located adjacent to the margin of the pupil. In bright light, this muscle contracts so as to decrease the pupil size (Plate 31B). The pupillary dilator muscles are radially oriented at the margin of the iris,

and contraction of these muscles increases the size or diameter of the pupil.

LENS

The lens is a biconvex, transparent, avascular structure posterior to the iris that is held in place by a system of zonule filaments or fibers (Fig. 13.3). Because of its elasticity, the lens can change its shape to a slight degree in response to the pull produced by the ciliary muscles. This slight change in shape is extremely important for the proper focus of objects onto the retina in accommodation. The adult lens is 9–10 mm in diameter and about 3.5–4.5 mm thick. Pull or tension on the zonule fibers flattens the lens. The capsule tends to compress the lens so that it is more spherical. Contraction of the circular muscles in the ciliary body relaxes the tension on the lens and permits the lens to accommodate to near vision. With aging, the lens hardens and loses its considerable elasticity. The lens is surrounded by a *lens capsule*, a carbohydrate-rich layer some 10–20 μm thick that is produced by and located on the outer surface of the epithelial cells (Fig. 13.11). It contains type IV collagen and glycoproteins. The lens is derived from surface ectoderm and is isolated after its formation. With age, the transparency of the lens is reduced such that vision may be affected in the condition called a lens *cataract*. A layer of cuboidal epithelial cells called the *lens epithelium* is located beneath the lens capsule on the anterior surface of the lens (Fig. 13.11). The apical surface of the epithelial cells faces the lens fibers, while the

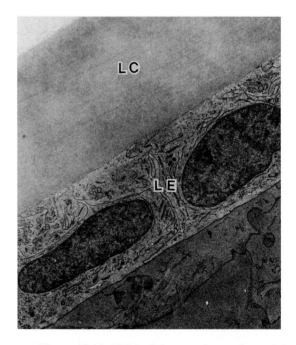

Figure 13.11. TEM of the anterior surface of the lens illustrates the lens capsule (LC), anterior lens epithelium (LE), and a few lens fibers. ×4885.

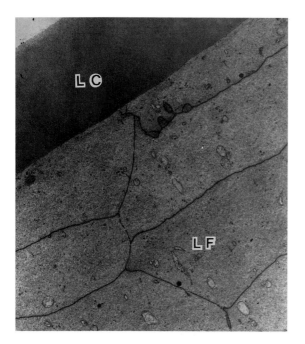

Figure 13.12. TEM of the posterior surface of the lens. A lens capsule (LC) and lens fibers (LF) are present, but no epithelial cells appear on the posterior surface of the lens. ×6045.

13.12). The adjacent fibers may show interlocking ball-and-socket-type connections, and there are many *gap junctions* between lens fibers (Fig. 13.13). New lens fibers are formed throughout life. The posterior lens surface lacks an epithelium (Fig. 13.12) because it is used up in the formation of the centrally located embryonic lens.

CILIARY ZONULE FILAMENTS (LIGAMENTS OF ZINN)

The zonules are filamentous structures that attach to the ciliary body at one end and to the margin of the lens at the other end (Plate 31D,E). They range from 7 to 10 mm in length and attach to the lens capsule just behind the equator of the lens. The opposite ends of the zonules attach to the basement membrane and basal portion of the inner, nonpigmented epithelium of the pars plica and pars plana of the ciliary body. The filaments stain with the PAS technique, have a diameter of 7–8 nm, and have a periodicity of 12 nm. The pull on circular and radial muscle fibers of the ciliary body reduces the tension on the zonule filaments such that the lens becomes more spherical.

RETINA

ORGANIZATION

The retina is a photosensitive layer about 0.5 mm thick that forms the inner layer of the eye (Plate 33A,C). Light must traverse the retina before reaching the photoreceptors. The isolated retina is reddish due to the presence of visual purple (*rhodopsin*) in the rod outer seg-

outer surface is covered by the lens capsule (Fig. 13.11). The anterior epithelial cells undergo division and marked shape changes at the margins of the lens. The epithelial cell elongates to form a lens fiber that may be 10–12 mm in length. The lens fibers lose nuclei and other organelles during differentiation and are filled with transparent proteins called *crystallins*. The fully differentiated lens fiber contains very few organelles (Fig.

Figure 13.13. SEM of stacked lens fibers. Note the ball-and-socket interdigitations between adjacent lens fibers. ×6955. (From R. Kessel and R. Kardon, *Tissues and Organs: A Text-Atlas of Scanning Electron Microscopy*, W. H. Freeman, New York, 1979, with permission)

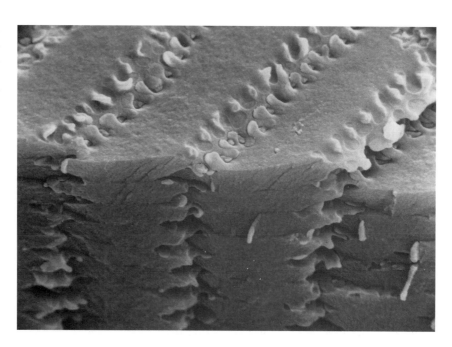

ments. A localized depression in the retina near the optic papilla, called the *fovea centralis* (Fig. 13.1), is located at a point approximately 2.5 mm lateral to the margin of the optic nerve papilla (Fig. 13.1). This region consists of a concentration of specific photoreceptors called *cone cells*, which are involved in color vision and visual acuity. The *optic papilla* or *disc* is the region of the retina where the optic nerve is attached (Plate 33D). There are no photoreceptors in the optic papilla; hence, this is the *blind spot* in the visual field. The anteriormost extent of the retina is the *ora serrata* (Fig. 13.1).

The fovea and a small area surrounding it have a yellow pigment and are called the *macula lutea*. The mac-

ula lutea contains only cone cells; therefore, it is the region in the retina with greatest visual acuity (resolution). Each cone cell synapses with a single bipolar neuron, which, in turn, synapses with a single ganglion cell; as a result, a high degree of resolution is produced in this region. The yellow color is due to a xanthophil pigment in ganglion cells in the fovea. The ganglion cells in the fovea are displaced so that light can impinge more directly on the cones without being appreciably dispersed. Blood vessels are usually absent from the center of the fovea, which contributes to its transparency.

There are three principal types of neurons in the retina: the *photoreceptors*, or rod and cone cells (Fig.

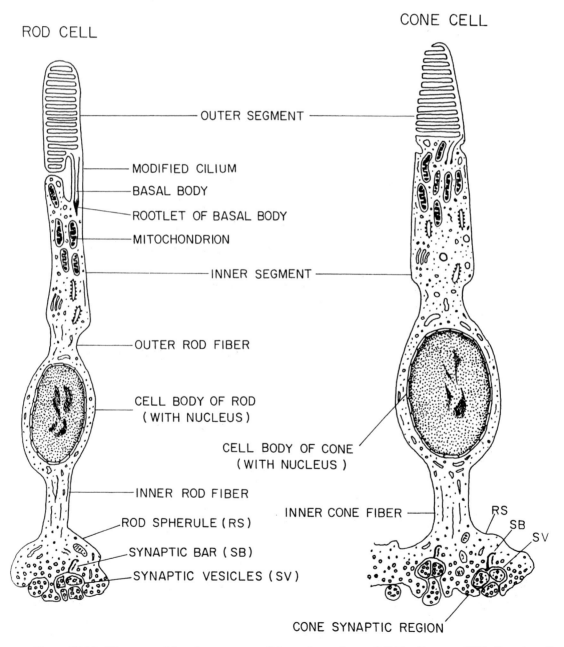

Figure 13.14. Diagrams of the ultrastructure of the rod and cone photoreceptors in the retina. (Modified from T.L. Lenz, *Cell Fine Structure.* **W.B. Saunders Company, Philadelphia, 1971, with permission)**

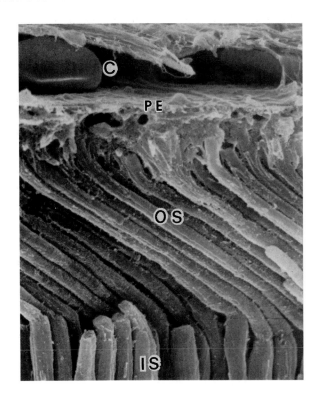

Figure 13.15. SEM of choriocapillaris (C. at top with RBC), pigmented epithelium (PE), rod outer segment (OS) and rod inner segment (IS) are identified. (From R. Kessel and R. Kardon, *Tissues and Organs: A Text-Atlas of Scanning Electron Microscopy*, W. H. Freeman, New York, 1979, with permission)

13.14), *bipolar neurons*, and *ganglion cells* (Fig. 13.17). Amacrine cells, horizonatal cells, astrocytes, and Müller cells are among the other cellular residents of the retina (Fig. 13.16). Ten layers of the retina have been identified (Figs. 13.16, 13.17).

PHOTORECEPTORS

Vision depends upon the response of specialized photoreceptor cells called *rods* and *cones*, which contain abundant light-absorbing receptor molecules that undergo various changes in response to light. The chemical changes that occur produce a polarization in the plasma membrane of the photoreceptors, creating an

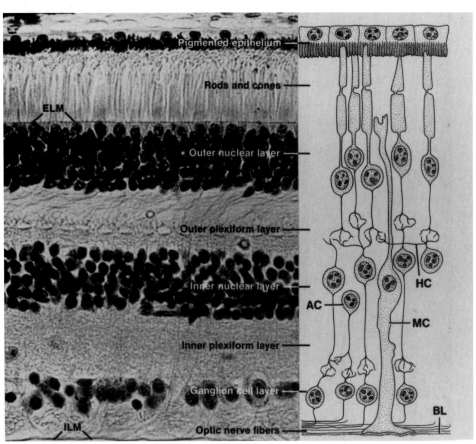

Figures 13.16, 13.17. LM of retina with layers identified and compared to the diagram of cell relationships in Figure 13.17. AC = amacrine cell; HC = horizontal cell; MC = Müller's cells; BL = basal lamina of Müller cells.

(From R.G. Kessel and R.H. Kardon, *Tissues and Organs: A Text-Atlas of Scanning Electron Microscopy*. W.H. Freeman, New York, 1979, with permission)

electrical signal that is transmitted along other cells in the retina through the optic nerve to a specific area in the brain. *Rod cells* are associated with *black*-and-*white vision* and function in *dim light*. The human retina has been estimated to contain 70–140 million rods and 7 million cones. The length of the elongated rod photoreceptor averages ~50 μm. Cone cells are slightly shorter than a rod, but their inner segment is wider. *Cone cells* are stimulated by *bright light* and are used in *color vision*. *Visual acuity* is also due primarily to cone cells. Nocturnal animals such as rats have mainly or exclusively rod cells. Cats and cattle also have numerous rod cells. Primates, as well as birds and bony fishes, have color vision.

Photoreceptors are highly elongated cells containing several specific regions (Figs. 13.14–13.16). The *outer segment* is specialized for light reception. The outer segment of a rod cell is a long cylinder, while the outer segment of a cone cell is more conical or pyramidal in shape. In both types of outer segments, there are many parallel membranes that have a stacked arrangement (Fig. 13.14). In the rod cell, the flattened, membranous

discs are stacked like c   nd are not continuous with the covering plasma i   rane; therefore, the membranous discs are said   "free-floating." In contrast, the membranous discs   he cone cell are continuous with the plasma membr. ie (Fig. 13.14). The rod and cone outer segments are joined by a narrow stalk with another cylindrical portion of the cell called the *inner rod* or *inner cone segments*. Mitochondria are numerous in the inner segments (Fig. 13.14). The connecting stalk between the inner and outer segments contains a modified cilium attached to one of a pair of basal bodies located adjacent to the stalk in the inner segment (Figs. 13.14, 13.18). The cilium has nine peripheral doublet microtubules, but there are no central microtubules. The function of the modified cilium is not clear.

The outer rod segment is known to arise developmentally from the inner segment. The outer rod segment contains approximately 600–1000 membranous discs that continually turn over, and the rate of production equals the rate of destruction. Shedding of rod membranous discs is especially prevalent in the morning after waking up. Phagocytosis of rod membranous

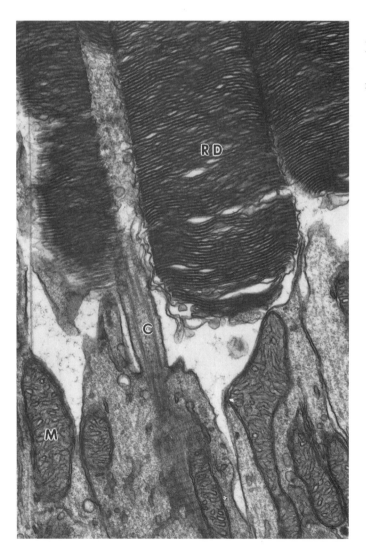

Figure 13.18. TEM of a rod outer segment shows flattened membranous disks (RD), the ciliary stalk (C), and mitochondria (M) in the inner rod segment. ×28,000

discs by pigmented epithelial cells (layer 1 of the retina) occurs primarily in the morning after initial exposure to light. Phagocytosis of cone discs is initiated by darkness and therefore occurs at night. It has been estimated that a single pigmented epithelial cell can phagocytose ~7500 shed discs per day. The new discs form as infoldings of the plasma membrane at the junction of the stalk and the outer segment. The infoldings detach from the plasma membrane and become flattened discs. Older discs are removed or shed at the tip of the outer segments. The phagocytosed discs are then digested intracellularly by the lysosomes and lysosomal enzymes produced by the pigmented epithelial cells (Fig. 13.7).

HORIZONTAL, AMACRINE, AND MÜLLER CELLS.

In addition to photoreceptors, other cell types present in the retina include (1) *horizontal cells*, which interconnect various photoreceptors; (2) *amacrine cells*, which are neurons that laterally interconnect ganglion cells and bipolar neurons; and (3) supporting neuroglia-type cells called *Müller cells* (Figs. 13.16, 13.19). Horizontal and amacrine cells provide for lateral integration of visual signals before they are sent to the brain. Signals arising in horizontal cells are carried from one rod or cone to other nearby receptors and then to several bipolar cells. Amacrine cells spread signals from one bipolar neuron to several ganglion cells. Müller cells are ex-

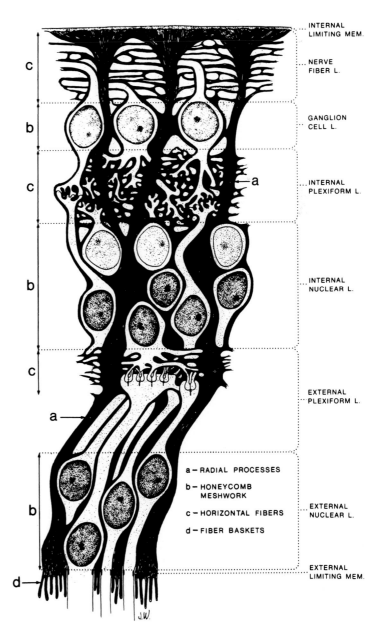

Figure 13.19. Diagram shows the highly irregular shape of the Müller cells and their relationship to other constituents of the retina. (From M. Hogan, J. Alvaredo, and J. Waddell, *Histology of the Human Eye. An Atlas and Textbook.* W.B. Saunders, Philadelphia, 1971, with permission)

a – RADIAL PROCESSES
b – HONEYCOMB MESHWORK
c – HORIZONTAL FIBERS
d – FIBER BASKETS

INTERNAL LIMITING MEM.
NERVE FIBER L.
GANGLION CELL L.
INTERNAL PLEXIFORM L.
INTERNAL NUCLEAR L.
EXTERNAL PLEXIFORM L.
EXTERNAL NUCLEAR L.
EXTERNAL LIMITING MEM.

tensively branched and extend into all layers of the retina, with the exception of layer 1 and part of layer 2 (Figs. 13.19, 13.20). The cells have a high metabolic rate and contain microfilaments and glycogen. They undoubtedly provide support to the retina and perhaps serve a nutritive function as well.

LAYERS OF THE RETINA

The layers of the retina are illustrated in Figures 13.15–13.17 and Figures 13.20–13.23.

Layer 1

The *pigmented epithelium* is a layer of cuboidal cells that contains melanin granules. These cells closely invest the tips of the rod outer segments and form a thin cytoplasmic flap that surrounds the tips of the outer rod segments (Figs. 13.15, 13.16). Adjacent pigmented epithelial cells have gap junctions, circumferential zonulae occludentes, and zonulae adherentes. The *circumferential zonulae occludentes* constitute the basis of the *blood-retina barrier*. The pigmented epithelial cells have plasma membrane infoldings adjacent to Bruch's membrane (Fig. 13.7). Since there are no specializations or anchoring devices between the pigmented epithelium and

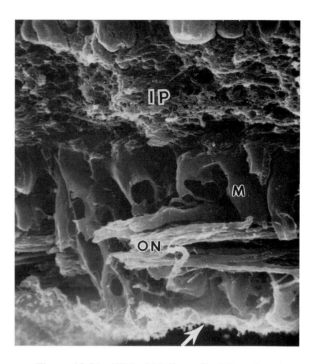

Figure 13.21. SEM of Müller cells (M) and optic nerve fibers (ON) or the axons of ganglion cells. The inner limiting membrane (arrow) and inner plexiform (IP) layer are denoted. ×1790. (From R. Kessel and R. Kardon, *Tissues and Organs: A Text-Atlas of Scanning Electron Microscopy*, W. H. Freeman, New York, 1979, with permission)

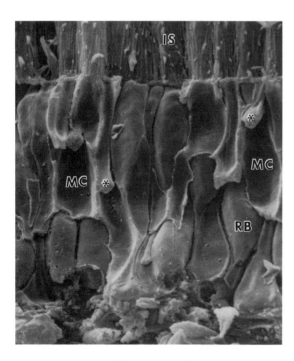

Figure 13.20. SEM of retina illustrates a small portion of rod inner segments (IS), rod cell bodies (RB), broken outer rod fibers (*), and thin pieces of Müller cells (MC), which form a packing around the rod cells ×3380. (From R. Kessel and R. Kardon, *Tissues and Organs: A Text-Atlas of Scanning Electron Microscopy*, W. H. Freeman, New York, 1979, with permission)

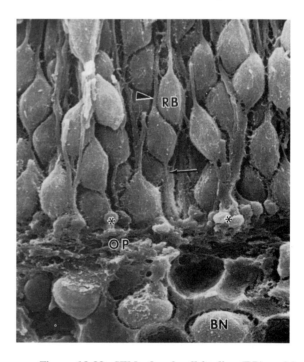

Figure 13.22. SEM of rod cell bodies (RB) and inner (arrow) and outer rod fibers (arrowheads) illustrates their shape without the surrounding Müller cells. Cell bodies of the bipolar neuron (BN) and outer plexiform layer (OP) are identified. Synaptic spherules (*) and synaptic region. ×2575. (From R. Kessel and R. Kardon, *Tissues and Organs: A Text-Atlas of Scanning Electron Microscopy*, W. H. Freeman, New York, 1979, with permission)

Figure 13.23. SEM of inner and outer rod segments. The ciliary connecting stalk is denoted by arrowheads. ×13,225. (From R. Kessel and R. Kardon, *Tissues and Organs: A Text-Atlas of Scanning Electron Microscopy*, W. H. Freeman, New York, 1979, with permission)

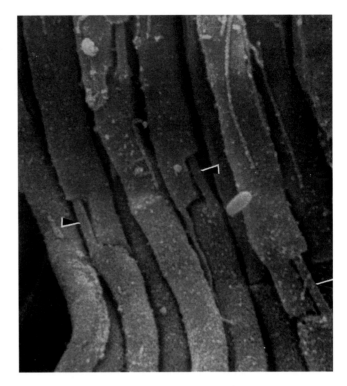

the tips of rod outer segments, these layers can become separated, as occurs in a detached retina. The cytoplasm of the pigmented epithelial cells contains lysosomes that are involved in the degradation of old photoreceptor membranous discs that are phagocytosed by the pigmented epithelium. In addition, the pigmented epithelium contains abundant smooth ER, which is thought to be involved in the esterification of vitamin A, which is then transported to the photoreceptors. The melanin granules in the pigmented epithelium produce a dark chamber for the eye, preventing reflection and glare (Fig. 13.7).

Layer 2

This layer consists of *rods and cones*, including the outer and inner segments, and is also called the *bacillary layer* (Figs. 13.14, 13.16). The inner segments of rods and cones can be separated into an *outer ellipsoid* and an *inner* portion called the *myoid*. As many as 100 rod cells converge on a single bipolar neuron. This arrangement accounts for the sharper, detailed, high-resolution view provided by cones.

Layer 3

The outer limiting membrane consists of a thin line with the LM. With the TEM, this line is revealed to be due to a precise alignment of desmosomes (maculae adherentes) between Müller cells and adjacent parts of rod and cone cells (Figs. 13.17; Plate 33A).

Layer 4

The *outer nuclear layer* consists of several layers of closely packed nuclei of rod and cone cells (Plate 33A; Fig. 13.17). The inner rod and cone segments narrow to become the outer rod and cone fibers before becoming continuous with the cell bodies, where the nuclei are located. The rod and cone cells narrow once again as the inner rod and inner cone fibers before terminating in a synaptic ending (synaptic spherules) (Fig. 13.14).

Layer 5

This layer is mainly composed of nerve processes and hence is called a *plexiform layer*, specifically the *outer plexiform layer* (Figs. 13.16, 13.17). This layer contains the synaptic endings of the rods and cones in relation to the dendrites of the bipolar neurons.

Layer 6

The *inner nuclear layer* contains primarily the cell bodies of *bipolar neurons* (Figs. 13.16, 13.17). The nuclei of Müller cells are located in this region as well, in addition to the nuclei of horizontal and amacrine cells. Extensions of the Müller cells fill all the spaces among the cellular residents and their processes.

Layer 7

The *inner plexiform layer* contains primarily nerve processes (Figs. 13.16, 13.17). Specifically, the layer contains the axons of the bipolar neurons and their synaptic connections with the dendrites of the ganglion cells.

Layer 8

This layer consists of *ganglion cell* bodies (Figs. 13.16, 13.17).

Layer 9

The layer of *optic nerve fibers* is formed by the axons of the ganglion cells (Figs. 13.16, 13.17). The nerves pass through openings in the Müller cells toward and into the optic nerve (Fig. 13.21). The nerves are unmyelinated until they reach the lamina cribrosa, where they acquire myelin. The optic nerve is surrounded by a sheath of the dura and an extension of the subarachnoid space. The optic nerve of the right eye transmits visual signals to the lateral geniculate body located in the left hemisphere. Conversely, the optic nerve of the left eye transmits visual signals to the lateral geniculate body located in the right hemisphere. These signals are then relayed from the geniculate bodies to the primary visual cortex of the occipital lobe on the same side of the brain.

Layer 10

This is the innermost layer of the retina and represents the boundary of Müller cells, together with the basal lamina covering the Müller cells (Figs. 13.16, 13.21).

MECHANISMS OF VISUAL EXCITATION

RODS

The visual pigment rhodopsin consists of two parts: an interior light-absorbing molecule called *retinal*, which is surrounded by and bound to a protein called *opsin*. Retinal is related to vitamin A, which is used to make retinal. When retinal is bound to opsin, retinal is in the *11-cis form*. Rhodopsin is sensitive to and absorbs light throughout the visible spectrum, but it absorbs green light maximally. When light interacts with rhodopsin, a series of rapid steps occur during which 11-cis retinal undergoes a conformational change to *all trans-retinal* and then dissociates from the opsin; this process is known as *bleaching* of the pigment. The dissociation of all trans-retinal and opsin initiates a transduction process that will be described subsequently. Once dissociated, the all trans-retinal enters the pigmented epithelium, where it is slowly converted to the 11-cis isomer form by ATP and enzymes present in the pigmented epithelium. When regenerated, the 11-cis retinal is rejoined to opsin and enters the disc membranes of the outer portion of the rod outer segments.

CONES

Cone visual pigments also consist of retinal and opsins. Three types of cones containing opsins of different color are present. These opsins differ from those in rods and they also differ from each other; thus, they are sensitive to different wavelengths. Blue cones respond maximally to wavelengths at around 420 nm, green cones to wavelengths at about 530 nm, and red cones to wavelengths at approximately 560 nm. There is, however, some overlap in the absorption spectra of the different cones. Perception of other colors results from the differential activation of different types of cones. For example, when all cones are equally stimulated, white is perceived. Further, yellow light stimulates both red and green cones; however, if the red cones are more strongly stimulated than the green cones, orange rather than yellow is perceived.

Color blindness is due to a recessive mutation in one of the genes concerned with the synthesis of the light-absorbing molecules; thus, there is a deficiency in one or more types of cone. The gene is carried on the X chromosome; thus it is inherited as a sex-linked trait. Approximately 1% of males are red-blind, and about 2% are green-blind.

LIGHT-DARK ADAPTATION

When one moves from a dark room into bright light, both rods and cones are stimulated and considerable amounts of photosensitive pigments are broken down; this results in a temporary glare. During this light adaptation, rod function is inhibited and cone functioning increases. During the next few minutes cone functioning improves, providing color vision and better visual acuity. Rhodopsin remains bleached in bright light, and eventually the rods become unresponsive. During dark adaptation, when one moves into a dark room, there is insufficient light to stimulate cones and a few minutes are required for the bleached rods to function as rhodopsin is regenerated and accumulates in the membranous discs. In dim light, the pupils also dilate to permit additional light to enter the eye.

TRANSDUCTION

The conversion of light into nervous impulses is called *transduction*; the primary step is a photochemical reaction in the outer segments of rods and cones. It is here that absorbed light energy produces conformational changes in visual pigment and concentration changes in ions and transmitters. A single photon of light appears to be sufficient to cause excitation of a single rod cell. While a single quantum of light may stimulate one rod, six rods may be required to discharge to produce a nervous impulse.

The outer rod segment contains about 1000 flattened membranous discs, each of which contains many closely packed, photosensitive rhodopsin molecules (Figs. 13.18, 13.24). The *rhodopsin* molecule consists of a transmembrane glycoprotein called *opsin* with a covalently attached prosthetic group in the interior called *ll-cis-retinal*. It is the ll-cis-retinal that is *light sensitive*, and a *single photon* of light almost instantaneously causes *isomerization* to all *trans-retinal*. This isomerization not only changes the shape of the retinal, but also produces a conformational change in the opsin protein. This is followed by dissociation of the trans-retinal from the opsin and its subsequent reversion to the ll-cis form. Müller cells and pigmented epithelial cells may be involved in the interconversion of retinal-retinol reactions required for rhodopsin resynthesis.

The plasma membrane of the rod *inner segment* contains many *sodium pumps* by means of which sodium molecules are pumped from the rod cell to the exterior (Fig. 13.25). The strong sodium pump in the inner segment operates under both light and dark conditions. Many mitochondria are present in the rod inner segment to provide the energy for sodium pumping. The plasma membrane covering the *outer segment*, in con-

trast, contains many *sodium channels*. In the dark, the sodium channels in the outer segment are open so that Na^+ ions enter the outer segments, only to be pumped out of the inner segments (Fig. 13.25). The conformational change in rhodopsin in the light is the event that causes sodium channels in the plasma membrane of the rod outer segment to close. However, a messenger system is required to couple the two events (Fig. 13.26).

In the dark, the sodium channels are open so that sodium pumped out of the cell can reenter the outer segments. It is the binding of *cyclic guanidine monophosphate* (*cGMP*) to the sodium channels in the dark that is responsible for keeping the channels open. In the *dark*, the *rod* cell is, paradoxically, *strongly depolarized* because of the many *open sodium channels* in the plasma membrane of the outer segment. The depolarized condition causes voltage-gated Ca^{2+} *channels* in the *synaptic region* of the cell to be held *open*. (Fig. 13.25). Thus, the influx of Ca^{2+} ions at the synaptic end of the rod cell results in a *steady state of discharge* of *neurotransmitter*. The neurotransmitter is *inhibitory* in its action and inhibits the postsynaptic neurons.

In the rod cell, a *G protein* called *transducin* couples the reception of a photon of light by a molecule of rhodopsin to the activation of a *phosphodiesterase enzyme* that *hydrolyzes cGMP* (Fig. 13.26). A decrease in *cGMP* (an intracellular mediator or messenger) causes an electrical change in the rod cell. Thus, illumination of the rod cell causes Na^+ channels in the plasma membrane of the outer segment to close, so that the cell becomes *hyperpolarized* and there is a *decrease in Ca^{2+} influx* at the *synapse* (Fig. 13.25). Therefore, there is a concomitant *decrease* in the rate of *transmitter release*. Since the neurotransmitter is inhibitory, in the light the postsynaptic neurons are less inhibited and therefore more excited. The rate of neurotransmitter release is graded with light intensity.

When a rod cell is exposed to *light*, there is a reduction in the intracellular concentration of both *calcium* and *cGMP*. However, it has been shown that cGMP causes the sodium channels to remain open. When the cGMP concentration falls, the channels close. Cyclic nucleotides typically work by activating a protein kinase to phosphorylate specific proteins, but this is not the case in the rod cell. Here the *cGMP* acts directly on the Na^+ channels to keep them open. The question remains: how does the conformational change in rhodopsin result in a decrease in the concentration of cGMP? The activated rhodopsin molecule rapidly catalyzes the activation of the G protein called *transducin*.

To summarize, in the light, rhodopsin is activated and binds to the G protein transducin. The α subunit of transducin, in turn, activates cGMP phosphodiesterase, which hydrolyzes cGMP, so that its level drops and the cGMP bound to the Na^+ channels dissociates, resulting in closure of the Na^+ channels and hyperpolarization of the rod cell. In addition, it should be mentioned that a

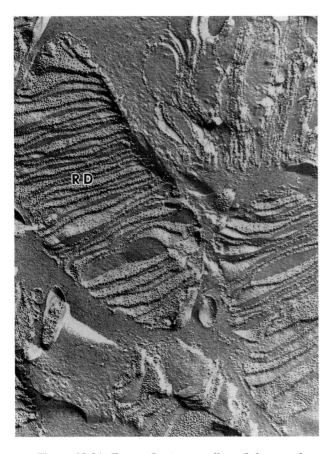

Figure 13.24. Freeze fracture replica of the membranous disks of the rod outer segment. The many small intramembranous particles in the rod disks (RD) represent rhodopsin molecules. ×38,595.

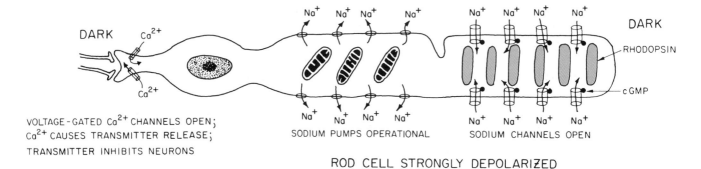

Figure 13.25. Diagrams of conditions that result in the rod cell's being strongly depolarized in the dark and hyperpolarized in the light.

rhodopsin kinase phosphorylates activated rhodopsin molecules, which can bind to an inhibitory protein called *arrestin* that blocks the ability of the rhodopsin molecules to activate the G protein transducin. This is one useful mechanism by which the photoreceptor can adapt to light. The region of phosphorylation is near the COOH end of the rhodopsin molecule.

DIABETIC RETINOPATHY

In the disease diabetes mellitus, the basement membranes of blood vessels in the retina thicken substan-

tially, and blood vessels may display local dilations (expansions) called *microaneurysms*. These vessels can then become leaky, especially in the macula, such that small focal areas of fluid appear as white spots. Hemorrhages from these microaneurysms are possible. If the blood supply to the retina is severely reduced, abnormal growth of new blood vessels is sometimes induced and retinal detachment can occur. *Diabetic retinopathy*, a disease that involves retinal blood vessels, is a common cause of blindness. Regulation of blood sugar levels may be beneficial in some cases. Use of lasers to prevent leakage of blood vessels may sometimes retard the disease process and prevent severe loss of vision.

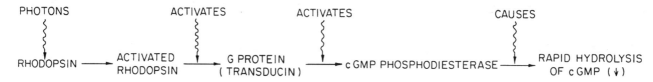

Figure 13.26. Diagram illustrates how photons interacting with rhodopsin can cause hydrolysis of cGMP during phototransduction.

NYCTALOPIA

Vitamin A deficiency can cause *night blindness* or *nyctalopia*. Prolonged vitamin A deficiency can result in degeneration of rod cells. Vitamin A supplements can restore rod cell function if administered prior to degeneration. Visual pigment in cones is also affected in night blindness, but the cones usually contain sufficient pigment to respond to very bright light.

SELECTED BIBLIOGRAPHY

Bloemendal, H., ed. (1981). *Molecular and Cellular Biology of the Eye Lens.* Wiley, New York.

Cunha-Vaz, J.G., ed. (1980). *The Blood-Retinal Barriers.* Plenum, New York.

De Valois, R.I., and De Valois, K.K. (1988). *Spatial Vision.* Oxford University Press, New York.

Hogan, M., Alvarado, J., and Weddell, J. (1971). *Histology of the Human Eye.* W.B. Saunders, Philadelphia.

Jacobs, G.H. (1981). *Comparative Color Vision.* Academic Press, New York.

Jakobiec, F.A., ed. (1982). *Ocular Anatomy, Embryology and Teratology.* Harper & Row, Hagerstown, MD.

Kistler, J., and Bullivant, S. (1989). Structural and molecular biology of the eye lens membranes. *Crit. Rev. Biochem. Mol. Biol.* **24**, 151–181.

Koretz, J., and Handelman, G. (1988). How the human eye focuses. *Sci. Am.* **259**, 92–99.

Land, M.F., and Fernald, R.D. (1992). The evolution of eyes. *Annu. Rev. Neurosci.* **15**, 1–30.

Masland, R. (1986). The functional architecture of the retina. *Sci. Am.* **255**, 102–119.

Nathans, J. (1989). The genes for color vision. *Sci. Am.* **260**, 42–49.

Rodieck, R. W. (1988). The primate retina. In *Comparative Primate Biology*, Vol. 4, *Neurosciences*, H.D. Steklis and J. Erwin, eds. Alan R. Liss, New York.

Schnapf, J., and Baylor, D. (1987). How photoreceptor cells respond to light. *Sci. Am.* **256**, 40–47.

Valberg, A., and Lee, B.B. (1991). *From Pigments to Perception.* Plenum, New York.

Yau, K.-W., and Baylor, D.A. (1989). Cyclic GMP-activated conductance of retinal photoreceptor cells. *Annu. Rev. Neruosci.* **12**, 289–328.

Nervous Tissue: The Ear

The ear consists of external, middle, and internal parts. The ears are located in cavities in the right and left temporal bones. The ear serves two functions: hearing and equilibrium. In hearing, sound is transmitted from air in the external ear to bone in the middle ear to fluid in the inner ear. The components of the external, middle, and inner ears and their functions are summarized in Table 14.1.

EXTERNAL EAR

The external ear consists of an *auricle* or pinna and the *external auditory meatus* (Fig. 14.1). The auricle contains a central piece of elastic cartilage covered with connective tissue and epidermis. Hairs, sebaceous glands, and sweat glands are present on the posterior surface of the pinna. The lobule of the external ear contains fat and connective tissue. The external auditory meatus is a canal in the temporal bone. The meatus extends from the exterior to the primary tympanic membrane or eardrum. The outer portion of the external auditory meatus contains some elastic cartilage that is continuous with cartilage in the pinna. The inner portion of the meatus is bony. Both parts of the meatus are lined with skin. Large, stiff hairs and sebaceous glands are present in the outer portion of the external auditory meatus. *Ceruminous glands*, which are simple coiled tubular glands, open onto the skin lining the meatus. These gland cells secrete by an apocrine method, and the cytoplasm contains many brown pigment granules and fat droplets. The secretions of the ceruminous glands and sebaceous glands together with desquamated epithelial cells collectively comprise the ear wax or *cerumen*.

MIDDLE EAR

TYMPANIC CAVITY AND EARDRUM

The middle ear includes the *primary tympanic membrane* or eardrum, a *small tympanic cavity* within the temporal bone that contains three small *auditory ossicles* or bonelets, and the *auditory* or *eustachian tube* (Fig. 14.1). The tympanic cavity is small, measuring 0.5 inch in height by 0.5 inch in length. The medial wall of the tympanic cavity has two potential openings to the inner ear: the oval window and the round window. The cavity communicates with the nasopharynx by means of the eustachian tube. The eustachian tube is open during swallowing and serves to equalize air pressure. The tympanic cavity also communicates posteriorly with blind-end mastoid air cells of the temporal bone. The lateral wall of the tympanic cavity is formed by the primary tympanic membrane. The main portion of the eardrum is called the *pars tensa*. The outer surface of the eardrum is covered with thin skin that is continuous with the epithelium of the external auditory meatus. The central portion, called the *substantia propria*, consists of fibrocytes, two layers of collagenic fibers, and elastic fibers. The inner surface of the eardrum is covered with a thin mucous membrane, consisting of simple squamous epithelium and connective tissue that is continuous with the mucous membrane lining the tympanic cavity. A small upper portion of the eardrum is loose because it lacks internal collagen fibers; this portion is called the *pars flaccida* or *Schrapnell's membrane*.

MALLEUS, INCUS, STAPES

The three ossicles or bonelets located in the tympanic cavity, from outside to inside, are the *malleus* (hammer),

Table 14.1 The Ear

Major Part	Components	Functions
External ear	Pinna	Collects sound waves and directs them into the ear
	External auditory meatus	Conducts sound waves to middle ear
	Hairs	Strain air
	Sebaceous glands	Produce sebum
	Ceruminous glands	Produce cerumen (ear wax)
Middle ear	Tympanic membrane (primary)	Eardrum forms the lateral wall of the tympanic cavity—transmits pressure waves to the malleus
	Tympanic cavity	Small space in temporal bone contains three bonelets (auditory ossicles) and two striated muscles
	Auditory ossicles	*Malleus* connects to inner surface of tympanic membrane and to incus; *incus* articulates with malleus and medially with stapes; *stapes* contain foot plate that is bound by an annular ligament into the oval window; transmit vibrations and amplify sounds to inner ear
	Stapedius muscle	Attaches to stapes, prevents stapes from moving too far into inner ear—protective
	Tensor tympani	Attaches to malleus; when contracts, makes tympanic membrane tense (accentuates high-pitched sounds)
	Eustachian (auditory) tube	Equalizes air pressure (opens during swallowing)
Inner ear	*Osseous (bony) labyrinth*	
	Vestibule	Contains perilymph for transmission of pressure waves developed at oval window; contains utricle and saccule of membranous labyrinth
	Semicircular canals	Contains perilymph, which bathes membranous semicircular ducts
	Osseous cochlea	Scala vestibuli and scala tympani contain perilymph
	Membranous labyrinth	
	Semicircular ducts	Contain endolymph and cristae ampullaris; involved in angular acceleration and deceleration
	Utriculus	Contains endolymph and macula utriculi; involved in static equilibrium, linear acceleration, and gravity reception
	Sacculus	Contains endolymph and macula sacculi; involved in static equillibrium, linear acceleration, and gravity reception
	Cohclear duct	Contains endolymph and organ of Corti; involved in hearing

incus (anvil), and *stapes* (stirrup) (Figs. 14.2–14.4). The vibration amplitude is enchanced about 10 times by the bonelets. The middle ear bonelets articulate with each other such that sound waves transmitted across them are increased in force due to the lever-type arrangement. They contain some compact bone with haversian systems. A small amount of hyaline cartilage (articular cartilage) is present on the articular surfaces of these bonelets. The handle of the malleus is attached to the primary tympanic membrane or eardrum, while the other end of the malleus articulates with the middle or central bonelet, the incus. Both the malleus and the incus may contain a small marrow cavity. The stapes is attached to the incus at one end, while the other end, called the *foot plate*, is positioned in the *oval window* and maintained in this position by an *annular ligament*. The annular ligament contains both elastic and collagen fibers.

STAPEDIUS AND TENSOR TYMPANI MUSCLES

Two small muscles, the *tensor tympani* and the *stapedius*, are associated with the bonelets. The tensor tympani muscle extends from the wall of the eustachian tube to the malleus. When the tensor tympani contracts, it makes the tympanic membrane tense and accentuates high-pitched sounds. It is innervated by a branch of the cranial nerve V. The stapedius muscle originates in the wall of the tympanic cavity and inserts on the stapes (Fig.

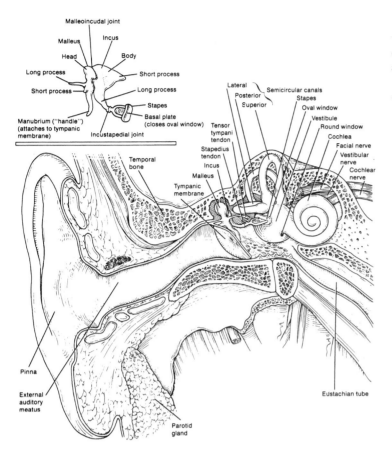

Figure 14.1. Diagram illustrates the organization of the external, middle, and inner ears. (From R. Kessel and R. Kardon, *Tissues and Organs: A Text-Atlas of Scanning Electron Microscopy*, W.H. Freeman, New York, 1979, with permission)

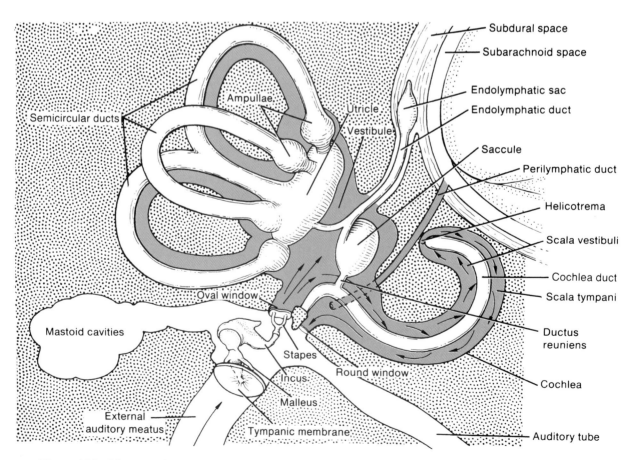

Figure 14.2. Diagram of the constituents of the external, middle, and inner ears. The parts of the osseous and membranous labyrinths are identified. (From T.H. Bast and B.J. Anson, *The Temporal Bone of the Ear*, 1949. Courtesy of Charles C. Thomas, Publisher, Springfield, IL)

Figure 14.3. SEM. The temporal bone was removed to show the tympanic cavity (TC) and vestibule (Ve). The foot plate (*) of the stapes (St), incus (In), and maleus (Ma) are also identified. ×30. (From R. Kessel and R. Kardon, *Tissues and Organs: A Text-Atlas of Scanning Electron Microscopy*, W.H. Freeman, New York, 1979, with permission)

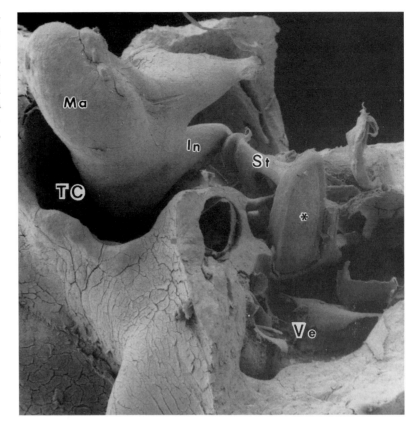

Figure 14.4. SEM illustrates a side view of the stapes. The foot plate (*) is bound into the oval window by an annular ligament, which was removed in this preparation. The ligament of the stapedius muscle is identified at the arrowhead. ×55. (From R. Kessel and R. Kardon, *Tissues and Organs: A Text-Atlas of Scanning Electron Microscopy*, W.H. Freeman, New York, 1979, with permission)

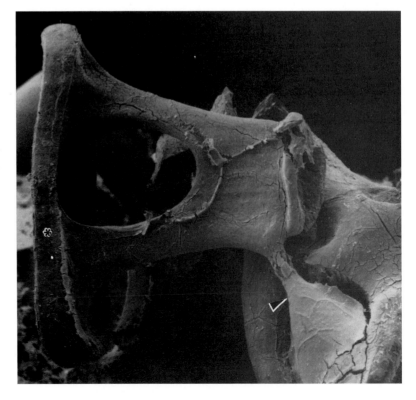

14.4). When it contracts, it moves the foot plate of the stapes slightly outward from the oval window to reduce the intralabyrinth pressure, that is, the pressure in the perilymph on the inner side of the foot plate. This reflexive contraction during loud noises probably plays a protective role, preventing the foot plate of the stapes from moving too far into the osseous labyrinth. The stapedius muscle is innervated by the cranial nerve VII.

The middle ear muscles are skeletal muscles but are *not* under voluntary control. They contract reflexively within about 1/10th of a second after exposure to loud external sounds. The middle ear muscles play an important role in muffling the lower frequencies of loud sounds, which improves hearing since human speech contains many high-frequency components. The middle-ear muscles are activated automatically during vocalization.

INNER EAR

GENERAL ANATOMY

The inner ear consists of several small, interconnected cavities and canals of different shapes in the temporal bone. Collectively, these cavities (semicircular canals, vestibule, cochlea) are called the *osseous labyrinth* (osseous, bone; labyrinth, maze) (Figs. 14.2, 14.5). The membranous labyrinth resides within the bony labyrinth. The *membranous labyrinth* consists of a series of very thin-walled compartments (sacs and ducts) of different sizes and shapes that are also interconnected (Figs. 14.2, 14.5). These communicating, thin-walled, fluid-filled compartments have names to distinguish them (semicircular ducts, utricle, saccule, cochlear duct) and are filled with a fluid called *endolymph*. The interconnected parts of the bony labyrinth also have names to designate them, and they contain a fluid called *perilymph*. The perilymph thus bathes the outer surface of the membranous labyrinth. It is important to understand that the components of the membranous labyrinth are contained *within* compartments comprising the osseous labyrinth, somewhat like a sac within a box situation. All parts of the membranous labyrinth are interconnected, and all parts of the osseous labyrinth are interconnected.

OSSEOUS LABYRINTH

The parts of the bony labyrinth are filled with perilymph. Perilymph is much like *extracellular fluid* in that

the concentration of Na^+ *ions* is relatively *high*. The parts include the *vestibule, osseous cochlea,* and three *osseous semicircular canals* (Fig. 14.6). These bony compartments are lined with a thin layer of connective tissue covered by a layer of simple squamous epithelial cells (a mesenchymal epithelium). The vestibule component of the osseous labyrinth has two potential openings to the middle ear cavity. They are potential openings because, under normal conditions, the openings are permanently covered. One of the potential openings is the *oval window,* which contains the *stapes foot plate* bound in this position by an *annular ligament.* The nearby second potential opening is called the *round window* (Fig. 14.5). It is covered by a *secondary tympanic membrane,* which provides pressure relief from the inner ear.

The *vestibule* is continuous with the *osseous semicircular canals* as well as the *osseous cochlea.* A thin, tubular structure called the *perilymphatic duct* extends from the vestibule toward the subarachnoid space of the brain. Because of this association, it has been suggested that the perilymph may somehow be derived from CSF. *Three semicircular canals* extend posteriorly from the vestibule: *superior, lateral (horizontal),* and *posterior.* The *superior* and *posterior* semicircular canals are *vertical* in orientation, and there is one horizontal semicircular canal. Close to their communication with the vestibule, the osseous semicircular canals are dilated; these dilated regions are called the *ampullae* of the semicircular canals. Since the superior and posterior semicircular canals share a common opening in one area, called the *crus communue,* there are only five openings from the vestibule into the semicircular canals.

The *cochlea* is a coiled, bony canal that is continuous with and extends from the vestibule. The cochlea is coiled 2 3/4 turns in humans, and this coiled shell has a central pillar of bone called the *modiolus.* Thin plates of bone extend laterally from the modiolus; these short, bony plates are called the *osseous spiral lamina.*

MEMBRANOUS LABYRINTH

The constituents of the interconnected and closed membranous labyrinth include both sacs (*utricle, saccule, endolymphatic sac*) and ducts (*semicircular ducts, endolymphatic duct,* and *cochlear duct*) (Figs. 14.5, 14.6). Two components of the membranous labyrinth, called the *utricule* and *saccule,* reside within the vestibule of the osseous labyrinth. These structures are very thin-walled and connected to each other, as well as to other components of the membranous labyrinth. The utricle is located uppermost, while the saccule is lower in position.

Figure 14.5. Summary diagram of the parts of the osseous labyrinth (above), the parts of membranous labyrinth (middle), and the neurosensory areas located within the

membranous labyrinth (bottom) (Redrawn from M. Ross, E. Reith and L. Romrell, *Histology, A Text and Atlas,* Williams and Wilkins, Baltimore, 1989)

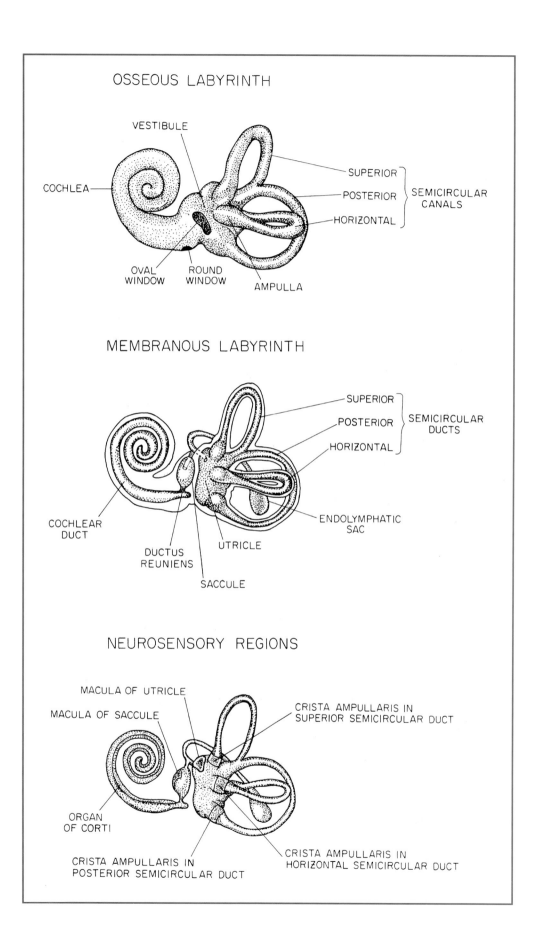

OSSEOUS LABYRINTH

VESTIBULE
COCHLEA
SUPERIOR
POSTERIOR } SEMICIRCULAR CANALS
HORIZONTAL
OVAL WINDOW
ROUND WINDOW
AMPULLA

MEMBRANOUS LABYRINTH

SUPERIOR
POSTERIOR } SEMICIRCULAR DUCTS
HORIZONTAL
COCHLEAR DUCT
DUCTUS REUNIENS
UTRICLE
SACCULE
ENDOLYMPHATIC SAC

NEUROSENSORY REGIONS

MACULA OF UTRICLE
MACULA OF SACCULE
CRISTA AMPULLARIS IN SUPERIOR SEMICIRCULAR DUCT
ORGAN OF CORTI
CRISTA AMPULLARIS IN POSTERIOR SEMICIRCULAR DUCT
CRISTA AMPULLARIS IN HORIZONTAL SEMICIRCULAR DUCT

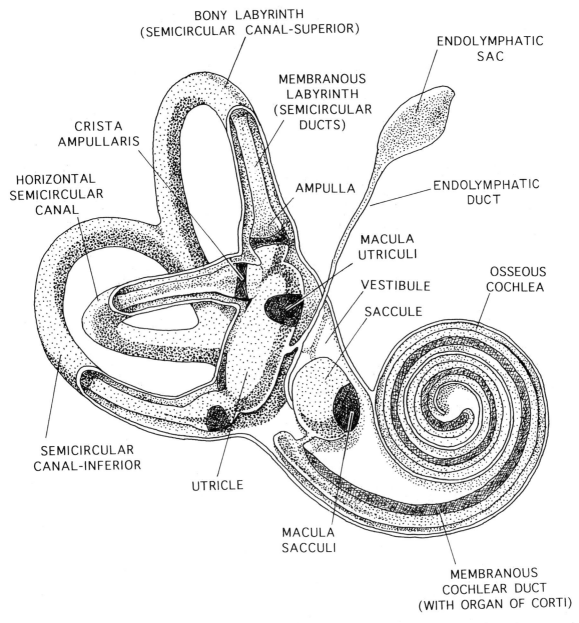

BONY LABYRINTH
(SEMICIRCULAR CANAL-SUPERIOR)

ENDOLYMPHATIC
SAC

MEMBRANOUS
LABYRINTH
(SEMICIRCULAR
DUCTS)

CRISTA
AMPULLARIS

HORIZONTAL
SEMICIRCULAR
CANAL

AMPULLA

ENDOLYMPHATIC
DUCT

MACULA
UTRICULI

VESTIBULE

OSSEOUS
COCHLEA

SACCULE

SEMICIRCULAR
CANAL-INFERIOR

UTRICLE

MACULA
SACCULI

MEMBRANOUS
COCHLEAR DUCT
(WITH ORGAN OF CORTI)

Figure 14.6. The diagram illustrates the relationship between the membranous labyrinth and the bony osseous labyrinth. Neurosensory areas are identified.

The utricle communicates in several places with the *membranous* semicircular ducts and is also connected to the saccule. The thin-walled, membranous semicircular ducts reside within the osseous semicircular canals. A long, coiled, thin-walled tube called the *membranous cochlea* or *cochlear duct* extends from the saccule (Fig. 14.6). The membranous cochlea or cochlear duct lies within a long, coiled bony canal called the *osseous cochlea*. Finally, a long, thin-walled tube extends from close to the junction of the utricle and saccule toward the subdural space. This tube is called the *endolymphatic duct* and terminates in a blind-end *endolymphatic sac* in relation to the *subdural space* of the brain (Fig. 14.6). This portion of the membranous labyrinth contains en-

dolymph and may play a role in its formation, circulation, and storage. *Endolymph* resembles *intracellular fluid* in that it has a relatively *high* concentration of K^+ ions.

NEUROSENSORY AREAS

Each part of the membranous labyrinth has important neurosensory areas (Fig. 14.6). In general, these areas contain neurosensory hair cells that are innervated, as well as supporting epithelial cells. The neurosensory areas are as follows:

1. *Macula utriculi.* This is a localized neurosensory region in the *utriculus.* It is concerned with *sta-*

tic equilibrium and is a *sensor of gravity* and *linear acceleration.*

2. *Macula sacculi.* This is a localized neurosensory area in a portion of the *sacculus.* It is also concerned with *static equilibrium*, and is a *sensor of gravity* and *linear acceleration.*

3. *Crista ampullaris.* These are three neurosensory areas located in the wall of the membranous ampullae of the semicircular canals. This structure detects *angular acceleration* and *deceleration.*

4. *Organ of Corti.* This specialized neurosensory area along the length of the membranous cochlea is involved in *hearing.*

The structure of these neurosensory areas will be investigated in more detail, followed by a consideration of functional mechanisms.

ORGANIZATION OF OSSEOUS AND MEMBRANOUS COCHLEA

The osseous portion of the cochlea is a coiled bony canal. The apex of the osseous cochlea is called the *cupula* or *hamulus.* There is an inner, conical axis of spongy bone to the cochlea called the *spiral modiolus*

(Fig. 14.7). The cochlea is also covered with additional bone of the skull. The modiolus is surrounded by a *spiral lamina* that is subdivided into an *osseous spiral lamina* and a *membranous spiral lamina.* The osseous spiral lamina consists of thin, bony plates that extend laterally at intervals from the modiolus. Blood vessels, nerves, and the *spiral ganglion* are located between the bony plates of the osseous spiral lamina. The spiral ganglion contains bipolar neurons, and the dendrites of these bipolar neurons extend into the organ of Corti to innervate the base of hair cells located there. The *membranous spiral lamina* extends as the resonant *basilar membrane* of the organ of Corti. The spaces within the osseous cochlea, called the *scala vestibuli* and *scala tympani*, are filled with perilymph. Further, the scala vestibuli and scala tympani are continuous at the end of the cochlea in a region called the *helicotrema.*

The membranous cochlea is called the *cochlear duct* and contains endolymph. The cochlear duct is pie-shaped or triangular in section and is bounded superiorly by Reissner's vestibular membrane, laterally by the *spiral ligament*, inferiorly by the *basilar membrane*, and medially by the *spiral limbus* (Fig. 14.8). The spiral ligament in the lateral cochlear wall consists of dense connective tissue. The spiral limbus is a thickened region overlying the osseous spiral lamina consisting of loose connective

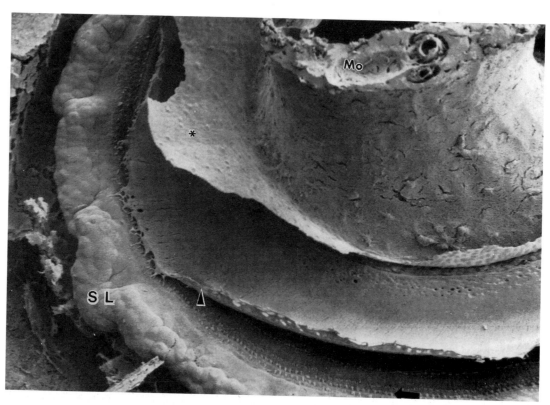

Figure 14.7. SEM of part of the coiled cochlea illustrates the bony modiolus (Mo), vestibular (Reissner's) membrane (*), tectorial membrane (arrowhead), and part of the spiral ligament (SL). ×250. The hair tufts of the hair cells are just visible (arrows). (From R. Kessel and R. Kardon, *Tissues and Organs: A Text-Atlas of Scanning Electron Microscopy*, W.H. Freeman, New York, 1979, with permission)

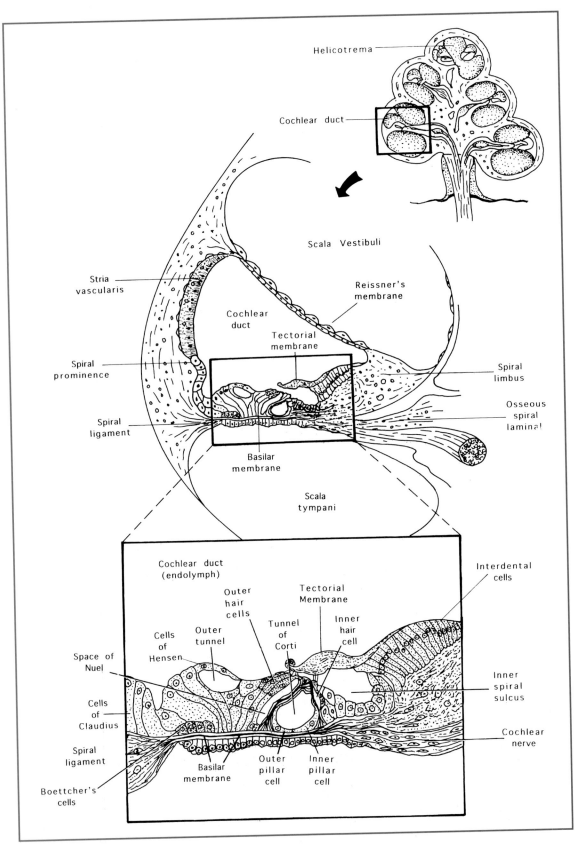

Figure 14.8. Diagrams illustrate the midsagittal section of coiled cochlea (top) and an enlargement of the fluid-filled chambers (cochlear duct, endolymph, scala vestibuli and scala tympani, perilymph) in the central diagram, as well as the organ of Corti, which is enlarged in the bottom figure (Redrawn from M. Ross, E. Reith and L Romrell, *Histology, A Text and Atlas*, Williams and Wilkins, Baltimore, 1989.)

tissue and blood vessels. The surface of the spiral lim-bus is covered by tall epithelial cells called *interdental cells* (Fig. 14.8). The tectorial membrane is anchored to the surface of the interdental cells. The spiral limbus branches into a *vestibular lip* that extends as the tector-ial membrane and a *tympanic lip* that extends as the basi-lar membrane. *Reissner's vestibular membrane* is only 2–3 μm thick (Fig. 14.7). On one side toward the scala vestibuli, it is lined by flattened mesothelial cells con-tinuous with those lining the scala vestibuli (Fig. 14.9). A flattened layer of epithelial cells lines the side of the Reissner's membrane adjacent to the cochlear duct, and the cells are linked by zonulae occludentes.

The neurosensory area of the membranous cochlea is called the *organ of Corti*, and it resides on the basilar membrane. The organ of Corti consists of special sen-sory cells, called *inner and outer hair cells*, and a number of nonsensory or supporting cells. The gelatinous tec-torial membrane extends from the vestibular lip of the spiral limbus over the internal spiral tunnel to cover the inner and outer hair cells (Figs. 14.8, 14.10). The lat-eral wall of the cochlear duct consists of a region called the *stria vascularis*, which is extensively vascularized (Fig. 14.8). The surface cells have numerous mitochondria and basolateral plasma membrane infoldings. The cells appear to play a role in ion and fluid regulation of the endolymph. The spiral prominence is lined by cuboidal cells that may play a role in the composition of the en-dolymph. The external spiral sulcus cells are believed to play a role in fluid absorption and phagocytosis.

ORGAN OF CORTI

The organ of Corti contains sensory hair cells as well as supporting cells, both of which reside on the basilar membrane and tympanic lip of the osseous spiral lam-ina (Fig. 14.11). There is a single row of *inner hair cells* that have *linear rows* of *stereocilia* extending from their free or apical margin. The single row of inner hair cells are supported by a single row of *inner phalangeal cells* (Fig. 14.11). Lateral to the inner hair cells is a space that is variously called the *inner tunnel* or *Corti's tunnel*. The tunnel of Corti is bounded by rows of tall cells that contain many internal microtubules and filaments called the *inner pillar cells* and the *outer pillar cells* (Fig. 14.12). The pillar cells reside on the basilar membrane, and their nucleus is located in this basal region. The in-ner pillar cells extend superficially to terminate on the surface of the organ of Corti. A smaller space called the *space of Nuel* is lateral to the tunnel of Corti. Just lateral to the space of Nuel are the outer rows of hair cells (Fig. 14.11). There are three rows of outer hair cells in hu-mans. However, one or two additional rows of hair cells may be added to the apex of the membranous cochlea. The hair cells have the form of tall cylinders that have a free or apical border with stereocilia extending from a cuticular plate (Figs. 14.13., 14.14). The tectorial membrane is a sheet of protein resembling keratin that forms a roof over the hair cells (Fig. 14.12). It is secreted by interdental cells and is usually shrunken and dis-torted by fixation. Nerve fibers from the spiral ganglion

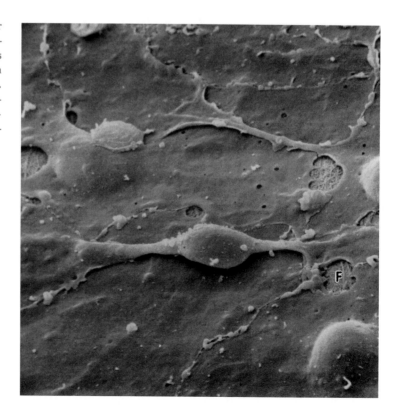

Figure 14.9. SEM of the upper surface of Reissner's vestibular mem-brane. There are intercellular spaces between the squamous cells in which fine fibrils (F) are apparent. ×2990. (From R. Kessel and R. Kardon, *Tis-sues and Organs: A Text-Atlas of Scan-ning Electron Microscopy*, W.H. Free-man, New York, 1979)

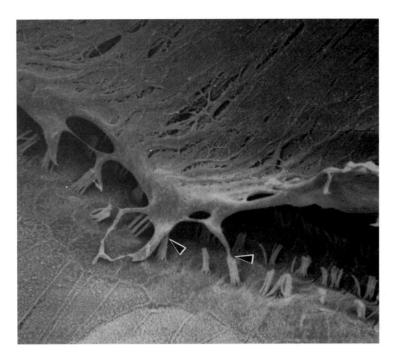

Figure 14.10. SEM of the tectorial membrane terminates as a net in relation to the hair tufts (arrowheads) of outer hair cells. ×1430. (From R. Kessel and R. Kardon, *Tissues and Organs: A Text-Atlas of Scanning Electron Microscopy*, W.H. Freeman, New York, 1979, with permission)

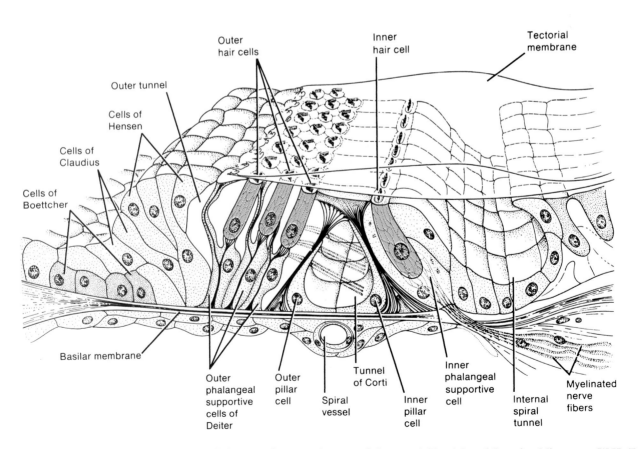

Figure 14.11. Diagram of the cellular constituents of the organ of Corti. (From R. Kessel and R. Kardon, *Tissues and Organs: A Text-Atlas of Scanning Microscopy*, W.H. Freeman, New York, 1979, with permission)

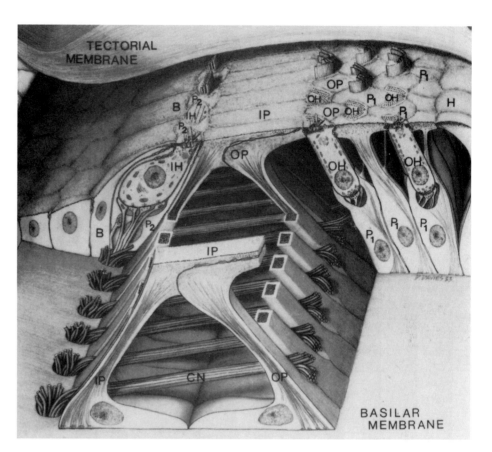

Figure 14.12. Diagram of the organ of Corti. Inner hair (IH) cell, inner pillar (IP), outer pillar (OP), outer hair (OH), phalangeal cells (P$_1$, P$_2$) and cochlear nerve (CN) are identified. H = Hensen's cells. (From D. Kelly, R. Wood, and A. Enders, *Bailey's Textbook of Histology*, 18th ed., Williams & Wilkins, Baltimore, 1984, with permission)

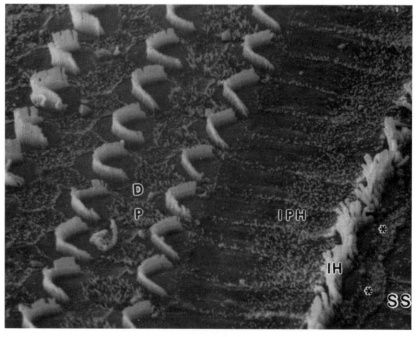

Figure 14.13. SEM of the organ of Corti shows the surface of inner spiral sulcus cells (SS), heads of inner phalangeal cells (*), inner hair cells (IH), inner pillar heads (IPH), and three rows of outer hair cells (V-shaped). Between the first row of outer hair cells are alternating outer pillar heads (P) and the phalangeal head of Deiter's cells (D). ×2365. (From R. Kessel and R. Kardon, *Tissues and Organs: A Text-Atlas of Scanning Electron Microscopy*, W.H. Freeman, New York, 1979, with permission)

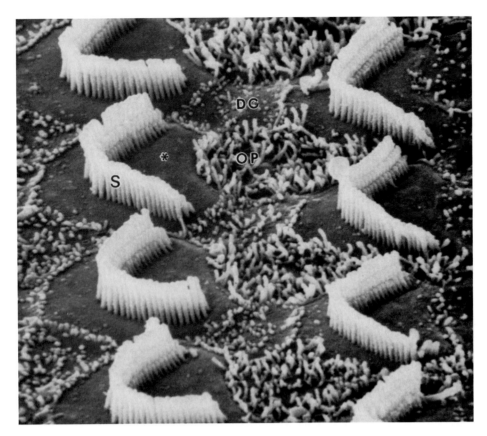

Figure 14.14. SEM of two rows of outer hair cells. Stereocilia (S) emerge from a cuticular plate (*) and have a V shape; there are three rows in this region. The phalangeal heads of Deiter's cells (DC) are smaller and have shorter microvilli than the outer pillar heads (OP). ×6300. (From R. Kessel and R. Kardon, *Tissues and Organs: A Text-Atlas of Scanning Electron Microscopy*, W.H. Freeman, New York, 1979, with permission)

cells extend across the tunnel of Corti and space of Nuel to innervate the base of each hair cell. Each row of outer hair cells is supported by similar rows of cells called the *outer phalangeal cells* or *Deiter's cells* (Fig. 14.15). Where the hair cells reside on phalangeal cells, the phalangeal cell extends a small, pencil-like extension between the hair cells to the surface of the organ of Corti. This extension of the phalangeal cell at the surface is called the *phalangeal head*. In the first row of outer hair cells, the phalangeal heads of the first row of phalangeal cells are interposed between the outer pillar heads (Figs. 14.11–14.15).

Lateral to the outer hair cell rows are several supporting type cells that have been given specific names (Fig. 14.11). Just lateral to the outer hair cells is another space called the *outer tunnel*. Cells lateral to the outer tunnel are called *cells of Hensen*, while cells of Claudius are even more laterally placed. The *cells of Claudius* reside on a layer of more eosinophilic-staining cells residing on the basilar membrane, and these are called *cells of Boettcher*. The functional role of these cells, other than acting as a supporting epithelium in the organ of Corti, has not been established.

HAIR CELLS

It is estimated that in the human organ of Corti, there are ~3500 inner hair cells and ~12,000 outer hair cells. While there is only a single row of inner hair cells, three to five rows of outer hair cells are possible, depending upon the organism and the location in the coiled cochlea. More than 100 stereocilia extend from an apical cuticular plate of each outer hair cell (Fig. 14.14). In contrast, inner hair cells contain 50–70 stereocilia. The height of stereocilia increases from inner hair cells to outer hair cells. Further, the height increases from the base of the cochlear duct toward the apex. The tuning function of stereocilia in the organ of Corti is related to height since stereocilia stiffness is inversely related to stereocilia length. A single long, nonmotile, modified cilium called a *kinocilium* may initially form on the hair cells, but it is lost during fetal development.

The stereocilia that extend from a cuticular plate at the apical end of the hair cells contain many longitudinally oriented filaments that contain actin in filamentous form. Immunofluorescence and EM studies indicate that the hair cells also have a prominent sub-

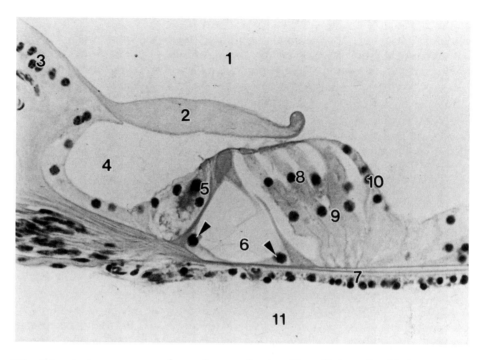

Figure 14.15. LM of the organ of Corti. 1 = Cochlear duct; 2 = tectorial membrane; 3 = interdental cells; 4 = inner spiral sulcus; 5 = inner hair cell; 6 = tunnel of Corti; 7 = basilar membrane; inner and outer pillar cells (arrowheads), basilar membrane; 8 = outer hair cells; 9 = outer phalangeal (Deiter's) cells; 10 = cells of Hensen; 11 = scala vestibuli. ×500.

plasmalemmal cytoskeletal lattice consisting of actin (6–7 nm thick) filaments that are cross-linked by spectrin-type filaments (3–4 nm thick). The stereocilia are in several rows of graded heights. Sometimes the stereocilia on the outer hair cells are arranged in the form of a V or W configuration rather than in linear rows, as occurs on the inner hair cells. Those stereocilia associated with the outer hair cells appear to be closely associated with the undersurface of the tectorial membrane. In fact, when the tectorial membrane is removed and the underside viewed in SEM, the broken ends of the tallest stereocilia from the outer hair cells are found to be embedded in the underside of the membrane. Thus, the tectorial membrane appears to be firmly attached to the tallest stereocilia on the outer hair cells. The inner hair cells, in contrast to the outer hair cells, do not appear to be attached to the tectorial membrane. It appears that the hair cells are capable of transmitting sound of different frequencies and are located in different regions of the cochlea. Hair cells that transmit high frequencies are located at the base of the cochlea, while those that transmit low frequencies are located at the apical end. Electrophysiologic evidence suggests that *inner hair cells*, which are unattached to the tectorial membrane, are *velocity sensitive* and are stimulated by the *drag on endolymph*. The *outer hair cells*, however, are attached and are *stimulated by the shearing action* of the tectorial membrane and basilar membrane; they can thus be considered as *displacement detectors*.

The inner and outer hair cells are supplied by both afferent and efferent nerve endings. Inner hair cells are primarily responsible for relaying sensory information to the auditory cortex. The inner hair cells have extensive *afferent* innervation, while the outer hair cells have many *efferent* fibers that appear to serve a motor function. The outer hair cells are able to generate high-frequency mechanical forces that can increase the sensitivity and frequency selectivity of the ear.

BASILAR MEMBRANE

The lower margin of the cochlear duct is separated from the scala tympani by the basilar membrane, on which resides the neurosensory organ of Corti (Plate 34A–C; 14.8, 14.11). The basilar membrane is the main resonant structure of the organ of Corti. It contains some 25,000 fibers, called the *auditory strings*, that are made of a toughened, collagen-like scleroprotein material. The surface of the basilar membrane adjacent to the scala tympani is only partially covered by scattered, highly modified epithelial (mesothelial) cells that have a bipolar shape. The basilar membrane is not uniform in thickness along its length; it tends to be narrowest and stiffest at the base of the cochlea, where high pitch discrimination is sensed. In contrast, the basilar membrane appears widest and most flexible at the tip, where low pitch discrimination appears to occur.

In order for sound to stimulate the hair cells, it must be transmitted to the inner ear. Sound waves transmitted through the external auditory meatus, primary tympanic membrane, middle ear ossicles, and foot plate of the stapes in the oval window, are changed from vibrations in air to vibrations in the perilymph. The movement of the foot plate inward on the perilymph of the vestibule creates the fluid vibrations that are transmitted through the perilymph of the osseous cochlea through Reissner's vestibular membrane to the endolymph-basilar membrane-organ of Corti complex of the membranous labyrinth.

Minute bending of the stereocilia produces a generator potential in the afferent sensory nerve terminals that synapse with the base of the hair cells (Figs. 14.12, 14.16). The more displacement occurs in the basilar membrane, the more the stereocilia are displaced and the greater is the frequency of action potentials in the afferent nerves associated with the hair cell base. Efferent fibers are also associated with the hair cell base. These fibers may play a role in controlling auditory input to the brain by enhancing or suppressing some afferent signals. The lower the frequency of vibration of the sound wave, the farther from the oval window is the site of displacement of the basilar membrane. Pitch de-

tection is related to the specific point or site of maximum displacement of the basilar membrane. When vibrations in the cochlear fluids cause displacement of the tectorial membrane-outer hair cell tuft-basilar membrane complex, electrochemical events are initiated within hair cells, with a consequent release of neurotransmitters and the generation of impulses (Fig. 14.16).

HAIR CELL TRANSDUCTION MECHANISMS

Tectorial membrane displacement causes movements of the stereocilia that can cause either stretching or compression of the thin interciliary strands of the hairs. When the sterocilia on the vestibular hair cells are displaced in an excitatory direction, that is, in the direction of increasing stereocilia height, the thin *interciliary strands* (also called *transduction links*) are *stretched* (Fig. 14.16). K^+ ions flow into these hair cells since the potassium concentration in the endolymph is very high. The

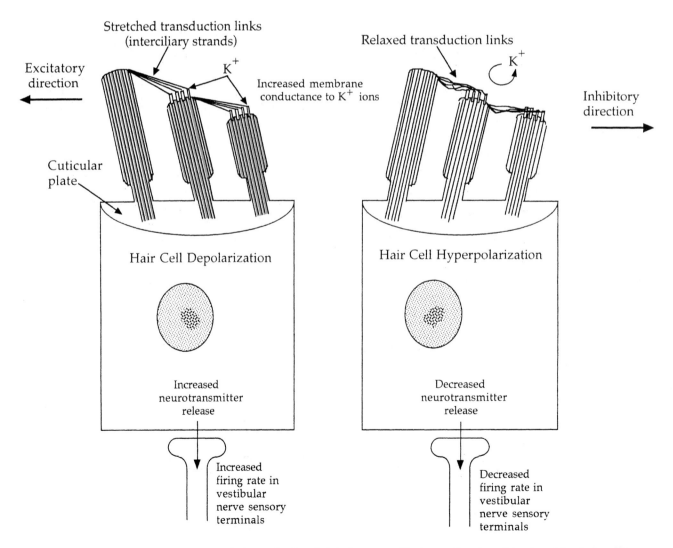

Figure 14.16. Diagram shows strands (transduction links) that extend between the sterocilia of cochlea hair cells.

K$^+$ ions enter the hair cell through ion channels in the membrane of the microvilli, and the resulting *depolarization* triggers transmitter release at the synapse at the base of the hair cell. Conversely, when the stereocilia are displaced in the opposite direction, the *interciliary strands* (transduction links) are compressed and *hyperpolarization* results.

The eighth cranial nerve has a vestibular division that innervates the sensory receptors in the maculae and cristae ampullaris and a cochlear division that innervates the sensory cells in the organ of Corti. The cell bodies of bipolar neurons of the vestibular division are present in the internal auditory meatus. Axons of these vestibular nerves enter the brain stem and terminate in vestibular nuclei located there. Large numbers of bipolar neurons comprising the cochlear nerve are present in the *spiral ganglion,* which is located in the membranous spiral lamina of the cochlea. The dendrites of the spiral ganglion cells extend to the organ of Corti, where they form synaptic terminations with the base of the inner and outer hair cells. Axons of the cochlear nerves (bipolar neurons) enter the brain stem and terminate in the cochlear nuclei located there. Nerve fibers from the cochlear nuclei pass to the thalamus and then to the auditory cortex of the temporal lobe. Prolonged loud noises can irreversibily damage the sensitive neurons of the spiral ganglion.

MACULA UTRICULI AND MACULA SACCULI

Microscopic organization

The *macula utriculi* is a localized neurosensory region in the utricle; the *macula sacculi* is also a localized neurosensory region but is located in the saccule (Fig. 14.17). In both cases, the maculae (macula, spot) are

Figure 14.17. Diagrams illustrate the morphology of the macula utriculi and macula sacculi. The hair tufts and polarity of kinocilia with respect to striola (dashed line) and otolithic membranes are illustrated. Cell bodies of some hair cells have a flask shape, while others are cylindrical. Hair cells have both afferent and efferent innervation. The macula utriculi is kidney-shaped, while the macula sacculi is comma-shaped. (From H. Lindeman, Studies of the morphology of the sensory regions of the vestibular apparatus. *Ergebn. Anat. EntroGesch.* 42, 1–113, 1969, Springer Verlag, New York, with permission)

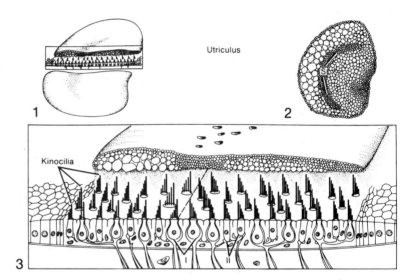

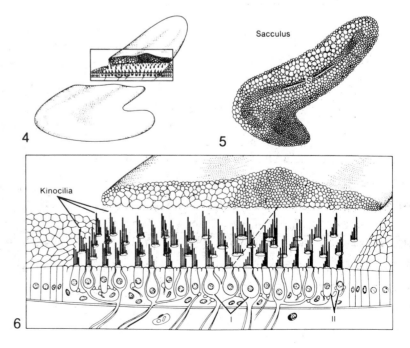

paired (one in each ear) and consist of both sensory hair cells and supporting cells. The plane of orientation of the *macula utriculi* is *horizontal*, and overall it has a *kidney shape*. Since there is one in each ear, they are approximately mirror images of each other. The *macula sacculi* has the overall shape of a *hook* or comma and is *vertical* in orientation, that is, perpendicular to the utricle. In both maculae, the hair tufts extend from the apical surface of the sensory cells into an overlying *otolithic membrane* that contains inorganic concretions (*otoliths*) of various sizes (Figs. 14.17–14.21). Both the macula utriculi and macula sacculi are concerned with detection of *static equilibrium*, with *gravity reception*, and in *sensing linear acceleration*. The supporting or sustentacular cells in the epithelium are columnar, have apical microvilli, and contain secretory granules. These cells appear to secrete the otolithic membrane and otoliths.

The flask-shaped type I sensory hair cells have a sensory nerve ending that ends in a chalice-like arrangement with the basal portion of the cell. Efferent nerve endings are also associated with the type I cell. Both afferent and efferent nerve endings are associated with the base of type II sensory hair cells. The sensory cells have a single modified cilium, called a *kinocilium*, and 50–100 *stereocilia* (modified microvilli). The stereocilia have graded heights, with the tallest ones located adjacent to the kinocilium (Fig. 14.22). The shorter stereocilia in the tufts are located farther from the kinocilium. The kinocilia and stereocilia extend into a sheet-like, gelatinous membrane (the *otolithic membrane*)

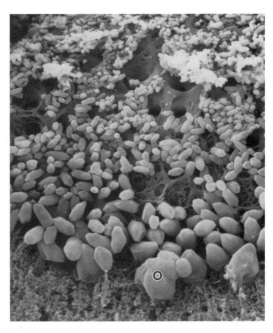

Figure 14.19. SEM of otoliths (O) of different sizes in the otolithic membrane. ×680. (From R. Kessel and R. Kardon, *Tissues and Organs: A Text-Atlas of Scanning Electron Microscopy*, W.H. Freeman, New York, 1979, with permission)

on which many *otoconia* or *otoliths* of different sizes are located. The *otoconia* or otoliths contain calcium carbonate and protein. As the otoliths are displaced by gravity, they move the kinocilium-stereocilia complex,

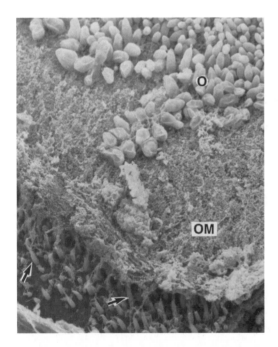

Figure 14.18. SEM of macula utriculi: Otoconia (O), otolithic membrane (OM) and hair tufts of hair cells (arrowhead). ×480. (From R. Kessel and R. Kardon, *Tissues and Organs: A Text-Atlas of Scanning Electron Microscopy*, W.H. Freeman, New York, 1979, with permission)

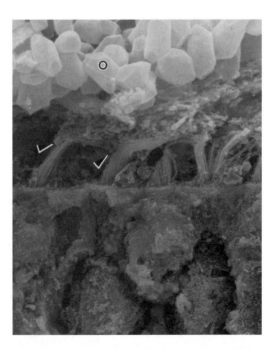

Figure 14.20. SEM of the otoliths (O) and otolithic membrane, which encloses (arrowheads) the tip of the hair tufts of hair cells. ×2300. (From R. Kessel and R. Kardon, *Tissues and Organs: A Text-Atlas of Scanning Electron Microscopy*, W.H. Freeman, New York, 1979, with permission)

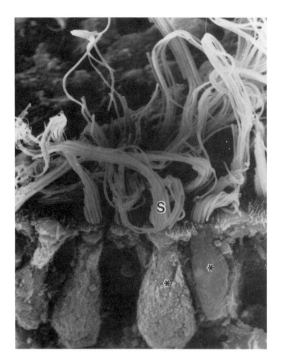

Figure 14.21. SEM of hair cell bodies (*) and hair tufts (stereocilia, S) in a section of the macula utriculi with the otolithic membrane removed. ×2040. (From R. Kessel and R. Kardon, *Tissues and Organs: A Text-Atlas of Scanning Electron Microscopy*, W.H. Freeman, New York, 1979, with permission)

either toward the kinocilium or toward the stereocilia side of the sensory hair tufts. Cells that surround the maculae contain basal infoldings and numerous mitochondria; they may play a role in the formation and modification of endolymph.

Hair tuft, otolithic membrane, striola

The sensory hair cells of the *macula utriculi* are morphologically polarized, so that the *kinocilium* of each cell faces *toward* a line or region termed the *striola*. The striola is identified by broken lines in Figures 14.17 and 14.23. The striola roughly divides the population of hair cells into two oppositely polarized groups. A very important difference in the *macula sacculi* is that the hair tufts are arranged such that the *kinocilia face away* from the *striola*. The precise orientation of hair tufts is important in vestibular function because the movement of the kinocilium-stereocilia complex causes changes in permeability and consequent ion movements in the apical end of the hair cells. This, in turn, results in increased or decreased firing of the afferent nerves innervating the base of the hair cell. During linear acceleration, gravity displaces the otoconia, with consequent displacement of the stereocilia. When the stereocilia are *bent* or displaced *toward* the *kinocilium*, there is *depolarization and excitation of the hair cell* (Fig. 14.24). Conversely, when the displacement of otoconia by gravity results in bending of the stereocilia *away from* the *kinocilium*, the sensory hair cells are then *hyperpolarized* and *inhibition* of the hair cell results (Fig. 14.24).

Hair tuft displacement

Positional changes in the head cause a shift of the endolymph and displacement of the otoconia-otolithic membrane such that a corresponding displacement of the kinocilium-stereocilia complex occurs. When mechanical shearing forces displace the kinocilium-stereocilia complex toward the kinociliary side of the cells,

Figure 14.22. SEM of hair cell tufts in the macula utriculi. The otolithic membrane was removed in order to illustrate the different hair tuft heights (*). The single kinocilium (arrow) on each hair cell is denoted. ×5300. (From R. Kessel and R. Kardon, *Tissues and Organs: A Text-Atlas of Scanning Electron Microscopy*, W.H. Freeman, New York, 1979, with permission)

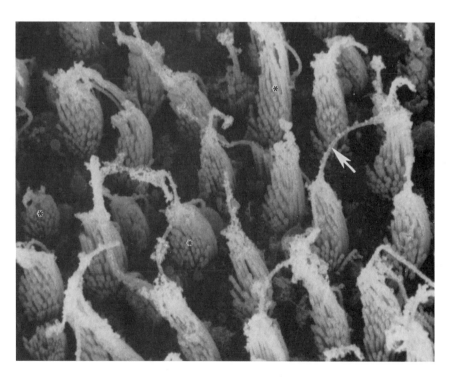

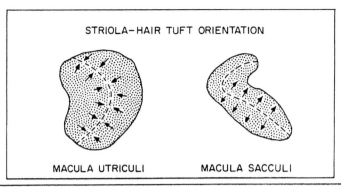

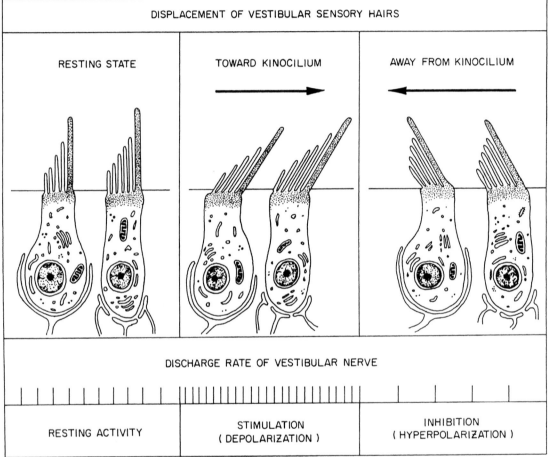

Figure 14.23. Diagrams (top) illustrate the hair tuft orientation with respect to the striola in the macula utriculi and macula sacculi. Diagrams of hair cells (bottom) illustrate different types of innervation. Both afferent and efferent nerves synapse with the base of the hair cells. The stereocilia are of graded heights, with the tallest being adjacent to the single kinocilium. When hair tufts are displaced toward the kinocilium, the hair cells are depolarized (stimulated). Conversely, when hair tufts are displaced away from the kinocilia (or toward the stereocilia), the hair cells are hyperpolarized (inhibited). When the hair tufts are upright, there is a low level of firing in the nerves innervating the hair cells. (Modified from J. Wersall, L. Gleisner, P–G. Lundquist. Ultrastructure of the vestibular end organs. In, A.V. DeReuck and J. Knight, eds., *Myotatic, Kinesthetic, and Vestibular Mechanism*, Little, Brown, Boston, 1967)

this causes depolarization and increased activity in the nerves innervating the cells (Figs. 14.23, 14.25). In contrast, when the displacement is toward the stereociliary side of the cell, that is, when displacement is away from the kinociliary side of the cell, this results in a hyperpolarization and decreased activity of the innervating vestibular nerve (Figs. 14.23, 14.25). There is always an

intermediate level of firing in the nerves innervating the hair cells.

Hair cell transduction

Recent studies on hair cell transduction mechanism in the maculae indicate that the tips of the kinocilia and

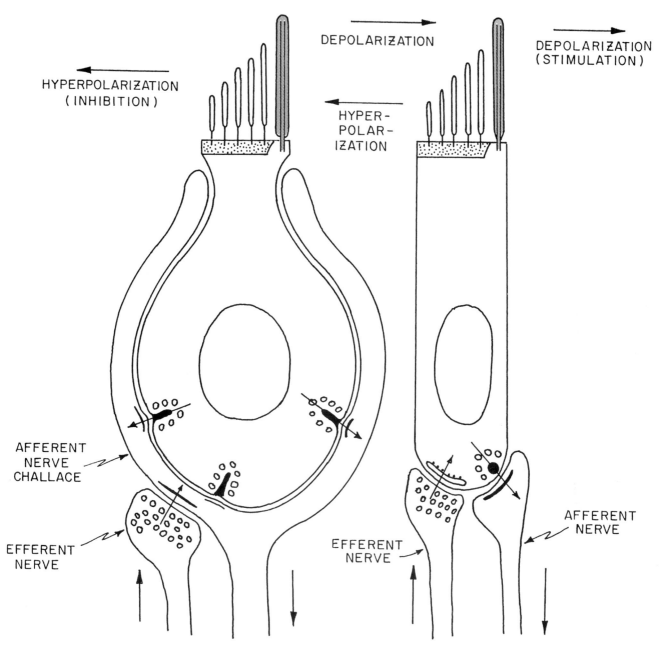

Figure 14.24. Diagram of type I and type II hair cells in maculae. Displacement of hair tufts and resulting depolarization or hyperpolarization are indicated.

adjacent stereocilia are important regions for this activity. EM studies show that thin filaments connect the tip of a kinocilium with the adjacent tall stereocilia. Because of this structural feature and because electrophysiologic recordings indicate that the region of inward current flow during a sensory response is at the tip of the cilia rather than at the base, the following sequence is considered likely. Movement of the ciliary tufts in the direction of increasing height (i.e., toward the kinociliary side of the cells) exerts a pull on the filaments connecting the ciliary tips. This pull causes a change in channel proteins sensitive to K^+ ions such that K^+ ions can now enter the tip of the cilia. An elec-

trochemical gradient is created because the endolymph surrounding the cilia has a high concentration of K^+ ions. The "current" thus generated spreads into the cell and outward across the membrane, resulting in a depolarizing receptor potential, and neurotransmitter is released at the synaptic region at the base of the hair cell at the vestibular nerve sensory terminals. Movement of the hair tufts toward the shorter ones (i.e., toward the stereociliary side of the cell) would not produce this effect and thus would provide direction to the response.

If the head is tilted to the left or right, some of the hair tufts in each macula utriculi will be depolarized, while others will be hyperpolarized because of the over-

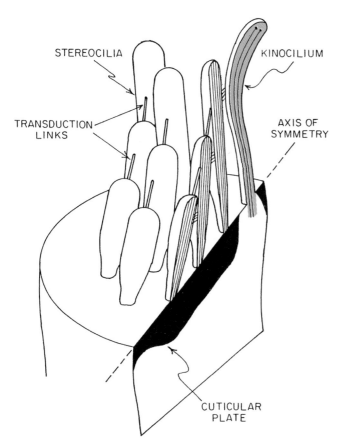

STEREOCILIA

KINOCILIUM

TRANSDUCTION
LINKS

AXIS OF
SYMMETRY

CUTICULAR
PLATE

Figure 14.25. Diagram illustrates hair tufts (kinocilium, stereocilia, and transduction links) of hair cells in maculae.

all shape of the maculae, their mirror images (thus 360° coverage) and the position or path of the striola. The same conditions pertain in the case of the macula sacculi if the head, for example, is tilted forward. It is the varying neural input; (i.e., increased or decreased activity in nerves innervating different hair cells, that is propagated over various pathways and through different nuclei in the CNS) that is interpreted differently in the cerebral cortex. The *macula utriculi* is primarily involved in providing information that the *head* is moved *forward* or *backward*. Conversely, the *macula sacculi* is mainly concerned with providing information that the *head* is deflected from *side* to *side*.

CRISTA AMPULLARIS (ANGULAR ACCELERATION AND DECELERATION)

General microscopic anatomy

The thin-walled, membranous semicircular ducts are filled with endolymph. The localized expansions of the ducts are called *ampullae*. Small patches of sensory hair cells and supporting cells are found in the wall of each ampulla, and each neurosensory structure is called a *crista ampullaris* (Figs. 14.26, 14.27). The crista am-

pullaris lies perpendicular to the plane of the duct, and is concerned with the sense of balance and with detecting angular acceleration and deceleration. The experience obtained in riding on a tilt-a-whirl is due to the activity of the crista ampullaris and associated nerves. The cristae contain supporting cells and sensory cells, as in the maculae. The sensory hair cells contain *apical tufts* or processes consisting of a *single kinocilium* and *many stereocilia* of graded heights (Figs. 14.28, 14.29). These processes extend into the lumen of the ampullae and are covered by a tall, gelatinous covering, called the *cupula*, that extends toward the wall opposite the crista ampullaris (Fig. 14.26). The cupula contains a jelly-like glycoprotein material that is more viscid than the endolymph surrounding the cupula. Because of its high water content, the cupula shrinks markedly during histologic preparation. Supporting cells surrounding the crista may be responsible for maintaining the high potassium concentration of the endolymph. The endolymph surrounds the cupula. When the head rotates, the *fluid* in the canal is *displaced*, causing a *shearing action* of the *hairs* that project into the *cupula*. This shearing action on the kinocilium-stereociliary tuft is converted into impulses in the nerves that form synapses at the bases of the hair cells.

Function of the cristae ampullaris

There are no otoconia or statoconia associated with the cupula. There is no striola in the crista ampullaris. While each hair tuft consists of a single long kinocilium and many long stereocilia of different lengths, the polarity of the hair tufts is the same in each crista. However, the hair cells are not all positioned in the ampullae in the same way. The cristae in the *horizontal semicircular ducts* have hair tufts in which the *kinocilia face toward the utricule*. In the two *vertical cristae* of the *superior* and *posterior semicircular ducts*, the *kinocilia* of all hair cells *face away from the utricle*.

The receptor hair cells are innervated by both afferent and efferent nerve endings. Movement of the head in space and angular acceleration and deceleration result in a displacement of the endolymph and cupula. This displacement translates into a shearing action on the kinocilium-stereociliary complexes.

Displacements cause either depolarization or hyperpolarization of hair cells. A *force* directing the *stereocilia toward* the *kinocilium* causes *increased activity* in the *vestibular nerve* that innervates the cells. *Conversely*, a *force displacing* the *kinocilium* toward the *stereocilia* causes a *decrease* in *activity* in the *vestibular nerve* innervating the hair cells. As long as the movement of the body is changing, that is, either accelerating or decelerating, the cupula will be displaced. However, when a constant velocity is achieved, the fluid in the canal moves at the same rate as the body and the cupula returns to its original orientation.

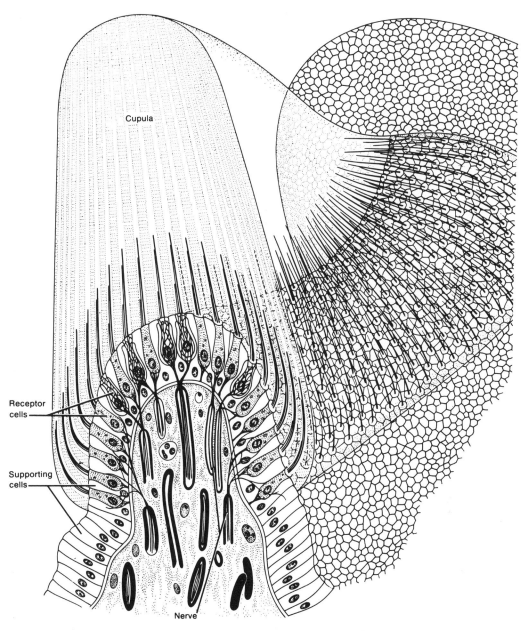

Cupula

Receptor
cells

Supporting
cells

Nerve

Figure 14.26. Diagram illustrates the organization of
the crista ampullaris. The neuroepithelium consists of hair
cells and supporting cells. The hair tufts extend into a gelatinous cupula, which is surrounded by endolymph in the membranous ampullae. (From L.C. Junqueira, J. Carneiro, and
A.N. Contopoulos, *Basic Histology*, (2nd ed., Appleton &
Lange Medical Publications, East Norwalk, CT, 1977, with
permission)

Movement of the head causes movement of the endolymph in the semicircular ducts, and this movement
causes displacement of the cupula. Thus, angular acceleration is detected by the crista ampullaris. It is important to recognize that semicircular ducts on opposite sides of the head, but in the same plane, are
functionally antagonistic to each other. For example,
when the head is turned to the right, the hair cells in
the crista of the right horizontal semicircular duct are
stimulated, while the hair cells in the crista of the left
horizontal semicircular duct are inhibited. These differences in hair tuft displacement in the horizontal and

vertical cristae ampullaris, and the consequent depolarization and hyperpolarization of the sensory cells and
the nerves innervating them, provide the appropriate
neural input to the CNS to permit us to know if we are
rotating or twirling in a left-handed or right-handed direction.

MEDICAL IMPLICATIONS

Otitis media is an inflammation of the middle ear. Bacterial infection can result when bacteria from the nose

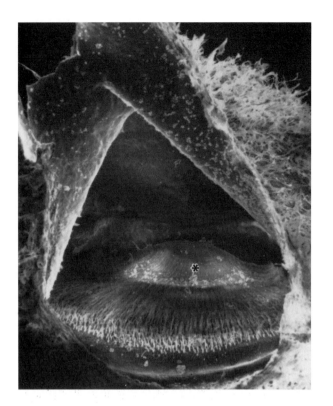

Figure 14.27. SEM. The membranous labyrinth of the ampulla was opened to illustrate the internally located crista ampullaris. The many small, light lines are hair tufts (stereocilia) of hair cells. The gelatinous crista (*) has shrunken markedly during tissue preparation. ×135. (From R. Kessel and R. Kardon, *Tissues and Organs: A Text-Atlas of Scanning Electron Microscopy*, W.H. Freeman, New York, 1979, with permission)

and throat invade the middle ear. The condition is common in young children because the eustachian tube does not drain properly. *Meniere's disease* is a condition of the inner ear that can result in vertigo (dizziness), hearing loss, and tinnitus (ringing in the ears). The cause is unknown, and therefore the disease is difficult to treat.

Otosclerosis is a condition in which the stapes foot plate may adhere to the oval window, as for example when new bone forms on the stapes foot plate. This interferes with sound reaching the inner ear.

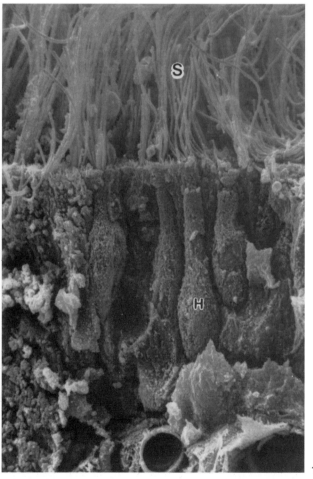

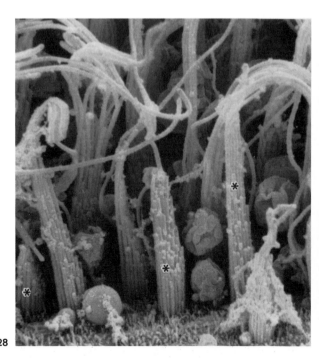

14.28

14.29

Figures 14.28, 14.29. SEM of crista ampullaris. The long hair tufts (S) of three different heights (*) are shown. Figure 14.29, ×3050; Figure 14.30, ×1750. (From R. Kessel and R. Kardon, *Tissues and Organs: A Text-Atlas of Scanning Electron Microscopy*, W.H. Freeman, New York, 1979, with permission)

SELECTED BIBLIOGRAPHY

Ashmore, J.F. (1991). The electrophysiology of hair cells. *Annu. Rev. Physiol.* **53**, 465–476.

Bredberg, G., Ades, H.W., and Engström, H. (1973). Scanning electron microscopy of the normal and pathologically altered organ of Corti. *Acta Otolaryngol.* (Stockh), **301** (suppl.), 3–48.

Corwin, J.T., and Warchol, M.E. (1991). Auditory hair cells: structure, function, development, and regeneration. *Annu. Rev. Neurosci.,* **14**, 301–333.

Edelman, G., Gall, W., and Cowan, W. (1988) *Auditory Functions.* Wiley, New York.

Engström, H., Bergström, B., and Ades, H.W. (1972). Macula utriculi and macula sacculi in the squirrel monkey. *Acta Otolaryngol.* **301** (suppl.), 75–126.

Hudspeth, A.J. (1989). How the ear's works work. *Nature* **341**, 397–404.

Hunter-Duvar, I.M., and Hinojosa, R. (1984). Vestibule: Sensory epithelia. In I. Frieman and J. Ballantyne, eds. *Ultrastructural Atlas of the Inner Ear,* Butterworths, London.

Karmody, D.S. *Textbook of Otoloaryngology.* Lea & Febiger, Philadelphia.

Lim, D.J. (1986). Functional structure of the organ of Corti: a review. *Hear. Res.* **22**, 117–146.

Lindeman, H.H. (1969). Studies on the morphology of the sensory regions of the vestibular apparatus. *Ergebn. Anat. EntwGesch.* **42**, 1–113.

Lindeman, H.H. (1973). Anatomy of the otolith organs. *Adv. Otorhinolaryngol.* **20**, 405–433.

Pickels, J., and Corey, D. (1992). Mechanoelectrical transduction by hair cells. *Trends Neurosci.* **15**, 254–259.

CHAPTER 15

The Vascular (Circulatory) System

All resident cells of the body are supplied with blood that contains nutrients (amino acids, sugars, fatty acids), enzymes, hormones, ions, metabolites, and oxygen essential for their survival and proper functioning. In addition, waste products that the resident cells generate, such as CO_2 and various nitrogenous wastes, are transported via the blood to the lungs and kidneys for elimination. A properly functioning circulatory system is critical for the harmonious interaction of billions of cells. The heart, which is a double pump, is required to propel and distribute the blood, nutrients, and wastes in two circuits: a systematic circuit and a pulmonary circuit. To keep these two circuits separate, the heart has two sides with two chambers (Fig. 15.1). The right side of the heart is concerned with pumping blood through the vessels comprising a *pulmonary circuit* for oxygenating blood in the lungs. The left side of the heart is concerned with pumping blood through vessels comprising the *systemic circuit.* The circulatory system is also responsible for the formation of substantial amounts of tissue fluid, which bathes the resident cells and serves as a vehicle or medium for the diffusion of both raw materials and waste products associated with the cells' activities.

The tubes or pipelines comprising the circulatory system are represented by arteries, veins, and capillaries. Each of these divisions has a special role to play in the proper functioning of the circulatory system. As a result of muscular contractions of the heart, blood flows through arteries of comparatively large diameter and low resistance to vessels of small diameter and high resistance. Blood flow in an adult at rest is approximately 5000 ml/min. The flow rate through smaller arteries (arterioles) is influenced by the diameter of the vessel, the number of vessels, and the degree of elasticity of the vessel wall. The resistance to blood flow in smaller arteries is due to active contraction of intramural smooth muscle. Most of the small arteries are partially constricted in vivo, and the level of tone in these small arteries in the resting animal is approximately proportional to their diameter. In the absence of this muscle tone, cardiac output would be insufficient to maintain the circulation in the vessels. The tone is due to a complex interplay of factors including nervous innervation and the nature and concentration of circulating and locally produced vasoactive materials. Substances produced by the endothelial cells lining the vessel lumen, as well as Na^+ and Ca^{2+} concentrations, are also important.

ORGANIZATION OF THE HEART

The heart is a pulsatile organ that exhibits alternate contractions (systole) and relaxations (diastole). The normal systolic pressure is about 120 mm Hg, and the normal diastolic pressure is about 80 mm Hg. However, the pressure is reduced to the point where it is near zero in the vena cavae that join the right atrium of the heart.

Since each half of the heart has an auricle and a ventricle, there are two auricles and two ventricles Fig. 15.2). Each side of the heart also has two valves: an intake valve and an exhaust valve (Fig. 15.2). Venous blood enters the right atrium from the inferior and superior vena cavae. Blood then flows through the tricuspid valve into the right ventricle, from which it is pumped, during ventricular contraction (systole), through a pulmonary semilunar *valve* into the pulmonary arteries to the lungs. Oxygenated blood returns from the lungs in the pulmonary veins to the left atrium. Blood then passes through the mitral or bicuspid valve to the left ventricle. From the left ventricle, blood passes through the aortic semilunar valve to the aorta, to be distributed throughout the body. The left ventricle functions as a one-cylinder pump and delivers blood in spurts into the aorta at a rate of about 70 spurts per minute.

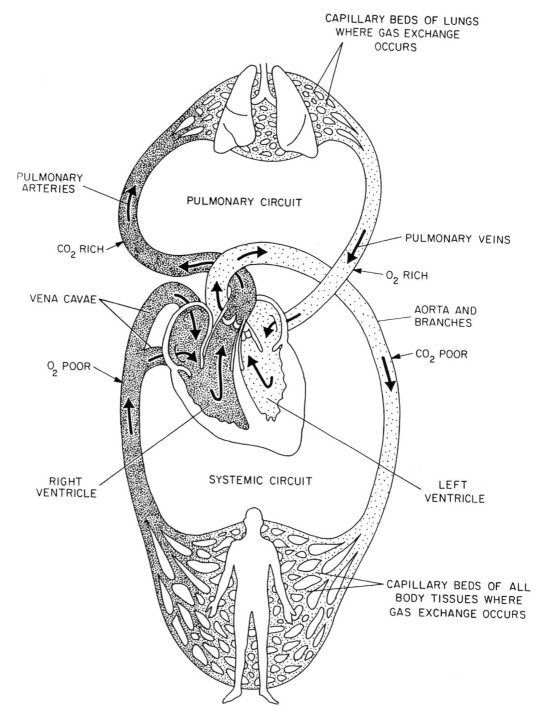

Figure 15.1. Diagram depicts the circulatory system, the heart, and the pulmonary and systemic circuits associated with the heart. (Redrawn and modified from E. Marieb, *Human Anatomy and Physiology*. Benjamin/Cummings Publishing Co., Menlo Park, CA, 1995, with permission)

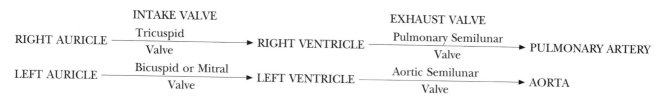

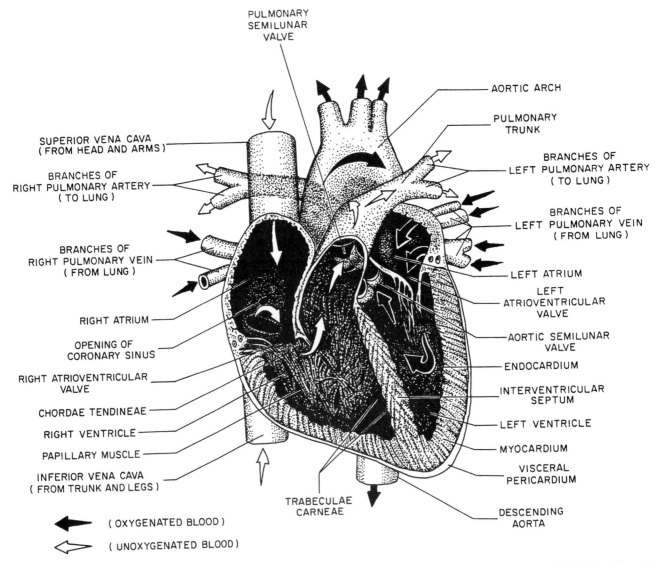

Figure 15.2. Diagram of the heart showing the chambers and their relationship to the vessels connected to the heart. (Redrawn from A.P. Spence and E.B. Mason, *Human* *Anatomy* and Physiology, 4th. ed. West Publishing Co., St. Paul, MN, 1992)

The heart has three layers: an inner *endocardium,* a middle *myocardium,* and an outer *epicardium.* The endocardium consists of endothelium and a small amount of subendothelial connective tissue. The heart valves are thin flaps of connective tissue covered by endothelium; thus they are extensions of the endocardium. The endothelium is continuous with the endothelium lining the interior of attached vessels, and this layer is continuous with the tunica intima of blood vessels. The myocardium is a thick layer of cardiac muscle that is thicker in the ventricles than in the auricles. This layer is continuous with the tunica media of attached blood vessels. The epicardium is a layer of fibroelastic connective tissue that is covered externally by a single layer of mesothelium (simple squamous epithelium). This layer is continuous with the tunica adventitia of attached blood vessels.

CONTROL OF HEARTBEAT: INNERVATION OF THE HEART

The stimulus for contraction arises within the heart and is propagated along specialized cells of a conduction system to the myocardium. The heartbeat originates from cells in the *sinoatrial (SA) node,* which is located in the heart wall near the junction of the superior vena cava and the right auricle. The muscle cells in this pacemaker region are smaller and have more poorly organized myofibrils than other atrial cells. Nerve endings are common in this region. From the SA node, the impulse travels to an *atrioventricular (AV) node.* The AV node is located in the right atrium near the junction with the right ventricle. The organization of the AV node is similar to that of the SA node. The SA and AV nodes are well innervated by both sympathetic and parasympathetic nerves. Impulses from sympathetic nerves tend to increase the rate of contraction, while impulses from parasympathetic nerves tend to slow the heart rate. From the AV node, the impulse travels to the AV bundle or bundle of His. The bundle of His contains modified cardiac muscle cells called *Purkinje cells* (or fibers).

VESSEL TYPES AND LAYERS

Histologic characteristics of the blood vascular system are summarized in Table 15.1. Arteries are often classified according to their principal function and principal tissue constituent. Therefore, the largest divisions of the arterial system are the *elastic* or *conducting arteries*; the intermediate-sized arteries are called *muscular* or *distributing arteries*, while the smallest divisions are called *arterioles*. The classification of veins is generally based solely on their size, including *small veins* or *venules*, *medium-sized veins*, and *large veins*.

A complete but very thin sheet of squamous epithelial cells called *endothelium* lines the interior of the heart (where it is called *cardiac endothelium*) and the interior of blood vessels (where it is called *vascular endothelium*). The venous and arterial divisions have variable amounts of smooth muscle and connective tissue (elastic fibers, collagen fibers, reticular fibers, and amorphous intercellular substances) arranged in specific layers that are variable in different divisions of the circulatory vessels.

The innermost layer of arteries and veins is the *tunica intima*. The innermost tunica intima layer always includes a continuous layer of endothelium (simple squamous epithelium). This layer may or may not include a thin layer of connective tissue (subendothelial connective tissue) adjacent to endothelium. There is sometimes a thick, fenestrated elastic fiber (*internal elastic lamina*) component to this layer. The middle layer, called the *tunica media*, is usually the thickest of the layers. The tunica media is the middle layer and typically consists of smooth muscle (especially in the arteries), as well as elastic fibers, collagenic fibers, amorphous intercellular substance, and cells that form these products. The outer layer, called the *tunica adventitia*, is an external layer or sheath of connective tissue. However, in large veins, smooth muscle may be present in this layer. The connective tissue components include collagen fibers (substantial amounts in veins), elastic fibers, amorphous intercellular substance, and the cells that form these components. The variations in these layers in different parts of the blood vessels will be examined. It should be emphasized that the transition in different kinds of arteries and veins is gradual; the changes are not abrupt.

FUNCTIONAL PROBLEMS OF THE CIRCULATORY SYSTEM

Between contractions, while the heart is relaxed (diastole), pressure in the arterial vessels may fall to *zero*; therefore, one problem is that of maintaining pressure in a system of pipes in which the taps are partly open. The problem is solved by the fact that arteries leading from the heart are composed of many elastic fibers that can be stretched when the heart contracts. Systolic pressure (systole, a contraction) is the pressure of blood in vessels during contraction of the heart. The many elastic fibers in the wall of the aorta are stretched at this time. Between contractions of the heart, the stretched elastic fibers in the wall of the aorta passively recoil (diastole), returning to their original length before stretching. In this way, it is possible to maintain diastolic pressure in the system.

Another problem faced by the circulatory system is how to selectively channel more or less blood to certain organs under different conditions of need (e.g., more blood to the right hand of a right-handed tennis player during a match). This problem is solved by having circular (spiral) smooth muscle in the wall of medium-sized or distributing arteries so that, by varying the degree of contraction, the arteries can supply more or less blood to a specific organ or body region.

Another problem is that in order to stand erect, considerable pressure must be generated in the circulatory system to overcome gravity. However, by the time blood reaches the capillary bed, the pressure must be greatly reduced so that it does not injure the delicate endothelium and so that transcapillary transport can occur. Pressure is reduced in a plumbing system by inserting pressure-reducing valves. The same effect is achieved in the body by the use of arterioles, which play the same role. Arterioles have relatively thick walls and small lumens. Because of the viscosity of blood, the narrow lumen of the muscular arteriole offers considerable resistance to the flow of blood. Thus, relatively high pressures can build up behind the arterioles. Therefore, pressure in the arterial system is regulated mainly by the degree of contraction (tonus) of smooth muscle cells in the walls of arterioles. If the degree of contraction is increased, hypertension can result. Veins are also faced with the problem of overcoming gravity; the longitudinal smooth muscle in some veins and the presence of valves play important roles. The extremely thin walls of capillaries solve the problem of gas and nutrient exchange between the circulatory system and resident cells.

UNIQUE FEATURES OF ARTERIES

Blood vessels and lymphatic capillaries are present only in the outermost layers of arteries; the reason is that

Table 15.1 Histologic Characteristics of the Blood Vascular System

Arterial-Venous Divisions	Approximate Diameter	Tunica Intima (Inner Layer)	Tunica Media (Middle Layer)	Tunica Adventitia (External Layer)
Elastic artery	~1 cm	Endothelium, basement membrane; elastic fibers, a few smooth muscle cells	Smooth muscle cells; fenestrated elastic laminae (~50 layers in aorta); reticular fibers; proteoglycans	Mainly elastic and collagenic fibers; vasa vasora; nervi vasora; thinner than tunica media
Muscular artery	0.5 mm–1 cm	Endothelium, basement membrane; elastic, collagenic, reticular fibers; prominent fenestrated internal elastic lamina—sometimes split; few smooth muscle cells	Smooth muscle layers (up to 30 or more); few reticular (IIII collagen) fibers, proteoglycans, external elastic lamina	Elastic, collagenic (type I) and reticular fibers; vasa vasora; nervi vasora; thinner than tunica media
Arteriole	30–400 μm (0.4 mm)	Endothelium, basement membrane; few elastic, collagenic fibrils; internal elastic lamina in larger arterioles	Smooth muscle layers (1–3 or 4); a few collagenic, elastic and reticular fibrils	Collagenic (I), elastic, reticular fibers; vasa vasora, nervi vasora, blends with connective tissue of organ
Capillary	5–15 μm	Endothelium, basal lamina; scattered pericytes	None	None
Veins Postcapillary venule	10–25 μm	Endothelium, basal lamina; scattered pericytes	None	None
Collecting venule	20–50 μm	Endothelium; continuous layer of pericytes	None	None
Muscular venule (small vein)	50–100 μm	Endothelium, basement membrane; pericytes	1–2 layers of smooth muscle cells	Elastic and collagenic fibers continuous with surrounding connective tissue
Small vein	0.1–1 mm	Endothelium, basement membrane; collagen fibers	2–3 layers of smooth muscle; vasa vasora; nervi vasora	Elastic, collagenic fibers; continuous with surrounding connective tissue
Medium vein	1–10 mm	Endothelium, basement membrane; circular smooth muscle; collagen and elastin fibers; internal elastic lamina possible	Smooth muscle (circular); collagen and elastin fibers; nervi vasora; vasa vasora	Collagen and elastin fibers; thicker than tunica media
Large vein	~1 mm–4 cm	Endothelium; basement membrane; collagen and elastin fibers; internal elastic lamina	~4–15 layers of smooth muscle in some large veins; collagen, elastin; vasa and nervi vasora	Elastin and collagen fibers; longitudinally oriented smooth muscle bundles in vena cava; much thicker than tunica media

blood pressure in the arteries would collapse them. Therefore, much of the arterial wall depends on diffusion from the vessel lumen, where blood is moving very rapidly, for its nourishment and oxygen. Further, if inert substances such as fatty substances build up in the vessel wall, this could interfere with diffusion, causing cell death in a localized region of the vessel wall.

Extensive use is made of the protein *elastin*, the major connective tissue fiber in arteries; these elastic fibers are often fenestrated, which facilitates diffusion. Collagen, which is more prevalent in veins, tends to cause blood platelets to agglutinate, as in thrombus formation.

Although both smooth muscle cells and connective tissue fibers are found in artery walls, there are not two distinct types of cells to produce them. In the walls of arteries, there is *one* kind of cell that is differentiated from a mesenchyme cell in the embryo through a *pericyte*-type cell, which can *form elastin, collagen,* and *reticular* fibers and is also capable of differentiating into a *smooth muscle cell.* Thus, the major cell type in the vascular system is unique because it retains broad capabilities for differentiation. It has been suggested that neural crest cells may also be present in the walls of blood vessels.

ARTERIAL DIVISIONS OF THE CIRCULATORY SYSTEM

ELASTIC ARTERIES

These large vessels conduct blood from the heart to muscular or distributing arteries and are characterized by the presence of large numbers of elastic fibers (Plate 35A). Such vessels include the aorta, pulmonary, innominate, common carotid, subclavian, and common iliac arteries. These vessels have a large lumen, but their wall is relatively thin, perhaps only 1/10th of the vessel diameter.

TUNICA INTIMA

The tunica intima is lined with a continuous sheet of endothelium, and the cells may be linked by different intercellular junctions. This layer comprises about one-fifth of the total wall thickness. The endothelium is surrounded mainly by loosely packed elastic fibers and perhaps a few collagenic fibers as well. The cells present in this layer secrete the elastic fibers and the amorphous (jellies) intercellular substances that surround the cells and fibers. This layer is called *subendothelial connective tissue.*

TUNICA MEDIA

The tunica media is the thickest tunic. The layer contains as many as 70 concentrically arranged, rather closely packed elastic fibers or sheets that are *fenestrated,* or have holes in them, to facilitate diffusion. Between the fenestrated elastic fibers are smooth muscle cells that produced the elastic fibers, a few fine collagenic fibers, and amorphous intercellular substance. Adjacent to the tunica adventitia may be one or more closely packed elastic fibers called the *external elastic lamina.*

TUNICA ADVENTITIA

This layer is relatively *thin* in elastic arteries compared to medium-sized arteries. The irregularly arranged connective tissue consists of collagen fibers, a few elastic fibers, and amorphous intercellular substance together with the cells that secreted these components. Nerves (*nervi vasora*) are largely restricted to the tunica adventitia in the wall of arteries. These nerves represent innervation from the ANS, both sympathetic and parasympathetic divisions.

MUSCULAR OR DISTRIBUTING ARTERIES

Muscular arteries include most of the named arteries, such as the femoral, renal, brachial, ulnar, and radial. While the main function of the elastic arteries is to conduct blood, the major function of the muscular arteries is to distribute blood to specific organs. While the major component of an elastic artery is the elastic fiber, which permits the vessels to expand with the force of blood from contraction of the heart, the major constituent of the muscular artery is the smooth muscle cell (Plate 36A–C). Blood flow is thereby regulated by smooth muscle, whose contraction and relaxation control the size of the vascular lumen. Since different parts of the body are under different conditions of activity, they require different amounts of blood. The arteries supplying these tissues and organs must then be capable of changing the size of their lumen such that different amounts of blood can be delivered to the organ at different times and under changing conditions.

TUNICA INTIMA

The tunica intima consists of a layer of endothelium that resides directly on a scalloped, thick elastic fiber called the *internal elastic membrane or lamina* (Plate 35B). In larger divisions of muscular arteries, there is usually a layer of subendothelial connective tissue between the endothelium and the internal elastic lamina. The subendothelial connective tissue consists of a few fine collagenic fibers and elastic fibers, amorphous intercellular substance, and the cells that synthesized and secreted this material. The internal elastic lamina, although considered part of the tunica intima, lies adjacent to the tunica media. In some vessels, a split or (double) internal elastic lamina is present.

TUNICA MEDIA

The tunica media is mainly muscular, consisting of ~5–30 helical layers of smooth muscle that are concentrically arranged. Among the smooth muscle cells may be fine reticular, collagenic, and elastic fibers, as well as some amorphous intercellular substance (Plate 36A,B). An external elastic lamina is located between the medial and adventitial layers and consists of several elastic fibers.

TUNICA ADVENTITIA

The tunica adventitia in a muscular artery is thick and is about one-half to two-thirds the width of the media. The layer consists primarily of longitudinally or helically arranged collagenic and elastic fibers, as well as amorphous intercellular substance and the cells that synthesized and secreted these connective tissue components (Plate 36A–C). Vasa vasora, lymphatics, and nerves are present in the tunica adventitia.

Comparison of Elastic Artery and Muscular Artery

Elastic Artery	Muscular Artery
Tunica intima width ~one-fifth of total wall; less elastin than in media	Tunica intima thinner in muscular artery (in many areas, endothelium lies directly on internal elastic lamina)
Tunica media comprises bulk of wall	Occasionally a split internal elastic lamina
Mainly elastic fibers in media; some smooth muscle cells.	Chiefly smooth muscle in media; relatively few collagenic, reticular, and elastic fibers
Tunica adventitia relatively thin; both collagenic and elastic fibers	Adventitia thick; approximately one-third to two-thirds of thickness of media; both collagenic and elastic fibers

ARTERIOLES

Arterioles are the pressure-reducing valves of the circulatory system. Pressure reduction is accomplished by constructing the arterioles such that they have relatively narrow lumens but relatively thick walls (Plate 36D; Fig. 37A). Since blood has viscosity, the narrow lumen of the arteriole, as well as its thick, muscular wall, offer considerable resistance to blood flow, permitting relatively high pressures to build up. The diameter of the arteriole lumen is regulated by the degree of contraction or tonus of the smooth muscle cells in the tunica media of the arteriole (Fig. 15.3).

Since the changes between the arterial divisions are quite gradual, how is the arteriole defined? This determination is made differently by various investigators. Some investigators define an arteriole as an arterial division that has a diameter of 300 μm or less and with one to three or four layers of circularly arranged smooth muscle cells in the tunica media. Other investigators indicate that arterioles range from 40 to 200 μm in diameter and use the thickness of the wall in relation to the lumen in defining an arteriole. The ratio of the thickness of the vessel wall to the diameter of the lumen is about 1:2 under normal conditions. However, in hypertension, arterioles have thicker walls in relation to the lumen.

Arterioles range from 40 to 200 μm in diameter (Plate 36D). When an arteriole is only about 40 μm in diameter, the muscular coat becomes a single layer. There is no internal or external elastic lamina, and the tunica adventitia merges imperceptibly into the surrounding connective tissue. Such a vessel, which has only a single layer of smooth muscle or a single smooth muscle cell in its wall, is called a *precapillary or terminal arteriole*. Thus, a precapillary or terminal arteriole is described as ranging from 30 to 50 μm, but with a continuous layer of smooth muscle (Fig. 15.4). In a *metarteriole*, the lumen is wider than that of a true capillary, but the smooth muscle cells are located only at intervals along its course.

LAYERS OF ARTERIOLES

The tunica intima of arterioles includes an endothelial lining that usually lies adjacent to an internal elastic lamina; in larger arterioles, a thin subendothelial connective tissue layer may be present. The internal elastic lamina is usually absent in smaller arterioles. The tunica media contains one to three or four layers of helically arranged smooth muscle (Plate 37A). A few fine collagenic and elastic fibers, as well as amorphous intercellular substance, may be present among the smooth muscle. Figure 15.5 is a specially prepared SEM that illustrates the smooth muscle and a nerve that is associated with a terminal arteriole. The tunica adventitia is approximately as thick as the tunica media. It consists of fine collagenic and elastic fibers, amorphous intercellular substance, and the cells that formed these connective tissue elements. This layer is often continuous with the surrounding connective tissue of the organ in which the arteriole is located.

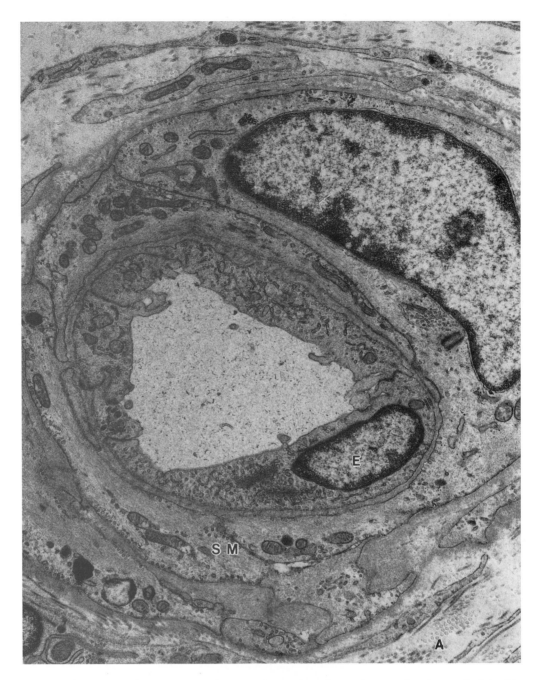

Figure 15.3. TEM of an arteriole. Endothelium (E), smooth muscle (SM) of media, and connective tissue of adventitia (A) are identified. ×20,800.

METARTERIOLES AND PERICYTES

Metarterioles are small vessels that have an incomplete smooth muscle layer. In addition, *pericytes or perivascular cells* are interspersed with the smooth muscle cells on these vessels. The pericytes are highly branched and reside on a capillary somewhat like a spider. They are not continuous as a layer, but intermittent in their distribution. The pericytes appear to be enclosed by the basal lamina of the endothelial cells in transmission electron micrographs. Pericytes are often associated with both capillaries and venules (Fig. 15.6). Pericytes can become phagocytic (and differentiate into macrophages). The cells can become smooth muscle cells during the growth of new veins from venules. Pericytes can assist in producing basement membrane (basal lamina) material for endothelium, and they reportedly are able to differentiate into reticular cells, fibroblasts, or adipocytes. They are difficult to distinguish in histologic sections.

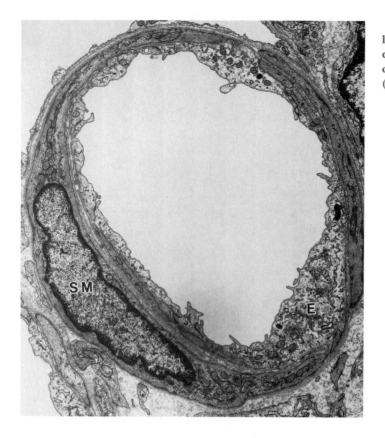

Figure 15.4. TEM of a precapillary (terminal) arteriole. The endothelium (E) is surrounded by a complete layer of smooth muscle (SM) cells. ×8400.

ARTERIOVENOUS ANASTOMOSES

In some regions, arteries and veins can be directly connected by means of *arteriovenous anastomoses*; there is no intervening capillary bed or sinusoidal connection. These vascular shunts are especially prevalent in the skin

on exposed regions of the body surface such as in the skin of hands, feet, lips, and nose. Smooth muscle cells are distributed along the arteriovenous anastomoses, so the shunts can be open or closed. When the shunts are open, blood passes directly into the veins and the capillary bed is bypassed. When the shunts are closed, blood

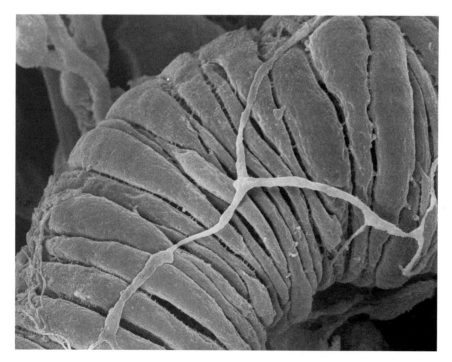

Figure 15.5. SEM of the smooth muscle and nerve associated with a terminal arteriole. ×5400. (From Fujiwara, T. and Uehara, Y., © 1984. The cytoarchitecture of the wall and the innervation pattern of the microvessels in the rat mammary gland: A scanning electron microscopic observation. *Am. J. Anat.* 170, 39–54. Reprinted by permission of John Wiley & Sons, Inc.)

Figure 15.6. SEM of the pericytes (highly branched cells) associated with the outer surface of a postcapillary venule. ×4400. (From T.
Fujiwara and Y. Uehara, The cytoarchitecture of the wall and the innervation pattern of the microvessels in
the rat mammary gland: A scanning
electron microscopic observation.
Am. J. Anat. 170, 39–54. © 1984).
Reprinted by permission of John Wiley & Sons, Inc.)

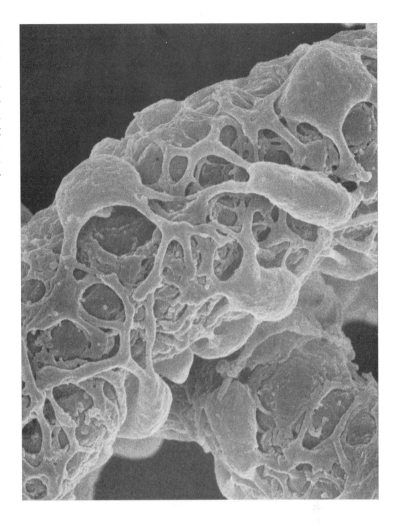

circulates through the capillary bed. The smooth muscles in the shunts are extensively innervated by the ANS.
A ring of smooth muscle cells, called a *sphincter*, has been
described at the point of origin of capillaries from
metarterioles.

CAPILLARIES

Capillaries are blood vessels that are denuded of all investing coats and persist as endothelial tubes (Figs. 15.7,
15.8). It has been estimated that most vertebrate cells

Figure 15.7. SEM microvascular
cast of thyroid. Each of the circular
capillary networks invests a thyroid
follicle. ×80. (From: R. Kessel and
R. Kardon, *Tissues and Organs: A Text-
Atlas of Scanning Electron Microscopy.*
W.H. Freeman, New York, 1979, with
permission)

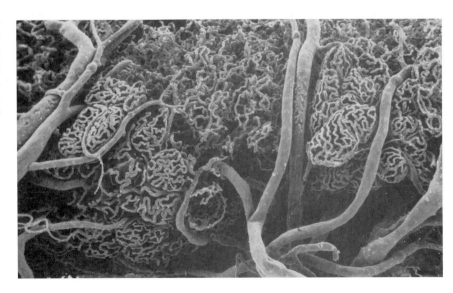

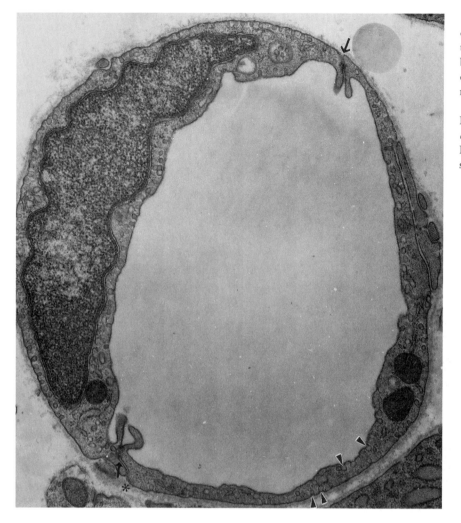

Figure 15.8. TEM of a continuous capillary; the junction between the two endothelial cells is denoted by arrows. Note the numerous micropinocytotic pits and vesicles (arrowheads) and basal lamina (*). ×30,000. (From: R. Roberts, R. Kessel, H. Tung. *Freeze Fracture Images of Cells and Tissues.* Oxford Univ. Press, New York, 1991, with permission)

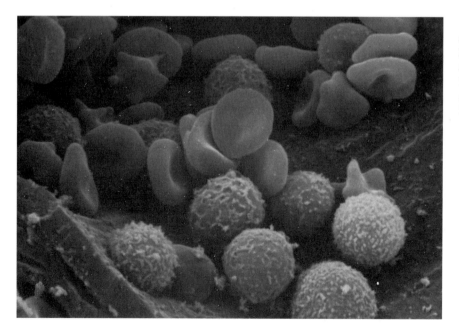

Figure 15.9. SEM of blood vessels filled with erythrocytes and leukocytes. ×6100. (From R. Kessel and R. Kardon, *Tissues and Organs: A Text-Atlas of Scanning Eecctron Microscopy.* W.H. Freeman, New York, 1979, with permission)

Figure 15.10. SEM of elongated leukocytes that adhere to endothelium in the interior of a blood vessel. The elongated shape of the leukocytes suggests that the cells were migrating along the endothelial surface when exposed to fixative. ×395. (From R. Kessel and R. Kardon, *Tissues and Organs: A Text-Atlas of Scanning Electron Microscopy.* W.H. Freeman, New York, 1979, with permission)

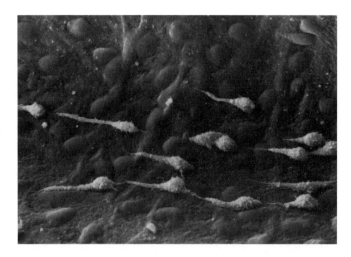

are no farther than 50 μm from a capillary. In humans, the surface area of capillaries is some 6000 m^2. Capillaries consist of endothelial cells that have a mesenchymal origin. Blood cells are in close proximity to the endothelium (Fig. 15.9), and sometimes adhere to the endothelium and migrate on the suface of these cells (Fig. 15.10). Capillaries usually range from 7 to 10 μm in diameter, which is just large enough for red blood cells and leukocytes to pass through the lumen. The total cross-sectional area of capillaries is approximately 800 times greater than that of the aorta. The rate of flow through the capillaries is about 0.4 mm/sec compared to about 320 mm/sec through the aorta. The pressure in the capillaries may approach 35 mm Hg at the arteriolar end but ranges down to about 10 mm Hg near the venous end.

There are several different types of capillaries based on the integrity of their endothelium. *Continuous capillaries* are those in which the endothelial cells are uninterrupted by pores or fenestrae (Figs. 15.8, 15.11). *Fenestrated or perforated capillaries* contain a number of pores ~60–70 nm in diameter that permit more rapid transcapillary transport than can occur by micropinocytosis (Figs. 15.12, 15.13). Some of these pores or fenestrae in side view (Figs. 15.12, 15.13) appear to be traversed by a thin, diaphragm-like structure (Fig. 15.13). However, special preparations that show the fenestrations in surface view (Fig. 15.14) demonstrate that a number of fibrils extend from the pore rim toward the center, re-

sulting in a sieve-like structure (Fig. 15.14). Fenestrated endothelium of glomerular capillaries in the kidney (Figs. 15.15, 15.16), however, lacks such structures. The most important mechanism by which materials pass between blood plasma and interstitial fluid is diffusion.

Sinusoidal (discontinuous) *capillaries* have a greatly enlarged diameter (e.g., 30–40 μm). In some regions, separations may occur between the endothelial cells in the wall of the sinusoid. The basal lamina surrounding the sinusoid may also be incomplete, and phagocytic cells are sometimes closely associated with the outer wall of the sinusoid. Sinusoidal capillaries are especially abundant in hematopoietic tissues (e.g., spleen and bone marrow) and in the liver.

THE ENDOTHELIUM

ORGANIZATION AND TRANSPORT

The endothelial cell is 25–50 μm long and 10–15 μm wide. The cells are oriented parallel to the long axis of the blood vessel (Figs. 15.17, 15.18). The shearing effect of blood flow affects the orientation of the endothelium. The endothelium is located between two major compartments of the body, the plasma in blood vessels and tissue fluid in the interstitial compartments. Therefore, endothelium is highly suited to mediate and regulate both unidirectional and bidirectional move-

Figure 15.11. Portion of an endothelial cell is enlarged to show micropinocytotic pits and vesicles (arrowheads) and basal lamina (*). ×90,000.

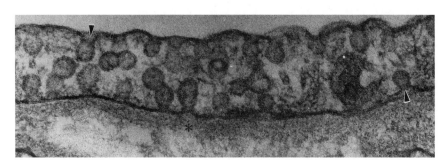

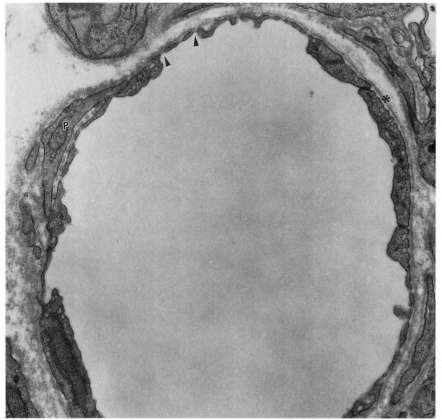

15.12

Figures 15.12, 15.13. TEM of a fenestrated capillary, part of which is enlarged in the lower figure. Fenestrations are denoted in both figures by arrowheads. Basal lamina (*). Portion of a pericyte (P). Figure 15.12, ×20,000; Fig. 15.13, ×100,000.

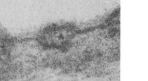

15.13

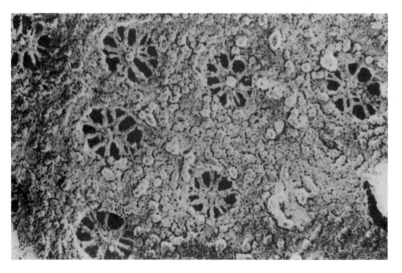

Figure 15.14. Several fenestral diaphragms on the etched luminal surface of a peritubular capillary in the rat kidney cortex. Note the numerous fibrils that arise from the pore rim and converge in the central region (preparation quick freeze, deep etch EM). (Reproduced from E. Baker and L. Orci, Endothelial fenestral diaphragms: A quick-freeze, deep-etch study. *Journal of Cell Biology* 1985, 100, 418–428, by copyright permission of The Rockefeller University Press)

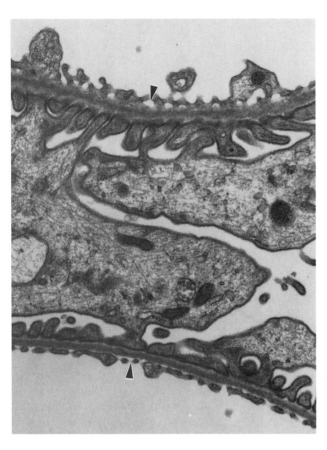

Figure 15.15. TEM of fenestrated endothelium of the renal glomerulus (arrowheads). ×17,500.

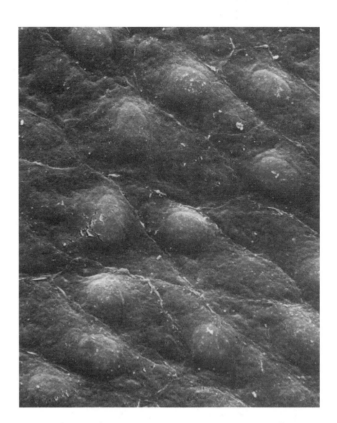

Figure 15.17. SEM of endothelial cells from rabbit endocardium. ×1430.

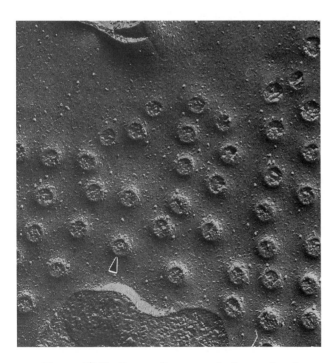

Figure 15.16. Freeze fracture of glomerular fenestrated endothelium; pores (arrowhead) are shown in surface view. ×35,000.

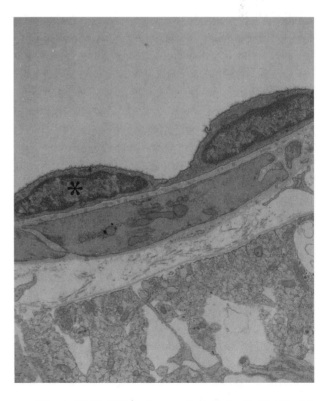

Figure 15.18. TEM of an endothelial cell (*). Nuclei cause bulging of cells seen with SEM. ×7825.

ment of diverse molecules, water, and ions that must be exchanged between these two large, significant compartments. In addition, endothelial cells may have perhaps as many as 10,000 small plasmalemmal vesicles per cell that are involved in transcellular transport or transcytosis (Figs. 15.8, 15.11). The plasmalemmal vesicles (60–70 nm) open to both the plasma front and tissue front of the endothelial cell, while some vesicles are located in the cytoplasm. Sometimes a group of vesicles exhibit continuity such that those attached to the plasma membrane and those in the cytoplasm are continuous, thus forming what has been called *thoroughfare channels*. The plasmalemmal vesicles are involved in the transendothelial transport of water-soluble molecules. The degree of transport can vary from single vesicle transport between plasma and tissue fronts to the more extensive transport indicated by the presence of patent thoroughfare channels traversing the endothelium.

JUNCTIONAL COMPLEXES

Endothelial cells are joined to each other by various types of junctions (Figs. 15.19, 15.20). Intracellular junctions play an important role in endothelial permeability. Possible endothelial junctions include tight junctions, adherens junctions, and syndesmos. A syndesmos is an adhering junction somewhat akin to a desmosome. However, while endothelial cells express plakoglobin and desmoplakin, endothelial cells do not express keratin, desmogleins, or desmocollins; hence true desmosomes are lacking in endothelium. Endothelial cells can rapidly change the type of junction to permit plasma

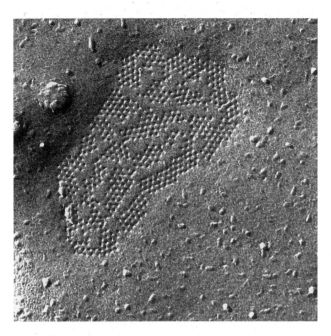

Figure 15.20. Freeze fracture of gap junction between endothelial cells. ×100,000.

and blood cells to exit the vessels (extravasation). Intercellular junctions are best developed in endothelium of large arteries but are largely absent in postcapillary venules, where cell extravasation and plasma exchange are particularly prevalent. In some areas where a barrier-type function is required, the endothelial cells are linked by *circumferential zonulae occludentes* (continuous tight junctions). These junctions are effective barriers to the movement of material through the intercellular space between endothelial cells. A basic feature of both the blood-brain barrier and the blood-retina barrier, for example, is the presence of circumferential zonulae occludentes in the endothelium. In terms of the development of tight junctions, the endothelia in the brain and retina are the tightest in the body. By contrast, endothelium in the bone marrow completely lacks tight junctions.

ENDOTHELIUM AS A SECRETORY CELL

The cytoplasm of the endothelial cell contains elements of the rER, free polyribosomes, a Golgi complex, mitochondria, some sER, centrioles, lysosomes, multivesicular bodies, and glycogen. Microfilaments and vimentin IFs are also present in the cell. The IFs are particularly prevalent in the perinuclear region, while the microfilaments are more concentrated in the peripheral cytoplasm. Endothelial cells can alter their shape and can shorten in response to histamine, for example. Rod-shaped granules (Weibel-Palade bodies ~0.1 μm in diameter and 3 μm in length) have been observed in the endothelial cytoplasm and appear to be the storage site

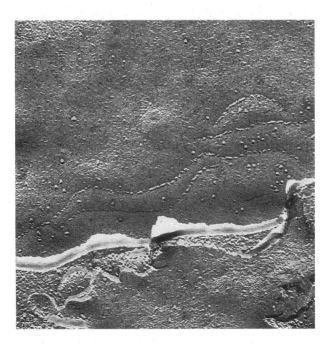

Figure 15.19. Freeze fracture of occluding junctions between endothelial cells. ×75,000.

of the von Willebrand factor, a major participant in platelet aggregation and adhesion. This factor serves as a carrier for factor VIII and is involved in platelet adhesion to the subendothelial extracellular matrix.

It appears that endothelial cells can divide, but at different rates. The endothelial cells lining the rabbit aorta appear to have a life span of 100 to perhaps 200 days, but the endothelium of veins divides more frequently. The luminal surface of the endothelial cells contains a cell coat containing a number of molecules. Some plasma proteins, such as α-2-macroglobulin, appear to be absorbed onto the surface of the endothelial cell and may protect the endothelium from proteolysis. The endothelium does not appear to be thrombogenic, as is the case for the subendothelial connective tissue, which attracts blood cells.

When endothelial cells are injured or the endothelial junctions are damaged or loosened (such as by a high concentration of histamine or serotonin), the platelets adhere to the area of vascular injury. The platelets in this region release serotonin, thrombospondin, thromboxane A_2 (this enhances platelet aggregation and thrombi formation), and *ADP*, and a platelet "plug" forms in the area. The thrombus enhances platelet aggregation since it results in the conversion of fibrinogen to fibrin. Heparin acts in an antagonistic manner by promoting thrombi neutralization by antithrombin III.

Endothelial cells are able to synthesize and secrete a variety of substances. Endothelial cells in the lung contribute to the metabolism of vasoactive substances. For example, a converting enzyme associated with lung endothelial cells is involved in the conversion of *angiotensin I* (a decapeptide) into an active octapeptide called *angiotensin II*. Endothelial cell enzymes are associated with the inactivation of norepinephrine, serotonin, and bradykinin. Endothelial cells also produce prostaglandins including prostacyclin, an antagonist of thromboxane A_2 that is produced by platelets. Endothelial cells also produce such coagulants as von Willebrand factor and plasminogen inhibitor. In addition, endothelium produces plasminogen activator and prostacyclin, which are anticoagulants. Plasminogen activator is a proteolytic enzyme that can activate plasmin, an active protease involved in tissue remodeling, as in wounds and inflammation. Plasminogen activator can degrade other proteins, either directly or indirectly; it also helps cells to dissolve their attachments and migrate through extracellular matrix. Endothelial cells can produce plasminogen activator, which permits the endothelial sprouts from capillaries to digest their way through the basal lamina of the parent capillary during angiogenesis. Endothelial cells have been described to produce other substances, including blood group antigens A and B, interferon A and B, and the constituents of its basal lamina (collagen IV, laminin, and entactin). Depending upon the specific location, endothelial cells can also express receptors; for example, insulin and transferrin.

Endothelial cells can also play important roles in the regulation and control of the contractile state of adjacent smooth muscle cells, in the proliferation of smooth muscle cells, and in the modulation of the function of white blood cells and platelets. It is now known that endothelial cells are able to synthesize and release substances that cause *vasorelaxation* [endothelium-derived relaxing factor (EDRF) or prostacyclin] or *vasoconstriction* [endothelium-derived contracting factor (EDCF)]. Thus, endothelial cells play an important role in cardiovascular homeostasis. The peptidergic EDCF has been isolated and identified as a 21-amino acid peptide called *endothelin* (*ET*). Endothelial-active molecules include proteins (e.g., platelet-derived growth factor and interleukins), peptides (e.g., endothelins), and smaller products (e.g., prostaglandins and EDRF). EDRF plays an important role in the regulation of vascular tone. For example, a primary effect of sympathetic stimulation of smooth muscle of coronary arteries is a contraction of this muscle. However, as a consequence of increased coronary blood flow, an EDRF is released, which causes a secondary effect of vessel dilation.

CAPILLARY BED-TRANSMURAL MIGRATION

Capillaries undergo extensive anastomoses in most organs, such as to form an extensive network of vessels for the microcirculation between the arterioles and venules. The enormity of the vascular capillary bed can be appreciated more fully when microvascular casts of the microcirculation are viewed in the SEM. For example, a portion of the circulatory system of the thyroid gland is illustrated in Figure 15.7. The rapid subdivision of vessels and their consequent decrease in size are evident.

Leukocytes can leave the bloodstream by passing between endothelial cells (*diapedesis*) to enter the tissue spaces. The movement of leukocytes into tissues involves specific leukocyte-endothelial cell interactions, with a number of cell adhesion molecules leading to attachment to and adhesion to endothelium followed by extravasation. A *selectin* family of cell adhesion molecules is associated with leukocyte attachment to endothelial cells that results in a rolling of leukocytes along the vessel wall. Another group of adhesion molecules called *integrins* are involved in the firm adhesion between leukocytes and endothelium prior to diapedesis. Increases in vascular permeability may be locally mediated by such agents as histamine and bradykinin. Capillaries that are involved in blood-tissue barriers (e.g., the blood-brain barrier) lack pores (fenestrations) or pinocytotic vesicles, but it is significant that continuous circumferential tight junctions are present.

ENDOTHELIUM-EPITHELIUM COMPARISONS

Endothelial cells differ from epithelium in several respects. Endothelium is derived from mesoderm and lacks epithelial cytokeratins. Rather, vimentin is the predominant *IF* in endothelium. Desmosomes, which are common in epithelia, are lacking in endothelium. Endothelial cells, like epithelia, have zonulae adherentes-type junctions and have a well-defined basement membrane or basal lamina. The endothelial tight junctions restrict pumps, channels, and transporters to the luminal (apical) or abluminal (basolateral) membrane, thus polarizing the endothelium. The circumferential tight junction is a barrier to diffusion, thereby permitting differences in the extracellular fluids on the inner and outer surfaces of the endothelial tubes.

VENOUS DIVISIONS OF THE CIRCULATORY SYSTEM

COMPARISON OF ARTERIES AND VEINS

Arteries and their companion veins of similar size and type are typically distributed throughout the body in close proximity to each other. This close spatial relationship frequently permits comparisons to be made in organization between the artery and its companion vein. In general, several differences in the companion vessels are apparent, including the following:

1. The lumen of an artery is smaller than its companion vein.
2. The wall of the artery is thicker and more rigid than its companion vein.
3. Arteries are generally better supplied with elastic fibers and smooth muscle cells than veins.
4. The tunica media of the artery is the thickest coat, while the tunica adventitia of veins is the thickest coat.
5. Veins tend to be more loosely constructed than arteries.
6. Collagen is more widely used in veins than in arteries, and
7. In general, the internal elastic lamina is better developed in arteries than in veins.

VENULES (SMALL VEINS)

Veins play an important role in storing extra blood and in the rapid control of cardiac output. Most of the extra blood in the circulation is stored in veins. When the veins constrict only slightly, extra blood is forced into the heart and causes the heart to pump much larger volumes. Veins exhibit much more variability than arteries. The smallest divisions beyond capillaries are usu-

ally called *postcapillary venules* and are some 10–30 μm in diameter. They are described to have increasing numbers of pericytes associated with them compared to the capillaries. The pericytes associated with a postcapillary venule are illustrated by the SEM in Figure 15.6. By the time these divisions approach 30–50 μm in diameter, they are called *collecting venules* and have collagen fibers and pericyte cells or fibroblasts associated with them. The collecting venules open into *muscular venules*, which are about 50–150 μm in diameter and have one or two layers of smooth muscle cells in their tunica media (Plate 37B). An internal elastic lamina may be present, and the tunica adventitia is quite well developed. These venules empty into collecting (medium-sized) veins that are some 100 to 300 μm in diameter and have several layers of smooth muscle in their tunica media. It is frequently difficult to distinguish histologically between postcapillary venules and collecting venules, as well as between muscular venules and small veins.

Venules are structurally quite variable. They have an endothelium, a tunica media with only one or two layers of smooth muscle, and an intervening internal elastic lamina. The adventitia layer is the thickest, consisting of connective tissue with abundant collagen fibers.

SMALL OR MEDIUM-SIZED VEINS

With the exception of the large main venous trunks, most of the veins in the body are small or medium-sized and are usually 1–9 μm in diameter. These vessels also have three tunics. The *tunica intima* consists of endothelium that resides directly on a poorly developed internal elastic lamina or a very thin layer of intervening connective tissue. The *tunica media* is much thinner than the companion artery. It is composed chiefly of spirally or circularly arranged smooth muscle cells, as well as a few collagenic and elastic fibers. The muscular media is well developed in the veins of limbs such as the saphenous vein. In a few veins of this type, the smooth muscle cells of the media have a longitudinal orientation. The tunica media is thicker and better developed in exposed veins than in deep veins; therefore the media is less muscular in deep veins of the limb, which are protected by muscles. The *tunica adventitia* is usually the thickest layer and consists chiefly of collagenic fibers. A few elastic fibers, and some amorphous intercellular substance and the cells that produced this material, are also present.

LARGE VEINS

The *tunica intima* is similar to the intima of medium-sized veins but usually has a thicker layer of subendothelial connective tissue (Plate 37D). The tunica intima consists of endothelium, subendothelial connective tissue, and an internal elastic lamina. The *tunica media* in most large veins has little smooth muscle. Thus, this layer is quite thin and contains principally fibrous connective tissue elements. The *tunica adventitia* is the thickest and best-developed layer of the three tunics. Longitudinally oriented smooth muscle bundles are commonly located in this layer. In the vena cava, the smooth muscle bundles are surrounded by both collagenic and elastic fibers.

Valves are widely distributed in veins of all sizes. The valves are folds of the tunica intima and consist of a layer of endothelium that encloses a small amount of subendothelial connective tissue. Valves are especially numerous in large veins of the arms and legs, and they assist in directing the flow of blood toward the right auricle when skeletal muscles surrounding these veins contract.

LYMPHATIC VESSELS

The walls of lymphatic vessels are constructed of an inner endothelial lining surrounded by a thin layer of connective tissue. In most lymphatic vessels, the layers found in the wall of the blood vessels are not well developed. The lymphatic vessels have funnel-shaped valves similar in construction to the valves located in the veins. The terminal lymphatic capillaries resemble blood capillaries; however, lymphatic capillaries do not show a well-developed basement membrane. Further lymphatic capillaries have no pericytes associated with them, and they originate as blind-end vessels. In addition, there are bundles of intercellular filaments about 5–10 nm in diameter associated with the outer surface of lymphatic capillaries. Some of these filaments appear to be collagen.

MEDICAL CONSIDERATIONS

Many blood vessels undergo gradual structural changes with increased age. Although the rate is variable, the coronary arteries tend to show early changes with aging. Weakening of the arterial wall occurs in certain diseases or other defects that can lead to a localized expansion, called an *aneurysm*, which might rupture. For example, individuals who exhibit a genetic deficiency of type III collagen production may be prone to rupture of the aorta. In *atherosclerosis* a thickening of the tunica intima occurs, with proliferation of smooth muscle cells and an increase in connective tissue. Smooth muscle cells and macrophages may become filled with cholesterol deposits. The thickened vessel wall may eventually become occluded, as commonly occurs in coronary arteries. Arteries in the heart, cerebrum, and kidneys, for example, are prone to develop local areas of necrosis or death with aging, and this can eventually result in vessel rupture. Angiotensin is a polypeptide that binds vascular endothelial cells. When this occurs, arterial smooth muscle cells contract, resulting in increased blood pressure.

SELECTED BIBLIOGRAPHY

Bearer, E.L., and Orci, L. (1985). Endothelial fenestral diaphragms: a quick-freeze, deep etch study. *J. Cell Biol.* **100**, 418.

Challice, C.E., and Viragh, S., eds. (1973). *Ultrastructure of the Mammalian Heart.* Academic Press, Orlando, FL.

Cliff, W.J. (1976). *Blood Vessels.* Cambridge University Press, Cambridge.

D'Amore, P.A. (1992). Capillary growth: a two-cell system. *Semin. Cancer Biol.* **3**, 49–56.

Davies, P.F., and Tripathi, S.C. (1993). Mechanical stress mechanisms and the cell. An endothelial paradigm. *Circ. Res.* **72**, 239–245.

Fujiwara, T., and Uehara, T. (1982). Scanning electron microscopical study of vascular smooth muscle cells in mesenteric vessels of the monkey. *Biomed. Res.* **3**, 649.

Johnson, P.C. (1978). *Peripheral Circulation.* Wiley, New York.

McEver, R.P. (1992). Leukocyte-endothelial cell interactions. *Curr. Opin. Cell Biol.* **4**, 840–849.

Mostov, K.E., and Simister, N.E. (1985). Transcytosis. *Cell* **43**, 389–390.

Palade, G.E. (1988). The microvascular endothelium revisited. In *Endothelial Cell Biology in Health and Disease*, N. Simionescu and M. Simionescu, eds. Plenum, New York.

Rubanyi, G.M. (1991). Endothelium-derived relaxing and contracting factors. *J. Cell. Biochem.* **46**, 27–36.

Shepro, D., and Morel, N. (1993). Pericyte physiology. *FASEB J.* **7**, 1031–1038.

Simionescu, M., and Simionescu, N. (1991). Endothelial transport of macromolecules: transcytosis and endocytosis. A look from cell biology. *Cell Biol. Rev.* **25**, 1–78.

Vanhoutte, P.M., Rubanyi, G.M., Miller, V.M., and Houston, D.S. (1986). Modulation of vascular smooth muscle contraction by the endothelium. *Annu. Rev. Physiol.* **48**, 307.

Zilla, P., von Oppel, U., and Deutsch, M. (1993). The endothelium: a key to the future. *J. Cardiol. Surg.* **8**, 32–60.

Zimmerman, G.A., Prescott, S.M., and McIntyre, T.M. (1992). Endothelial cell interactions with granulocytes: tethering and signaling molecules. *Immunol. Today* **13**, 93.

The Integument

The integumentary system consists of skin and its derivatives and is the human body's largest organ. The integument forms the external covering of the body and is made up of a cellular but avascular epidermis derived from ectoderm and a connective tissue dermis that is vascularized and derived from mesoderm (Plate 38A–D). The outer *epidermis* consists of tiers of cells that are constantly being replaced from the inside toward the outside. Blood vessels do not penetrate the basement membrane that forms the boundary between the dermis and epidermis. The thickness of both epidermis and dermis can vary from approximately 0.5 mm to 3 or 4 mm. The undersurface of the dermis is attached to *subcutaneous tissue*, also called *hypodermis* or *superficial fascia* (Fig. 16.1). The hypodermis is often heavily infiltrated with adipocytes.

Derivatives of the epidermis can be produced by cell proliferation in its basal layer, followed by downgrowth of these cells into the dermis and by cellular differentation. In humans, these epidermal derivatives include *sweat* (sudoriferous) *glands, hair follicles, sebaceous glands, fingernails,* and *toenails.*

DEVELOPMENT

In the third and fourth months of fetal life, the palms of the hands and soles of the feet, as well as the tips of fingers and toes, are covered by epidermal ridges and grooves and look somewhat like a field "plowed by contour." The epidermal ridges are caused by the epidermis following the scalloped contour of the underlying dermal ridges. During subsequent development, the epidermis grows down (downgrowths are called *inter-*

papillary pegs) into the primary dermal ridge such that each primary dermal ridge is divided into secondary dermal ridges. However, in regions that become thin skin, the epithelial downgrowths are more numerous and restricted in their extent, producing secondary dermal papillae rather than ridges. Eccrine sweat gland ducts open at the tips of the interpapillary pegs.

The development of the skin thus begins very early in the embryo, and early on the epidermis begins to differentiate its derivatives including hair, nails, sebaceous glands, and sweat glands. Hair begins to form on the head of a fetus at about 3 months. By the time of birth, all the hair follicles that the infant will ever possess are present. However, many of the hairs do not begin to grow until puberty. Also, in humans, the female has roughly the same number of hair follicles as a male, but many follicles in the female are very small and colorless, so they frequently are not noticed. With adolescence, the sweat glands and sebaceous glands change from a rather dormant state to a state of full activity.

DIAGNOSIS

The integument is a useful organ for the diagnosis of many diseases and constitutes the basis for the branch of medicine called *dermatology.* The integument is a visible structure that requires no exploratory operations. Its texture and color are frequently useful in the diagnosis of circulatory impairments (cyanosis, blue lips); vitamin deficiency (skin is rough and scaly in vitamin A deficiency); and specific skin eruptions associated with allergies and childhood diseases such as scarlet fever, chicken pox, and measles.

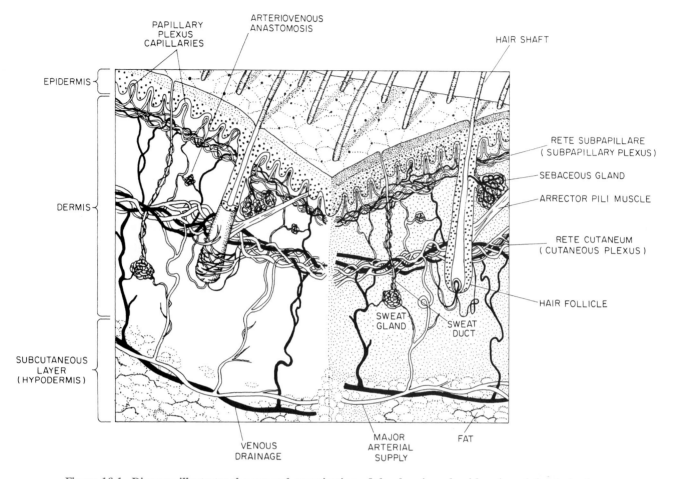

Figure 16.1. Diagram illustrates the general organization of the dermis and epidermis and the derivatives.

FUNCTIONS

The integument serves a variety of functions, among the most important of which is protection of the body from physical, chemical, and biological insults. The epidermal cells (keratinocytes) differentiate into keratin. This outer layer of the epidermis is particularly thick and more resistant to friction on the surface of the hands (palmar surfaces) and feet (plantar surfaces). The very inert protein keratin serves as a barrier to water loss and bacterial invasion. The melanin in epidermal melanocytes serves, within limits, to protect from the harmful ultraviolet component of sunlight. In addition, vitamin D is manufactured in skin that is exposed to ultraviolet rays. Vitamin D is irradiated ergosterol, which is a derivative of cholesterol. Vitamin D is necessary for proper mineral metabolism, and the lack of sufficient vitamin D in children can produce rickets. In addition, the integument contains structures that permit detection or reception of stimuli such as pain, deep pressure, touch, and temperature. The presence of sweat glands permits the body to regulate its temperature, and some substances are excreted in sweat. The dermis contains dense, irregular connective tissue that is somewhat re-

sistant to physical injury. When large areas of the integument are injured, as in burns, many adverse effects are produced including severe dehydration and electrolyte imbalance. The individual may be unable to regulate body temperature, and such external factors as chemicals and microorganisms can produce infection or other toxic phenomena. In addition, various sensations such as those for touch, pressure, and temperature are lost.

ORGANIZATION OF EPIDERMIS

LAYERS

Mitotic cells occur in the basal layer of epidermal cells, the *stratum basale* (*germinativum*). Melanocytes are intermixed with the mitotic cells in this layer (Fig. 16.2). As the cells divide, they are pushed more superficially and become polygonal in shape. In this region, called the *stratum spinosum* (stratum Malpighii), the cells develop numerous maculae adherentes or spot desmosomes that anchor the cells and prevent their mechanical separation (Plate 38D). As the cells move farther

Comparison of Soft and Hard Keratin

	Location	Physical and Chemical Characteristics
Soft keratin	Stratum granulosum of epidermis; called *kerato*hyaline; basophilic	More reactive, less permanent than hard keratin
	Inner root sheath of hair (Henle's layer, Huxley's layer, and cuticle of inner root sheath) and hair medulla; called *trichohyalin*; acidophilic	Continuous desquamation, no increase in size
Hard keratin	Cuticle of hair, hair cortex fingernails, and toenails	Does not desquamate; more permanent; chemically unreactive; S—S chemical bonds; contains cystine

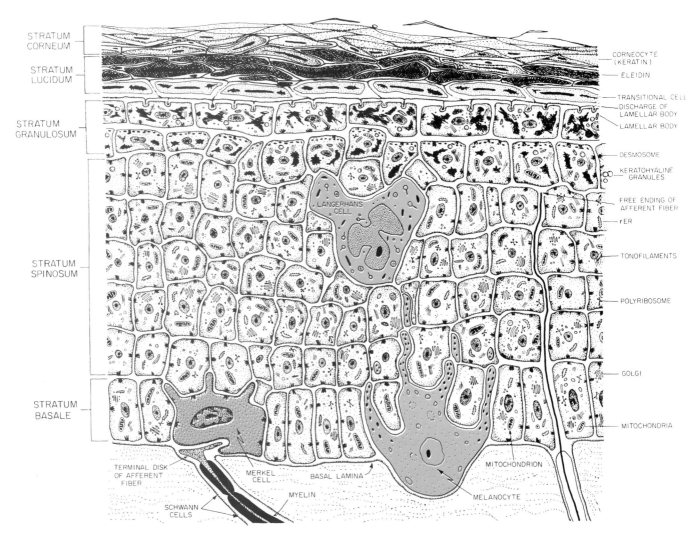

Figure 16.2. Diagram of the epidermis illustrating the layers and cell types present.

from the blood vessels in the dermal papillae or ridges, they initiate a transformation into keratin that leads to their death. These cells, called *keratinocytes*, comprise about 85% of the epidermal cells. During keratinization, keratohyalin (soft keratin) granules (Figs. 16.2, 16.3) appear within cells of the *stratum granulosum*, which is only one to three cell layers thick. The basophilic keratohyalin is converted into eleidin, which is present in a layer of thick skin called the *stratum lucidum* (Plate 38B; Fig. 16.3). A few pyknotic nuclei may be present in this layer (Plate 38B). The most superficial part of the epidermis is a layer of corneocytes (transformed keratinocytes) called the *stratum corneum*, which consists of the tough, impermeable, albuminoid protein called keratin (Figs. 16.2–16.4).

Keratin covers the outer layer of the epidermis in thick and thin skin. Keratin is *not* a secretory product of the cells, but results instead from the tranformation of cells called *keratinocytes*. As the cells move from the base of the epithelium, they change in shape from columnar, to polygonal, to flattened or squamous, to scales. On the superficial surface of the epidermis, the keratin scales are worn away from the surface. They are said to *desquamate*, and the process of this shedding is called *desquamation*. The keratin scales (squames) are replaced by underlying living cells that become keratinized. The keratin on the human plantar epidermis is completely replaced in about 1 month.

KERATINOCYTES

The keratinocyte is so named because its most abundant protein is keratin. The inner part of the epidermis contains living cells, principally the *keratinocyte* (Fig. 16.2). The outer part of the epidermis contains skeletons of cells called *corneocytes* (Fig. 16.2). During differentiation the living keratinocyte is transformed into a dead corneocyte. While the corneocytes are not living, they function to prevent dessication, provide resistance to chemical and physical injury, and resist attack by microorganisms. It is quite unusual that this cellular transformation results in a dead cell that is much more able to carry out its functions than the living cell from which it developed! Keratinocytes are generated in the basal layer of the epidermis and prepare to become corneocytes through increased specialization (terminal differentiation) followed by programmed death. Several

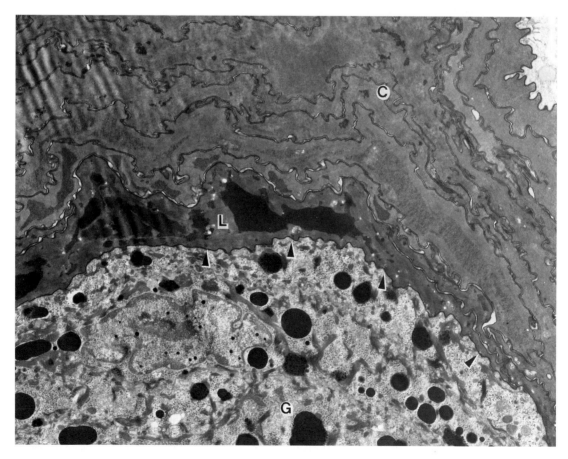

Figure 16.3. TEM of the stratum granulosum (G) with keratohyalin granules, stratum lucidum (L), and the corneocytes (C) of the stratum corneum. Note the thickened membrane (arrowhead) between the granulosum and lucidum. ×7500.

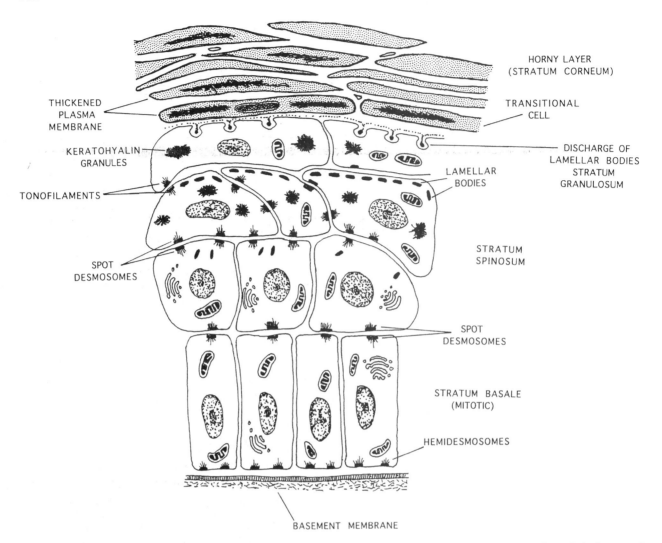

Figure 16.4. Diagram of the formation and extrusion of lamellar bodies and the development of a relatively water-impermeable portion of the epidermis.

weeks may be required for a recently formed keratinocyte to move through the layers of the epidermis and to be shed (desquamate) from the outer surface as a corneocyte. The keratinocyte contains rER, mitochondria, Golgi complex, free polyribosomes, 10-nm filaments (keratin), and lysosomes. The functions ascribed to the keratinocyte are diverse.

1. Surface keratinocytes synthesize a glycolipid (acylglucosylceramide molecules) in lamellar bodies, which then undergo exocytosis to form a waterproof barrier (see the later discussion).
2. The cells synthesize soft keratin, called *keratohyalin* (basophilic), by free polyribosomes (keratohyalin + tonofilaments rapidly give rise to keratin). Surface keratinocytes have thickened plasma membranes. The surface cells produce an acid phosphatase that is thought to cause exfoliation or sloughing.
3. The cells may produce a thymulin or thymopoietin-like substance to enhance T-lymphocyte proliferation.
4. Keratinocytes ingest and digest melanin granules from melanocytes in Caucasians.
5. The cells are thought to release *IL-1*, which is also released from Langerhans cells. The binding of IL-1 to appropriate T4 helper cell receptors causes the T4 helper cells to produce *IL-2* receptors and to release IL-2. When these interact or combine, the T4 cells are activated to proliferate and produce α-IFN, which can stimulate the cytotoxic activity of T killer cells.

    The Langerhans cell (Fig. 16.2) is an antigen-presenting cell (APC) that is able to process antigen and present it in conjunction with MHC proteins. This process may activate appropriate T4 (helper) cells to produce IL-2 receptors, release IL-2, and, after combination, stimulate lymphocyte proliferation.
6. Keratinocytes are also able to synthesize and se-

crete several polypeptide growth factors, such as *epidermal growth factor* and *transforming growth factor-α* (*TGF-α*). TGF-α is a polypeptide that stimulates proliferation and migration of keratinocytes. Therefore, keratinocytes are autocrine since the growth factors that they produce and release stimulate their own growth. In addition, fibroblasts in the connective tissue of the dermis produce substances that are necessary for optimal proliferation of keratinocytes.

The keratinocyte begins the synthesis of *keratohyaline granules* and *lamellar bodies* near the border of the stratum spinosum and stratum granulosum (Fig. 16.4). The keratohyaline granules appear to be synthesized by free polyribosomes, and the cells become virtually filled with these granules. The keratohyaline granules contain a material that combines with the tonofilaments to become *soft keratin.* During this process, the nucleus and organelles degenerate and the plasma membrane becomes thickened (Fig. 16.4). At the time that the keratohyaline bodies are formed, the cells produce lamellar bodies that are rich in *glycolipid*, which functions as a water barrier. The lamellar bodies are formed intracellularly and are discharged into the extracellular space of the stratum granulosum to form a waterproof layer (Fig. 16.4). Intercellular fluids between the epidermal cells and tissue fluid in the connective tissue of the papillary layer of the dermis would be lost, constituting a life-threatening situation, were it not for the waterproofing glycolipid released from the cells in the stratum granulosum.

The *integrins* are cell surface molecules that play important roles in cell-cell and cell-matrix interaction. Integrins are transmembrane glycoproteins and consist of noncovalently associated α and β subunits. Integrins are expressed by basally located keratinocytes in the epidermis but are not associated with more superficially located cells. Thus, the keratinocytes lose adhesive properties as they move away from the basement membrane.

MELANOCYTES

Melanocytes are derived from neural crest cells that separate from the neural tube during its closure in the early embryo. The cells then undergo massive migration to the basal layer of the epidermis (Fig. 16.5). The melanocytes number about 1 in 4 to 1 in 10 of the basal cells. The melanocytes have several long, thin branches that extend among the keratinocytes in the epidermis.

Melanin is an endogenous integument pigment produced by the melanocytes (Fig. 16.5). *Tyrosinase* is synthesized in the rER of melanocytes and is packaged in the Golgi apparatus into premelanosomes. The tyrosinase appears to be used to produce *dihydroxyphe-*

nylalanine (*dopa*) from *tyrosine*. When melanin appears in the premelanosomes, they are called *melanosomes.* The melanin granules move into the dendritic processes and are phagocytosed by the surrounding keratinocytes. This cell-to-cell transfer (i.e., from melanocytes to keratinocytes) is called *cytocrine secretion.*

$$\text{Tyrosine} \xrightarrow[\text{tyrosinase}]{\overset{\text{oxidized}}{\underset{}{\text{by}}}} \text{Dopa} \xrightarrow[\text{tyrosinase}]{\overset{\text{oxidized}}{\underset{}{\text{by}}}} \text{Dopaquinone} \xrightarrow[\text{intermediates}]{\text{several}} \text{Melanin}$$

The melanin produced in melanocytes is ingested into surrounding keratinocytes by phagocytosis (Fig. 16.5). In Caucasians the melanin is degraded by lysosomes in the keratinocytes. However, in Negroids the melanin granules are more stable and are not degraded.

When skin is exposed to ultraviolet light, increased amounts of melanin are produced and suntan results. In some individuals, melanin may form in patches, which is the basis of freckles. To some degree, the effect of the ultraviolet light of sunlight on skin is beneficial because it irradiates ergosterol, a cholesterol derivative. Vitamin D is irradiated ergosterol. Overexposure to ultraviolet light (from about 280 to 320 nm) appears to be closely associated with the development of epithelial skin cancers. Melanin tends to scatter excessive ultraviolet rays, thereby protecting the deepest cells in the epidermis. Ultraviolet irradiation is necessary to cause a moderate sunburn because the capillaries and venules in the papillary and subpapillary regions dilate. In more severe cases of sunburn, tissue fluid leaks from the capillaries and venules, and the fluid accumulates between the epidermis and dermis to form a blister. When severe burns occur, epithelial cells in the deep regions of the hair follicles proliferate and form a new layer at the interface between the living and nonliving regions of the dermis. Gray hair may be due to the inability of melanocytes to make tyrosinase.

IMMUNITY AND LANGERHANS CELLS

The skin appears to be an important site where certain types of lymphocytes, particularly *T helper cells*, undergo maturation. Thus, a major T-cell population is present in the epidermis. There is some evidence that keratinocytes are capable of producing a substance similar to the hormone thymopoietin (thymulin), which is produced in the thymus and which influences T-cell maturation. Cultured epidermal keratinocytes can synthesize *IL-1*, which is also produced by APCs such as macrophages. IL-1 binds to responsive T-cell receptors, and these particular T cells release *IL-2*. IL-2, in turn, promotes T-cell proliferation in response to the specific

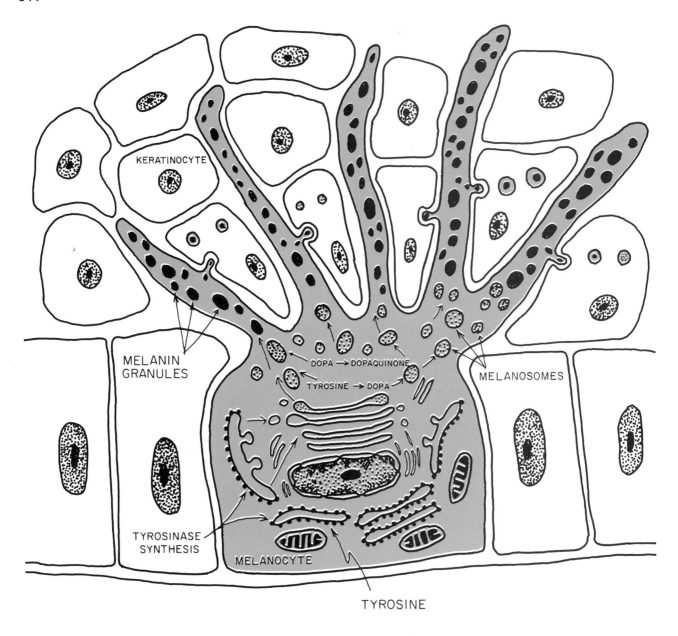

KERATINOCYTE

MELANIN
GRANULES

DOPA → DOPAQUINONE

TYROSINE → DOPA

MELANOSOMES

TYROSINASE
SYNTHESIS

MELANOCYTE

TYROSINE

$$\text{TYROSINE} \xrightarrow{\text{TYROSINASE}} \text{DOPA}$$

Figure 16.5. Diagram of a melanocyte and its role in the synthesis of melanin.

immunologic challenge to produce α-IFN, which stimulates the cytotoxic activity of T cells.

Langerhans cells represent another cell type in the epidermis (Fig. 16.2). Special staining methods are required to demonstrate these cells, but they are thought to be a type of macrophage. The cells originate in the bone marrow and are transported to the integument in the vascular system. Langerhans cells possess dendritic processes and contain racket-shaped cytoplasmic granules that are not evident in H&E-stained sections. It has been suggested that the cells may be involved in antigen recognition (immunity) in the skin. Langerhans cells are thought to be important in processing and presenting antigen to T-helper cells.

In terms of the coordinated responses to immunologic reactions in the skin, the following events are presently considered likely to occur. If a foreign antigen penetrates the stratum corneum, it encounters Langerhans cells, which present this antigen, together with an MHC protein, to T cells in the epidermis that might be programmed to respond to the particular antigen that entered. The T cells become activated and expose a receptor for IL-1 that can be produced by keratinocytes. The binding of the IL-1 to receptors activates the T cell, so that it produces and releases IL-2. IL-2 binds to receptors on other responsive T cells in various lymphoid tissues and causes proliferation, thus forming a large population of T cells able to react to the antigen.

DERMIS

Two layers of the dermis are usually distinguished: (1) a *papillary layer* adjacent to the epidermis and (2) a *reticular layer* that consists of more densely arranged connective tissue. The reticular layer of the dermis is attached to or continuous with the hypodermis, which is mainly loose areolar connective tissue with accumulations of fat. Fat is stored (as paniculus adiposus) in many regions of the hypodermis but is never found in the eyelids, scrotum, or penis.

TYPES OF SKIN

Skin is commonly classified as (1) *thick skin*, which is found on the fingers, palms, and bottom of the feet and toes, and (2) *thin skin*, which covers the remainder of the body (Plate 38A–C). The terms *thick* and *thin* refer only to the width of the epidermal layer. When sections of thick and thin skin are compared histologically, the stratum germinativum or basale is found to be similar in both types. The stratum spinosum is usually thinner in thin skin. The stratum granulosum is not as prominent in thin skin and may not be a continuous layer. The stratum lucidum is not found in thin skin. The stratum corneum is very much thinner in thin skin.

CIRCULATORY SYSTEM

A flat layer of vessels is located in the papillary layer of the dermis, and these vessels comprise the *rete subpapillare* (Fig. 16.1). Capillary loops extend into the connective tissue papillae, and these capillary plexuses supply tissue fluid to the basal layer of cells in the epidermis. Another flat plexus of vessels is located in the middle region of the reticular dermis, and this network is called the *rete cutaneum* (Fig. 16.1). Subcutaneous arteries and veins are also located in the hypodermis. Branches of the plexuses supply a rich capillary bed to the papilla of the hair follicle and to sebaceous and sweat glands, as well as to accumulations of adipose tissue.

The circulatory system of the integument is very extensive and provides the skin with more blood than is needed simply to nourish the cells there. The extensive system of blood vessels cools the body. During rigorous activity, the sweat glands pour water onto the skin surface, and the evaporation of this water cools the blood circulating through the capillaries of the dermis. At high temperatures, blood vessels in the dermis dilate and there is increased secretory activity of sweat glands; both activities are important in temperature regulation. Conversely, at low temperatures, blood vessels in the dermis constrict and the sweat glands become more inactive. When the temperature is high and during vigorous exercise, the smooth muscle in the walls of the blood vessels relax so that more blood flows through the integu-

ment; hence, a "flushed" appearance is noted. In contrast, during cold weather, the smooth muscles in the blood vessel walls contract markedly, reducing the flow of blood through the skin and thereby conserving body heat. In addition, blood vessels in the skin assist in regulating blood pressure. There are arteriovenous shunts in the blood vessels such that blood may bypass capillaries and flow directly from small arteries into veins. Such a mechanism serves as a safety valve against marked blood pressure elevation.

NERVES AND SENSORY RECEPTORS

The integument contains an abundant supply of nerves that innervate the many blood vessels present, as well as sweat glands, hairs, sebaceous glands, and arrector pili muscle. The presence of a vast array of sensory receptors attests to the importance of the integument in mediating the interaction of the organism with its environment. Sensory receptors present in the integument include both free and encapsulated nerve endings.

MERKEL'S DISK

Merkel's disk or ending is a modified epidermal cell in the stratum basale whose base is flattened and a free nerve ending is flattened against the base of this cell (Fig. 16.2). The apical part of the cell extends several broad, finger-like projections into the keratinocyte layer, and desmosomes anchor the Merkel cell and the surrounding cells. Merkel endings are able to transduce stimulus energy into an afferent nerve impulse. This receptor is thought to be a mechanoreceptor that responds to displacement due to touch, pressure, or stretch. Two other types of cutaneous sensory receptors are *thermoreceptors* and *nociceptors*.

FREE NERVE ENDINGS

Some afferent nerve fibers lose their Schwann cells and myelin and either enter the epidermis, where they are located among the keratinocytes, or are present in the papillary layer of the dermis. The function of these nerve endings is unknown, but they are thought to be thermoreceptors or nociceptors. A network of free nerve endings also envelopes the hair follicles, and branches extend into the external root sheath of the hair follicle. These nerves appear to be sensitive to hair displacement and are thus mechanoreceptors.

PACINIAN CORPUSCLES

Pacinian corpuscles (corpuscles of Vater-Pacini) are encapsulated mechanoreceptors that are located in the dermis and subcutaneous tissue, including a distribution in mesenteries, wall of the urinary bladder, external genitalia, and joint capsules (illustrated in Chapter 10). The oval corpuscles may range up to 1 or 2 mm in length. The myelinated nerve loses the myelin just inside the corpuscle but extends to the area near the opposite pole of the corpuscle. The nerve is surrounded by numerous highly flattened cells whose function is unknown. The Pacinian corpuscle is sensitive to vibrations as well as deep pressure, but the exact mechanism by which the sensations are detected is unclear.

MEISSNER'S CORPUSCLES

These touch receptors are located in the papillae of the papillary layer of the dermis, especially in thick skin. They are also located in the eyelid, external genitalia, nipples, and lips, as well as on the plantar surface of the feet. The corpuscle is an oval structure; the nerve extends in a spiral throughout its length, and stacks of flattened cells surround the nerve. The flattened cells surrounding the nerve are considered to be modified Schwann cells (illustrated in Chapter 10).

RUFFINI CYLINDERS (CORPUSCLES)

These sensory endings are located deep in the dermis and in the subcutaneous tissue and are particularly numerous on the plantar surface of the feet. The myelinated afferent nerve loses its myelin, and the nerve branches extensively to surround collagen fibers bundles in the center of the corpuscle. The receptors appear to be mechanoreceptors that are stimulated by the displacement of the collagen fibers with which they are closely associated. Structurally, the Ruffini corpuscles are similar to the Golgi tendon organs. It is thought that the nerves are responsive to the degree of tension in the collagen fibers in the dermis.

KRAUSE END BULBS

In these receptors, the afferent myelinated fiber branches repeatedly inside the capsule to form a network of unmyelinated nerve processes. The function of these receptors is unclear, but they are considered to be some type of mechanoreceptor. They are distributed in the papillary layer of the dermis of the conjunctiva,

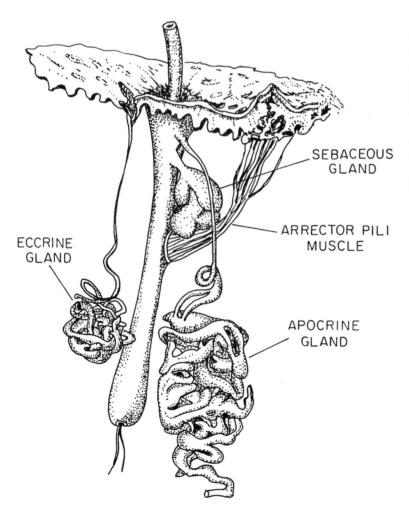

Figure 16.6. Relationship of apocrine and eccrine sweat glands to epidermis. Apocrine sweat glands open into hair follicles while eccrine sweat gland open into epidermis. Note the arrector pili smooth muscle and its attachment to hair follicle and the undersurface of epidermis. (Redrawn from W. Montagna and P. Parakkal. The Structure and Function of Skin, Academic Press, Orlando 1974)

SEBACEOUS GLAND

ARRECTOR PILI MUSCLE

ECCRINE GLAND

APOCRINE GLAND

and are also present in the connective tissue of the tongue, mouth, pharynx, and external genitalia.

GERMINATION OF HAIR

Hair follicles begin to differentitate during the third month of fetal life and are marked by localized downgrowths of epidermis into the dermis and hypodermis (Fig. 16.6). In 5- and 6-month-old embryos, delicate hairs called *lanugo* cover the fetus. This hair is shed, but the hairs in the eyebrows, eyelids, and scalp are not. Hair follicles are not formed after birth. At puberty in males, coarse hairs develop in the axilla, pubic region, and face because of the influence of testosterone.

Germination of a hair involves the formation of two types of keratin. *Hard keratin* is present in the *cuticle* of the *hair* and the *hair cortex* (Figs. 16.7, 16.8). It also occurs in the *nails* of both fingers and toes. Hard keratin is quite unreactive and contains considerable amounts of S-S (disulfide) bonds and cystine. Its production does not involve the formation of keratohyalin (or trichohyalin) granules. Hard keratin does not desquamate, which explains the necessity for haircuts and the need to trim fingernails and toenails. *Soft keratin* is present in the epidermis of skin. Its formation does involve the formation of keratohyalin and trichohyalin granules. Soft keratin desquamates and is less permanent than hard keratin.

During the formation of a hair follicle, the epidermis grows into the dermis in the form of a long, solid column of cells that are collectively called the *external root sheath*. The deepest part of the external root sheath is called the *germinal matrix* or *hair matrix*, for it is these epithelial cells that will subsequently cause the hair to germinate. The proliferative cells in the germinal matrix are closely associated with a *connective tissue papilla* that is derived from the dermis and contains a network of blood capillaries. The connective tissue papilla is richly vascularized so that nutrients and wastes can easily diffuse between the vessels and the cells in the germinal matrix.

Growth of the hair is initiated when proliferation of cells in the germinal hair matrix commences. As the cells divide, the progeny are pushed up the center of the epithelial downgrowth. As the cells become pushed farther and farther away from the capillaries in the connective tissue papilla, they begin to transform into keratin. Initially, the proliferating cells develop into *hard keratin* and form the *cuticle* of the *hair* and the *hair cortex*. Following this burst of activity, another extensive proliferation occurs by the cells in the proliferating germinal matrix. These cells comprise an *internal root sheath* that extends upward to surround the previously formed hair cuticle and hair cortex. The internal root sheath, however, extends only partially up the forming follicle.

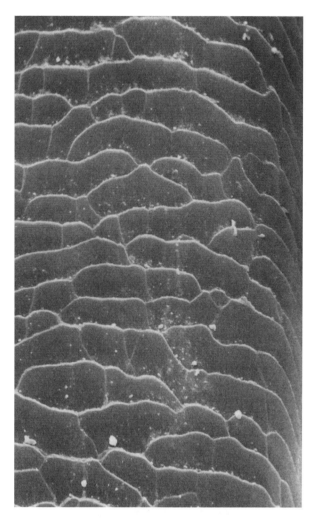

Figure 16.7. Human hair (SEM) showing the shingle-like appearance of the cuticle of the hair cells. ×1425. (From R. Kessel and R. Kardon. *Tissues and Organs: A Text-Atlas of Scanning Electron Microscopy.* W.H. Freeman, New York, 1979, with permission)

The internal root sheath differentiates into three distinct layers, each of which is only one cell thick. From inside the follicle to outside, the layers are *the cuticle of the inner root sheath, Huxley's layer,* and *Henle's layer.* All cell layers comprising the internal root sheath contain *soft keratin.* However, the soft keratin granules in Henle's and Huxley's layers stain acidophilic rather than basophilic, as is the case for the stratum granulosum in the epidermis. The acidophilic-staining soft keratin is called *trichohyalin,* to distinguish it from the basophilic soft keratin in the stratum granulosum layer, which is called *keratohyalin.* Not all hairs contain a central *medulla.* However, when the hair medulla is present, the cells contain trichohyalin granules of soft keratin. The remainder of the original cellular downgrowth persists as the external root sheath. The terminal hairs that extend above the epidermis may or may not consist of a central medulla of soft keratin surrounded by a cortex

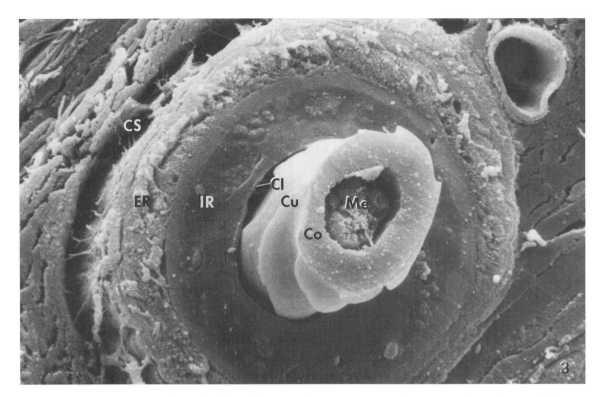

Figure 16.8. Section of hair. SEM. Medulla (Me), hair cortex (Co), cuticle of hair (Cu), cuticle of inner root sheath (Cl), inner root sheath (IR), external root sheath (ER), and connective tissue sheath (CS) are identified. ×4200. (From R. Kessel and R. Kardon. *Tissues and Organs: A Text-Atlas of Scanning Electron Microscopy.* W.H. Freeman, New York, 1979, with permission)

and cuticle of hard keratin. Some hairs contain only a poorly developed medulla. Layers of the hair follicle are illustrated and identified in Plate 39A–C.

The hair cuticle consists of thin, overlapping scale-like cells whose free edges are directed toward the tip of the hair (Figs. 16.7, 16.8). The cuticles of the inner root sheath cells are also flattened, and their free margins are directed downward; hence, they interlock with cuticle of the hair cells. This arrangement makes it difficult to pull hairs out of the follicle without removing a portion of the adjacent internal root sheath that joins it farther down in the hair follicle.

COLOR

The color of hair is due to the amount and kind of melanin present in the hair cortex layer. Although hair can be of different colors, the pigment in hair as observed with a microscope can be *black, brown,* or *yellow.* Yellow melanin is called *pheomelanin,* while brown and black melanins are called *eumelanin.* The amount of eumelanin and pheomelanin and the type of eumelanin are genetically determined.

GROWTH

Hair growth is a cyclic phenomenon, and different hair follicles commonly alternate between phases of activity and inactivity. Periodically, new hairs are germinated to replace old ones. In some animals, almost all hair is shed at one time, which necessitates the acquisition of a completely new crop of hair. In humans, hair growth is more asynchronous, with hair follicles on an individual existing in different states of growth and resting periods.

BALDNESS

Genetic factors are responsible for baldness. However, genetic factors that tend to cause *baldness* can be fully effective only if male sex hormones (androgens) are present in sufficient quantity. Castration, and hence the lack of male sex hormone production, would tend to hold in check any hereditary tendency to develop baldness. Eunuchs have a deficiency of male sex hormones and they rarely are bald. Aristotle, who was bald, noted this situation in eunuchs. The loss of hair occurs early in humans. Even in the fetus, the entire head, including the forehead, is covered by hair. After about the fifth month of fetal life, the hair follicles in the forehead involute and are normally absent at birth. However, there are some cases on record of individuals who have a bushy growth of hair on the forehead like that on the scalp. It has been stated that, evolutionarily speaking, humans are becoming increasingly bald, which has broad and significant ramifications, if true. Reports are on record of scalp hair growing to a length of 12 feet if not cut. Androgens not only affect hair growth but are also responsible under certain genetic conditions for the loss of scalp hair.

EPIDERMAL REPAIR

While hair in humans is not very important to keep the body warm, it is important in repair of the epidermis necessitated by burns, for example. The proliferative cells remaining in the germinal matrix can participate in some regeneration and also are useful in split-skin grafting. Human hair grows at a rate of approximately one third of a millimeter per day. The follicle is set in the integument at an angle so that the hair lies generally upon the skin, except when smooth muscle cells attached to the hair follicle contract.

ARRECTOR PILI

In thin skin especially, each hair follicle has a bundle of smooth muscle associated with it that is called the *arrector pili muscle* (Fig. 16.6). The arrector pili muscle is attached to the connective tissue sheath near the hair base and extends to the papillary layer of the dermis. The arrector pili muscle is located on the same side of the hair follicle as the sebaceous gland (Fig. 16.7). When the muscle contracts, the hair follicle is straightened or becomes more upright, and the contraction causes pressure on the sebaceous gland so as to assist in expressing secretion (sebum) into the hair follicle. The arrector pili muscles are innervated by the sympathetic division of the ANS. Cold is a common stimulus for the reflex activity that leads to contraction of the smooth muscle, leading to a condition known as "goose bumps" or "goose pimples." The epinephrine that is released during flight or fear may also cause contraction of the arrector pili muscles. The arrector pili muscles are much better developed in cats than in humans.

SEBACEOUS GLANDS

There are two major kinds of secretory glands in the integument of humans. One of these, the sebaceous gland, develops as an outgrowth of the cellular downgrowth that will ultimately form the hair follicle (Fig.

16.6). As a consequence, the sebaceous gland retains a connection to the hair follicle. The gland produces *sebum*, which is an oily mixture of fatty acids, cholesterol, triglycerides, and cell debris. The cells proliferate at the base of the sebaceous gland and begin to accumulate the secretory product. As the cells synthesize and fill up with sebum, they tend to move farther from the basement membrane bordering the dermis where blood vessels are located. Thus, the cells eventually die and degenerate (*holocrine secretion*) as they spill their contents around the hair follicle and onto the skin surface. Several sebaceous glands are associated with each hair follicle. The glands are simple alveolar in type and open into the upper part of the hair folicle. The cells are large, rounded, and pale-staining because the secretory granules are readily dissolved. This secretion tends to waterproof and soften the hairs of the scalp. While most sebaceous glands develop from the external root sheath of hair follicles, it is possible to find sebaceous glands in areas that have no hairs. Such sebaceous glands are located in the eyelids, nipples, and labia minora, for example. The increased level of sex hormones at puberty tends to cause increased proliferation of the basal cells in sebaceous glands and increased secretion. Occasionally, the glands can bulge into the dermis to form pimples or acne.

SWEAT GLANDS

Sweat glands or sudoriferous glands present in mammals are coiled tubular glands and are of two types: *apocrine* and *eccrine* (Fig. 16.6). Apocrine sweat glands are associated with hair follicles, and eccrine sweat glands are not associated with hair follicles but open onto the skin surface by piercing the epidermis. Eccrine and apocrine sweat glands are intermixed, for example, in the armpit or axilla in humans.

Most human sweat is produced by eccrine sweat glands. Eccrine sweat glands secrete water, which cools the body by evaporation. The secretion also tends to moisten areas such as the palms and soles, which are exposed to friction. Different eccrine sweat glands produce sweat in response to heat, as well as various psychic stimuli. The number of eccrine sweat glands on a human is said to range from 2 to 5 million. The fact that some individuals sweat more profusely than others is due to a difference not in the number of sweat glands but in their relative activity. The ill effects of sweating include loss of water and sodium, which can have deleterious effects if not replaced.

ECCRINE SWEAT GLANDS

The eccrine sweat glands are rather widely distributed but are not associated with hair follicles (Fig. 16.6). The glandular secretory portion of the eccrine sweat glands contains clear cells, dark cells, and myoepithelial cells. The secretory cells are arranged into a stratified cuboidal epithelium, with the dark cells positioned next to the lumen and the light cells located basally adjacent to the myoepithelial cells and the basement membrane. The dark cells contain numerous secretory granules with a glycoprotein content. The cells also contain substantial amounts of rER. The clear cells lack secretory granules but contain numerous mitochondria and glycogen, as well as some sER. The free surface of these cells contains microvilli and microplicae. The clear cells are believed to produce sweat, a watery secretion that contains little protein but instead such constituents as urea, uric acid, ammonia, and sodium chloride. Sweat appears to move through intercellular channels to the lumen of the gland. The evaporation of sweat results in

cooling and is, therefore, important in temperature regulation of the body.

In some disease conditions, the components of sweat may be altered. Specifically, under certain conditions of renal insufficiency, the concentration of urea in sweat may increase to the point that urea crystals may appear in the sweat on the surface of the skin, especially the upper lip. The myoepithelial cells aid in moving the sweat through the coiled sweat gland. The duct consists of stratified cuboidal epithelium and spirals through the dermis and epidermis. The duct cells stain darker or more acidophilic in H&E-stained sections than the secretory cells.

The *eccrine sweat glands* increase their secretion in response to heat and nervous stress and strain. As a result, perspiration may appear in quantity on the forehead and palms of the hands. The glands are innervated by the sympathetic division of the ANS but uniquely are

Table 16.1 Sweat Glands

	Eccrine Sweat Glands	*Apocrine Sweat Glands*
Location	Wide distribution, especially on palms, and soles, scalp, forehand and axilla; ducts open onto skin surface (secretory portion in dermis)	Located in anal, genital, axillary, and areolar regions; ducts open into hair follicles
Type of Gland	Simple coiled tubular with secretory and ductal portions	Simple coiled tubular with both secretory and ductal portions; larger in diameter than eccrine sweat glands
Secretory Cell Types	Dark mucous cells not in contact with basement membrane (glycoprotein secretory granules) clear serous cells, no secretory granules; contain glycogen, basal plasma membrane infoldings; myoepithelial cells	Single layer of granular epithelial cells, some variation in shape; surrounded by myoepithelial cells
Ducts	Stratified cuboidal epithelium; inner row of cells somewhat hyalinized because of tonofilaments; duct epithelium resorbs sodium and chloride; scattered myoepithelial cells	Stratified cuboidal (in places, there may be three layers of epithelial cells); inner layer of cells has keratinized cytoplasmic border resembling a cuticle; scattered myoepithelial cells
Secretion	Water, Na^+, Cl^-, K^+, urea, lactate, ammonia, uric acid (hypotonic solution)	Viscous secretion; contains proteins, carbohydrates, ammonia, lipids, ferric iron, chromogens, fatty acids
Innervation	Cholinergic nerve endings; eccrine secretion persists for duration of stimulus	Adrenergic nerve endings primarily (but some cholinergic stimuli)
Function	Major source of evaporative heat loss (in adult male, under severe heat stress, 1–2 liters of sweat may be secreted in 1 hour)	Unclear if secretion has a pheromone function Example of modified apocrine sweat glands: Glands of Moll—eyelids Ceruminous glands—external auditory meatus Areolar glands of Montogomery—around nipple

stimulated by cholinergic transmitters that are usually associated with the parasympathetic division of the ANS. The eccrine and apocrine sweat glands are compared in Table 16.1.

APOCRINE SWEAT GLANDS

In humans, apocrine sweat glands have a more limited distribution than eccrine sweat glands. The apocrine sweat glands are located in the axilla, the circumanal region, and the region of the external genitalia, and are associated with the areola and nipple of the mammary glands. The glands are coiled and tubular. There is only a single type of secretory cell; it is cuboidal or columnar and stains acidophilic (Plate 40B,C). *Myoepithelial cells* are also associated with the base of the secretory cells. The duct portion of the gland contains stratified cuboidal epithelium like the eccrine duct cells (Plate 40A). The duct, however, opens into the hair follicle near the location of the sebaceous gland. The *apocrine sweat glands* develop at puberty in response to sex hormones. The secretory product is proteinaceous and may also contain steroids. In some mammals, the secretion of these glands may contain pheromones that may be involved in such activities as courtship, maternal behavior, and social interactions. In certain animals, the secretion from apocrine sweat glands is used to identify specific territories. The apocrine sweat glands do not respond to heat, but they do increase secretion in response to emotional and certain other sensory stimuli.

FUNCTIONS OF THE INTEGUMENT

The functions of the integument are summarized in Table 16.2.

MEDICAL ASPECTS OF THE INTEGUMENT

Dandruff is due to an increased rate of keratinization of localized regions of the scalp, producing localized flaking and itching of the skin. Eczema involves enhanced cell division in the epidermis caused by sensitivity to various substances (e.g., soaps, fabrics) and environmental conditions (e.g., heat or dryness). Psoriasis also results from localized overactive areas of cell division in the epidermis, but its cause is presently unclear. Factors such as stress and infections may initiate the condition, which appears to be hereditary. Uticaria or hives is an allergic reation in which localized areas of itching develop. Athlete's foot is a fungal infection that usually occurs on the toes and soles of the feet. Impetigo is a contagious bacterial infection especially prevalent in young children; encrusting pustules may be formed. Common causes of infectious skin diseases include bacteria, viruses, fungi, and parasites. A carbuncle is an infection of the skin and subcutaneous tissue that results in pustules. Erysipelas is a surface cellulitis of the skin caused by the *Streptococcus* bacterium. Inflammation of the hair follicle (boil) caused by the *Staphylococcus* bacterium is called a *furuncle*. *Seborrhea* is the increased discharge of sebum from the sebaceous glands.

Table 16.2 Functions of the Integument

I. PROTECTION	
1. Barrier to physical, chemical, and biological insults	Stratified squamous epithelium, keratin, collagen in dermis
2. Barrier to water and electrolyte loss (terrestrial existence)	Keratinocytes produce keratin, transform into corneocytes
	Keratinocytes secrete impermeable glycolipid layer
3. Barrier to bacterial invasion	Keratinocytes produce keratin, become corneocytes
4. Ultraviolet irradiation	Melanocytes in epidermis contain melanin granules
II. SYNTHESIS	
1. Vitamin D synthesis (for proper mineral metabolism)	Ergosterol (skin) $\longrightarrow$ vitamin D
2. Keratin (impermeable albuminoid protein)	Keratinocyte → corneocyte (keratohyalin → eleidin → keratin)
3. Keratinocyte synthesizes glycolipid; packaged in lamellar bodies	Discharge of lamellar bodies results in waterproofing layer

(continued)

Table 16.2 (continued)

III.	IMMUNOLOGIC FUNCTION (skin-associated lymphatic tissue)	
	1. Keratinocyte	Synthesizes IL-1 and factor affecting lymphocyte maturation
	2. Langerhans cell	Antigen-presenting cell in epidermis
	3. T lymphocytes	Helper (T4) and cytotoxic (T8) lymphocytes
IV.	REGULATION—BODY TEMPERATURE	
	1. Sweat glands	Cooling by evaporation of sweat
	2. Capillary plexuses (rete subpapillare)	Cooling of blood in plexuses adjacent to epidermis
	3. Arteriovenous shunts	Closed in cold weather to prevent heat loss
	4. Hairs (in some animals)	Maintain warmer body temperature
V.	REGULATION—WASTES	
	1. Elimination of metabolic wastes and ingested or absorbed substances in secretion of sweat	Sweat glands
VI.	EPIDERMAL DERIVATIVES	
	1. Sebaceous glands, hairs, nails, claws, hoofs	Sebum protects skin and hairs; hairs involved in temperature regulation in some animals; nails, claws, hoofs have a variety of functions in protection, food getting, locomotion
VII.	SENSORY RECEPTION	
	1. Meissner's corpuscle, encapsulated mechanoreceptor	Tactile reception, located in dermis
	2. Vater-Pacini corpuscle, encapsulated mechanoreceptor	Deep pressure reception, located in dermis
	3. Free nerve endings in epidermis	Thermal reception and pain (nociceptors) receptors
	4. Krause's end bulbs	Mechanoreceptor in dermis
	5. Ruffini cylinders	Mechanoreceptor in dermis
	6. Merke cell (disk)	Mechanoreceptor in epidermis
VIII.	MEDICAL DIAGNOSIS	Integument important in diagnosis of circulatory impairments, allergies, vitamin deficiencies, many childhood diseases, etc.
IX.	ECONOMIC IMPORTANCE	Leather produced by tanning and drying of collagen in the dermis; pelts used in making garments

A *neoplasm* is an abnormal growth. Skin neoplasms may be benign or malignant. Malignant melanoma is a malignant tumor of melanocytes and is the most dangerous form of skin cancer. Squamous cell carcinoma is a malignant condition of the squamous epithelial cells. Basal cell carcinoma is the most common type of malignant tumor of epithelial cells.

SELECTED BIBLIOGRAPHY

Achten, G., and Parent, D. (1983) The normal and pathologic nail. *Int. J. Dermatol.* **22**, 556–569.

Bommannan, D., Potts, R.O., and Guy, R.H. (1990). Examination of stratum corneum barrier function *in vivo* by infrared spectroscopy. *J. Invest. Dermatol.* **95**, 403–408.

Braathen, L.R., Bjercke, S., and Thorsby, E. (1984). The antigen-presenting function of human Langerhans cells. *Immunobiology* **168**, 301–317.

Brod, J. (1991). Characterization and physiological role of epidermal lipids. *Int. J. Dermatol.* **30**, 84–90.

Dlugosz, A.A., and Yuspa, S.H. (1993). Coordinate changes in gene expression which mark the spinous to granular cell transition in epidermis are regulated by protein kinase. *C. J. Cell Biol.* **120**, 217–225.

Edelson, R.L., and Fink, J.M. (1985). The immunologic function of the skin. *Sci. Am.* **252**, 46–58.

Fuchs, E., and Coulombe, P.A. (1992). Of mice and men: genetic skin diseases of keratin. *Cell* **69**, 899–902.

Goldsmith, L.A., ed. (1983) *Biochemistry and Physiology of the Skin.* Oxford University Press, New York.

Millington, P.F., and Wilkinson, R. (1983). *Skin.* Cambridge University Press, Cambridge.

Price, M.L., and Griffiths, W.A. (1985). Normal body hair— a review. *Clin. Exp. Dermatol.* **10**, 87–104.

Prota, G. (1992). *Melanins and Melanogenesis.* Academic Press, San Diego, CA.

Roop, D. (1995). Defects in the barrier. *Science* **267**, 474–475.

Sato, K., Kang, W.H., Saga, K., and Sato, K.T. (1989). Biology of sweat glands and their disorders. I. Normal sweat gland function. *J. Am. Acad. Dermatol.* **20**, 537–563.

Streilein, J.W. (1983). Skin-associated lymphoid tissues (SALT): origins and function. *J. Invest. Dermatol.* **280**(suppl), 12s–16s.

The Respiratory System

17

All resident cells in the body require oxygen to carry out metabolic processes and then produce carbon dioxide as one waste product of this biologic oxidation. A separate circulatory system, called the *pulmonary circuit*, delivers deoxygenated, carbon dioxide-rich blood from the right ventricle to the lungs by way of the pulmonary artery. Oxygenated blood from the lungs returns to the left auricle (see Chapter 15). The respiratory system is adapted to facilitate not only the oxygenation of blood, which is then distributed to all resident cells of the body, but also the exchange of carbon dioxide, which is subsequently exhaled. Since the air in the lung air sacs must be changed frequently to accommodate the needs of gas exchange, the air in the system must be changed at least 15 times per minute, depending upon the intensity of body activity. Therefore, inspiratory and expiratory movements are required for the ventilation of the lung alveoli. Oxygen diffuses from the air in the alveoli into the capillaries surrounding the alveoli and forms a complex with hemoglobin (oxyhemoglobin) in the erythrocytes. Carbon dioxide, carried as reduced hemoglobin by the erythrocytes, diffuses from the blood into the alveolar sacs and alveoli.

Knowledge of the relationships between the lungs and surrounding bony skeletal cage is necessary in order to understand inspiration and expiration. The lungs are located in a thoracic cage that, from posterior to anterior, consists of the vertebral column, ribs, costal cartilages, and sternum (Fig. 17.1). The bottom of this cage is formed by a diaphragm that is a musculotendinous sheet of smooth muscle and collagen fibers. The lungs are covered by two thin layers that are continuous with each other at the root or hilum of the lung. The outermost of these layers is the *parietal pleura* and the in-

nermost layer, immediately adjacent to the lungs, is the *visceral pleura*. The free or serosal surface of both parietal pleura and visceral pleura consists of a layer of simple squamous epithelial cells called *mesothelial cells*. A thin layer of fluid is located between the parietal and visceral pleura, and this region is a potential space called the *pleural cavity*. The thin fluid film reduces friction of these surfaces during inspiratory and expiratory movements.

The *hilum* or root of the lung is the point where the extrapulmonary bronchus, pulmonary artery, and vein, as well as lymphatic vessels and nerves, enter or exit the lung. It is also in this region that the parietal and visceral pleura are continuous. Therefore, the lungs lie in the thoracic cavity but outside the pleural cavities. During fetal life, the lungs fill the thoracic cage and are attached at many points to the inner surface of the cage by elastic fibers. During subsequent growth, therefore, the lungs tend to be stretched in all directions as the thorax increases in size and since the lungs are attached to the thorax by the elastic fibers.

VENTILATION OF THE LUNGS

When the intercostal muscles that extend between the ribs of the thoracic cage contract, the thoracic cage tends to enlarge, especially to deepen in its anterior-posterior plane because of the nature of the articulation between the ribs, vertebrae, and sternum. In addition, contraction of the diaphragm, which lowers the diaphragm, and relaxation of abdominal muscles elongate the thoracic cage. Thus, during inspiration, the thoracic cage is enlarged through the contraction of some muscles and the relaxation of others. Since the

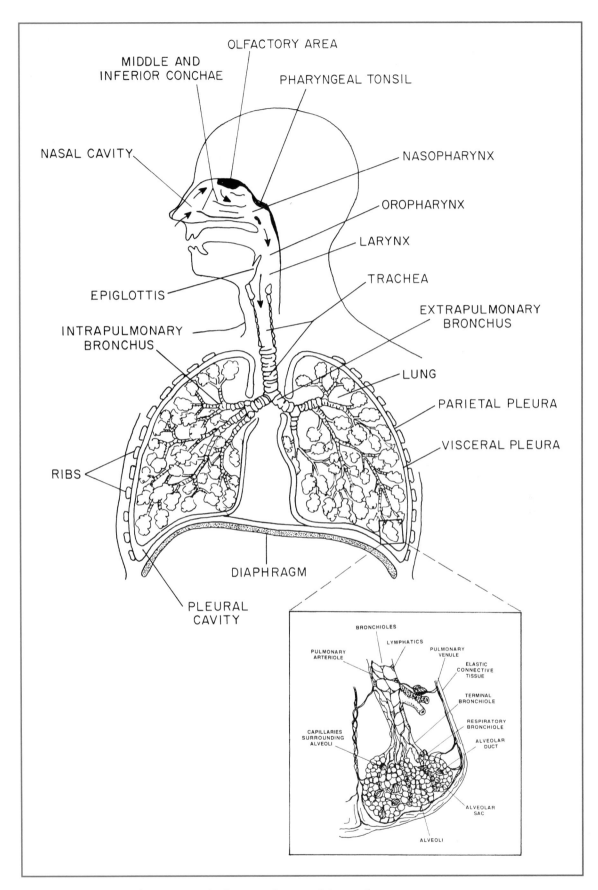

Figure 17.1. Schematic diagram of parts of the respiratory system.

lungs fill the thoracic cage and are attached by elastic fibers and since there is only one opening into the lungs through the trachea and bronchi, the lungs become more inflated as the thoracic cage is enlarged, similar to the situation of inflating a bellows. Expanding the cage and enlarging the lungs during inhalation results in a decrease in air pressure in the lungs relative to the outside; thus, air enters to equalize the pressure difference. Inhalation causes elastic fibers in the lungs to become stretched. The enlargement of the thoracic cage also aids in drawing blood into the pulmonary vessels. During inspiratory movements, the air enters the nostrils and nasal cavities or mouth and passes through the nasopharynx, oropharynx, larynx, trachea, and divisions of the bronchial tree en route to the extremely thin-walled alveoli, whose outer surfaces are covered by extensive capillary plexuses where the actual exchange of carbon dioxide and oxygen occurs.

For individuals at rest, expiration may be a passive event resulting from the recoil of the stretched elastic fibers and the relaxation of the intercostal muscles. During more strenuous activity, the abdominal muscles contract to force the viscera against the undersurface of the diaphragm, thus compressing the thoracic cage and causing expiration of air from the lungs. As indicated, the lungs fill the thoracic cage early in development and are attached at numerous places to the inner surface of the thoracic cage by elastic fibers, resulting in a stretching of the entire lung. Even at the end of expiration at rest, the elastic fibers are still stretched. Inspiration, therefore, increases the tension on the stretched elastic fibers.

CONDUCTING PORTION OF THE RESPIRATORY SYSTEM

The paired nasal cavities, single nasopharynx, oropharynx, larynx, trachea, and branched bronchi comprise the conducting portion of the respiratory system. The two main functions of this portion are to conduct air to the lungs and condition the air. The air is conditioned by being cleaned, humidified, and warmed or cooled. Because a gas is contained within the conducting portion of the respiratory system, it is essential that this portion be prevented from collapsing, as might occur during violent inspiratory movements. Protection is provided by selected deposits of cartilage and bone in the walls of the conducting passageways. The conducting portion of the system also strains the incoming air of particles and other foreign objects. This function is performed by the hairs located in the vestibule of the nasal cavities and by the presence of numerous ciliated cells, goblet cells, and glands in these passageways. The mucus traps small particles and some microorganisms. These constituents are moved by cilia on the surface of

epithelial cells toward the pharynx, where they are removed from the system by the cough reflex. In the nasal cavities, the cilia beat so as to propel trapped substances posterior to the pharynx, whereas those cilia on cells in the trachea, for example, propel the mucus-trapped particles superiorly or anteriorly toward the pharynx. Not only does the mucus trap particulate material, it also plays a role in absorbing such water-soluble gases as sulfur dioxide and ozone. Most of the conducting portion of the respiratory system contains mucous or seromucous glands in the lamina propria, and the glands communicate with the cavities by ducts (Plate 41A).

The conducting portion of the respiratory system warms or cools the inhaled air by the presence of large, thin-walled blood vessels in the lamina propria immediately adjacent to the epithelium lining the nasal cavities (Plate 41A). The secretion of seromucous glands in the lamina propria and many goblet cells in the epithelium humidifies the air that is inhaled.

NASAL CAVITIES

The paired nasal cavities communicate with the outside by nares or nostrils and are continuous posteriorly with the nasopharynx. Each nasal cavity consists of an anterior portion called the *vestibule* and a larger region called the *nasal fossa*. The integument covering the outer surface of the nose continues through the nostrils to line the vestibule, which contains nonkeratinized stratified squamous epithelium. Sebaceous and sweat glands and thick, short hairs (vibrissae) are present in the outer part of the vestibule. The hairs strain the incoming air of coarse particles. The paired nasal fossae are separated by a bony *nasal septum*. In addition, three bony shelves, the *superior concha, middle concha*, and *inferior concha*, extend from the nasal septum into the nasal cavities. The superior part of both nasal cavities, as well as the superior nasal conchae in the nasal cavities, are covered by *olfactory epithelium*, which functions in the perception of smell. The middle and inferior conchae as well as the remainder of the nasal cavities are lined by *respiratory epithelium (Schneiderian membrane)*, which will be described in more detail subsequently. The nasal conchae create turbulance in the air such that the direction of air movements is continually and rapidly changing. The particles carried in this air do not change direction as rapidly and therefore tend to continue forward, striking the conchae and falling forward, to be trapped in the mucous sheet. The removal of particulate material during this process is called *turbulent precipitation* and may effectively trap small particles. The turbulence caused by the conchae and the increased surface area allow for warming of the air as it passes over the epithelium warmed by the "swell bodies."

OLFACTORY EPITHELIUM: ORGANIZATION

The olfactory mucosa consists of a modified, pseudo-stratified columnar epithelium that is thicker than the surrounding respiratory epithelium lining the remainder of the nasal cavities (Plate 41B). The olfactory mucosa covers the superior nasal conchae and part of the middle conchae as well. The olfactory epithelium consists of bipolar neurons, sustentacular or supporting cells, and basal cells (Figs. 17.2–17.4). The olfactory bipolar neurons taper to a thin dendrite at one end that terminates as a modified cilium (Figs. 17.4, 17.5, 17.6). At the other end, the bipolar olfactory cell extends as an axon that exits the nasal cavity to become the olfactory cranial nerve, which connects to the olfactory lobes of the brain. The long, thin dendrite terminates as a small knob called the *olfactory bulb* (Fig. 17.5). The olfactory bulb, in turn, extends as several cilia, called *olfactory cilia*, which then narrow and extend for long distances on the surface of the olfactory mucosa (Figs. 17.4, 17.5). The cilia that extend from the bulb contain nine doublet and two central microtubules, but where the cilia narrow, only two microtubules extend into the narrow part of the cilia. The olfactory cilia extend from basal bodies located in the olfactory bulb.

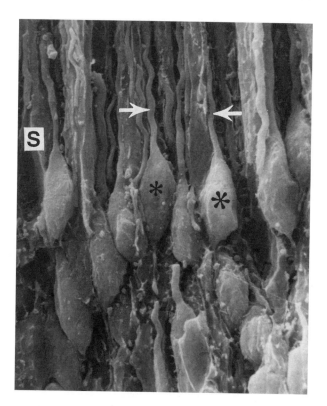

Figure 17.3. SEM of the enlarged region of an olfactory epithelium showing cell bodies (*) of bipolar neurons. Dendrites are denoted by arrows. Bipolar neurons are surrounded by supporting cells (S). ×1795. (From R. Kessel and R. Kardon, *Tissues and Organs: A Text-Atlas of Scanning Electron Microscopy*, W.H. Freeman, New York, 1979, with permission)

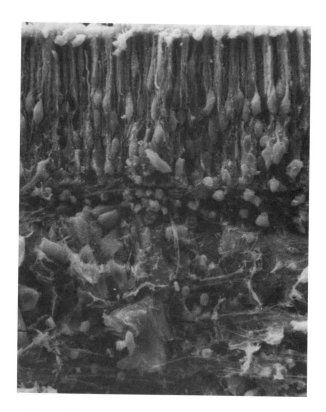

Figure 17.2. SEM of olfactory epithelium; the epithelium is located at the top of the figure and connective tissue lamina propria in the lower half of the figure. ×470. (From R. Kessel and R. Kardon, *Tissues and Organs: A Text-Atlas of Scanning Electron Microscopy*, W.H. Freeman, New York, 1979, with permission)

The olfactory cilia are kept moist by the secretion of glands, called the *tubuloalveolar glands of Bowman*, that are located in the lamina propria beneath the epithelium. The watery secretion of these glands is important in preventing dessication of the olfactory cilia and in dissolving odors so that they can be perceived by the modified ciliary dendrites of the olfactory cell. At the apical region of the olfactory dendrite and adjacent sustentacular (supporting) cells, circumferential tight junctions (zonulae occludentes) are present. The *basal cells* in the olfactory epithelium in some animals can differentiate into new olfactory receptor cells. This represents a unique case in which neurons are replaced in postnatal life.

MECHANISMS OF SMELL

Odor molecules stimulate receptors in the olfactory receptor cells after initially being absorbed into the mucus and subsequently diffusing to the receptors located in the plasma membrane of the olfactory cilia. During the transduction process, channels in the plasma membrane open, permitting inward flow of cations and giv-

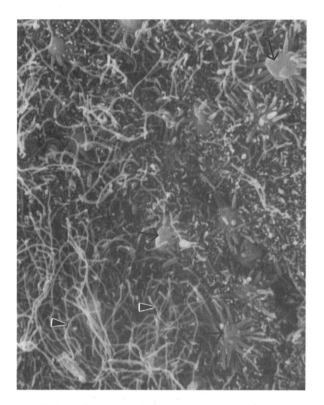

Figure 17.4. View of olfactory epithelium from the surface by SEM. Olfactory bulbs (arrows) and olfactory cilia (arrowheads) are identified. ×3200. (From R. Kessel and R. Kardon, *Tissues and Organs: A Text-Atlas of Scanning Electron Microscopy*, W.H. Freeman, New York, 1979, with permission)

ing rise to a *depolarizing receptor potential*. Thus, it now appears that odors are detected when the odorants, which are small, volatile, lipid-soluble molecules, bind to receptor proteins on the surface of the olfactory cilia, generating electrical signals to the brain. It has been estimated that a large family of genes, perhaps 100 to 300 genes, code for odor receptor proteins. It is presently estimated that as many as 1000 different receptors exist and that much of the odor discrimination occurs at the receptor level rather than in the brain. When an odor molecule binds to its receptor, it appears to trigger a G protein that activates adenylate cyclase so as to produce cAMP, which, in turn, opens ion channels in the membranes of these sensory neurons.

RESPIRATORY EPITHELIUM

The mucous membrane or mucosa of the nasal cavities consists of an epithelium that is pseudostratified, ciliated, and columnar. It contains goblet cells and an adjacent layer of loose connective tissue containing mucous and serous glands (Plate 41A). Depending upon its location, the lamina propria is anchored to the periosteum of bone or the perichondrium of cartilage. The secretions of glands and goblet cells keep the surface of the epithelium moist, and the secretions may inactivate certain bacteria. The connective tissue may contain numerous plasma cells, as well as fibroblasts,

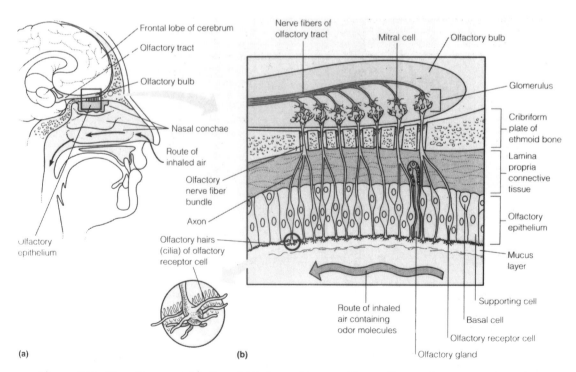

Figure 17.5. The olfactory epithelium (b) is located in the superior portion of the nasal cavity (a). The structure of the bipolar olfactory cells and their connections with the mitral cells (neurons) in the olfactory bulb are shown in (b).

(From *Human Anatomy and Physiology*, 3rd ed. by E.N. Marieb. © 1995 by The Benjamin/Cummings Publishing Company, Inc., Redwood City, CA. Reprinted by permission.)

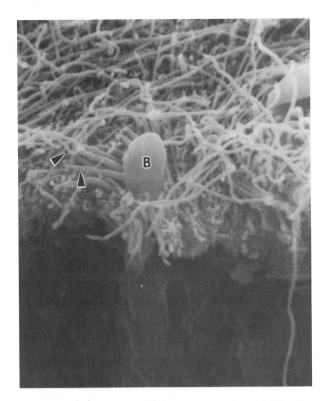

Figure 17.6. SEM of olfactory bulb (B) and cilia (arrowheads). ×6420. (From R. Kessel and R. Kardon, *Tissues and Organs: A Text-Atlas of Scanning Electron Microscopy*, W.H. Freeman, New York, 1979, with permission)

macrophages, and elastic and collagenic fibers. Large blood vessels called *venous plexuses* are also present in the connective tissue. Periodically, the venous plexuses in different nasal fossae become engorged with blood and distended such that air flow in a fossa may be reduced for a time. For this reason, these venous plexuses have been called *swell bodies*. The venous plexuses may act to prevent dessication of both the respiratory and olfactory epithelia.

An extensive capillary bed is also located in the connective tissue of the nasal cavities, and blood flows from a posterior to an anterior direction in these vessels. The direction of air flow, however, is opposite to the direction of blood flow, and the resulting countercurrent flow system that is created is more effective in warming the incoming air in cold weather and in cooling the incoming air in hot weather. The thin-walled veins that are present in the inferior and middle nasal conchae may become sufficiently engorged with blood to slow the passage of air through the nasal cavities, resulting in a "stuffed-up nose."

PARANASAL AIR SINUSES

Paranasal sinuses are four small, air-filled spaces that are named for the bones in which they are located: frontal,

ethmoidal, sphenoidal, and maxillary sinuses. These sinuses communicate with the nasal cavity so that the lining of the paranasal sinuses is continuous with that of the nasal cavities. However, the epithelium is not as thick in the sinuses. The lamina propria is thinner in the sinuses, and the number of goblet cells is reduced.

NASOPHARYNX

The pharynx serves in part to connect the nasal cavities and larynx and is divided into the nasopharynx, oral pharynx, and laryngeal pharynx. The epithelium in this region is highly variable; it may be stratified squamous-nonkeratinized, pseudostratified ciliated columnar, or stratified columnar. The epithelium is located adjacent to a connective tissue layer that may in some places contain glands. The connective tissue layer is surrounded by striated muscle that is surrounded by another connective tissue layer that anchors the pharynx to nearby structures.

LARYNX

The larynx is responsible for sound production and also serves as a sentinel for the lungs. It is located between the pharynx and trachea. The wall of the larynx contains several named hyaline and elastic cartilages that prevent collapse. These cartilages are connected by ligaments, as well as by intrinsic and extrinsic voluntary muscles. The mucosa consists of epithelium and connective tissue that may contain seromucous glands. The *epiglottis* is a modified region of the superior portion of the larynx, consisting of a plate of elastic cartilage that is surrounded by lamina propria and stratified squamous epithelium. During swallowing, the larynx is raised and forced against the epiglottis to prevent food from entering the larynx. In cases of drowning, no water is usually found in the lungs; the individual dies from asphyxiation caused by laryngeal spasms.

In many areas, the mucosa of the larynx is lined by respiratory epithelium, but in some regions, including the epiglottis, the epithelium is stratified squamous in type. The underlying connective tissue contains a number of named cartilages, as well as tendons, intrinsic muscles, and occasional glands. The larger cartilages are hyaline and include the thyroid, cricoid, and much of the arytenoid cartilages. The remainder of the arytenoid cartilages, as well as the cunieform and corniculate cartilages and the cartilage plate in the epiglottis, are elastic cartilages. The tendons present interconnect the cartilages, and the intrinsic muscles are striated skeletal in type.

The wall of the larynx has two pairs of mucosal folds that extend into the lumen. The upper pair of folds are the *false vocal cords*. The lower pair of folds are the *true vocal cords.* The true vocal cords contain a number of elastic fibers, as well as skeletal muscle, and are covered by stratified squamous epithelium. As a result, tension in the ligaments of the true vocal folds or true vocal cords can be varied so that sound of different frequencies can be generated as air is forced between them. Sounds are produced by the vibrations of the true vocal folds due to the passage of air across the free margins of the vocal folds.

TRACHEA

The trachea is a tubular structure ~11 cm long and ~2 cm in diameter. It extends from the base of the larynx to the point where the trachea bifurcates into two short primary extrapulmonary bronchi, which then enter the lungs. The trachea is supported and prevented from collapsing by some 15–20 horseshoe-shaped cartilages whose open end faces posteriorly (Plate 41C; Fig. 17.7). The cartilages can be felt by drawing the finger along the exterior throat region. The gap between the ends of each cartilage posteriorly is filled with smooth muscle and connective tissue. In addition, connective tissue

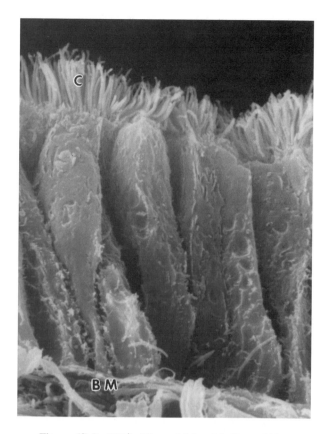

Figure 17.8. SEM of bronchial epithelium. Cilia (C) of ciliated columnar cells and basement membrane (BM) are identified. ×3445. (From R. Kessel and R. Kardon, *Tissues and Organs: A Text-Atlas of Scanning Electron Microscopy*, W.H. Freeman, New York, 1979, with permission)

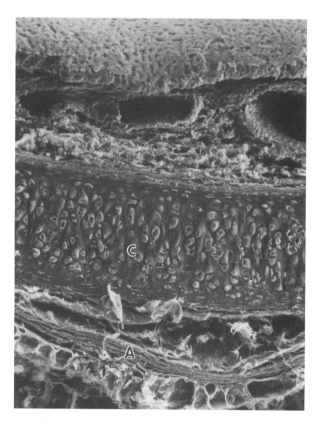

Figure 17.7. SEM of the trachea wall. Epithelium is at the top; lamina propria contains several empty blood vessels; cartilage (C) and connective tissue adventitia (A) are identified. ×195. (From R. Kessel and R. Kardon, *Tissues and Organs: A Text-Atlas of Scanning Electron Microscopy*, W.H. Freeman, New York, 1979, with permission)

is located between the adjacent cartilage pieces and is continuous with the perichondrium of the hyaline cartilage. The inner epithelial surface of the trachea is lined by pseudostratifed, ciliated columnar epithelium containing goblet cells. The cilia beat toward the pharynx. The basement membrane of the trachea is quite thick, and the connective tissue lamina propria contains numerous elastic fibers. There is such a large aggregation of elastic fibers that a distinct region called the *membrana elastica interna* is usually evident in the lamina propria (Figs. 17.8, 17.9). Seromucous glands are present in a submucosal layer, and the ducts of these glands open onto the epithelial surface. Lymphocytes, mast cells, plasma cells, and solitary lymphatic nodules may be pres-ent in the lamina propria and submucosa of the trachea. The organization of the tracheal wall permits some extension when the head is tilted backward and allows it to elongate during inspiration. The presence of smooth muscle (the trachealis muscle) between the ends of the cartilages permits contraction and narrowing of the tracheal lumen to increase the velocity of expired air during coughing, which may aid in clearing the passageway of an obstruction. The trachea and

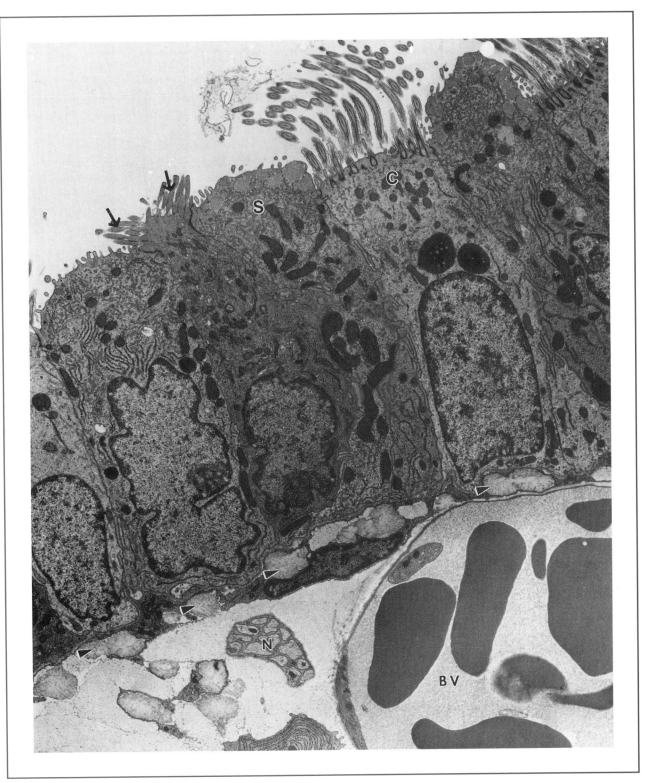

Figure 17.9. TEM of trachea epithelium. Ciliated (C) cells, secretory (S) cells, and cells with short, broad microvilli (arrows) with characteristics of brush cells are identified. Groups of elastic fibers (arrowheads) are located at the base of the epithelium. Nerves (N) and blood vessels (BV) are present in the lamina propria connective tissue. ×9000.

bronchi are quite sensitive to light pressure, so foreign substances can easily initiate the cough reflex.

In addition to ciliated cells, the tracheal epithelium contains goblet cells and a brush cell named for the tuft of microvilli that extends from the apical surface somewhat like the bristles of a brush (Fig. 17.9). The function of the brush cell is not clear, but it may function as a chemoreceptor (Fig. 17.10). A fourth cell type is a small, rounded cell in the basal portion of the epithelium. These basal cells appear to be stem cells that can differentiate into ciliated cells or mucus-producing goblet cells. Neuroendocrine cells, perhaps comparable to enteroendocrine cells of the gastrointestinal tract, known as *Kulchitsky* or *K cells*, are also present in the epithelium. Dense-core secretory granules are present in the cytoplasm of these cells. Several substances have been described in the secretory granules of the K cells, including *serotonin, calcitonin* (a polypeptide hormone), and the gastrin-releasing peptide called *bombesin.* Afferent nerve fibers synapse with the base of some epithelial cells. Migratory lymphoctyes and mast cells may sometimes be present in the epithelium.

THE BRONCHIAL TREE AND THE RESPIRATORY PORTION

The bronchi branch off the trachea, enter the lungs, and then branch repeatedly into various grades of bronchioles, the smallest of which open into alveolar ducts and alveoli (Fig. 17.11). The trachea thus divides into two short primary extrapulmonary bronchi that enter the lungs at the hilum to become intrapulmonary bronchi. Upon entering the lung, the primary bronchi branch into three bronchi in the right lung and two bronchi in the left lung, each branch supplying a unit of lung structure called a *pulmonary lobe* (Fig. 17.11). The intrapulmonary bronchi exhibits several differences in histologic organization compared to the trachea and extrapulmonary bronchi. In intrapulmonary bronchi, the cartilages are no longer C-shaped or U-shaped plates; instead, there are a number of smaller individual pieces of hyaline cartilage (Plate 41D; Plate 42A). In addition, two bands of smooth muscle completely surround the intrapulmonary bronchus (Plate 42A). One of the bands is helically wound in a left-hand

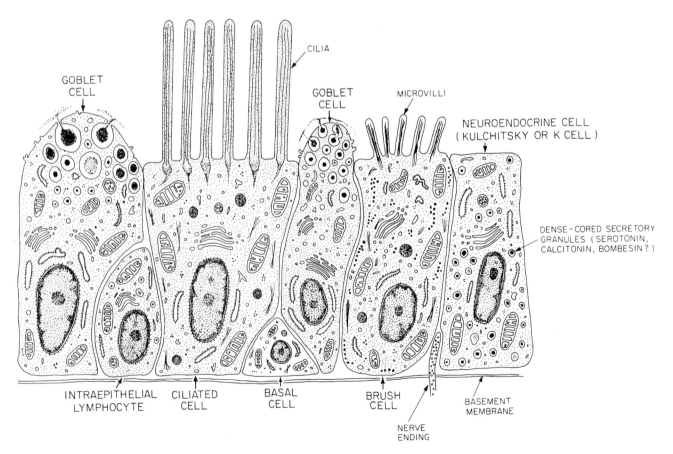

Figure 17.10. Diagram of cell types in the epithelium of trachea and bronchi.

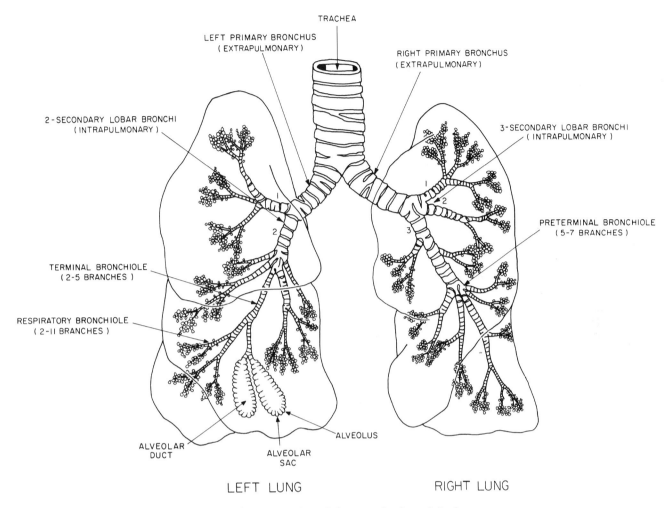

TRACHEA

LEFT PRIMARY BRONCHUS
(EXTRAPULMONARY)

RIGHT PRIMARY BRONCHUS
(EXTRAPULMONARY)

2-SECONDARY LOBAR BRONCHI
(INTRAPULMONARY)

3-SECONDARY LOBAR BRONCHI
(INTRAPULMONARY)

PRETERMINAL BRONCHIOLE
(5-7 BRANCHES)

TERMINAL BRONCHIOLE
(2-5 BRANCHES)

RESPIRATORY BRONCHIOLE
(2-11 BRANCHES)

ALVEOLUS

ALVEOLAR
DUCT

ALVEOLAR
SAC

LEFT LUNG

RIGHT LUNG

Figure 17.11. Drawing of the organization of the lung.

spiral, while the other band is helically wound in a right-hand spiral. Because of contractions of the smooth muscle in bronchioles, the mucous membrane is thrown into longitudinal folds. Histamine causes contraction of the smooth muscles. Stimulation of the *vagus* nerve (parasympathetic innervation) results in *constriction* of the *bronchi.* Conversely, *sympathetic* stimulation of the bronchi results in *dilation.* During asthmatic attacks, drugs that mimic sympathetic neurotransmitters, like *isoproterenol,* may be used to cause *bronchial dilation.* The intrapulmonary bronchi are lined by pseudostratified, ciliated columnar epithelium, and goblet cells are present (Plate 42A). Seromucous glands are present in the submucosa. These glands are innervated by the ANS, and evidence indicates that sympathetic stimulation elicits mucus secretion. Parasympathetic stimulation via ACh appears to elicit secretion by both mucous and serous cells. Solitary lymphatic nodules are present in the lamina propria of bronchi and appear a few days after birth. In addition, B lymphocytes of both the IgA and IgE classes are located in the lamina propria of the bronchi. Further, IgA-secreting plasma cells can be observed in the lamina propria and in close proximity to

glands. These lymphatic cells constitute the *bronchus-associated lymphatic tissue.*

The bronchi exhibit dichotomous branching, and the branches eventually give rise to bronchioles, which have a diameter of only 1 mm or less (Plate 42B–D; Figs. 17.12, 17.13). A *primary bronchiole* supplies a unit of lung structure called a *lobule.* Thus, the primary bronchiole supplies a lobule and is ~1 mm in diameter. There are no cartilages in the wall of a bronchiole since they are no longer needed as the bronchioles are sufficiently deep within the lung not to collapse (Plate 42B–D; Plate 43). There are no glands in bronchioles. The epithelium of the primary bronchiole is ciliated simple columnar, with nonciliated, dome-shaped *Clara cells* interspersed (Fig. 17.13). Clara cells contain numerous mitochondria, sER, and electron-dense serous secretory granules (Fig. 17.13). It has been suggested that the cells contribute a surface active component to the surfactant. A thin lamina propria is located adjacent to the epithelium of bronchioles and the two helically wound bands of smooth muscle are still present, similar to the situation described for bronchi.

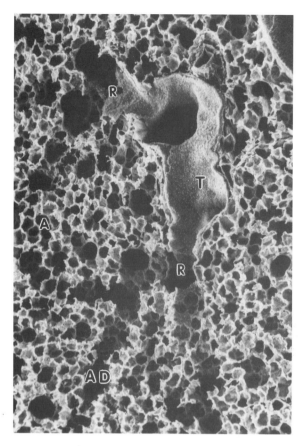

Figure 17.12. Low-magnification SEM view of the lung. Terminal bronchiole (T) respiratory bronchiole (R), and alveolar duct (AD) are denoted. ×70. (From R. Kessel and R. Kardon, *Tissues and Organs: A Text-Atlas of Scanning Electron Microscopy*, W.H. Freeman, New York, 1979, with permission)

Terminal bronchioles branch to form two to five (usually four) short *respiratory bronchioles* (Figs. 17.11, 17.12). The respiratory bronchioles are characterized by the presence of some alveolar outpocketings in their walls. The cilia are lost in the respiratory bronchioles, so that the lining is provided by simple cuboidal epithelial cells. Communicating pores occur between adjacent respiratory bronchioles and serve to equalize air pressure in the lung. These communicating pores are called *Lambert's sinuses.*

BRONCHUS-ASSOCIATED LYMPHOID TISSUE

The lower respiratory tract contains scattered lymphatic nodules that are primarily distributed under the epithelium of the bronchi. Collectively these nodules comprise the bronchus-associated lymphoid tissue (BALT). The B lymphocytes, macrophages, and T lymphocytes that are present in nodules under the epithelium of the bronchial tree are favorably distributed to detect in-

haled antigens. IgA is the principal immunoglobulin that is produced by plasma cells to interact with the inhaled antigens.

ALVEOLAR DUCTS (ALVEOLI)

Each respiratory bronchiole can branch to form 2–11 *alveolar ducts* (Figs. 17.11, 17.12, 17.14, 17.15). When alveolar ducts are sectioned longitudinally, they tend to be long and narrow; they have been likened to a long hallway of a hotel. The alveoli have been likened to hotel rooms off the hallway that lack doors (Plate 43). The term *alveolus* comes from the Latin meaning "little hollow." It has been estimated that there are some 300 million alveoli in both lungs and that they provide more than 80 m^2 of surface. The alveolar ducts, alveolar sacs, and alveoli have a similar histologic structure, differing only in their shape and location (Fig. 17.11). The alveoli of adjacent alveolar ducts are positioned close to an extensive capillary plexus that closely surrounds all of the alveoli associated with the alveolar ducts (Plate 43; Fig. 17.16). The thin partitions between alveoli are called *interalveolar septa* or walls (Figs. 17.16, 17.17). Small pores about 8–12 mm in diameter extend between adjacent alveolar ducts (Fig. 17.18). These pores are called the *interalveolar pores of Kohn* and permit alternate routes for movement of air should obstruction occur.

ALVEOLAR EPITHELIUM

The alveoli have an epithelium that consists of two cell types joined by tight junctions and desmosomes.

ALVEOLAR TYPE I PNEUMOCYTES

The most numerous and thinnest of the alveolar epithelial cells are *type I pneumocytes* (also called *small alveolar cells* or *alveolar type I cells*) (Figs. 17.19–17.21). Type I pneumocytes are unable to divide and contain numerous micropinocytotic vesicles. It has been proposed that the type I pneumocytes play a role in the removal of surfactant produced by type II pneumocytes. In some places, the cytoplasm of the type I pneumocyte is so thin that electron micrographs are required to visualize this part of the cell.

ALVEOLAR TYPE II PNEUMOCYTES

A second, less numerous alveolar epithelial cell is variously called the *type II pneumocyte, alveolar type II cell, granular pneumocyte, septal cell, corner cell, niche cell,* or *great alveolar cell* (Fig. 17.13). These important cells of the in-

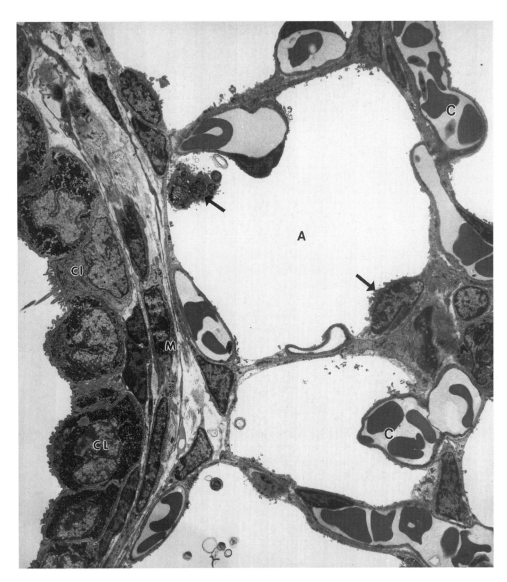

Figure 17.13. TEM of the lung. A bronchiole is located at the left, with ciliated (CI) cells, Clara (CL) cells, and smooth muscle (M). Alveoli (A), type II pneumocyte (arrows), and capillaries with erythrocytes (C) in the interalve- **olar septa are denoted. ×6000 (From R. Roberts, R. Kessel, and H. Tung,** *Freeze Fracture Images of Cells and Tissues,* **Oxford Univ. Press, New York, 1991, with permission)**

teralveolar septum are more rounded, and their apical surface has short, stubby microvilli (Fig. 17.22). Following destruction of the alveolar epithelium by, for example, inhalation of nitrous oxide, increased mitotic activity of the remaining type II cells is observed, followed by their differentiation into type I pneumocytes. Continuous renewal of the alveolar epithelium occurs through the division of the pneumocyte type II cells. The cytoplasm of pneumocyte II cells contains rER, Golgi complex, mitochondria, multivesicular bodies, and many prominent membrane-bound bodies that internally contain many lamellae (Fig. 17.23). These multilamellar bodies or cytolysomes contain a surface active substance called *surfactant*. Thus, the cells have two im-

portant functions: serving as stem cells and producing surfactant.

SURFACTANT

Surfactant is a complex surface active substance containing phospholipids, proteins, *GAGs*, and ions that greatly reduce surface tension in the lung alveoli. The phospholipid dipalmitoyl lecithin is an important constituent that is responsible for reducing the surface tension. Pneumocyte type II cells are believed to constitute about 3% of the surface of all alveoli, while pneumocyte type I cells constitute ~97% of the alveolar surface.

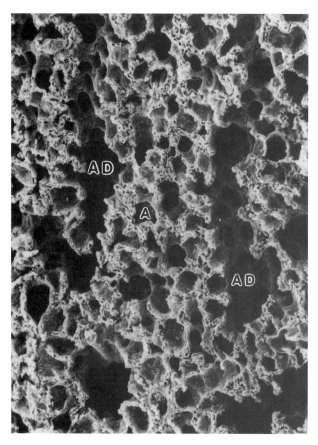

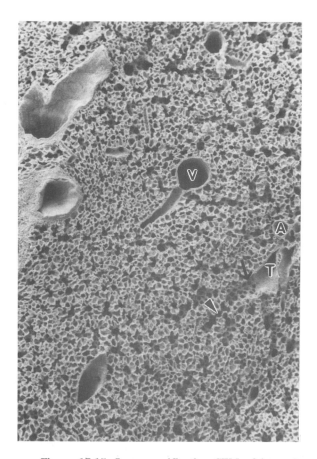

Figure 17.14. SEM of lung. Alveolar ducts (AD) and alveoli (A) are illustrated. ×130. (From R. Kessel and R. Kardon, *Tissues and Organs: A Text-Atlas of Scanning Electron Microscopy*, W.H. Freeman, New York, 1979, with permission)

Figure 17.15. Low-magnification SEM of lung. A terminal bronchiole (T) is continuous with the respiratory bronchiole (arrow) and alveolar duct (arrowhead). Pulmonary vein (V) and pulmonary artery (A). ×27. (From R. Kessel and R. Kardon, *Tissues and Organs: A Text-Atlas of Scanning Electron Microscopy*, W.H. Freeman, New York, 1979, with permission)

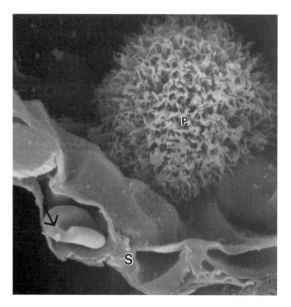

Figure 17.16. SEM of two alveoli, one of which has an alveolar phagocyte (P) and an intervening interalveolar septum (S) that has been fractured to reveal capillaries and erythrocytes (arrow). ×4990. (From R. Kessel and R. Kardon, *Tissues and Organs: A Text-Atlas of Scanning Electron Microscopy*, W.H. Freeman, New York, 1979, with permission)

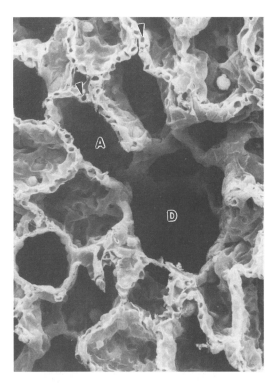

Figure 17.17. SEM of the lung. The alveolus (A) is continuous with a transversely sectioned alveolar duct (D). Interalveolar septa have many empty blood capillaries (arrowheads) ×800 (From R. Kessel and R. Kardon, *Tissues and Organs: A Text-Atlas of Scanning Electron Microscopy*, W.H. Freeman, New York, 1979, with permission)

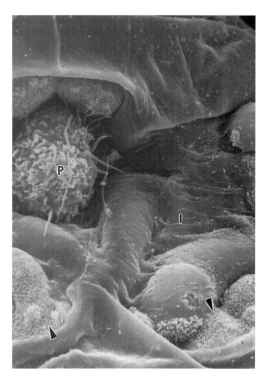

Figure 17.19. SEM of the alveolar surface. An alveolar phagocyte (P), alveolar type II pneumocytes (arrowheads), and smooth alveolar type I cells (I) are identified. ×3470. (From R. Kessel and R. Kardon, *Tissues and Organs: A Text-Atlas of Scanning Electron Microscopy*, W.H. Freeman, 1979, with permission)

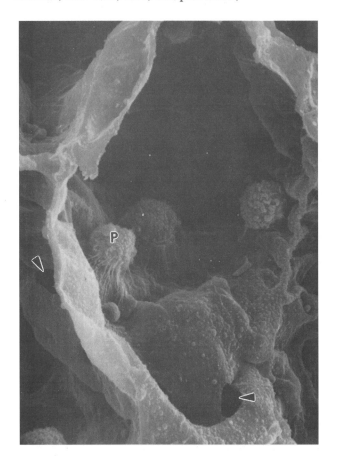

The cytolysomes are discharged by exocytosis into the alveoli, resulting in a thin surface active film of material that covers the alveolar surface. The material is called *surfactant* and is rich in dipalmitoyl phosphatidylcholine. As a result, not as much inspirational force is required to inflate the lungs. Furthermore, the surfactant-coated alveolar epithelial cells resist the tendency to round up and alter the alveolar surface. Moreover, surfactant facilitates the transport of gases between an air-liquid interphase. Finally, surfactant reportedly has some bactericidal effects that would be useful in counteracting airborne microorganisms that might be inspired in the air. Both alveolar epithelial cells reside on a basal lamina (Fig. 17.24). In some areas, the epithelial basal lamina may touch or fuse with the basal lamina of the endothelial cells that comprise the extensive capillary plexuses surrounding each of the tiny alveoli. In areas where alveoli communicate with the alveolar

Figure 17.18. SEM of an alveolus. Interalveolar pores (arrowheads) and three alveolar phagocytes (P) are identified. ×1795. (From R. Kessel and R. Kardon, *Tissues and Organs: A Text-Atlas of Scanning Electron Microscopy*, W.H. Freeman, New York, 1979, with permission)

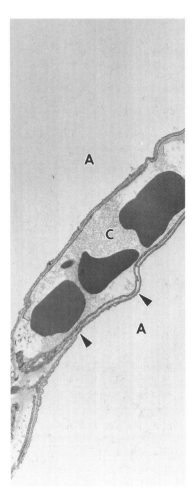

Figure 17.20. Low-magnification view of an interalveolar septum. The capillary (C) contains an erythrocyte. Alveolar type I cells of the alveolus are denoted by arrowheads. Alveolus (A). ×3875. (From R. Roberts, R. Kessel, H. Tung. *Freeze Fracture Images of Cells and Tissues.* Oxford Univ. Press, New York, 1991, with permission)

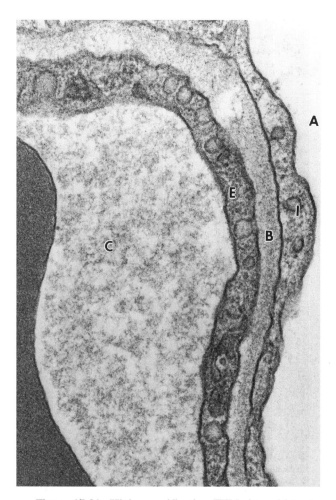

Figure 17.21. High magnification TEM view of blood-air barrier. Alveolus (A) with air, type I pneumocyte (I), basal laminae (B), endothelium (E), and capillary (C) with a portion of an erythrocyte. ×62,000. (From R. Roberts, R. Kessel, H. Tung. *Freeze Fracture Images of Cells and Tissues.* Oxford Univ. Press, New York, 1991, with permission)

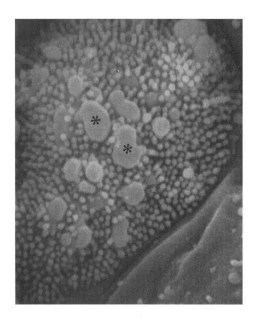

Figure 17.22. SEM of an alveolar pneumocyte type II cell with short, stubby microvilli and regions of surfactant (*) that have been released by exocytosis from the cell. ×15,600. (From R. Kessel and R. Kardon, *Tissues and Organs: A Text-Atlas of Scanning Electron Microscopy*, W.H. Freeman, New York, 1979, with permission)

duct, groups of several smooth muscle cells may be present.

INTERALVEOLAR SEPTUM

The interalveolar septum forms a very thin barrier between air in alveoli and blood in capillaries. The cells that form the barrier are the flattened type I pneumocytes, the capillary endothelial cells, and basal laminae. The very thin barrier facilitates diffusion and exchange of oxygen and carbon dioxide.

Scattered fibroblasts, elastic fibers, and fine collagenic fibrils, as well as macrophages, contractile interstitial cells, and an occasional mast cell, may be present in the interalveolar septum (Figs. 17.23, 17.24). About 20% of the lung mass consists of collagen (type I and II) and elastic fibers. Type I collagen is primarily present in the walls of bronchi and bronchioles and in the

pleura. In some places, the interalveolar septum may be occupied only by the alveolar epithelial cell, the endothelial cell, and the basal laminae of these two cell types (Fig. 17.25). As a consequence, the diffusion distance between air in the alveolus and the capillary lumen, called the *alveolar-endothelial barrier*, may be reduced to ~0.2 μm (Figs. 17.20, 17.21). In the disease emphysema, there is progressive destruction of the alveolar wall and a consequent reduction in respiratory surface.

ALVEOLAR PHAGOCYTES

Alveolar macrophages are widely distributed in the lungs and are highly phagocytic, hence their designation as alveolar phagocytes or *dust cells* (Figs. 17.16–17.19). These macrophages apparently arise initially from monocytes that leave the bloodstream and popu-

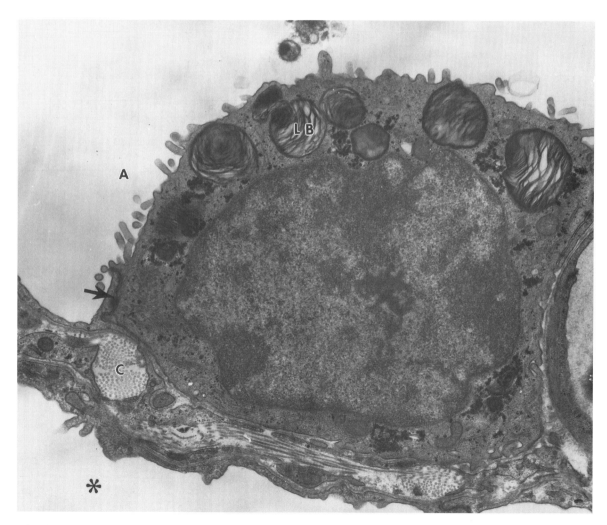

Figure 17.23. TEM of an interalveolar septum. Alveolus (A). The type II pneumocyte contains lamellar bodies (LB). The junction with thin alveolar type I cells is denoted by the arrow. Collagenic fibrils (C). Capillary (*). ×15,500.

(From R. Roberts, R. Kessel, H. Tung. *Freeze Fracture Images of Cells and Tissues.* Oxford University Press, New York, 1991, with permission)

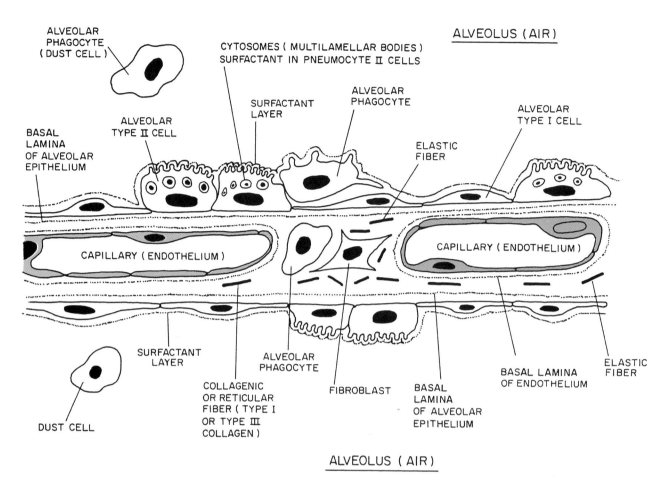

Figure 17.24. Diagram of an interalveolar septum illustrating its components.

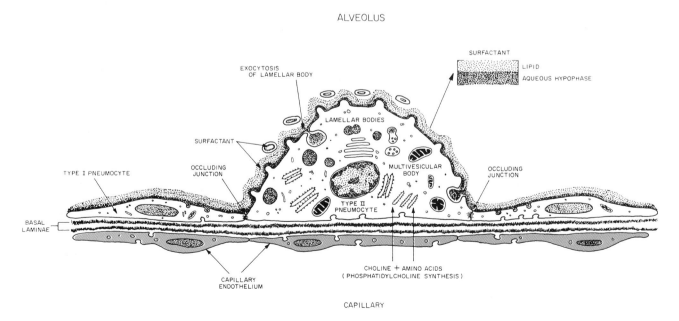

Figure 17.25. Diagram of the blood-air barrier.

late the lungs. However, the alveolar macrophages resident in the lungs can divide to form a partially self-propagating population of cells.

MEDICAL CONSIDERATIONS

Normally, the consistency of mucus is such that it is easily propelled by the cilia, which tend to move the mucus as a sheet; this movement has been referred to as a *mucociliary escalator*. However, in individuals with cystic fibrosis, the mucus is unusually thick or viscous, and it is difficult to move the mucous sheet and clear the passageways of mucus. Consequently, such individuals commonly suffer more frequent respiratory infections.

Fluid that passes into the pleural cavity is called a *pleural effusion*. Blood in the pleural cavity is called *hemothorax*; pus in the pleural cavity is called *pyothorax* or *emphysema*; *pneumothorax* is air in the pleural cavity; and *hydrothorax* is a watery fluid in the pleural cavity.

Pleurisy is an inflammation of the pleura in which adhesions may occur between the visceral and parietal layers, making breathing painful. *Asthma* involves reversible bronchospasm that can obstruct the small airways and produce shortness of breath. *Hyaline membrane disease* (respiratory distress syndrome) results from a lack of surfactant, which is required for alveolar inflation. When surfactant is deficient, alveoli collapse and entry of air is reduced, resulting in respiratory distress.

In certain cases of severe heart disease, erythrocytes may extravasate from the endothelium into the alveolus, where alveolar macrophages engulf the erythrocytes and produce hemosiderin from the hemoglobin. Such cells, when coughed up with sputum, give a positive histochemical test for iron and for this reason are called *heart-failure cells.*

It appears that particles more than approximately 10 mm in diameter are strained or otherwise retarded in the nasal passages. Particles ranging from about 2 to 10 mm are usually trapped in the mucociliary escalator and directed to the pharynx, where they are either swallowed or expectorated. Still smaller particles that enter the lung appear to be engulfed by the alveolar phagocytes. Chronic smoking results in the transformation of respiratory epithelium (pseudostratified, ciliated columnar epithelium) into stratified squamous epithelium.

Each ciliated epithelial cell may have as many as 200 cilia up to 6 μm long. Some abnormal ciliary conditions are now known to exist, such as lack of dynein, lack of radial spoke linkages, and aberrant positioning of the outer ciliary doublet microtubules. Such abnormal variants of ciliary structure cause defective motility; the result is abnormal clearing of the mucous sheet and various forms of respiratory distress. Specifically, in the genetic defect known as *Kartagener's syndrome*, the cilia are unable to move because dynein (ATPase) is lacking. As a consequence, the cilia are not functional and chronic respiratory infections occur. Such male individuals are sterile because of nonmotile sperm.

The important role of surfactant in reducing surface tension in the alveoli is apparent in cases of respiratory distress syndrome in infants born prematurely. If the surfactant has not been formed, or is incapable of being formed, or is found in reduced amounts, there is marked inability to expand or inflate the alveoli, resulting in severe respiratory distress.

SELECTED BIBLIOGRAPHY

Barnes, P.J. (1989). Airway neuropeptides: roles in fine tuning and in disease? *News Physiol. Sci.* **4**, 116–120.

Bates, D.V. (1989). *Respiratory Function in Disease*, 3rd ed. W.B. Saunders, Philadelphia.

Crouch, E., Parghi, D., Kuan, S., and Persson, A. (1992). Surfactant protein D: subcellular localization in nonciliated bronchiolar epithelial cells. *Am. J. Physiol.* **263**, L60–L66.

Fink, B. (1975). *The Human Larynx: A Functional Study.* Raven Press, New York.

Fisherman, A.P., ed. (1988). *Pulmonary Diseases and Disorders*, 2nd ed. McGraw-Hill, New York.

Gross, I. (1990). Regulation of fetal lung maturation. *Am. J. Physiol.* **259**, L337–L344.

Haagsman, H.P., and Van Golde, L.M.G. (1990). Synthesis and assembly of lung surfactant. *Annu. Rev. Physiol.* **53**, 441–464.

Hawgood, S., and Shiffer, K. (1991). Structures and properties of the surfactant-associated proteins. *Annu. Rev. Physiol.* **53**, 375–394.

Holian, A., and Scheule, R.K. (1990). Alveolar macrophage biology. *Hosp. Pract.* **25**, 49–58.

Karczewski, W.A., et al. (1988). *Control of Breathing During Sleep and Anesthesia.* Plenum, New York.

Massaro, D., ed. (1988). *Lung Cell Biology.* Marcel Dekker, New York.

Nicholas, T. (1993). Control of turnover of alveolar surfactant. *NIPS.* **8**, 12–18.

West, J.B. (1987). *Pulmonary Pathophysiology—The Essentials*, 3rd ed. Williams & Wilkins, Baltimore.

Widdicombe, J.G., and Webber, S.E. (1990). Airway mucus secretion. *News Physiol. Sci.* **5**, 2–5.

Wright, J.R., and Dobbs, L.G. (1991). Regulation of pulmonary surfactant secretion and clearance. *Annu. Rev. Physiol.* **53**, 395–414.

The Digestive System

ORGANIZATION AND GENERAL FUNCTIONS

The digestive system consists of distinct organs involved in the ingestion, digestion, and absorption of foodstuffs necessary for the life of all resident cells in the body (Fig. 18.1). The digestive tube is structurally and functionally differentiated for a division of labor in the digestive process. During embryonic development, outgrowths from the tube occur that then differentiate into digestive glands, permitting further specialization in the digestive process. A variety of cell types present in the digestive tract produces the multitude of enzymes, hormones, and other factors necessary for digestive functions. Numerous enzymes are produced to cleave proteins, carbohydrates, and fats into simpler molecules that may be transported to and into cells for use as raw materials. In addition, the digestive system is one of the largest endocrine "organs" in the body. Lymphatic nodules are present throughout the digestive tract and comprise the gut-associated lymphatic tissue (GALT). T and B lymphocytes, macrophages, and plasma cells are widely distributed in the connective tissue of the system.

Several parts of the digestive tube share a common plan in their histologic organization. This basic plan will be described, with an explanation of how each region is structurally modified to carry out specific functions. Before the basic plan of the digestive tract is presented, however, the organization and function of the oral cavity and pharynx will be described since they deviate significantly from the basic plan of the digestive tube.

ORAL CAVITY

LIPS AND CHEEKS

The oral cavity is formed, in part, by the lips and cheeks. The lips consist of skeletal muscle called the *orbicularis* *oris* that is surrounded by connective tissue and externally by thin skin. The outer surface of the lips contains hair follicles, sebaceous glands, and sweat glands. The red portion of the lips is covered by keratinized, stratified squamous epithelium that is somewhat transparent. There are also deep connective tissue papillae adjacent to this transparent epidermis, and blood vessels are brought close to the surface of the lips and are responsible for the red color. Since very little keratin is associated with the red portion of the lips, they must be periodically moistened with saliva by the tongue to prevent chapping. Just inside the free margin of the lips, the epithelium is thicker, nonkeratinized, stratified squamous. The connective tissue lamina propria beneath the epithelium contains mucus-secreting *labial* *glands*. The inner lining of the cheeks consists of nonkeratinized, stratified squamous epithelium and a connective tissue lamina propria. The lamina propria is continuous with a submucosa layer. Since both layers contain loose connective tissue, this boundary is not sharply delineated. Bundles of skeletal muscle are closely associated with the loose connective tissue in the cheeks.

TONGUE

The tongue consists of a central region of skeletal muscle fibers arranged in all possible orientations. The muscle is surrounded by a layer of loose connective tissue lamina propria and externally by an epithelial layer that is highly modified by the formation of several types of papillae. The papillae located on the dorsal surface of the tongue are folds of epithelium that contain a core of lamina propria connective tissue. The undersurface of the tongue is covered by stratified, squamous, nonkeratinized epithelium. The dorsal surface of the tongue is covered by stratified, squamous, keratinized epithelium.

Figure 18.1. Major parts of the alimentary canal. (Redrawn and modified from G. Bevelander, *Outline of Histology*. 7 ed. Mosby-Yearbook, 1971, with permission)

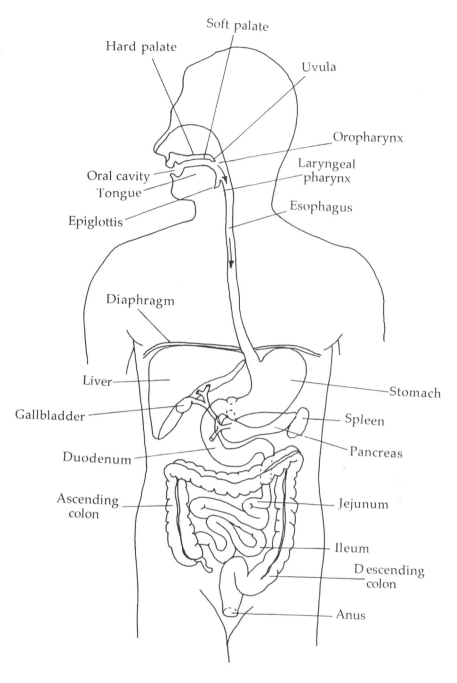

However, the degree of keratinization is variable in different organisms and reflects to some degree the extent to which the epithelium is maintained in a moistened condition.

FILIFORM PAPILLAE

The most numerous of the papillae are *filiform papillae*, which are narrow, taper to a point, and are covered by stratified squamous epithelium (Plate 44C; Fig. 18.2). A white coating on the tongue is sometimes evident and is due to a reduced rate of desquamation of keratin squames from the tips of the papillae. These papillae have a mechanical function and are useful in licking ice cream cones, for example.

FUNGIFORM PAPILLAE

Fungiform papillae are broader than filiform papillae (Fig. 18.2). Fungiform papillae are rounded at their free end and narrow somewhat at their base. The name is derived from the similarity of their shape to small fungi. Fungiform papillae are generally much less numerous than filiform papillae and are more concentrated on the anterior portion of the tongue. The stratified squamous epithelium convering these papillae is not usually

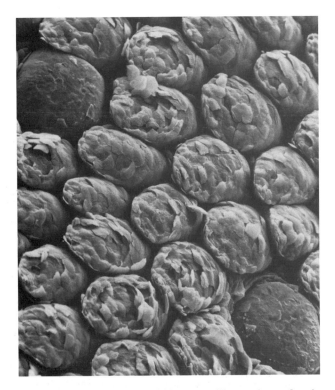

Figure 18.2. SEM of filiform papillae and two fungiform papillae (rat). ×190. (From R. Kessel and R. Kardon, *Tissues and Organs: A Text-Atlas of Scanning Electron Microscopy,* **W.H. Freeman, 1979, New York, with permission)**

keratinized. Infrequently, taste buds may be located within the epithelium of these papillae (Fig. 18.3).

CIRCUMVALLATE PAPILLAE

Circumvallate papillae consist of 8–12 large papillae that are distributed along and just posterior to the sulcus terminalis. Each papilla is surrounded by a vallum or rampart equivalent to a moat around the papilla (Plate 44A; Fig. 18.4). The surface of these papillae may be covered with lightly keratinized, stratified, squamous epithelium, but the walls of the papillae have nonkeratinized epithelium. Many taste buds are located along the lateral wall of these papillae (Plate 44A). Groups of serous glands, called the serous glands of von Ebner, are present in the connective tissue at the base of the papillae (Plate 44A). The secretion of these glands passes through ducts that open at the base of the valla or ramparts surrounding the papillae. The secretion keeps the epithelium moist and facilitates the taste process since substances to be tasted must be in solution.

FOLIATE PAPILLAE

Foliate papillae are well developed in some animals, such as rabbits, but are rudimentary in humans (Plate

44B). These papillae are associated with the lateral and basal portions of the tongue. They are broad, somewhat similar to fungiform papillae, but have a number of long epithelial downgrowths into the connective tissue lamina propria in the core of the papillae; therefore, in longitudinal section, these papillae have a folded appearance. Taste buds are frequently associated with these papillae.

TASTE BUDS

Taste buds are epithelial differentiations that are associated with sensory nerve endings. They have a bowed or barrel shape and are orientated perpendicular to the free margin of the epithelium in which they reside. Internally, the taste bud consists of highly elongate, tapering cells of two main types: *taste receptors* (chemoreceptors) and *supporting* or *sustentacular cells* (see Chapter 4). The free surface of the taste bud contains a small depression called the *taste pore*. The receptor and supporting cells both have microvilli associated with the tapered end adjacent to the taste pore. Basal cells in the epithelium are capable of differentiating into both sensory and supporting cells. In addition, the basal cells proliferate to maintain a pool of cells that replace cells in the taste bud, which reportedly have a life span of about 10 days. The basal plasma membrane of the taste receptor cells synapses with nerve terminals. Substances to be tasted must be in solution and enter the interior

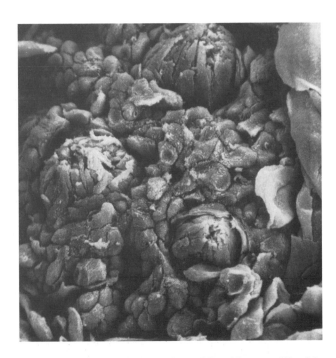

Figure 18.3. SEM of a surface of fungiform papilla with surface cells removed to illustrate three taste buds. ×950. (From R. Kessel and R. Kardon, *Tissues and Organs: A Text-Atlas of Scanning Electron Microscopy,* **W.H. Freeman, New York, 1979, with permission)**

Figure 18.4. SEM of a circumvallate papilla from the surface. ×850. (From R. Kessel and R. Kardon, *Tissues and Organs: A Text-Atlas of Scanning Electron Microscopy,* **W.H. Freeman, New York, 1979, with permission)**

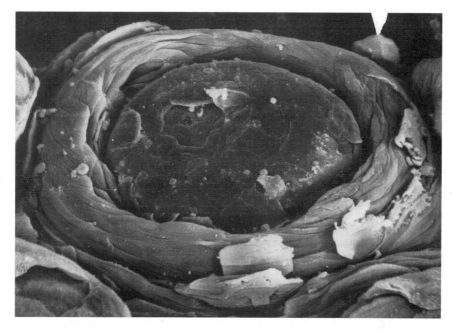

of the taste bud through the taste pore. Here the substances reduce the negative resting potential of the chemoreceptor cells and generate afferent impulses in the nerves that synapse with the cell at its base. Different regions of the tongue are better able to appreciate or recognize certain tastes than others (Fig. 18.5). While the basic tastes include *salty, bitter, sweet,* and *sour,* the ability to appreciate other, more subtle tastes involves different combinations of the four basic tastes.

LINGUAL TONSIL

The posterior portion or root of the tongue contains many small protuberances comprising the lingual tonsils. In the region of these tonsils, the stratified squamous epithelium is folded into a number of crypts. Many solitary lymphatic nodules are located in the connective tissue lamina propria just beneath these epithelial folds. The crypts have a tendency to fill with desquamated cells, but mucous glands in the region have ducts that open into the crypts; thus the crypts can be cleaned or flushed of debris. In the palatine tonsils, the crypts are not cleaned by glandular secretions; thus they may become obstructed and infected, requiring removal.

PHARYNX

Food passes from the oral cavity into the esophagus via the oropharynx. The oropharynx is lined with stratified squamous epithelium that is surrounded by a lamina propria layer of loose connective tissue. The connective

tissue is surrounded by striated muscles that may be used to constrict and elevate the pharynx. The vagus nerve provides the principal innervation to the muscles of the pharynx. Swallowing can be either involuntary or voluntary. Once food is in the pharynx, however, further movement is involuntary and is automatically regulated by a swallowing center in the medulla and lower pons of the CNS.

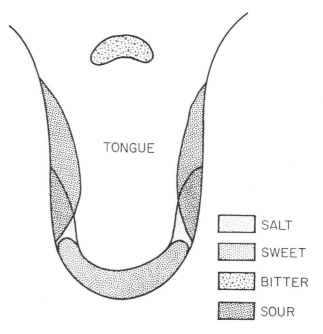

Figure 18.5. Taste perception on the dorsum of the tongue.

TEETH

DENTITION

The human initially has 20 deciduous (baby, milk) teeth; 10 are present in each jaw, 5 in each quadrant. These are lost and replaced by 32 permanent teeth: 16 in each jaw, 8 in each quadrant (Table 18.1). The deciduous teeth appear at approximately 6 months, and all 20 teeth are present by ~2 years, but they begin to be lost at approximately 6 years. On either side of the midline in either jaw are central and lateral incisors, canines, and two primary molars. The permanent teeth also include central and lateral incisors. Next to the incisors are the canine and premolars. The premolars replace the primary molars of deciduous (primary) dentition. Lateral to the premolars are three molars.

ORGANIZATION OF THE TEETH

The interior of the tooth has a *pulp cavity* consisting of a broader pulp chamber and a narrow root canal. The bulk of the tooth consists of *dentin*, which surrounds the pulp cavity but is covered by *enamel* and *cementum* (Fig. 18.6). The anatomic crown is that dentin covered by enamel. The part of the tooth that extends above the gingiva is the clinical crown. The anatomic root of the tooth consists of a central pulp cavity surrounded by dentin, which, in turn, is covered by cementum. The teeth are set in sockets or aveoli and anchored by a periodontal ligament that consists of collagen fibers. These collagen fibers extend from bone to the cementum of the tooth root.

TOOTH DEVELOPMENT

Tooth development begins at about the sixth week of embryonic development (Plate 45A). The initial stage, called the *bud stage*, is a thickening of the oral ectodermal epithelium and a slight condensation of the cranial neural crest mesoderm. It is believed that clusters of neural crest mesoderm (neural ectoderm) accumulate in different regions where tooth development is to occur and induce the overlying epithelial cells of the oral ectoderm to proliferate. With continued division, these cells grow down into the underlying mesoderm and carry with them the basement membrane. A thin stalk called the *dental lamina* connects the epithelial downgrowth to the overlying epithelium (Plate 45B; Fig. 18.7). The downgrowth then flattens and expands, followed by a shallow invagination that results in a *cap stage* (Plate 45B). A proliferation of cells from the dental lamina results in the formation of the *bud* for the *permanent tooth*, which typically remains dormant for a considerable period. When viewed in section, the cap stage is surrounded completely by the basement membrane and the internal two layered structure is lined by the outer enamel (dental) epithelium and inner enamel (dental) epithelium, which are continuous with each other (Fig. 18.7). The outer dental epithelium reflects around the rim of the bell to become the inner dental epithelium. The rim of the bell where the two epithelial sheets join is called the epithelial *sheath of Hertwig* and marks the point between crown and root of the future cement-enamel junction.

With additional growth, the tooth bud assumes the shape of a bell and is called the *bell stage*. The mesenchyme that fills the bell is collectively called the *dental papilla* and will develop into the pulp cavity. At about this time, the bell stage formation loses its connection

Table 18.1 Human Dentition

	Deciduous (Milk, Baby) Teeth	*Permanent Teeth*
Total Number of Teeth	20	32
	10 in each jaw	16 in each jaw
	5 in each quadrant	8 in each quadrant
Kinds of Teeth in Each Quadrant	1 central incisor	1 central incisor
	1 lateral incisor	1 lateral incisor
	1 canine	1 canine
	2 primary molars	2 premolars
		3 molars
Time of Appearance	~6 months	First premolars at ~age 6
	All present by ~2 years	Second premolars at ~age 12
	Begin to disappear at ~6 years	Third molars at ~age 18

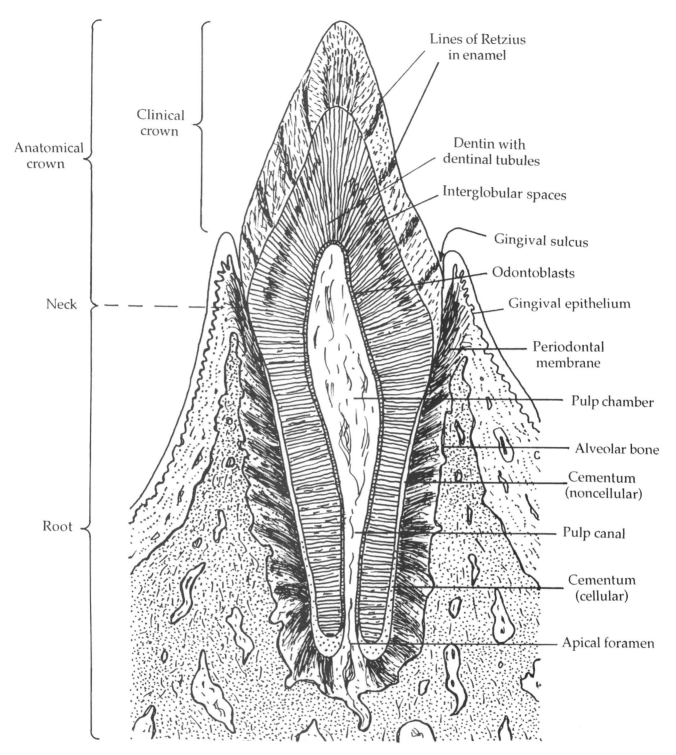

Figure 18.6. Diagram of a section of an incisor identifying its parts. (Redrawn and modified from C.R. Leeson and T.S. Leeson, *Histology*, 3rd ed., W.B. Saunders, Philadelphia, 1976)

with the oral epithelium. Two calcified extracellular substances, dentin and enamel, will be secreted in a polarized fashion by two facing layers of cells (odontoblasts and ameloblasts) that have different embryologic origins. The *enamel-secreting ameloblasts* (or *ganoblasts*) and the *dentin-secreting odontoblasts* are aligned in a row and are initially separated only by a basement membrane. Both cells will subsequently synthesize and export extracellular product toward the basement membrane. The developing tooth is called an *enamel organ* during secretion of this calcified substance. The inner dental (enamel) epithelium becomes a single layer of tall

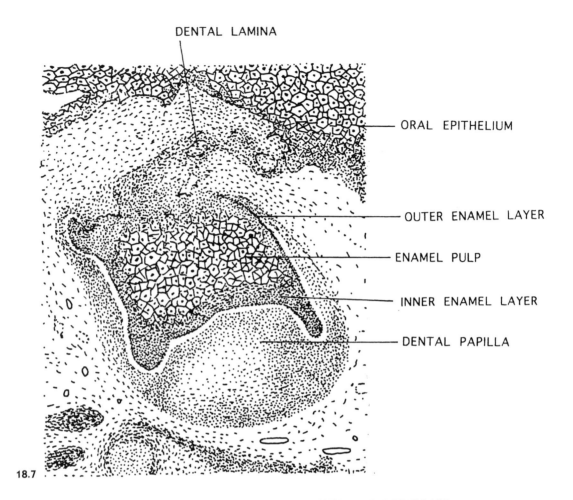

DENTAL LAMINA

ORAL EPITHELIUM

OUTER ENAMEL LAYER

ENAMEL PULP

INNER ENAMEL LAYER

DENTAL PAPILLA

18.7

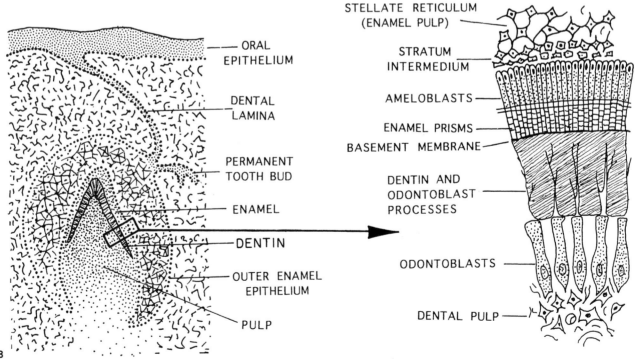

ORAL EPITHELIUM

DENTAL LAMINA

PERMANENT TOOTH BUD

ENAMEL

DENTIN

OUTER ENAMEL EPITHELIUM

PULP

18.8

STELLATE RETICULUM (ENAMEL PULP)

STRATUM INTERMEDIUM

AMELOBLASTS

ENAMEL PRISMS

BASEMENT MEMBRANE

DENTIN AND ODONTOBLAST PROCESSES

ODONTOBLASTS

DENTAL PULP

Figures 18.7, 18.8. Drawings of a developing tooth at approximately 3 months and at 7 months. Figure 18.8 illustrates the ameloblasts and odontoblasts of the enamel organ during initial secretion of dentin and enamel.

378

columnar cells—the ameloblasts. The intervening cells between the inner and outer enamel (dental) epithelium become organized into a *stratum intermedium* and a *stellate reticulum* (Fig. 18.8). The stratum intermedium is a layer one to three cells thick adjacent to the inner enamel epithelium. The remainder of the cells are irregular in shape and loosely packed into what is called the *stellate reticulum.*

Columnar ameloblasts form at the tip of the dental papilla and progressively extend along the side of the papilla that will be the future crown. The ameloblasts induce the formation of columnar odontoblasts from neural crest cells among the mesenchyme cells. Thus, inductive molecules pass from the ameloblasts across the basement membrane and cause the odontoblasts to secrete the initial layer of predentin adjacent to the basement membrane at the tip of the dental papilla. Predentin becomes dentin after calcification. The secretion of this predentin triggers the adjacent ameloblasts to extend a process that comes in contact with a process from the odontoblast. The ameloblasts also appear to phagocytose the basement membrane in this area. The initial predentin that is secreted becomes calcified or mineralized and converted to dentin. Shortly thereafter, the apposing ameloblasts begin the secretion of enamel (Plate 45C,D; Figs. 18.8,

18.9). As a result of the polarized secretion by both ameloblasts and odontoblasts, the cells do not become trapped by their secretory product; instead, they are displaced by this product. The odontoblasts move inward toward the pulp cavity, while the ameloblasts are displaced outward toward the surrounding mesenchyme (Fig. 18.9). As the odontonblast secretes dentin in a polarized manner toward the basement membrane, it leaves a small, slender extension of the cell, called an *odontoblast process*, at the region of the basement membrane (Fig. 18.8). The odontoblast process is located within a narrow channel or canal in dentin called the *dentinal tubule* (Plate 46A). With continued deposition of dentin, the odontoblast process and dentinal tubule become progressively longer. Dentin is thereby riddled with many tissue fluid-filled channels (a number equal to the number of odontoblasts). These channels represent a potential avenue by which bacteria can reach the pulp cavity should pronounced damage occur to the enamel.

Eventually, during formation of the cementum and the tooth root, cells of Hertwig's epithelial root sheath induce mesenchyme cells in the root area to form dentin. The epithelial root sheath then breaks down, and *cementoblasts* originating from *mesenchyme* secrete *cementum* on the outer surface of the dentin. Sufficient

Figure 18.9. Later stage of tooth development.

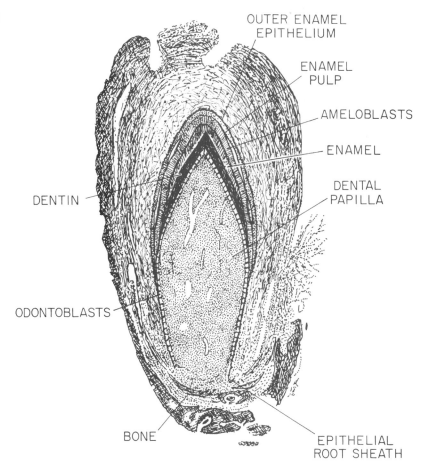

OUTER ENAMEL EPITHELIUM

ENAMEL PULP

AMELOBLASTS

ENAMEL

DENTAL PAPILLA

DENTIN

ODONTOBLASTS

BONE

EPITHELIAL ROOT SHEATH

space for root development is available only after eruption of the tooth. Therefore, root formation plays an important role in tooth eruption. During secretion of cement, collagen fibers are trapped in the cement matrix. These fibers (called *fibers of Sharpey*) are important in anchoring the tooth in its socket.

ODONTOBLASTS AND DENTIN

Odontoblasts are held together in a sheet by junctional complexes. The cell contains rER, a prominent Golgi complex, and mitochondria. The odontoblastic process contains secretory granules, microfilaments, and microtubules. The odontoblasts do not divide, but persist throughout life and are capable of secreting additional dentin under appropriate stimuli such as loss of a portion of a tooth. Predentin contains type I collagen, phosphoprotein, and small amounts of GAG and glycoprotein. During calcification, hydroxyapatite crystals form and grow in the matrix. Dentin is harder than bone and consists of 80% inorganic matter. However, enamel is much harder than dentin and consists of 96% minerals.

AMELOBLASTS AND ENAMEL

Enamel is a secretory product of the ameloblast. It has such a high mineral content and is so hard that it is typically removed in decalcified preparations necessary for sectioning teeth and staining for LM study. Enamel is composed of enamel rods or prisms. The ameloblast has a cone or truncated process, called the *Toomes process*, extending from the apical end; it is from this process that enamel is released by exocytosis. A single ameloblast produces a single enamel prism as a secretory product (Fig. 18.9). The ameloblast contains rER, mitochondria, a prominent Golgi complex, secretory granules of different sizes, and a cytoskeleton consisting of microtubules, microfilaments, and IFs. Junctional complexes are located between adjacent ameloblasts. The ameloblast secretory granule contains enamel matrix, which consists of *calcium phosphate* (as *hydroxyapatite*) in an organic matrix consisting of protein and polysaccharide. There is also a water-binding protein called *amelogenin*. In addition, an acidic glycosylated protein *enamelin* comprises part of the organic matrix. Enamel is calcified rapidly and is approximately 96% mineral. As the tooth erupts, the ameloblasts degenerate and are no longer associated with the erupted tooth. Thus, no more ameloblasts are present to synthesize replacement enamel. Acids in food may produce small pits in the enamel surface. These surfaces may then harbor food, on which acid-producing bacteria can act to cause loss of enamel, such as occurs in dental caries.

CEMENTUM

Cementum is a calcified intercellular substance containing collagen. It is avascular and resembles bone in many respects (Plate 46B; Fig. 18.6). The organic matrix that is secreted by cementoblasts is not initially calcified but becomes calcified later. Cementum is acellular in the upper portion of the root, but the lower part of the root consists of cellular cementum. The *cementocyte* resides in a lacuna and has processes that reside in canaliculi of the cement. Cementum can be formed in adult life by appositional growth (Plate 46B).

TUBULAR DIGESTIVE TRACT

GENERAL PLAN

The wall of the tubular portion of the digestive tract (esophagus, stomach, small intestine, large intestine, appendix, rectum, and anal canal) (Fig. 18.1) is organized into four principal layers. From inside to outside, the layers are a *mucous membrane* or *mucosa*, a *submucosa*, a *muscularis externa*, and a *serosa* (or, in limited regions, an *adventitia*) (Fig. 18.10).

MUCOSA

The mucosa or mucous membrane consists of three layers: an inner layer of *epithelium*, a middle layer of loose connective tissue called the *lamina propria*, and an outer *muscularis mucosa* consisting of smooth muscle. The greatest diversity or variability in the organization of the four basic layers occurs in the mucosa.

EPITHELIUM

The epithelium varies from stratified squamous in the esophagus and anal canal to simple columnar. The simple columnar epithelium is also somewhat variable. In the stomach, columnar cells of the gastric pits secrete mucus directly. However, in the small and large intestine, unicellular mucous gland cells called *goblet cells* are differentiated. The simple columnar epithelium lining the small intestine serves a major absorptive function, and these cells contain many long microvilli on their free apical surfaces. Glandular cells differentiate from the epithelial layer; examples are the parietal and chief cells in gastric glands of the stomach. In addition, cells that have an endocrine or paracrine secretory function are widely distributed throughout the epithelium of the digestive mucosa. Further, the epithelium of the mucous membrane may proliferate, invade the underlying lamina propria or submucosa, and differentiate into exocrine glands in this region. For example, mucous

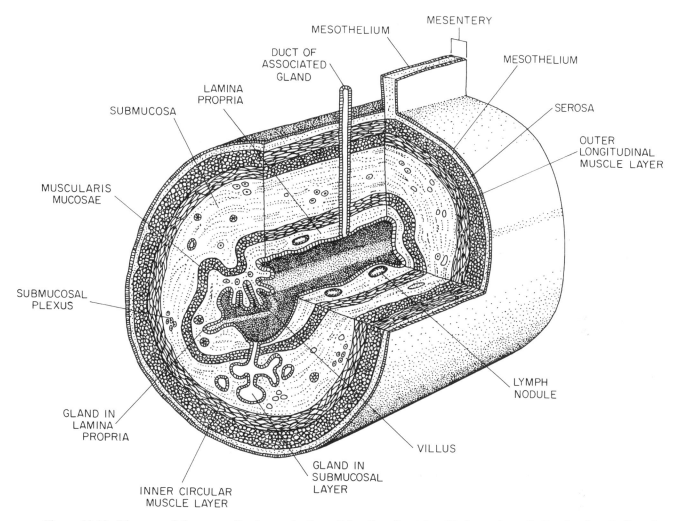

Figure 18.10. Diagram of the generalized organization of the digestive tube. (Redrawn from G. Bevelander, *Outline of Histology*, 7th ed., C.V. Mosby, St. Louis, 1971)

glands (*esophageal glands*) are located in the *submucosa* of the lower *esophagus*. In addition, *Brunner's glands* are located in the *submucosa* of the *duodenum* but communicate by ducts with the lumen of the duodenum by piercing the epithelial layer. The epithelial lining of the embryonic digestive tube proliferates to form major digestive glands including the salivary glands, pancreas, liver, and gallbladder.

LAMINA PROPRIA

The lamina propria is a thin layer of loose connective tissue that forms a packing or support for the epithelium and its glandular derivatives. Fibroblasts, macrophages, mast cells, and plasma cells are usually quite prevalent in the lamina propria, as are blood vessels, nerves, and lymphatic vessels. Scattered lymphatic nodules are commonly found under the moist epithelium of the digestive tract; these nodules comprise the GALT.

MUSCULARIS MUCOSA

The third layer of the mucosa is a muscularis mucosa that consists of two thin layers of smooth muscle. The *inner* layer of smooth muscle is arranged in a *circular* or *helical* configuration, while the *outer* layer of smooth muscle is *longitudinal* in orientation. The contraction of the muscularis mucosa causes independent movements of the mucosa such as folding, which facilitates digestion and absorption. Some smooth muscle cells extend the length of the villi in the cores of connective tissue, and the degree of contraction of the smooth muscle cells can alter the villus length.

SUBMUCOSA

The submucosa consists of a thick layer of moderately dense *connective tissue* that contains fibroblasts, macrophages, plasma cells, and mast cells, as well as collagenic, reticular, and elastic fibers. Many blood vessels, nerves, and lymphatic vessels are also present in the submucosa since these structures are distributed throughout an organ in the loose connective tissues. Mucous glands are present in the submucosa of the *duodenum* (*Brunner's glands*) and esophagus (*esophageal glands*).

MUSCULARIS EXTERNA

This layer consists of two relatively thick layers of smooth muscle with different orientations. The *inner* layer is *cir-*

cular in orientation, while the *outer* layer is *longitudinal*. It is by peristaltic contractions of these two layers that the contents of the digestive tract are moved along its length.

AUTONOMIC INNERVATION

The *submucosal plexus of Meissner* represents *postganglionic fibers* of the *sympathetic* division of the ANS, as well as *preganglionic fibers, postganglionic neurons,* and *postganglionic*

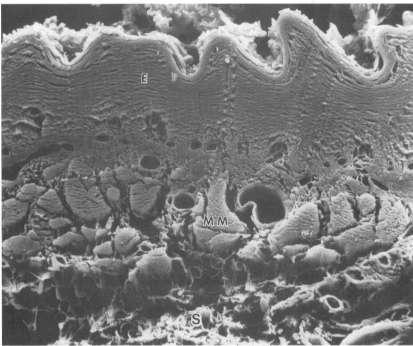

18.11

Figures 18.11, 18.12. SEM of the esophagus. Epithelium (E), muscularis mucosa (MM), submucosa (S), and muscularis externa (E) are identified. Figure 18.11, ×435; Figure 18.12, ×155. (From R. Kessel and R. Kardon, *Tissues and Organs: A Text-Atlas of Scanning Electron Microscopy*, W.H. Freeman, New York, 1979, with permission)

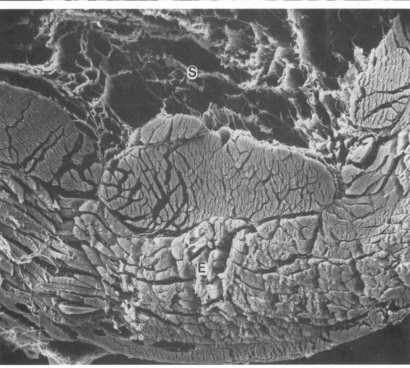

18.12

fibers of the *parasympathetic* division. These nerves innervate epithelium and glands, the smooth muscle in the blood vessels, and the muscularis mucosa (Plate 47C). The *myenteric plexus* of *Auerbach* consists of *sympathetic postganglionic fibers*, as well as *preganglionic parasympathetic fibers* (vagus), *postganglionic parasympathetic neurons*, and *postganglionic parasympathetic fibers* that innervate the smooth muscle cells. *Parasympathetic* stimulation tends to *increase peristalsis*, while *sympathetic stimulation* tends to *slow* it. The plexus is located between the circular and longitudinal layers of the muscularis externa (Plate 48E).

SEROSA AND ADVENTITIA

The thinnest and outermost layer of the digestive tract is called the *serosa*. It consists of a layer of simple squamous epithelium to which a thin layer of loose connective tissue is attached (Plate 50A). In some selected regions, the outer layer consists only of connective tissue; such a layer is called an *adventitia*.

ESOPHAGUS

The esophagus or gullet is a tubular structure approximately 10 inches long that extends from the pharynx to the stomach (Figs. 18.11, 18.12). It serves principally to conduct masticated food from the mouth to the stomach. The mucosa or mucous membrane consists of the epithelial layer, a lamina propria, and, in some areas, a muscularis mucosa. In primates the epithelium is stratified, squamous, nonkeratinizing epithelium, which is useful for protecting against abrasive food particles in transit from the mouth to the stomach. In the upper part of the esophagus and near the stomach, the lamina propria may contain cardiac glands that secrete mucus. The muscularis mucosa is absent in the upper part of the esophagus but is thickest in that part of the esophagus nearest the stomach. Furthermore, the smooth muscle comprising the muscularis mucosa has a longitudinal orientation.

The submucosa of the esophagus consists of loose areolar connective tissue that contains blood vessels, nerves, and lymphatics. Fibroblasts, mast cells, macrophages, and plasma cells may be present in the mucosa, as well as collagenic, elastic, and reticular fibers. Esophageal glands may be present in the submucosa in parts of the esophagus. These glands are compound tubuloalveolar in type and produce mucus. The mucus is conducted through ducts that penetrate the epithelium and open into the lumen of the esophagus.

The muscularis externa is variable in its organization in different regions of the esophagus. In the upper third of the esophagus, the muscle present is usually all striated. In the middle third of the esophagus, the muscularis externa consists of an inner circular smooth muscle layer and outer longitudinal striated muscle layer. In the lower third of the esophagus, all of the muscle is usually smooth. An adventitia layer surrounds most of the esophagus. However, after the esophagus pierces the diaphragm, the remaining short portion is surrounded by a serosa.

STOMACH

The stomach is an expanded reservoir of the digestive tube that is located between the esophagus and small intestine (Fig. 18.13). The anatomic regions of the stomach include a *fundus*, which is the superior portion that lies above a horizontal line extending from the esophageal-gastric junction. The major portion of the stomach, approximately two-thirds, is called the *body* or *corpus*. The lower *pyloric region* of the stomach consists of a *pyloric antrum*, *pyloric canal*, and *pyloric sphincter*. The capacity of the stomach is approximately 1–1.5 quarts,

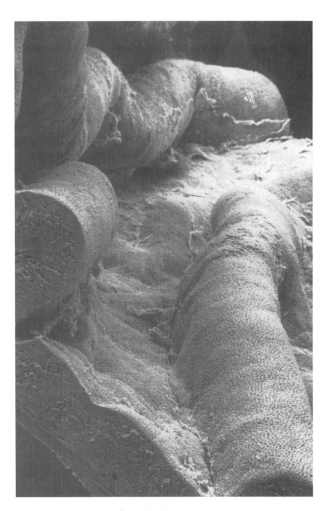

Figure 18.13. SEM of the stomach shows folds or rugae. ×40. (From R. Kessel and R. Kardon, *Tissues and Organs: A Text-Atlas of Scanning Electron Microscopy*, W.H. Freeman, New York, 1979, with permission)

and food remains in this region of the digestive tract for about 3.5–4 hours. The stomach contents can be retained by a prominent *pyloric sphincter* muscle located at the junction of the pylorus and duodenum.

The *mucosa* or *mucous membrane* of the stomach is relatively thick and structurally highly modified (Figs. 18.14–18.16). The simple columnar epithelium is invaginated so as to form tubular *gastric pits* that are variable in length in different regions of the stomach (Plate 47A,B). Each gastric pit is continuous with one to three tubular glands called *gastric glands*. The gastric glands may be simple or branched tubular glands (Fig. 18.17). The gastric glands also vary in different regions of the stomach.

In the *cardiac* stomach, the gastric pits may be nearly one-half the width of the mucosa. The gastric glands in this region are small and contain mucus-secreting cells and a few parietal cells. In the *corpus* and *fundus* portions of the stomach, the gastric pits or foveolae are shortest, but the glands in these regions are tall, well developed, and contain *mucous neck cells*, *chief cells*, and *parietal cells* (Fig. 18.17). Regions of the gastric glands in the corpus and fundus are divided into a *base*, near the muscularis mucosa, a middle *neck* region, and a more superficial part called the *isthmus* that is continuous with the gastric pit (foveola) (Plate 47D). In the *pylorus*, the gastric pits are deeper than those of the fundus and body, but the gastric glands

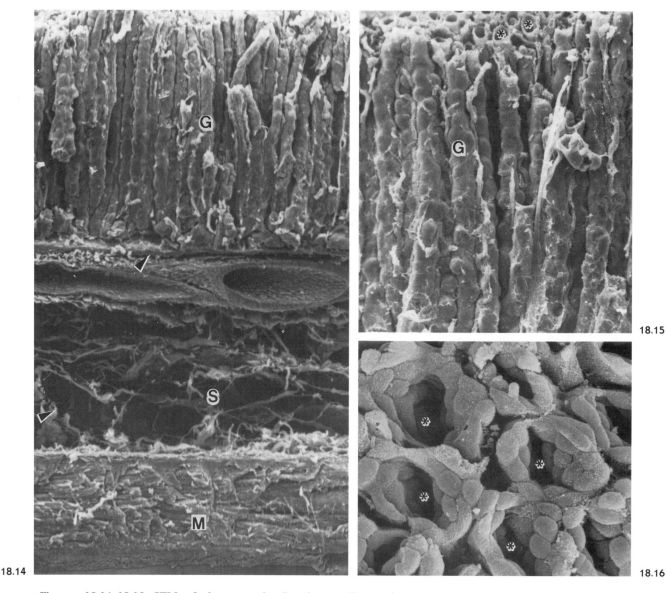

18.14

18.15

18.16

Figures 18.14–18.16. SEM of the stomach. Gastric glands (G) and openings (*) into gastric pits or foveolae. The muscularis mucosa (arrowheads), submucosa (S), and muscularis externa (M) are identified. Figure 18.14, ×120; Figure 18.15, ×240; Fig. 18.16, ×800. (From R. Kessel and R. Kardon, *Tissues and Organs: A Text-Atlas of Scanning Electron Microscopy*, W.H. Freeman, New York, 1979, with permission)

Figure 18.17. Diagram of a gastric gland with cell types.

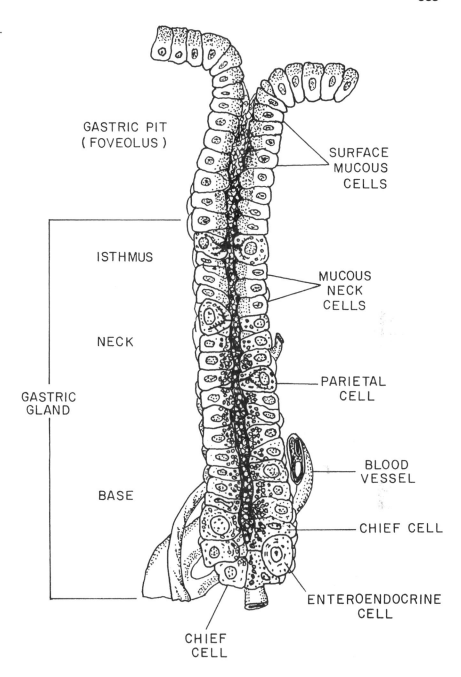

GASTRIC PIT
(FOVEOLUS)

SURFACE
MUCOUS
CELLS

ISTHMUS

MUCOUS
NECK
CELLS

NECK

PARIETAL
CELL

GASTRIC
GLAND

BLOOD
VESSEL

BASE

CHIEF CELL

ENTEROENDOCRINE
CELL

CHIEF
CELL

in this region consist mainly of *mucous neck cells* with a few parietal cells.

A thin lamina propria layer forms a packing among the many gastric glands. This connective tissue layer contains an extensive capillary plexus (Figs. 18.18, 18.19), nerves, and lymphatic vessels. Fibroblasts, macrophages, plasma cells, and mast cells may also be present in this layer. The muscularis mucosa at the base of the gastric glands may consist of three rather than two layers of smooth muscle. The mucosa is surrounded by a submucosa layer of loose connective tissue containing blood vessels, nerves, and lymphatic vessels. In some regions, solitary lymphatic nodules may be present in the submucosa. The muscularis externa layer consists of three layers

rather than the usual two. The middle layer of the muscularis externa is circular in orientation, the inner layer is oblique in its distribution, and the outer layer of smooth muscle is longitudinal. Through muscular contractions of the muscularis externa, the contents of the stomach are mixed with digestive juices prior to moving into the duodenum. A thin serosa layer forms the outer covering of the stomach. It consists of a single layer of simple squamous mesothelial cells and a narrow layer of attached loose connective tissue. When the stomach is empty, a number of branching longitudinal folds of the mucosa and submucosa called *rugae* (Fig. 18.13) are present. The rugae are transient, however, for they are absent in the full stomach.

EPITHELIAL CELL FUNCTION

Absorption of simple molecules such as water, salts, sugar, alcohol, and some drugs occurs across the epithelium into the blood vessels in the lamina propria. Considerable cell diversity is found in the epithelium of the gastric pits and glands; this diversity is related to the diverse function of cell products. *Hydrochloric acid, mucus, three enzymes, intrinsic factor,* and *hormones* are products produced and released by these epithelial cells. The turnover rate of cells in the gastric pits and glands is quite rapid, undoubtedly reflecting the presence of a proteolytic enzyme and a strong concentration of hydrochloric acid (pH 0.8) in the gastric secretion. The entire epithelial cell population turns over every 3–6 days. Gastrin has a proliferative effect on the gastric mucosa.

SURFACE EPITHELIUM (SURFACE MUCOUS CELLS)

The epithelial cells that line the stomach lumen and the gastric pits are simple columnar in type (Plate 47B). These cells are tall and lack microvilli, but the cytoplasm stains faintly in H&E preparations due to the presence of numerous mucigen granules. The columnar epithelial cells synthesize, package, and export mucus directly; therefore, goblet cells are not differentiated for mucus production in the stomach, as they are in the small and large intestines. The surface mucous cells continuously secrete carbohydrate-rich glycoproteins that constitute a thick mucous layer to protect the mucosa from the high acidity of the gastric fluid. Without the surface mucous layer, ulceration of the mucosa would occur.

MUCOUS NECK CELLS

Other cells that can synthesize and secrete mucus are present in the stomach mucosa, especially in the middle and upper portions (isthmus and neck) of the gastric glands. The mucous neck cells are interspersed among the parietal cells in this region of the gastric gland. The mucous neck cells produce acidic glycoproteins rather than the more neutral mucus produced by the surface epithelium. The mucous neck cells contain more rER and exhibit greater basophilia in staining than the surface mucous cells.

PARIETAL (OXYNTIC) CELLS

The parietal or oxyntic cells are large, rounded, acidophilic-staining cells that secrete 0.1 N hydrochloric acid (Plate 47D; 48A–C). This concentration of hydrochloric acid is lethal to living cells. The hydrochloric acid and pepsin in the gastric juice are thereby able

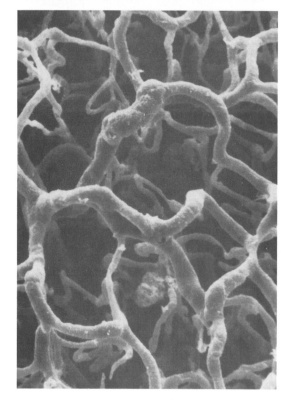

18.18

18.19

Figures 18.18, 18.19. SEMs of vascular replicas showing the microvasculature surrounding the gastric glands in the stomach mucosa. Figure 18.18, ×150; Figure 18.19, ×900; (From R. Kessel and R. Kardon, *Tissues and Organs: A Text-Atlas of Scanning Electron Microscopy,* W.H. Freeman, New York, 1979, with permission)

to kill cells and uncooked foods such as oysters. The pH inside the parietal cell, however, is nearly neutral. The acidophilic staining of parietal cells is due to the presence of extensive numbers of mitochondria and a prominent sER. In addition, the cells are characterized by the presence of an intracellular canaliculus (Plate 48C). The intracellular canaliculus is a deep invagination into the cell by means of which the plasma membrane is additionally folded into a number of microvilli that further increase the plasma membrane surface area (Fig. 18.20). This unique and prominent plasma membrane specialization is associated with the function of hydrochloric acid secretion by these cells. The basolateral plasma membrane contains *receptors* for *gastrin, histamine,* and *ACh,* all of which can stimulate the secretion of *H*⁺ *ions* into the *lumen* of the *intracellular*

canaliculus and *bicarbonate ion secretion* into the *intracellular spaces* and lamina propria.

HYDROCHLORIC ACID SECRETION

The enzyme *carbonic anhydrase* is abundant in the parietal cell and catalyzes the formation of *carbonic acid. Carbon dioxide* and *water* in the presence of *carbonic anhydrase produce carbonic acid,* which dissociates into *hydrogen ions* and *bicarbonate ions. Hydrogen ions* are actively transported across the membrane into the intracellular canaliculus by H^+,K^+-ATPase, and the energy required is provided by the many mitochondria in the cell. *Chloride ions* absorbed into the cell from the capillaries in the adjacent lamina propria are also transported

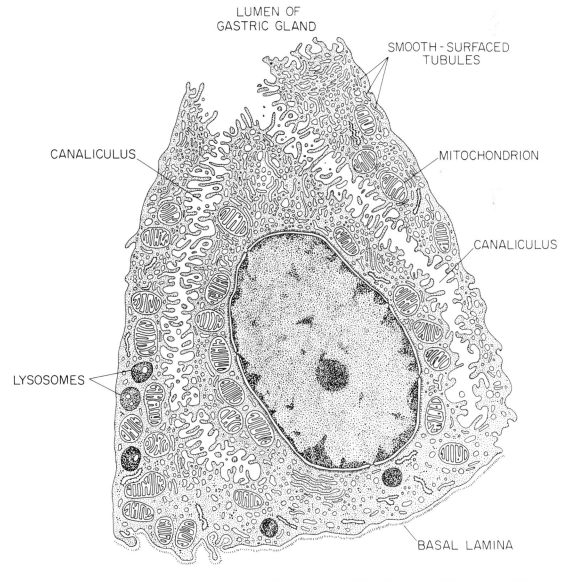

LUMEN OF
GASTRIC GLAND

SMOOTH-SURFACED
TUBULES

CANALICULUS

MITOCHONDRION

CANALICULUS

LYSOSOMES

BASAL LAMINA

Figure 18.20. Diagram of the ultrastructure of a parietal (oxyntic) cell. (Redrawn and modified from T.L. Lentz. *Cell Fine Structure.* **W.B. Saunders, Philadelphia, 1971, with permission)**

through the canalicular membrane. Thus, the hydrogen and chloride ions join to produce hydrochloric acid in the canaliculus outside the cell.

INTRINSIC FACTOR

Parietal cells also synthesize and secrete the *glycoprotein instrinsic factor*. Intrinsic factor binds to vitamin B$_{12}$, which is a necessary requirement for the absorption of this vitamin. Vitamin B$_{12}$ is an important coenzyme required for *erythropoiesis*. Pernicious anemia can result when parietal cells are reduced in number such that insufficient gastric factor is produced for vitamin B$_{12}$ absorption to occur. Therefore, the gastric intrinsic factor is also referred to as the *antipernicious anemia factor*.

CHIEF (ZYMOGENIC) CELLS

The chief cells are concentrated in the basal portion of the gastric glands in the corpus and fundus (Plate 48A,B). The chief cells produce *pepsinogen*, an inactive form of the proteolytic enzyme *pepsin*. The cells stain basophilic since they contain significant amounts of rER for the synthesis of the protein pepsinogen. In an *acid* environment, pepsinogen is converted to pepsin, which initiates protein digestion by cleaving the proteins into proteoses and peptones. The chief cells also produce a *lipase* that participates in the splitting of fats. Still another enzyme, called *rennin*, acts to curdle milk in some organisms.

ENTEROENDOCRINE CELLS

The epithelium of the digestive tract contains numerous widely distributed enteroendocrine cells not easily identified in routine H&E sections that produce a variety of hormones and other factors. Several types of enteroendocrine cells have been described in the stomach and are listed in Table 18.2. They tend to be most concentrated in the pyloric antrum. The cells were initially identified on the basis of staining with heavy metal salts. The granules of some cells precipitate silver from a solution of ammoniacal silver nitrate and were therefore called *argentaffin cells*. Some of the cells stain with solutions of potassium dichromate and were therefore called *enterochromaffin cells*. Still other cells contain granules that precipitate silver in the presence of a reducing agent and were called *argyrophil*(ic) *cells*. As it became apparent what specific substances were produced by these cells, using mainly immunocytochemical methods, the term *enteroendocrine* was introduced to characterize this diffuse neuroendocrine system. Many cells have granules containing polypeptide hormones, but other cells have granules containing biogenic amines

(norepinephrine, epinephrine, serotonin, or 5'-hydroxytryptamine). Some of the cells can incorporate amine precursors and have amino acid decarboxylase activity. Therefore, these cells were called *APUD cells* (for *a*mine *p*recursor *u*ptake *d*ecarboxylase). Since it is now apparent that not all of the cells concentrate amine precursors, the term APUD has largely been replaced by *DNES* (*d*iffuse *n*euro*e*ndocrine *s*ystem). While a number of DNES cells produce hormones that are distributed to target cells via the blood vascular (endocrine) system, other DNES cells are paracrine since they produce and release substances (polypeptides) that diffuse through the intercellular spaces to neighboring cells that are regulated by the secretory product. Some of the DNES cells produce polypeptides and amines that can also act as chemical mediators of the nervous system (neurocrine).

SMALL INTESTINE

The human small intestine extends between the stomach and the colon and is approximately 20 feet long. The initial segment is called the *duodenum* and is approximately 12 inches long. The pancreatic duct and common bile duct pierce the wall of the duodenum at the *ampulla of Vater*. The *jejunum* constitutes approximately two-fifths of the total length of the small intestine. The *ileum* connects the jejunum and colon.

GENERAL ORGANIZATION

The major functions of the small intestine are digestion and absorption of food. The small intestine contains a number of structural specializations to increase the effective surface area for digestive and absorptive functions. Circularly arranged folds of both the mucosa and submucosa, called *plicae circulares* or *valves* of *Kerckring*, are especially prevalent in the jejunum, but they are also present in the duodenum and ileum. The valves of Kerckring are permanent structures since they are present regardless of whether the small intestine is empty or full. They increase the absorptive surface. The surface area of the small intestine is also markedly increased by the presence of over 4 million *villi*. The villi are evaginations of the mucosa into the gut lumen (Fig. 18.21). Each villus is covered by an epithelium enclosing a core of lamina propria connective tissue. The lamina propria contains extensive capillary plexuses (Fig. 18.22), nerves, and a large lymphatic vessel called a *lacteal*. The villi vary in shape and concentration throughout the small intestine (Figs. 18.23–18.25). In general, the length and surface area of the villi are maximum at the beginning of the small intestine and decrease to a minimum height toward the end of the ileum. Villi are described to be broadest and leaf-like in the duodenum. They have a tongue-shaped configuration in the upper

Table 18.2 Enteroendocrine Cells and Products of the Digestive Tube

Name	Product(s)	Location	Nature of Molecule	Mechanism of Action	Functions	Factors Causing Release
G	Gastrin	Pyloric antrum, duodenum	Peptide	Endocrine, paracrine	Stimulate hydrochloric acid, pepsinogen secretion; stimulate growth of gastric mucosa	Vagus stimulation, distention of stomach, caffeine, alcohol
D	Somatostatin	Gastric antrum, duodenum	Polypeptide	Endocrine, paracrine, neurocrine	Inhibits release of hormones (gastrin, insulin, glucagon, GH)	
EC	Serotonin	Stomach, intestines	Amine	Endocrine, paracrine,	Increases intestinal peristalsis	
	Substance P	Stomach, intestines			Increases intestinal peristalsis	
	Endorphin	Intestine	Peptide	Neurocrine	Alleviates pain	
	Motilin	Small intestines	Peptide	Endocrine	Increases intestinal peristalsis	
S	Secretin	Duodenum, jejunum	Peptide	Endocrine, paracrine	Stimulates bicarbonate secretion by pancreatic ducts (acts on duct system via cAMP)	Acid chyme in duodenum
C	Cholecystokinin/ pancreozymin (CCK)	Duodenum Jejunum	Peptide	Endocrine	Stimulate secretion of pancreatic enzymes; causes gallbladder contraction; stimulates enterokinase secretion	Food in small intestine
K	GIP (gastric inhibitory peptide)	Duodenum Jejunum (crypts)	Peptide	Endocrine	Inhibits gastric secretion and motility; stimulates insulin secretion	Fat and glucose in duodenum
D₁	VIP (vasoactive intestinal peptide)	Stomach, intestine	Peptide	Neurocrine, endocrine, paracrine	Stimulates ion and water secretion, gut motility; increase intestinal secretion	
P	Bombesin	Pylorus, duodenum (crypts)	Peptide	Neurocrine, paracrine	Causes release of gastrin	
	Glucagon	Stomach, duodenum			Stimulates glycogenolysis by hepatocytes	
	Glicentin	Stomach, intestines			Stimulates glycogenolysis by hepatocytes	
	Neurotensin	Small intestine			Decreases peristalsis, stimulates epithelial blood supply to ileum	
	Urogastrone	Duodeum (Brunner's glands)			Inhibits hydrochloride acid secretion, stimulates epithelial cell proliferation	

jejunum and tend to be finger-like in shape in the lower jejunum. There are approximately 160 million tubular invaginations of the intestinal mucosa located at the base of the villi, and they are called the *crypts or intestinal glands of Lieberkuhn* (Fig. 18.21). These also increase the surface area of the small intestine. The crypts of Lieberkuhn are usually shorter and narrower than the villi and are approximately 0.3 to 0.5 mm in length. These tubular invaginations also markedly increase the secretory and absorptive surface of the small intestine. The bases of the crypts of Lieberkuhn extend to the muscularis mucosa but do not penetrate this layer of the mucous membrane (Plate 49A,B). Some alteration in villus shape is possible by contraction of smooth muscle cells from the muscularis mucosa that extend the length of the villus. Cells in the crypts of Lieberkuhn

proliferate to renew the cell population lining the crypts and covering the villi. This is an enormous function since it appears that the entire epithelial cell population of the small intestine is replaced every 5 or 6 days.

MUCOSA

Epithelial cell types

The principal cell type covering the villus is the *intestinal absorptive cell* or *enterocyte*, which is columnar in shape (Figs. 18.26–18.29). The apical end of the enterocyte contains long, slender *microvilli* (1.4 μm high), approximately 3000 per cell (Figs. 18.26–18.29). The microvilli increase the surface area enormously. The microvilli tips contain a prominent glycocalyx (Figs. 18.30,

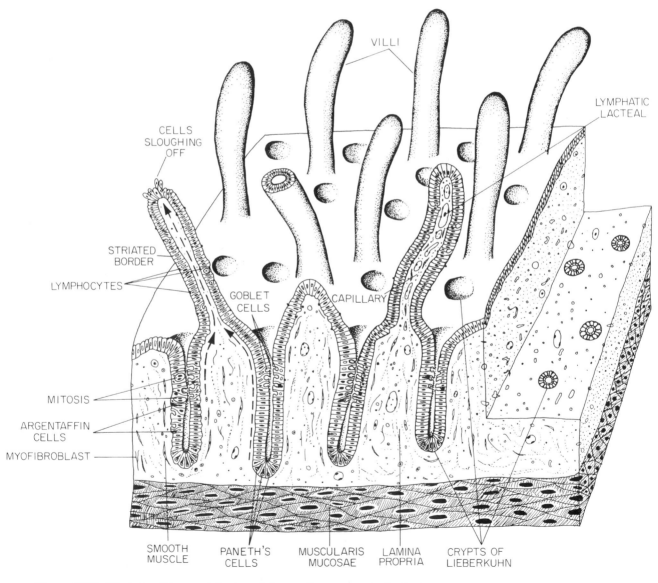

Figure 18.21. Diagram of the organization of the small intestine and the relationship of villi and crypts of Lieberkuhn. (Redrawn and modified from A. Ham, *Histol- *ogy*, **6 ed. Lippincott-Raven, Philadelphia, 1969, with permission)**

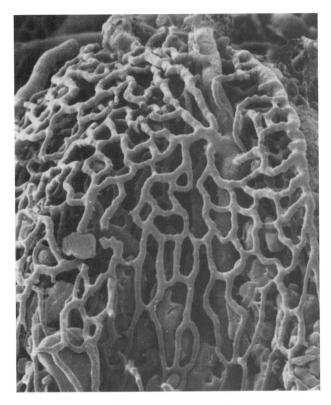

Figure 18.22. SEM of the microvasculature of a single villus. The capillary plexus is present under the epithelium in lamina propria and absorbs digested food products. ×440. (From R. Kessel and R. Kardon, *Tissues and Organs: A Text-Atlas of Scanning Electron Microscopy*, W.H. Freeman, New York, 1979, with permission)

18.31). Several enzymes are associated with the microvilli of enterocytes, including *ATPase, alkaline phosphatases, peptidases, disaccharidases,* and *enterokinase* (enteropeptidase) (Table 18.3). Pancreatic enzymes present in the intestinal lumen are absorbed into the glycocalyx of the enterocytes. It is here that intestinal enterokinase cleaves and activates the trypsinogen from the pancreas to active trypsin. Trypsin then activates other pancreatic hydrolases. The monosaccharides and amino acids resulting from the digestive process in the microvilli then enter the enterocyte through the microvillous membrane by transport proteins. The sugars and amino acids absorbed into the enterocytes are released at the base of the cells and enter the capillaries of the lamina propria. The enterocyte also manufactures a secretory protein called *protein J*, which binds to and protects secretory immunoglobulin A (IgA), which is associated with microvilli in the intestinal lumen.

Lipids are also hydrolyzed by pancreatic lipase absorbed into the glycocalyx of the enterocyte brush border. The resulting fatty acids and monoglycerides diffuse across the apical plasma membrane and accumulate in the apical cytoplasm. Fatty acids that are longer than 12 carbon atoms must be reesterified into triglycerides by enzymes in the *sER* in the apical cytoplasm of the enterocyte. The triglycerides are then bound to glycoprotein (apoprotein) in the Golgi apparatus. The lipoprotein droplets thus formed, called *chylomicrons*, are released from the cell and enter a lymph vessel (lacteal) in the lamina propria.

Figure 18.23. Low-magnification SEM of the small intestine. Note the villi (V), and muscularis layer (M); the latter has contracted. ×30. (From R. Kessel and R. Kardon, *Tissues and Organs: A Text-Atlas of Scanning Electron Microscopy*, W.H. Freeman, New York, 1979, with permission)

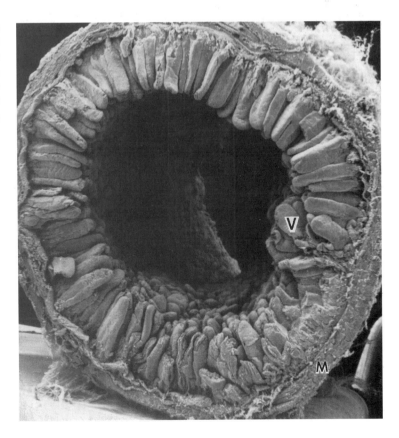

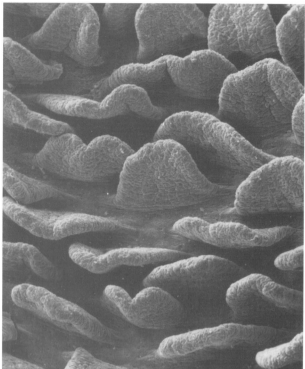

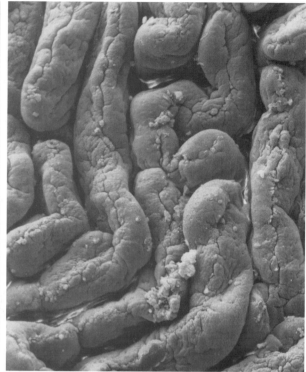

18.24

18.25

Figures 18.24, 18.25. SEMs of the small intestine from within the lumen. Note the tongue-shaped villi in the left illustration and the broad villi in the right illustration. Figure

18.24, ×70; Figure 18.25, ×155. (From R. Kessel and R. Kardon, *Tissues and Organs: A Text-Atlas of Scanning Electron Microscopy*, W.H. Freeman, New York, 1979, with permission)

Zonulae occludentes, zonulae adherentes, and maculae adherentes are prominent junctional complexes between associated enterocytes. Gap junctions are also common among enterocytes. The basolateral plasma membrane of the enterocyte contains *Na,K-dependent ATPase*, which is involved in pumping *sodium* into the *intercellular space*. Water is passively drawn out of the cell into the intercellular space as well and is absorbed into capillaries (Fig. 18.22) in the lamina propria. This system makes possible the retrieval and removal of water from the gut lumen.

Paneth cells

Paneth cells are located at the base of the crypts of Lieberkuhn and have a life span of about 1 month (Plate 49D). Paneth cells contain extensive rER, a prominent Golgi complex, and large, acidophilic-staining secretory granules that are discharged into the crypt lumen by exocytosis. The acidophilic secretory granules contain *lysozyme*, which digests the cell walls of certain bacteria. *Zinc* is present in the secre-

tory granules, but its functional significance is not clear. Paneth cells appear to be phagocytic and can ingest and digest certain microorganisms, thus assisting in the regulation of microbial flora in the small intestine.

Goblet cells

The villus epithelium is covered and lubricated by a protective layer of mucus that lies external to the glycocalyx of the enterocytes. The mucus is produced by goblet cells that are widely distributed throughout the small and large intestines (Plate 49C; Figs. 18.26, 18.27). Mucigen granules accumulate in the distal or apical ends of the rounded goblet cells prior to discharge. The goblet cells have a 4- to 6-day life span.

Caveolated cells

Caveolated cells are located in the crypts of the small and large intestines and on the villi of the small intestine. They are characterized by many invaginations

Figures 18.26–18.29. SEMs of the intestinal epithelium and goblet (G) cells. Note the numerous long microvilli (M) associated with the apical ends of the intestinal epithelial cells. Figure 18.26, ×4375; Figure 18.27, ×7800; Figure

18.28, ×9600; Figure 18.29, ×17,500. (From R. Kessel and R. Kardon, *Tissues and Organs: A Text-Atlas of Scanning Electron Microscopy*, W.H. Freeman, New York, 1979, with permission)

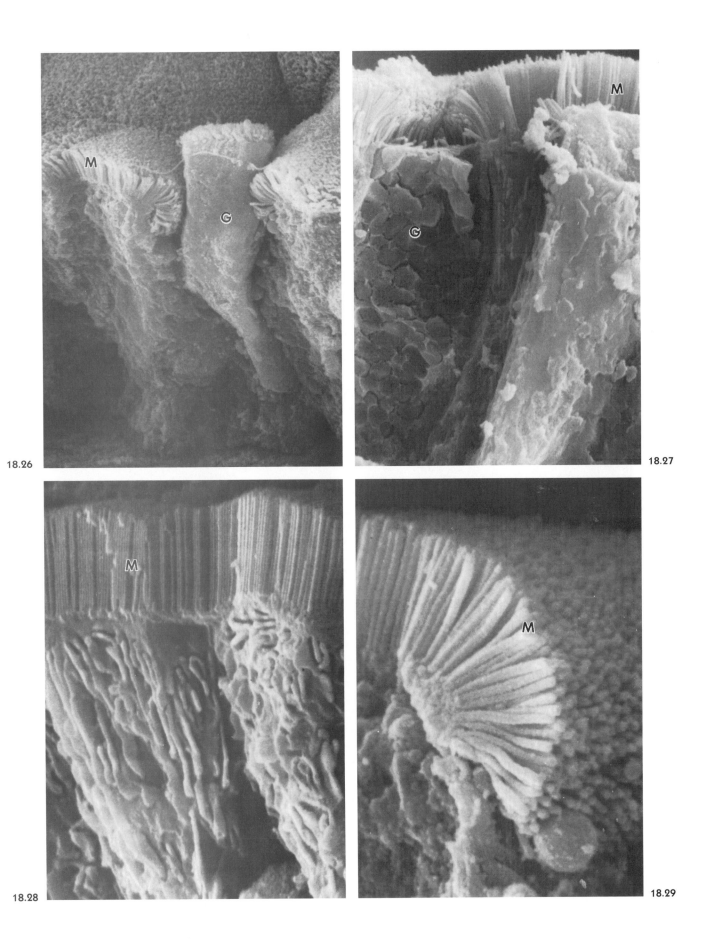

18.26

18.27

18.28

18.29

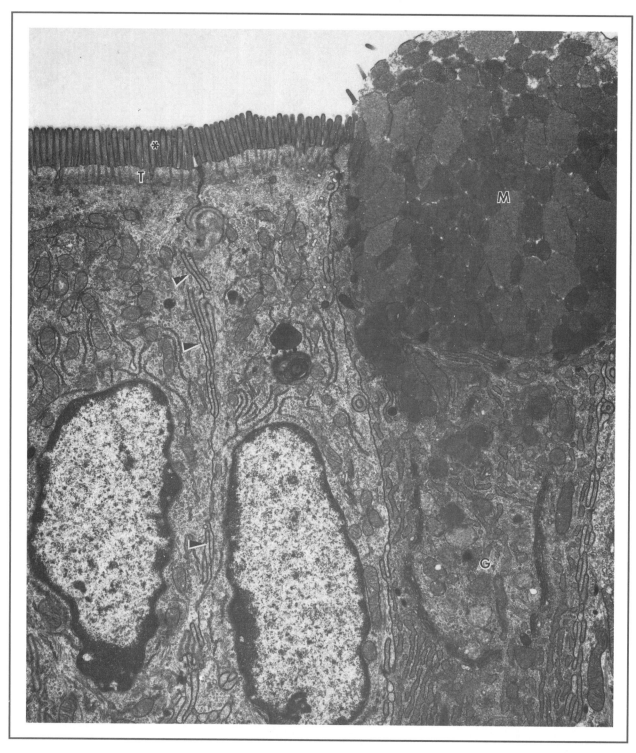

Figure 18.30. TEM of an intestinal epithelial cell and a goblet cell. The goblet cell is filled with mucigen granules (M) and has a prominent Golgi (G) complex. Note the microvilli (*) and terminal (T) web of intestinal absorptive cells and interdigitating plasma membranes (arrowheads). ×10,000. (From R. Roberts, R. Kessel, R. Tung. *Freeze Fracture Images of Cells and Tissues*. Oxford University Press, New York, 1991, with permission)

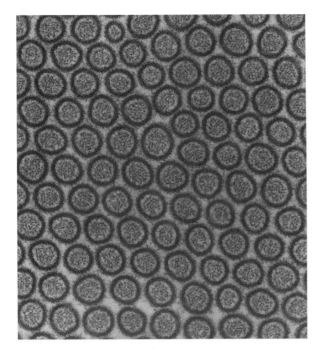

Figure 18.31. TEM shows microvilli in cross section and intestinal epithelial cells. A glycocalyx surrounds the microvilli, and actin microfilaments are present in the microvilli. ×54,600.

(caveolae) of the apical plasma membrane. Their function is unknown, but it has been suggested that they may be chemoreceptors.

Enteroendocrine cells

Enteroendocrine cells are widely distributed throughout the intestines (Plate 50B,C; Fig. 18.32). In the small intestine, the secretory product of these cells may be released and diffuse into the lamina propria, where it enters the blood vessels in this region, to be distributed to other parts of the body. In other cases, the cell product is released and diffuses to other cells in the region (Table 18.2).

MUSCULARIS EXTERNA

The muscularis externa is one of the thickest layers of the digestive tube, consisting of sheets of smooth muscle cells that are usually arranged into an inner circular layer and an outer longitudinal layer (Fig. 18.33). This smooth muscle is primarily responsible for movement of material through the digestive tube by peristalsis. By the alternate contraction and relaxation of these layers, peristalsis conducts the contents of the digestive tube toward the anus. Between the two layers of the muscularis externa, clusters of neuronal cell bodies comprising the myenteric plexus of Auerbach can be observed. These nerve cell bodies are actually postganglionic neurons of the parasympathetic division of the ANS. The constituents of the myenteric plexus of Auerbach were identified earlier. The submucosal plexus of Meissner consists of the same components as Auerbach's plexus but is located in the submucosa. Hormones that affect digestive tract motility are listed in Table 18.4.

REGIONAL DIFFERENCES IN THE SMALL INTESTINE

Brunner's glands

The basic histologic organization of the small intestine is the same in the duodenum, jejunum, and ileum. However, certain regional characteristics constitute important landmarks. The upper duodenum contains branched tubuloalveolar glands of Brunner that produce an alkaline mucus (pH 8.2–9.3), as well as bicarbonate ions (Plate 49A). The secretion has a buffering

Table 18.3 Microvillus-Associated Enzymes in Intestinal Epithelial Cells		
Class	*Enzyme*	*Functional Significance*
Peptidase	Aminopeptidase	Produces free amino acids, dipeptides, and tripeptides
	Entoerokinase	Activates trypsinogen to trypsin (trypsin activates other proenzymes)
Disaccharidase	Maltase	Digests maltose to glucose
	Sucrase	Digests sucrose to glucose and fructose (lack of sucrase results in malfunction of gastrointestinal tract)
	Lactase	Digests lactose to glucose and galactose (deficiency of lactase results in malfunction—lactose intolerance)
Phosphatases	Alkaline phosphatase	Removes phosphate groups from organic-linked phosphates (enzyme activity may be regulated by vitamin D)
	Ca^{2+}, Mg^{2+}-ATPase	Required for absorption of dietary calcium; enzyme activity regulated by vitamin D

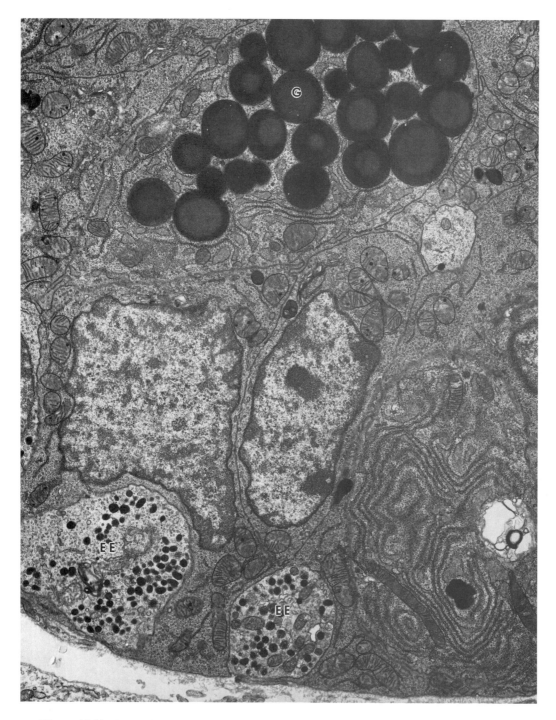

Figure 18.32. TEM of the base of an intestinal gland (crypt of Lieberkuhn) illustrating the granules (G) in a Paneth cell and the granules in two enteroendocrine (EE) cells. ×9900.

action for the acid gastric contents that enter the duodenum. Brunner's glands secrete in response to feeding and in response to parasympathetic stimulation by the vagus nerve. Brunner's glands have also been described to contain *urogastrone*, a peptide that inhibits hydrochloric acid secretion by parietal cells and stimulates epithelial proliferation in the small intestine.

GUT-ASSOCIATED LYMPHATIC TISSUE (GALT)

The interior of the gastrointestinal tract is lined by a moist epithelial membrane. The gut lumen contains a variety of antigens, microorganisms, and other potentially harmful foreign molecules. In view of the short

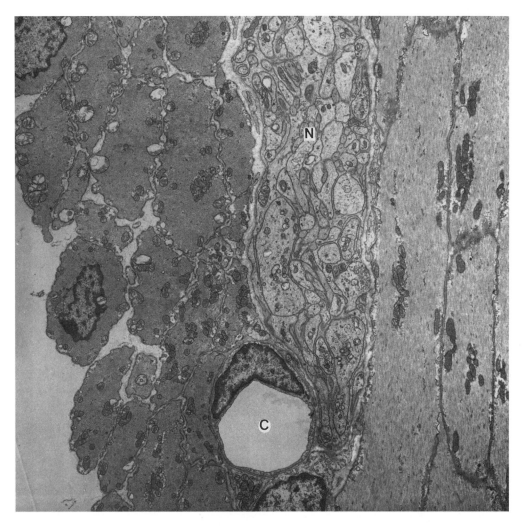

Figure 18.33. TEM of the smooth muscle of the muscularis externa. The smooth muscle cells are sectioned transversely at the left and longitudinally at the right. Unmyelinated nerves (N) of the autonomic nervous system (Auerbach's plexus) are identified. Capillary (C). ×3700.

	Hormone	Where Produced
Increased Intestinal Motility	Motilin	Small intestine
	Serotonin	Stomach, small intestine, colon
	Substance P	Stomach, small intestine, colon
	Vasoactive intestinal peptide	Stomach, small intestine, colon
Decreased Intestinal Motility	Neurotensin	Small intestine

Table 18.4 Hormones Affecting Digestive Tract Motility

distance between the lumen and the blood vascular system in the lamina propria beneath the basement membrane of the epithelium, it is not surprising that a variety of immune cells are located in the epithelium and lamina propria of the entire digestive tract. It is common to find solitary lymphatic nodules located beneath the moist epithelial membrane of the digestive tract. Scattered lymphocytes and plasma cells, as well as antigen-presenting macrophages, are also present in the connective tissue of the lamina propria, and lymphocytes are able to migrate into and between the epithelial cells.

PEYER'S PATCHES

Peyer's patches are closely packed lymphatic nodules that are present in the wall of the ileum. The nodules occupy approximately one-half of the circumference of the submucosa in the ileum. Although lymphatic tissue

may be distributed throughout the small intestine, it progressively increases in amount from proximal to distal regions. The lymphatic nodules of Peyer's patches contain principally B lymphocytes and some T lymphatocytes, as well as plasma cells and macrophages. Peyer's patches comprise part of the *GALT*.

M CELLS

A specialized type of epithelial cell, called the *M cell*, occurs in the epithelial layer of the intestine (Fig. 18.34). This cell is so called because its apical surface, when viewed by SEM, is populated by a number of microfolds. The basal portion of the cells is often deeply indented, forming a large concavity in which lymphocytes and even part of a macrophage may be located. The apical surface of the M cell contains many micropinocytotic pits and vesicles, both smooth and coated. M cells appear to sample antigens from the gut lumen by incor-

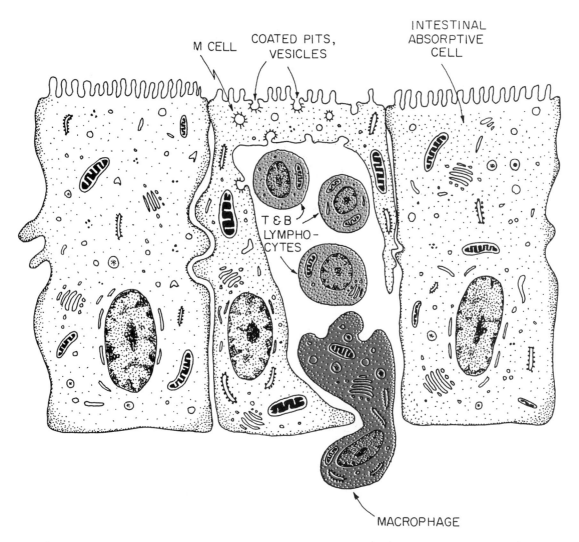

Figure 18.34. Diagram of the relationship of T and B lymphocytes and macrophages with the M cell in the intestinal epithelium.

porating the antigen into vesicles, which may then fuse with the plasma membrane and release their content to intraepithelial lymphocytes and macrophages. It is of interest that the M cells appear to be more concentrated in the epithelium overlying Peyer's patches in the ileum. The intraepithelial lymphocytes may then migrate into the lamina propria, where helper T lymphocytes can eventually reach lymphatic nodules in Peyer's patches or in mesenteric lymph nodes. B-cell proliferation could then take place in the lymphatic nodules.

Plasma cells are scattered throughout the lamina propria of the digestive tract and produce the dimeric secretory IgA, while other plasma cells produce IgM, which is a polymeric secretory immunoglobin. Some IgE that binds to mast cells may be produced, as well as some IgG, which mediates general humoral immunity. The lamina propria thus constitutes an immunologic battleground, with T and B lymphocytes, macrophages, plasma cells, and mast cells particpating in the battles. Foreign proteins, or antigens, may be presented to macrophages and lymphocytes in this region. It is also of interest that intestinal epithelial cells produce a glycoprotein that carries a dimeric form of secretory IgA to the microvillous border and protects it from proteolytic enzymes in the intestinal lumen. This IgA is strategically positioned to interact with antigens in the intestinal lumen.

LARGE INTESTINE (COLON AND LARGE BOWEL)

The large intestine begins at the ileocecal valve. An initial segment consists of a blind end pouch called the *cecum*. From the cecum extends a finger-like process called the *vermiform appendix*. Other parts of the large intestine include the ascending colon, transverse colon, descending colon, sigmoid colon, and rectum. The rectum is continuous with the anus. The principal functions of the colon include resorption of water and elimination of undigested food products (feces). No digestive enzymes are secreted by the colon. Enzymes that are added in the small intestine may sometimes continue to act on food as it enters the colon. Some digestion may also be accomplished by putrefactive bacteria in the colon.

The mucosa of the large intestine lacks villi and plicae but contains crypts of Lieberkuhn (Plate 50D). The crypts are approximately 0.5 mm long and extend to the muscularis mucosa (Figs. 18.35–18.37). The crypts are longer in the large intestine than in the small intestine. The lamina propria forms a packing among the intestinal crypts of Lieberkuhn. The principal epithelial cell type in the large intestine or colon is a simple columnar epithelium of columnar absorptive cells. The apical ends of the cells have short microvilli. Many goblet cells are differentiated in the crypts of Lierberkuhn, and the mucus released from these cells lubricates for the feces and protects the epithelium from the luminal contents. The basolateral membranes of the absorptive cells contain Na^+,K^+-dependent ATPase, which is involved in the transport of sodium and chloride into the lamina propria; water passively follows the transported ions. Potassium and bicarbonate are transported in the opposite direction into the lumen. In addition to columnar absorptive cells and goblet cells, the crypts in the colon contain a few Paneth cells, enteroendocrine cells, and generative cells that can proliferate and differentiate into other epithelial cell types.

The lamina propria may contain solitary lymphatic nodules that sometimes locally displace the crypts in the region. Many lymphocytes, macrophages, and plasma cells are located in the nodules and elsewhere in the lamina propria. The plasma cells can locally produce IgA.

The muscularis externa of the colon and cecum has a unique arrangement in which the longitudinal smooth muscle fibers in the outer layer of the muscularis are organized into three longitudinal bundles of equal size called *taeniae coli*. Because of tonus in the muscles of the taeniae coli, the wall of the colon may have sacculations or *haustra*.

The serosa is incomplete because the ascending and descending portions of the colon are located in a retroperitoneal position. Lobules of fat (called the *appendices epiploicae*) are commonly draped from the outer surface of the colon.

The cecum and vermiform appendix have a histologic organization similar to that of the remainder of the colon. However, the cecum and appendix do not have the longitudinal muscle bands or taeniae coli. Crypts of Lieberkuhn in the vermiform appendix are usually less numerous and therefore less concentrated than elsewhere in the large intestine. In addition, the lymphatic nodules are more numerous and form a nearly complete layer in the appendix. An extensive system of lymphatic vessels is also present in the appendix.

RECTUM AND ANUS

The sigmoid colon continues as the rectum, which is continuous with the anal canal. The anal canal continues as the anus. The mucosa of the rectum is similar to that of the colon. There are no taeniae coli in the muscularis externa of the rectum. The upper portion of the rectum contains a number of circular semilunar folds called the *plicae transversales recti*. The rectum has an outer adventitia layer rather than a serosa. The anal canal is only 2–3 mm in length. It also has a number of longitudinal folds of the inner wall called the *rectal columns* of *Morgagni*. The simple columnar epithelium of the anal canal abruptly changes to stratified squamous epithelium approximately 2 mm above the anal

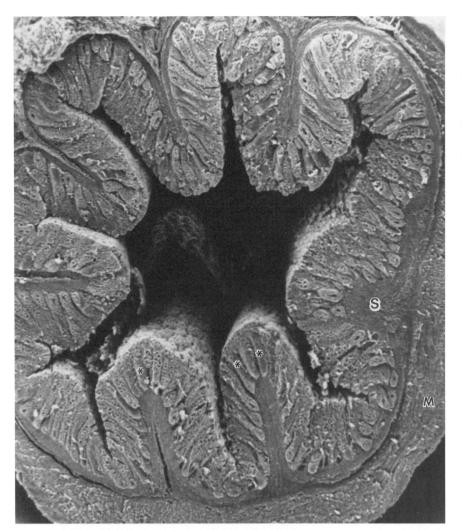

Figure 18.35. SEM of a large intestine. The mucosa is folded. Note the many intestinal glands (crypts of Lieberkuhn) (*), the submucosa (S), and the muscularis (M) externa. ×60. (From R. Kessel and R. Kardon, *Tissues and Organs: A Text-Atlas of Scanning Electron Microscopy*, W.H. Freeman, New York, 1979, with permission)

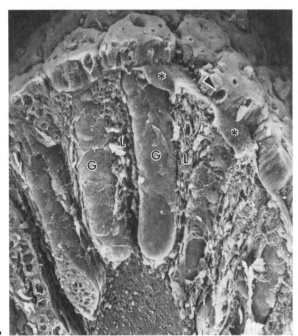

18.36

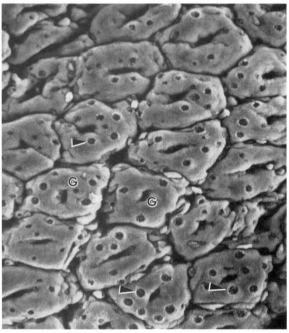

18.37

Figures 18.36, 18.37. SEMs of the colon. Intestinal glands (G) are observed from the side in the left figure and from the lumen in the right figure. The lamina propria (L), basement membrane (*) of the epithelium, goblet cells (arrowheads), and openings into the crypts are identified. Figure 18.36, ×280; Figure 18.37, ×500. (From R. Kessel and R. Kardon, *Tissues and Organs: A Text-Atlas of Scanning Electron Microscopy*, W.H. Freeman, New York, 1979, with permission)

Table 18.5 Digestive Enzymes

Source	Enzyme	Activator	Substrate	Catalytic Function and/or Product
Salivary glands	Salivary α-amylase		Starch	Hydrolyzes 1.4 α linkages, producing α-limit dextrins, maltotriose, and maltose
Stomach	Pepsin (pepsinogens)	Hydrochloric acid	Proteins and polypeptides	Cleave peptide bonds adjacent to aromatic amino acids
Exocrine Pancreas	Trypsin (trypsinogen)	Enterokinase	Proteins and polypeptides	Cleave peptide bonds adjacent to arginine or lysine
	Chymotrypsins (chymotrypsinogens)	Trypsin	Proteins and polypeptides	Cleave peptide bonds adjacent to aromatic, hydrophobic amino acids
	Elastase (proelastase)	Trypsin	Elastin	Cleaves bonds adjacent to alanine, glycine, or serine
	Carboxypeptidase A (procarboxypeptidase)	Trypsin	Proteins and polypeptides	Cleaves carboxy-terminal amino acids with aromatic or branched aliphatic side chains
	Carboxypeptidase B (procarboxypeptidase)	Trypsin	Proteins and polypeptides	Cleaves carboxy-terminal amino acids with basic side chains
	Pancreatic lipase	Emulsifying materials	Triglycerides	Di- and monoglycerides and fatty acids
	Pancreatic α-amylase	Chloride ions	Starch	Similar to salivary α-amylase
	Ribonuclease	—	RNA	Nucleotides
	Deoxyribonuclease	—	DNA	Nucleotides
	Phospholipase A (prophospholipase A)	Trypsin	Lecithin	Lysolecithin
Intestinal Mucosa	Enterokinase	—	Trypsinogen	Trypsin
	Aminopeptidases	—	Polypeptides	Cleave N-terminal amino acid from peptide
	Dipeptidases	—	Dipeptides	Two amino acids
	Glucoamylase	—	Maltose, maltotriose	Glucose
	Lactase	—	Lactose	Galactose, glucose
	Sucrase	—	Sucrose	Fructose, glucose
	α-Dextrinase	—	α-Limit dextrins	Glucose
	Nucleases and related enzymes	—	Nucleic acids	Pentoses, purine and pyrimidine bases
	Intestinal lipase	—	Monoglycerides	Glycerol, fatty acids

opening. This stratified squamous epithelium is continuous with the epidermis of the integument. The submucosa in the anal canal contains many blood vessels, nerves, and Pacinian corpuscles. Veins in this region form large hemorrhoidal plexuses that are susceptible to varicosities. The circular layer of the muscularis externa is thickened near the end of the anal canal and forms the internal anal sphincter. Skeletal muscle fibers that surround the lower portion of the anal canal form an external anal sphincter, which can be controlled voluntarily.

MEDICAL CONSIDERATIONS

Asprin, bile salts, and high concentrations of alcohol are among the substances that can be extremely damaging to the stomach mucosa. When epithelial cells are lost through damage of various kinds, some of the persisting cells change shape and rapidly cover the basement membrane exposed by the dead cells that are sloughed from the epithelium. This is followed by rapid proliferation of stem cells located in the gastric glands to replace the lost epithelial cells.

Pockets (diverticula) can occur in the mucous membrane in the digestive tract, often in the sigmoid colon, duodenum and jejunum. When bacteria and food become trapped in these pockets they become inflamed, as in *diverticulitis*. *Hemorrhoids*, or piles, results from dilation of the veins in the anal canal. In peptic ulcers the mucous membrane may be eroded, resulting in an open sore that can extend to the muscularis mucosa. *Ulcers* may occur in the distal esophagus, stomach, pyloric antrum, duodenum, and jejunum, but most are duodenal. A bacterium, *Helicobacter pylori*, appears to be the cause of many peptic ulcers. Inflammation of the bowel is called *colitis* when the large intestine is involved and *ileocolitis* when both the small and large intestines are involved.

The major enzymes involved in digestive system function are summarized in Table 18.5. The variety of substances that affect digestive tract function are summarized in Table 18.6.

Table 18.6 Substances Affecting Digestive Tract Function

Gastrin	Stimulates gastric secretion (stimulated by food in stomach; inhibited by acid in stomach lumen)
	Produced by G cells in gastric antrum
	Causes release of histamine from EC cells in stomach
	Release locally inhibited by somatostatin
Gastric inhibitory peptide (GIP)	Inhibits gastric acid secretion (like enterogastrone)
	Potent stimulant of insulin release
	Immunoreactive GIP cells in duodenum and jejunum
Cholecystokinin (CCK)	Stimulates gallbladder contraction
	Stimulates secretion of exocrine pancreas
	Produced by EC cells in intestinal mucosa
	Neurotransmitter in some peripheral and CNS nerves
Vasoactive intestinal Polypeptide (VIP)	Stimulates intestinal epithelial cell secretion
	Role in blood flow control in GI tract
	Role in GI tract motility; pancreatic secretion
	VIP expressed in neurons in myenteric and submucosal plexus
Motilin	Causes contraction of GI tract smooth muscle
	22-amino acid polypeptide
Somatostatin	Inhibits various physiologic functions
	Inhibits GH release
	Tetradecapeptide
Glucagon	Most produced in islets of Langerhans in humans
	Glucagon gene is expressed in some Enteroendocrine cells of the digestive tract
Pancreatic polypeptide (PP)	Inhibits secretion of exocrine pancreas; causes gallbladder relaxation
	PP released after food ingestion due to vagal stimulation
	PP cells concentrated in islets of head of pancreas; scattered in exocrine pancreas and pancreatic ducts

SELECTED BIBLIOGRAPHY

Bhaskar, K.R., Garik, P., Turner, B.S., Bradley, J.D., Bansil, R., Stanley, H.E., and LaMont, J.T. (1992). Viscous fingering of HCl through gastric mucin. *Nature* **360**, 458–461.

Bongiovanni, G.L., ed. (1988). *Essentials of Clinical Gastroenterology*, 2nd ed. McGraw-Hill, New York.

Fort, J.G. (1980). Mechanism of gastric H^+ and Cl^- transport. *Annu. Rev. Physiol.* **42**, 111.

Gaudin, A.J., and Jones, K.C. (1989). *Human Anatomy and Physiology*. Harcourt Brace Jovanovich, San Diego, CA.

Gitnick, G., ed. (1988). *Handbook of Gastrointestinal Emergencies*, 2nd ed. Elsevier, New York.

Grube, D. (1986). The endocrine cells of the digestive system: amines, peptides, and modes of action. *Anat. Embryol.* **175**, 151.

Hayworth, M.F., and Jones, A.L. (1988). *Immunology of the Gastrointestinal Tract and Liver*. Raven Press, New York.

Ito, S. (1981). Functional gastric morphology. In *Physiology of the Gastrointestinal Tract*, Vol. 1, L.R. Johnson, ed. Raven Press, New York.

Lamont, J.T. (1992). Mucus: the front line of intestinal mucosal defense. *Ann. N.Y. Acad. Sci.* **664**, 190–201.

McHugh, P., and Moran, T. (1986). The stomach, cholecystokinin, and satiety. *Fed. Proc.* **45**, 1384–1390.

Moog, F. (1981). The lining of the small intestine. *Sci. Am.* **245**, 154.

Owen, D. (1986). Normal histology of the stomach. *Am. J. Surg. Pathol.* **10**, 48.

Roper, S. (1992). The microphysiology of peripheral taste organs. *J. Neurosci.* **12**, 1129–1134.

Schubert, M.L., and Shamburek, R.D. (1990). Control of acid secretion. *Gastroenterol. Clin. North Am.* **19**, 1–25.

Selsted, M.E., Miller, S.I., Henschem, A.H., and Ouellette, A.J. (1992). Enteric defensins: antibiotic peptide components of intestinal host defense. *J. Cell Biol.* **118**, 929–936.

Shaffer, E., and Thomson, A.B.R. (1989). *Modern Concepts in Gastroenterology*. Plenum, New York.

Targan, S.R. (1992). The lamina propria: a dynamic, complex mucosal compartment. *Ann. N.Y. Acad. Sci.* **664**, 61–68.

Ten Cate, A.R. (1985). *Oral Histology: Development, Structure, and Function*, 2nd ed. C.V. Mosby, St. Louis.

Walsh, J., and Dockray, G., eds. (1994). *Gut Peptides: Biochemistry and Physiology*. Raven Press, New York.

The Glands of Digestion

SALIVARY GLANDS

ORGANIZATION

The salivary glands consist of several glands associated with the oral cavity that produce a fluid called *saliva*. The major salivary glands include the *parotid, submandibular* (formerly called *submaxillary*), and *sublingual* glands.

The major salivary glands consist of *parenchyma*, which includes the soft cellular elements consisting of secretory alveoli or acini, as well as the duct system. In addition, the connective tissue elements form a packing for the parenchyma and comprise the *stroma* of the glands. The connective tissue stroma divides the parenchyma into lobules. The connective tissue within a lobule is called *intralobular connective tissue*, and the ducts located here are called *intralobular ducts* (see Chapter 4). The connective tissue that separates the lobules of salivary glands is called *interlobular septa*, and the ducts present in the *interlobular septa* are called *interlobular ducts* (see Chapt. 4). The connective tissue present between the lobes of larger glands is called *interlobar septum*, and the ducts located in this connective tissue are called *interlobar ducts*. Minor salivary glands in the oral mucous membrane include the *labial* glands, *buccal* glands, and *molar* glands. The *serous glands* of *von Ebner* are associated with the *circumvallate papillae*.

CELLS OF SECRETORY UNITS

The cells of the secretory units that comprise the parenchyma of the salivary glands are of two main types: (1) *serous secreting cells* and (2) *mucous secreting cells* (Plate

51A–C). In a serous alveolus the cells have more prominent, centrally located nuclei. The extensive rER is located in the basal portion of the cells, and the protein-rich secretory granules are usually retained in the apical cytoplasm since they are less soluble than mucous droplets (Plate 51B,C). The lumen of a serous alveolus is quite small, and cell boundaries are indistinct in LM preparations. In contrast, the mucous-secreting alveoli contain cells that synthesize and package mucus, a glycoprotein-rich secretion. The cells usually appear clear in routine histologic LM preparations since the secretory material is soluble and tends to be dissolved during processing. The cell boundaries in mucous alveoli are distinct, the nuclei are more compressed at the base of the cells, and a lumen in the alveolus is usually quite prominent. Both mucous and serous secretory alveoli are surrounded by highly branched cells called *basket* or *myoepithelial cells*, which surround the alveoli much like a hand surrounds a baseball (Fig. 19.1). These cells are contractile and assist in discharge or movement of secretions from secretory alveoli and small branches of intralobular ducts.

Plasma cells in the connective tissue of the salivary glands produce IgA. A protein called the *secretory piece* is apparently produced by epithelial cells of the acini and combines with IgA to form *secretory IgA*, which is resistant to proteolysis and is released into the saliva, where it is important in defense against pathogens.

COMPOSITION OF SALIVA

The seromucous secretion of the salivary glands includes an α-amylase that breaks the 1–4 glycoside bonds of carbohydrates. Saliva contains an antibacterial enzyme called *lysozyme*. Saliva also moistens food, thus aiding in stimu-

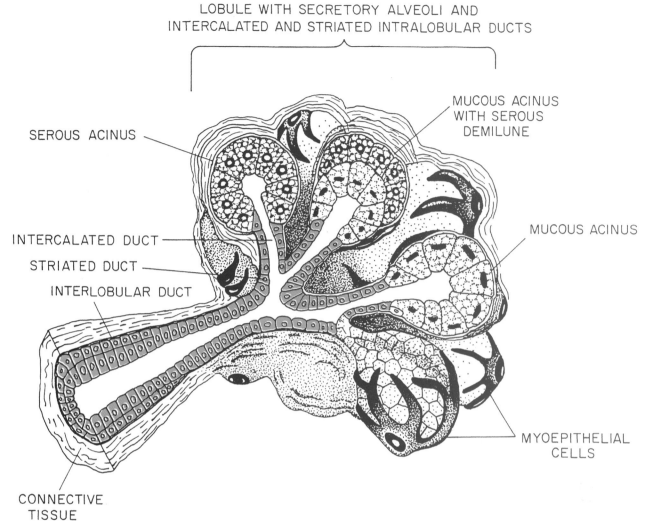

Figure 19.1. Diagram of the organization of salivary glands. Mucous alveoli, serous alveoli, and mucous alveoli capped with serous demilunes are connected with intercalated ducts and striated intralobular ducts. Branched myoepithelial cells are closely associated with the periphery of the secretory alveoli. (Redrawn and modified from S.L. Erlandsen and J.L. Magney, *Color Atlas of Histology*, Mosby Year Book, St. Louis, 1992, with permission)

lating taste buds and moistening dry food. Saliva also contains IgA produced by plasma cells in the connective tissue surrounding the secretory units. Additional organic substances present in saliva in variable quantity include glucose, urea, uric acid, creatinine, and cholestrol. Inorganic constituents present in saliva include sodium, potassium, calcium, phosphate, and chloride ions.

The saliva produced by the acini is modified by ducts as it travels through them. In the case of glands containing serous-secreting cells, the *intercalated ducts* are prominent and the duct cells secrete bicarbonate into the duct lumen, but chloride ions are reabsorbed from the secretion (Fig. 19.2). In glands like the sublingual gland, in which mucus-secreting cells predominate, the intercalated ducts are shorter and not easily observed. *Striated ducts* are present in all salivary glands. These cells reabsorb sodium from the secretion, while potassium is added to the secretion (Fig. 19.2). Under normal rates of secretion, more sodium is reabsorbed than potassium is secreted; thus the secretion becomes *hypotonic*. However, during increased rates of secretion, more sodium and less potassium is present in the salivary secretion; thus the saliva may be isotonic or even hypertonic under these conditions.

DUCT SYSTEM

The smallest intralobular ducts located within a lobule are called *intercalated ducts* and connect directly to the secretory alveoli (Plate 51A,B). These epithelium-derived cells are simple squamous or cuboidal (Fig. 19.1). They are readily apparent in the parotid and submandibular glands. They are very short and difficult to

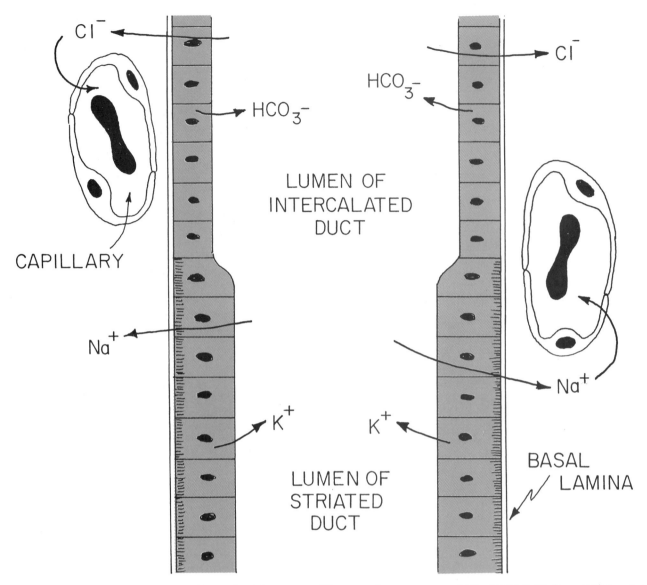

Figure 19.2. Diagram of the salivary gland duct system illustrates the movement of Cl^-, HCO_3^-, Na^+, and K^+ ions into and out of the salivary gland duct system.

observe in the sublingual glands. The larger *striated intralobular ducts* connect with intercalated ducts, are simple columnar epithelial cells and have basal plasma membrane infoldings, hence the name *striated ducts* (Plate 51A,B). The striated intralobular ducts modify the secretion by the selective transport and resorption or secretion of additional materials. Larger interlobular ducts may be lined with low stratified columnar epithelium. The smaller divisions of the interlobular ducts may have simple columnar or pseudostratified epithelium. If a gland is large enough and contains large lobes, the interlobar septa may contain interlobar ducts with a stratified columnar epithelium (Fig. 19.1).

Salivary glands are controlled mainly by signals from parasympathetic nerves. A variety of taste stimuli, including sour taste and the presence of smooth objects in the mouth, elicit marked secretion of saliva. Salivation is

also stimulated or inhibited by smelling foods that an individual likes or dislikes. A liter or more of saliva may be produced in 1 day. While saliva is a dilute aqueous fluid, it is not simply an ultrafiltrate of blood. Saliva differs significantly from blood plasma, particularly in its concentration of H^+, Cl^-, glucose, and proteins. Among its other functions, saliva flushes the oral cavity of bacteria. Saliva is important in keeping the taste buds moist and is necessary for proper voice articulation.

PANCREAS

ORGANIZATION AND FORMATION

The pancreas begins to develop at approximately the fourth week of fetal life in humans from two outpocketings from the dorsal and ventral aspects of the embryonic duodenum, which subsequently fuse to form the head, body, and tail of the adult pancreas (Fig. 19.3). The endodermal epithelial cells then proliferate extensively to form large numbers of rounded secretory units that are all interconnected by a highly branched duct system. During proliferation, the epithelial cells come into contact with the mesenchyme, which induces the epithelial cells to differentiate into serous-producing secretory units (acini) and duct cells. During embryonic origin, groups of cells bud from the epithelial masses and become the islets of Langerhans, the endocrine portion of the pancreas. Since the islet cells separate from the remainder of the proliferating epithelial cells, which remain connected with ducts (exocrine pancreas), they must release their secretory products into the surrounding capillaries (endocrine pancreas) (Plate 51D). The pancreas is both exocrine and endocrine and, unlike the liver, the two functions are carried out by distinct populations of cells. The exocrine pancreas consists of secretory alveoli and acini that are connected

to ducts, while the endocrine pancreas consists of clusters of vascularized cells without ducts that are scattered throughout the exocrine pancreas.

The exocrine portion of the pancreas is a serous, compound acinar, or tubuloacinar gland. The gland consists of *parenchyma* (cellular elements) and *stroma* (connective tissue elements). The parenchyma consists of many *serous-producing alveoli* or acini that are supplied by *interlobular* and *intralobular ducts*. Acinar cells produce digestive enzymes (e.g., trypsin, chymotrypsin) that are synthesized in an inactive form called a *proenzyme*. The secretory alveoli are subdivided into lobules by the connective tissue stroma. The connective tissues present between the lobules comprise *interlobular septa*. Interlobular ducts, blood vessels, nerves, and lymphatic vessels are present in the interlobular septa. Smaller amounts of connective tissue, as well as smaller branches of blood vessels, nerves, lymphatic vessels, and ducts (intralobular), extend into the substance of each lobule within connective tissue called *intralobular septa*.

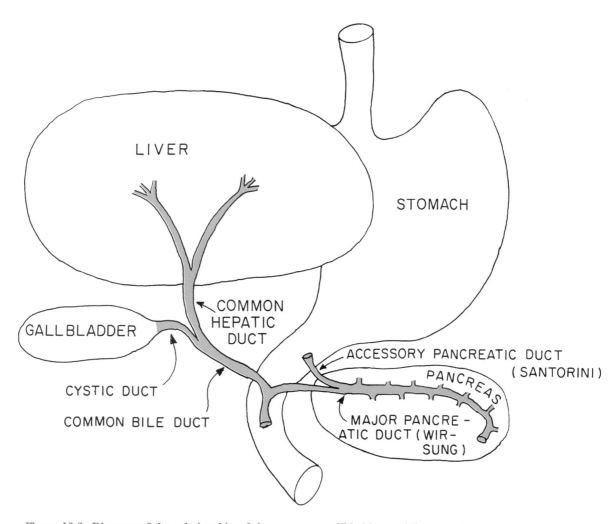

Figure 19.3. Diagram of the relationship of the pancreas, gallbladder, and liver and the major ducts.

EXOCRINE PORTION

Acini of the exocrine portion of the pancreas secrete the pancreatic juice, which contains a number of enzymes (zymogens) that are capable of digesting major food constituents, including carbohydrates, proteins, lipids, phospholipids, and nucleic acids. In addition, large quantities of bicarbonate ions produced by the duct cells aids in neutralizing the acid chyme that enters the duodenum from the stomach.

Extensive amounts of rER are located in the base of the exocrine cells. The Golgi complex is located in a supranuclear region, and many membrane-bound secretory (zymogen) granules are often packed in the apical ends of the cells (Figs. 19.4, 19.5). Amino acids incorporated into the exocrine cells from adjacent capillaries are synthesized into proteins in the rER, move to the Golgi complex for packaging, and become located in the secretory granules, which are subsequently discharged by exocytosis at the apical ends of the cells (Figs. 19.4–19.7).

Trypsin is secreted in an enzymatically inactive form called *trypsinogen*, chymotrypsin as inactive *chymotrypsinogen*, and carboxypeptidase as inactive *procar-*

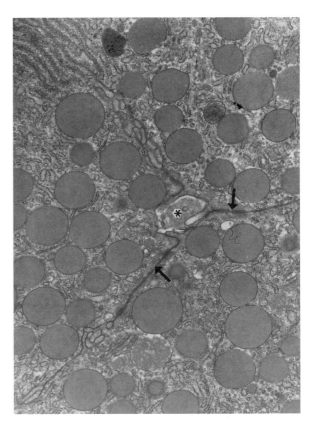

Figure 19.5. TEM of the apical end of several pancreatic exocrine cells. The lumen (*) and the region of junctional complexes (arrows) are identified. ×12,090.

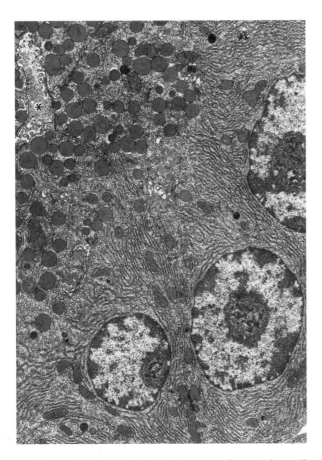

Figure 19.4. TEM of several pancreatic exocrine cells. The apical secretion or zymogen granules discharge into the beginning of a duct system (*). ×4650.

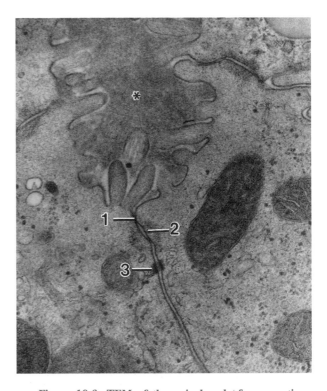

Figure 19.6. TEM of the apical end of pancreatic exocrine cells. The lumen (*) contains secretory product. The zonula occludens (1), zonula adherens (2), and macula adherens (3) are identified. ×38,595.

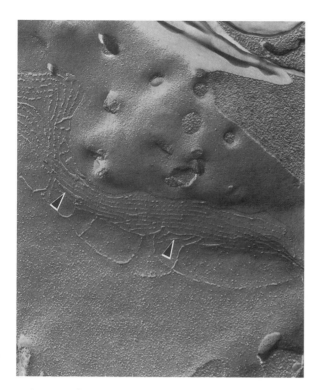

Figure 19.7. Freeze fracture EM of the zonula occludens shows several sealing strands (arrowheads) between the alveolar secretory cells. ×38,750.

boxypeptidase. These substances become activated only after they arrive in the duodenum. *Trypsinogen* is activated by *enterokinase*, which is secreted by the duodenal mucosa (Brunner's glands) when chyme contacts the mucosa. *Chymotrypsinogen* and *procarboxypeptidase* are subsequently activated by *trypsin*. To prevent the pancreas from digesting itself, it is important that the proteolytic enzymes be inactive until they reach the small intestine. The pancreatic acinar cells also secrete a *trypsin inhibitor* that prevents trypsin activation inside the secretory cells, as well as in the acinar and duct lumens.

Because of its dual embryologic origin, the pancreas has two ducts. The major duct (*duct of Wirsung*) joins with the common bile duct just prior to entering the duodenum at the ampulla of Vater. A minor or accessory duct (*duct of Santorini*) branches from the major duct and opens into the duodenum independently of the major duct (Fig. 19.3). The sphincter of Oddi near the ampulla of Vater controls the entry of pancreatic secretion and bile into the duodenum. The head of the pancreas lies in the curvature of the duodenum. The pancreas lies posterior to the stomach, and the tail lies in close proximity to the spleen.

HORMONAL EFFECTS ON THE EXOCRINE PANCREAS

The pancreas is affected by a number of hormones. The major ones are listed here together with their functional relationships. *Secretin*, a polypeptide with 27 amino acids, is synthesized by S cells located in the mucosa of the duodenum and upper jejunum in an inactive form called *prosecretin*. When acid enters the duodenum from the stomach, it causes release and activation of secretin, which is absorbed into the blood. Secretin then causes the secretion of large quantities of fluid with a high concentration of bicarbonate ions and a low concentration of chloride ions. In the duodenum, bicarbonate reacts with the acid to neutralize it, as shown in the following reaction:

$$HCl + NaHCO_3 \rightarrow NaCl + H_2CO_3 \rightarrow H_2O + CO_2$$

(chyme)   (pancreas)

The protective buffering by the bicarbonate is important in preventing duodenal ulcers. Bicarbonate secretion by the pancreas also provides an optimum neutral or slightly alkaline medium for the action of the pancreatic digestive enzymes.

Another hormone that influences pancreatic exocrine activity is the polypeptide *cholecystokinin (CCK).* The presence of food (such as proteoses, peptones, and long chain fatty acids) in the duodenum causes the discharge of cholecystokinin from mucosal epithelial cells in the duodenum and upper jejunum. CCK travels via the bloodstream to the pancreas and stimulates the pancreatic acinar secretory cells to release digestive enzymes.

ENDOCRINE PORTION (ISLETS OF LANGERHANS)

The islets of Langerhans are 100–200 μm in diameter and consist of aggregations of cells that are separated from the exocrine pancreas by a thin aggregation of reticular fibers (Plate 51D). It has been estimated that the human pancreas contains 500,000 to 1 million islets of Langerhans, and they are more concentrated in the tail region. All cells in the islets are in contact with fenestrated capillaries and are supported by fine reticular fibers. The cells in the islets are coupled by gap junctions. The cell types present in the islets of Langerhans, their secretory products, and their actions are described in detail in Chapter 20. Beta (β) cells comprise about 75% of all cells in the islets and produce *insulin*, which *reduces the blood sugar level.* Insulin is released from cells in response to elevated blood glucose and amino acids. The reduction in blood sugar level by insulin is accomplished by stimulating glucose transport into liver and muscle for storage in the form of glycogen. Insulin also stimulates anabolic processes including glycogen, lipid, and protein synthesis. Insulin regulates the activity of target cells by binding to insulin receptors located in the plasma membrane.

GALLBLADDER

ORGANIZATION

The gallbladder is a sac-like structure about 10 cm long suspended from the posterior surface of the liver (Fig. 19.3). It consists of a body, neck, and cystic duct. The gallbladder wall consists of several layers similar to those of the digestive tube. The gallbladder stores and concentrates bile in response to neurologic and humoral stimuli.

The gallbladder is not a gland since it only stores, concentrates, and releases a product (bile) that is synthesized by the liver. The inner layer, the mucosa or *mucous membrane*, consists of a *simple columnar epithelium* and a layer of connective tissue *lamina propria* (Figs. 19.8–19.10). The epithelium and lamina propria are so extensively folded that the layer appears to be "glandular." The term *Rokitansky-Aschoff sinuses* was earlier applied to the anastomosing folds of the gallbladder mucosa. There is no true submucosa layer in the gallbladder. The *muscularis externa* consists of a thin layer of irregularly arranged smooth muscle. When dietary fats enter the duodenum, CCK is released from intestinal crypts, causing sphincters to relax and the muscularis layer to contract, expelling *bile* into the duodenum for the *emulsification* of *fats*. A *serosa* layer consisting of mesothelial cells and a thin layer of loose connective tissue surrounds most of the gallbladder, but an *adventitia* is present in the region where the gallbladder is attached to the liver.

FUNCTION

The gallbladder secretes 600–1200 ml of bile per day. Bile contains cholesterol, lecithin, fatty acids, and bile salts. The bile salts are synthesized from cholesterol and emulsify fat in the digestive tract, which facilitates the absorption of fatty acids and monoglycerides. Bile is important in the process of fat digestion and absorption because bile acids help to emulsify large fat particles into much smaller ones that can be acted on by lipase from the pancreatic juice. Bile acids also facilitate the transport and absorption of the end products of fat digestion through the intestinal epithelium. Bile also plays a role in excretion of waste products in the blood including bilirubin, an end product of hemoglobin degradation, and excess cholesterol synthesized by hepatocytes. Bilirubin is a pigment resulting from the degradation of hemoglobin of erythrocytes removed from the circulation by macrophages in the spleen and Kupffer cells in the liver. The hepatocytes take in the bilirubin and conjugate it with glucuronide in the ER. The resulting bilirubin glucouronide conjugate is largely excreted into the bile.

The strongest stimulus for gallbladder contraction is provided by CCK, which is released from the duode-

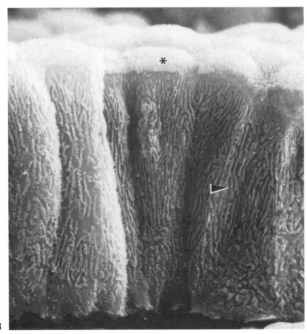

19.8

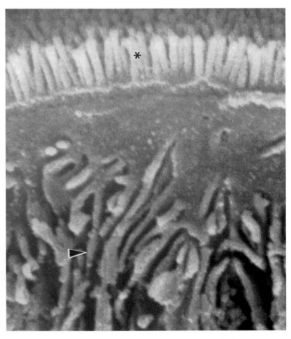

19.9

Figures 19.8, 19.9. Both figures illustrate gallbladder epithelium by SEM. The columnar cells have short apical microvilli (*) and many lateral plasma membrane folds (arrowheads). Figure 19.8, ×3250; Figure 19.9, ×16,250. (From R. Kessel and R. Kardon. *Tissues and Organs. A Text-Atlas of Scanning Electron Microscopy.* W.H. Freeman, New York, 1978 with permission)

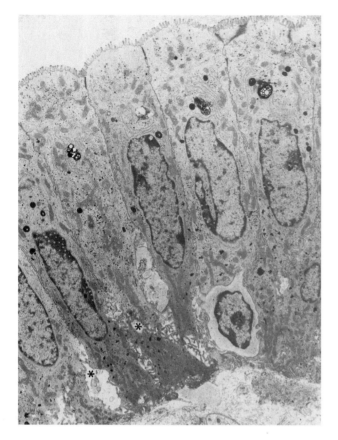

Figure 19.10. TEM of columnar epithelium of the gallbladder. Short, stubby microvilli populate the apical surface (top). The cytoplasm contains numerous mitochondria. The basolateral plasma membrane borders the intercellular spaces (*); the plasma membrane in this region contains many sodium pumps. ×3,100.

nal mucosa in response to the entry of fatty foods into the duodenum. The salts of bile acids have a detergent action on fat particles that decreases surface tension and permits the breakup of the fat globules. Bile salts also

participate in the absorption of fatty acids, monoglycerides, cholesterol, and other lipids across the intestinal epithelium into lacteals located in the lamina propria of intestinal villi. The constituents and functions of bile are summarized in the Table 19.1.

Bile acids and cholesterol, which are synthesized by the liver hepatocytes, and bilirubin are secreted into bile canaliculi and then travel through intrahepatic bile ducts to extrahepatic bile ducts. The common *hepatic duct* joins with the *cystic duct* from the *gallbladder* to become the *common bile duct*. Bile may travel to the duodenum in the common bile duct or be directed to the gallbladder by way of the cystic duct. As bile passes from the gallbladder through the cystic duct and the common bile ducts, *sodium* and *bicarbonate ions* are added to bile under the influence of *secretin*.

CONCENTRATION OF BILE

In order for bile to be concentrated by the gallbladder, sodium ions are actively pumped from the epithelial cells into the intercellular spaces of the basolateral compartment (Figs. 19.10, 19.11). Mitochondria in the epithelial cells provide the energy to actively pump the sodium ions. This activity increases the osmotic pressure in the basolateral compartment such that water in the bile is drawn by osmosis into the blood vessels in the lamina propria adjacent to the base of the epithelial cells. Continuous circumferential zonulae occludentes are located at the apices of the epithelial cells and effectively seal off the intercellular space, isolating the concentrated bile in the lumen of the gallbladder so as to form a blood-bile barrier (Fig. 19.12). Under normal conditions, bile undergoes a fivefold increase in concentration in the gallbaldder, but an even greater concentration gradient is possible.

Table 19.1 Constituents and Functions of Bile

Constituent	*Function*
Electrolytes: Na^+, Cl^-, HCO_3^-, K^+, Ca^{2+}, Mg^{2+}	Keep bile isotonic; largely reabsorbed by intestinal epithelium
Bile salts (e.g., glycoholic, taurocholic acids)	Assist in digestion and absorption of lipids from digestive tract by emulsifying them
Bile pigments (mainly the glucuronide of bilirubin produced in spleen from hemoglobin breakdown)	Bilirubin is detoxified and eliminated in digestive tract
Cholesterol, phospholipids (e.g., lecithin)	Contained in bile but largely reabsorbed by digestive tract; used in membrane and steroid biosynthesis
Water	Vehicle in which other constituents are suspended; reabsorbed by digestive tract

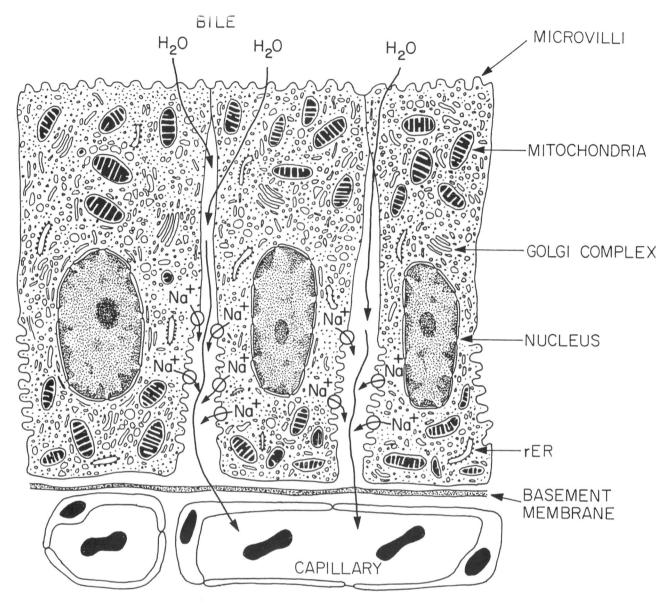

Figure 19.11. Diagram of gallbladder epithelial cells. Sodium ions are actively transported across the basolateral plasma membrane, which creates an osmotic gradient that draws water from the bile into the intercellular spaces and into capillaries adjacent to the basement membrane. This results in the concentration of bile in the lumen of the gallbladder.

LIVER

GENERAL ORGANIZATION

The liver is the largest gland in the body and the second largest organ after the integument. The liver secretes *sugar* and other useful substances into the circulatory system and is therefore considered an *endocrine gland.* The liver also secretes *bile* into a system of ducts; this represents its primary *exocrine function.* The liver is located beneath the diaphragm in the abdominal cavity. It has four lobes and is surrounded by a connective

tissue capsule called the *capsule of Glisson,* which is covered by a peritoneal mesothelium over most of its surface.

That region of the liver where the portal vein, hepatic artery, bile duct, nerves, and lymphatic vessels enter or leave the organ is called the *hilum* (porta hepatis). Once inside the liver, the branches of the *portal vein, hepatic artery,* and *bile ducts* travel together as *portal triads* (Figs. 19.13–19.17). A nerve and a small lymphatic vessel also travel in the portal triads. The elements of the portal triads branch repeatedly on their way to supply the more than 1 million basic structural units of the liver

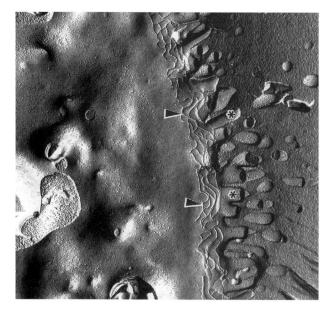

Figure 19.12. Freeze fracture replica of the apical region of gallbladder epithelium. Microvilli (*) and sealing strands of the zonula occludens (arrowheads) are identified. ×24,000.

called the *hepatic lobules.* Replicas made of the liver microcirculation and viewed in the SEM show the vascular relationships clearly (Fig. 19.16).

HEPATIC LOBULES

The liver is derived in the embryo as an epithelial outgrowth of the endodermally lined digestive tract. The proliferating epithelial cells develop *hepatic lobules* (Figs. 19.14, 19.15). A lobule is shaped roughly like a polyhedral prism (about 0.7 by 2.0 mm). A cross section of a lobule has the shape of a polygon, usually a hexagon. In such a section, the *center* of a *lobule* is marked by a *central venule* that extends through the long axis of the polygon, while the *portal triads* or *tracts* are located at the *angles* of the *polygon* or hexagon (Figs. 19.17, 19.18). Numerous plates of hepatocytes (a muralium) radiate from the central venule toward the portal areas that contain the portal triad (Plate 52A–D). These regions at the apices of the portal triad, which includes the connec-

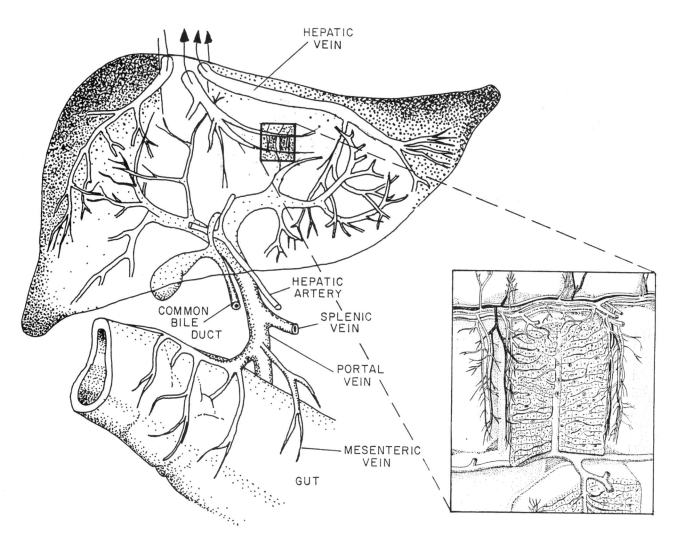

Figure 19.13. Diagram illustrates blood supply to the liver.

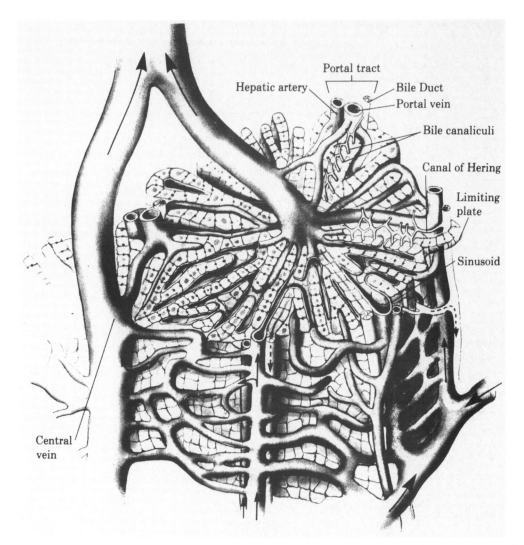

Portal tract

Hepatic artery ———— Bile Duct
———— Portal vein

———— Bile canaliculi

———— Canal of Hering

———— Limiting plate

———— Sinusoid

Central vein

Figure 19.14. Diagram of a portion of a single liver lobule. (From R. L. Bacon and N. R. Niles, *Medical Histology.* *A Text-Atlas with Introductory Pathology*, **Springer-Verlag, New York 1983. Reproduced by permission)**

tive tissue, are variously called a *portal canal, portal tract, portal area,* or *portal radicle* (*Kiernan's space*) (Plate 52C). The connective tissue stroma comprising the portal canal carries branches of the portal triad, which includes the hepatic artery, hepatic portal vein, and bile duct (Fig. 19.18). Lymphatic vessels are also located in these regions.

Since the pig liver has relatively large amounts of connective tissue to demarcate the boundaries of the hepatic lobules, the extent of the lobules is clear. In humans, however, the boundary of the lobule can be approximated by locating a central venule in cross section with radially disposed plates of hepatocytes and intervening sinusoids and then noting the position of the portal triads with respect to the central venule. If an imaginary line is then drawn to interconnect the portal triads, the approximate boundary of the lobule can be discerned. The number of portal tracts per lobule in humans ranges from three to six.

CIRCULATORY SYSTEM

The liver is unique in that it receives not only a supply of arterial blood from the *hepatic arteries* but also a supply of venous blood from veins originating in digestive organs (Fig. 19.13). Capillaries in the digestive system form the *hepatic portal vein,* which courses to the liver, where it again breaks down into an extensive capillary system within the substance of the liver (Fig. 19.16). Roughly 75% of the blood to the liver is carried in the hepatic portal vein. Oxygen-laden blood in much smaller quantity is conveyed to the liver in the hepatic artery, which is a branch from the coeliac trunk of the abdominal aorta.

The hepatic portal (or portal) vein branches repeatedly as it courses through the parenchyma of the liver. The small branches that supply the portal triads are portal venules (interlobular veins). The portal venules then branch into distributing veins that extend around

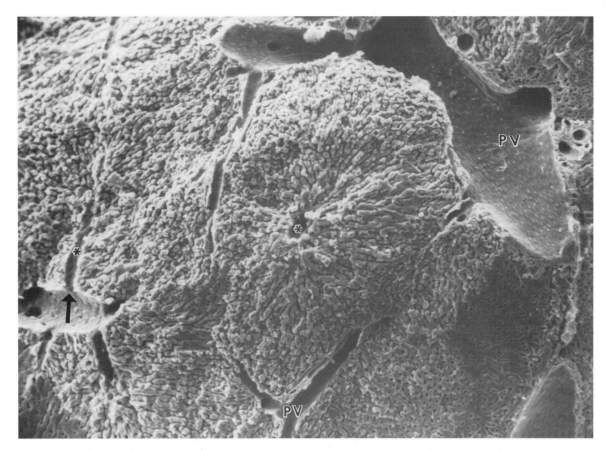

Figure 19.15. SEM of a liver that was cut to display the internal parts. The numerous interconnecting plates of hepatocytes in a liver lobule radiate toward a central venule (*) located in the middle of the lobule. The classic liver lobule is bounded on the periphery by groups of ducts and vessels, the most prominent of which are the conducting and distributing portal veins (PV). Blood flows from the periphery of the lobules through the many sinusoids to the central venule and into a sublobular vein (arrows). ×110. (From R. Kessel and R. Kardon. *Tissues and Organs: A Text-Atlas of Scanning Electron Microscopy.* W.H. Freeman, New York, 1978 with permission)

Figure 19.16. Liver microvasculature cast. Several lobules with a central vein (CV) and radiating sinusoids (S) are apparent. Portal areas containing a conducting portal vein (CPV), distributing portal vein (DPV), and arterial divisions (Ar) are identified. Arrowheads at the periphery of a classic lobule identify regions where distributing portal veins communicate with sinusoids. ×95. (From R. Kessel and R. Kardon, *Tissues and Organs: a Text-Atlas of Scanning Electron Microscopy.* W.H. Freeman, New York, 1979, with permission)

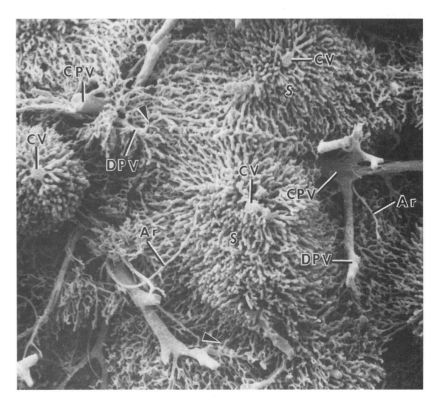

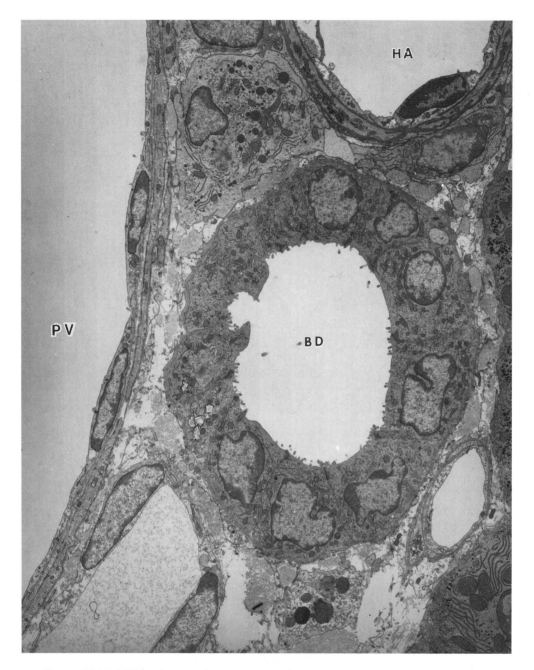

Figure 19.17. TEM of a portal tract or portal area. Structures identified include the hepatic portal vein (PV), hepatic artery (HA), bile ductule (BD), and edge of hepatocytes. ×15,145. (From: R. Roberts, R. Kessel, H. Tung. *Freeze Fracture Images of Cells and Tissues.* Oxford University Press, 1991, with permission)

the periphery of the lobule (Fig. 19.17). From the distributing branches of the portal vein, small inlet venules open directly or communicate with the *sinusoids* (Figs. 19.16, 19.18). Blood then travels in the system of sinusoids toward the central venule of the liver lobule (Plate 52A,B). The *central venules* of adjacent lobules drain into sublobular veins. The *sublobular veins* converge as the *hepatic vein*, which subsequently joins the *inferior vena cava.*

The hepatic artery also branches repeatedly as it courses through the liver parenchyma. The small branches that supply the portal triads (interlobular ar-

teries) branch to extend around the periphery of the lobule. From these branches, small inlet arterioles extend to and become continuous with the sinusoidal capillaries. As a consequence, both arterial and venous blood empty into the sinusoidal system of the lobule.

ENDOTHELIAL CELLS, SPACE OF DISSE, KUPFFER CELLS

The hepatic lobule consists principally of radiating plates of heptocytes and intervening sinusoids through

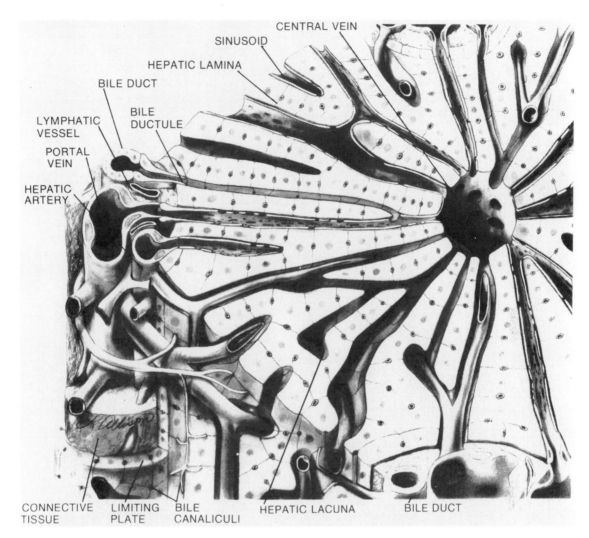

CENTRAL VEIN
SINUSOID
HEPATIC LAMINA
BILE DUCT
BILE DUCTULE
LYMPHATIC VESSEL
PORTAL VEIN
HEPATIC ARTERY
CONNECTIVE TISSUE
LIMITING PLATE
BILE CANALICULI
HEPATIC LACUNA
BILE DUCT

Figure 19.18. Diagram of part of a hepatic lobule shows branches of the hepatic artery and hepatic portal vein and their relationship to sinusoids that communicate with the central vein (venule). The bile canaliculi, bile ductule, and bile duct are illustrated. Sinusoids lined by fenestrated en- **dothelium, which is shown in some of the sinusoids. (From T.S. Leeson and C.R. Leeson, *Histology*, 4th ed., Philadelphia, W.B. Saunders Company, 1981. Reprinted by permission)**

which blood travels from the periphery of the lobules to the center where the central venule is located (Fig. 19.18). It is important to emphasize that in the hepatic lobule, every hepatocyte is in contact with another hepatocyte and a sinusoid (Fig. 19.19). This arrangement is important for liver function because bile will be released into a canaliculus between two liver cells, and contact with the sinusoid is important for the endocrine secretion and for the interchange with blood. The sinusoids are lined by a thin layer of *endothelial cells* that are unusual in the presence of numerous and quite large holes or *fenestrations* (Plate 52D; Figs. 19.20–19.23). The walls of the sinusoids have discontinuities between endothelial cells, as well as transcellular fenestrations (Fig. 19.21). The fenestrations may be 100 nm in diameter. The fenestrated endothelium is separated from the hepatic plates by a subendothelial space called the *space of Disse* (Fig. 19.20). The perisinusoidal space

(of Disse) is present between the sinusoidal endothelium and adjacent hepatocytes that extend small microvilli into this space (Fig. 19.23). Networks of reticular fibers, an occasional unmyelinated nerve, fat-storing cells, and pit cells are present in the space of Disse (Fig. 19.19). The significance of the fat-storing cell is unclear, but they may be involved in storing vitamin A. The pit cells may represent granule-containing lymphocytes, perhaps NK cells, similar to those observed in the small intestine, mammary gland, lung, and epididymis. The function of the many large fenestrations in the endothelial cells is to facilitate contact between the sinusoidal blood and the hepatocyte surface so that uptake of substances into the hepatocytes and release of substances from the hepatocytes can easily occur.

Another cell type present in the sinusoids is the *stellate cell* of *von Kupffer* (Plate 52D; Figs. 19.22, 19.23). This large, branched cell is phagocytic. Kupffer cells ap-

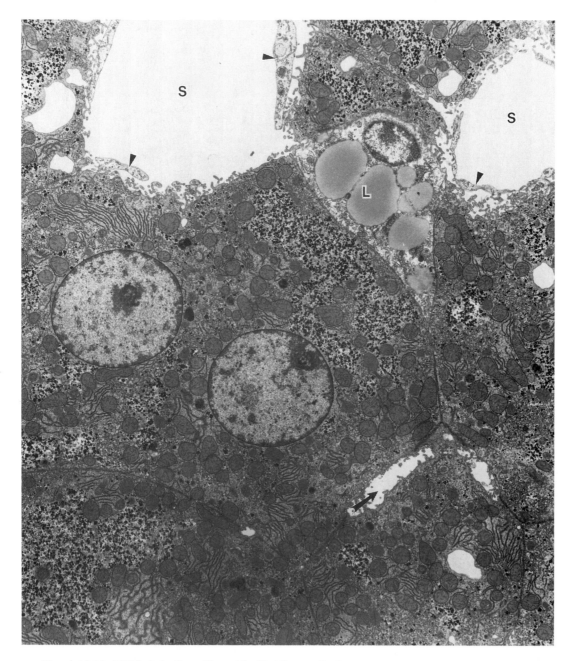

Figure 19.19. TEM of the liver. Sinusoids (S), bile canaliculus (arrows), sinusoidal endothelium (arrowheads), and a lipid-storing cell (L) are shown. ×5000.

parentaly are derived from circulating monocytes, and there is evidence that they can undergo mitotic division in the liver. The cytoplasm of the cells contains lysosomes and vacuoles, and they exhibit a positive histochemical reaction to peroxidase. Kupffer cells can phagocytize damaged erythrocytes. Kuppfer cells are also located at branches of the sinusoids. Although they have a number of functions related to their phagocytic activity, they can metabolize worn-out erythrocytes and digest the hemoglobin. Kupffer cells are involved in immunologic reactions since they have surface receptors for immunoglobulins and complement, and they secrete IL-1 and TNF. The cells can also phagocytize cel-

lular debris, particulate material, and certain microorganisms.

BILE PASSAGEWAYS

The liver cells or hepatocytes are organized into interconnected plates of cells that form a layer one or two cells thick. The sinsuoids are present between the plates. The hepatocytes range from 20 to 30 µm in diameter and have six or more surfaces. The surface of each liver cell is in contact with a sinusoid via the space of Disse (Figs. 19.20, 19.23). Some hepatocytes may contact

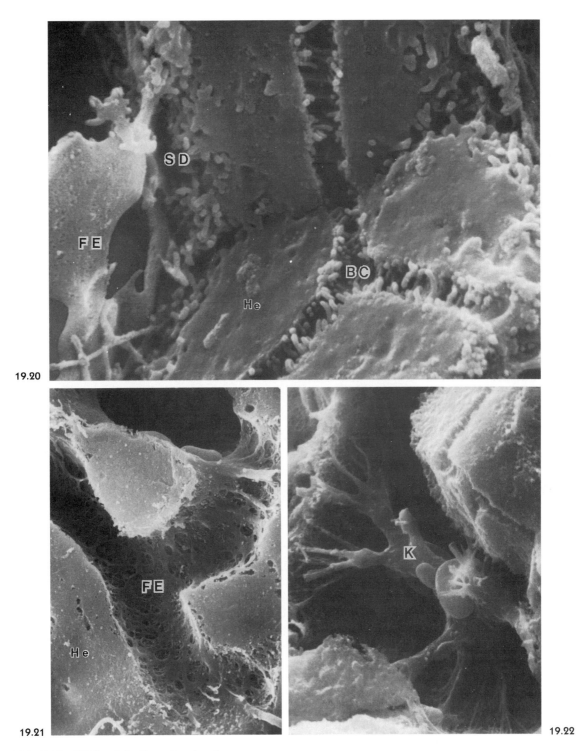

Figures 19.20–19.22. SEMs of the liver showing fenestrated endothelium (FE), space of Disse (SD), bile canaliculus (BC), hepatocytes (He), and a stellate cell of von Kupffer (K). Figure 19.20, ×15,925; Figure 19.21, ×3600; Figure 19.22, ×4810. (From R. Kessel and R. Kardon. *Tissues and Organs: A Text-Atlas of Scanning Electron Microscopy.* W.H. Freeman, New York, 1978, with permission)

more than one sinusoid. Whenever two hepatocytes are in contact, a small tubular intercellular space called a *bile canaliculus* is formed (Figs. 19.20, 19.24). Such canaliculi are precisely formed in all of the hepatocytes in a plate so that the bile can travel within the canali-

culi from the central region of the lobule to the bile ducts at the periphery of the lobule in the portal areas (Fig. 19.19). The intercellular canaliculus is prevented from leaking bile by the presence of *circumferential zonula occludentes* and is stabilized by *spot desmosomes* (Figs.

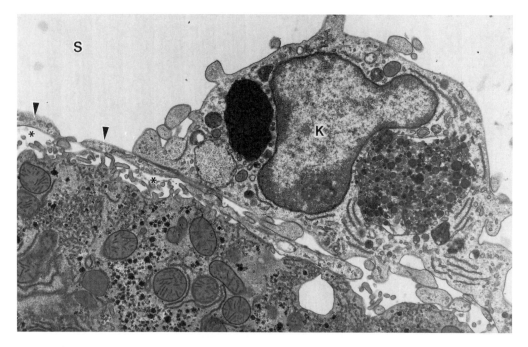

Figure 19.23. TEM of a liver sinusoid. The Kuppfer cell (K), endothelium (arrowheads), sinusoid (S), and space of Disse (*) are shown. ×12,000 (From: R. Roberts, R. Kessel, H. Tung. *Freeze Fracture Images of Cells and Tissues.* Oxford University Press, 1991, with permission)

19.25–19.26). The hepatocyte plasma membranes may be folded into short microvilli and extend into the lumen of the canaliculus. *Bile canaliculi* can be identified in LM preparations by staining for the enzyme alkaline phosphatase, which is present in bile. The canaliculi extend from near the central venule toward the periphery of the lobule, and they anastomose extensively.

Bile flows in the canaliculi to the periphery of the classic lobule and enters small terminal bile ductules called *canals of Hering* (preductules) (Fig. 19.14). The canals of Hering are short channels that conduct bile from the canaliculi through the limiting plate into the interlobular bile ducts of the portal area (portal tract, portal canal) (Fig. 19.18). Interlobular (*intrahepatic*) *bile ducts* in the portal areas form a continuous network of passageways that gradually increase in size as they approach the porta hepatis. The cells of these passageways are lined by cuboidal or columnar epithelial cells that have microvilli on their luminal surface. The system of intrahepatic bile ducts eventually converges into right and left hepatic ducts that exit the liver (Fig. 19.3).

HEPATOCYTES

The hepatocyte comprises about 80% of the total cell population in the liver and is one of the most versatile cells since it performs many vital functions for other resident cells in the body. Like other epithelial structures, the hepatocytes have the capacity for turnover, although

at a slow rate. The liver possesses regenerative capabilities. When a portion of the liver is surgically removed or diseased, the liver cells begin to divide; this process continues until the original liver mass is restored. This capacity is more pronounced in some mammals, such as the mouse, but is more restricted in humans.

All cytoplasmic organelles are represented in the hepatocyte (Figs. 19.19, 19.24). Hepatocytes may be binucleate, while other nuclei may be polyploid. The cytoplasm contains rER, sER, lysosomes, peroxisomes, mitochondria, Golgi complexes, microfilaments and microtubules. The rER synthesizes a number of important proteins such as albumin, fibrinogen, and prothrombin. The sER is also a prominent organelle in the liver cell and is involved in carbohydrate synthesis and degradation, as well as synthesis of bile acids, cholesterol, and lipoproteins. The sER also contains enzymes involved in detoxification of lipid-soluble drugs. Each hepatocyte contains well over 1000 mitochondria. Hepatic lysosomes are involved in autophagy and in the processing of materials taken into the cell by receptor-mediated endocytosis. The hepatocyte commonly contains lipid droplets and extensive stores of glycogen, depending on the nutritional state.

Among the important conversions possible in the hepatocyte cytoplasm is the ability to convert lipids and amino acids into glucose through a complex metabolic process called *gluconeogenesis*. The hepatocyte also plays an important role in *deamination* of *amino acids*. The *urea* resulting from this process is released into the blood and transported to the kidney for excretion.

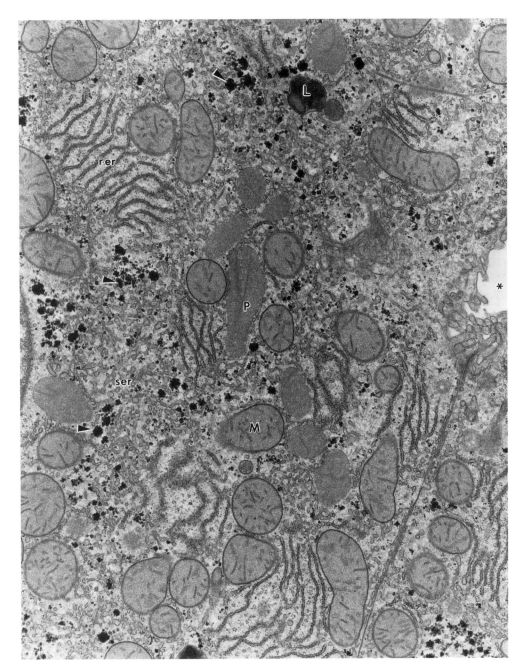

Figure 19.24. TEM of a hepatocyte. Mitochondria (M), peroxisome (P), lysosome (L), sER (ser), rER (rer), glyco- gen (arrowheads), and bile canaliculus (*) are shown. ×19,500.

FUNCTIONS OF HEPATOCYTES

The hepatocyte can perform endocrine and exocrine functions, while in the pancreas, exocrine functions are carried out by distinct cell types. The liver constantly produces bile. Some of the bile is conveyed to the duodenum via the common bile duct, but most of it is sent to the gallbladder for concentration until it is released in response to the presence of food in the digestive tract. Bile acts by emulsifying fats into micelles, which facilitates

their digestion and absorption into the intestinal epithelium. Another important function of the liver is the storage of carbohydrate as glycogen, as well as the mobilization and release of glucose as an energy source for distribution by the blood vascular system to all resident cells of the body. Fatty acids are synthesized into triglycerides in the sER and joined in this region with protein synthesized in the rER to form VLDL particles. The sER is also involved in cholesterol synthesis. It has been estimated that the liver performs several hundred functions.

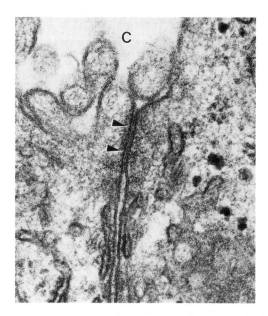

Figure 19.25. TEM of two adjacent hepatocytes in the region of the bile canaliculus (C). Arrowheads denote the circumferential zonula occludens, which seals off the canaliculus. ×62,000.

ALTERNATIVE VIEWS OF LIVER ORGANIZATION: CLASSIC LIVER LOBULE, PORTAL LOBULE, LIVER ACINUS

Although the liver has only a single organizational plan, histologists have used different terms in viewing its organization, each term emphasizing different features of its structure or function (Fig. 19.27). The organization of the classic hepatic lobule is based on a central vein surrounded by radiating plates of sinusoids and hepatocytes and triads at the periphery. Blood flow is from periphery to center in these lobules, and bile flow is from center to periphery. This view of the organization of the liver does not emphasize the exocrine function of the liver because exocrine lobules are usually defined as a group of acini all emptying into a centrally located duct. In the portal lobule concept, the exocrine secretion is collected in the center of the structural unit. Still another way of viewing liver organization is the liver acinus concept, which relates the type of blood that hepatocytes are exposed to during flow through the lobule. Thus, in this case, the liver cells encounter different blood compositions.

The term *portal lobule* is used to describe portions of those lobules whose bile *canaliculi drain* into the *same bile duct* (an intralobular duct) of a portal tract (Fig. 19.27). This unit of liver organization functionally includes all of the canaliculi that supply bile secreted by hepatocytes into a single bile duct. In a portal lobule, the boundaries are the central venules of three classic hepatic lobules, while the center of the portal lobule is

the portal tract with its contained bile duct. The boundaries of the portal lobule thus differ markedly from those of the classic hepatic lobule.

The blood supply to the plates of hepatocytes is important because as blood circulates through the liver, the hepatocytes are not all exposed to the same type of blood, as reflected in the concentration of dissolved oxygen and the quantity of nutrients present. In addition, the concentration of possible toxic substances to which the hepatoctes are exposed is variable, depending upon their position relative to the flow of blood.

The concept of a *portal acinus* has evolved to reflect the position of hepatocytes in relation to their blood supply. The vascular supply to an acinus, via distributing branches of the portal vein, is important in the concept of an acinus. The acinus has an oval- to diamond-shaped region that includes the hepatocytes of two neighboring classic lobules, with a *central region* that is occupied by *branches* of the *distributing portal veins* and hepatic *arteries* at the boundaries of the two classic lobules. Figure 19.27 delineates the boundary of a portal acinus, the peripheral landmarks of which are the central venules of adjacent classic lobules. Zones in the portal acinus are used to denote the relative distance of hepatocytes in the acinus from their blood source in branches of the distributing portal veins and distributing branches of the hepatic arterioles. Hepatocytes located closest to the blood supply, in zone 1 of the acinus, are exposed to blood of highest quality, that is, blood that is richest in both oxygen and nutrients. Hepatocytes located farther away from their blood supply, in zones 2 and 3 of the acinus, are

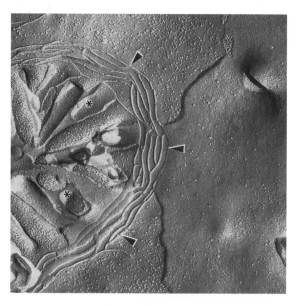

Figure 19.26. Freeze fracture preparation illustrates the sealing strands (arrowheads) of the zonula occludentes, which is the basis of the blood-bile barrier. Microvilli (*) extend into the bile canaliculus. ×70,000.

Figure 19.27. Diagram of the structural boundaries of the classic hepatic lobule, portal lobule, and portal acinus. PS = portal space (tract or radicle); CV = central venule. (Redrawn from T.S. Leeson and R.S. Leeson, *Histology*, 2nd ed., W.B. Saunders, Philadelphia, 1970)

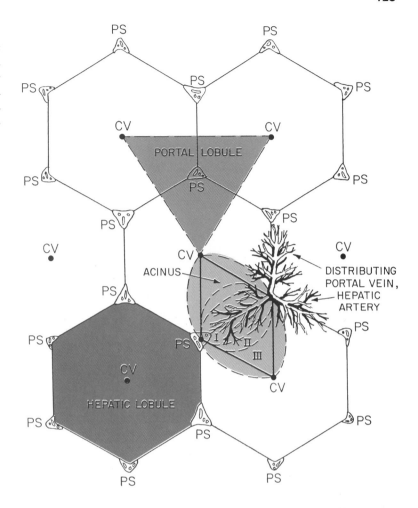

exposed to significantly fewer nutrients and less oxygen, as well as a higher concentration of waste products. Thus, in zone 3, the hepatocytes are exposed to a blood supply virtually exhausted of oxygen and nutrients but with a high concentration of metabolic wastes. Zone 3 is the principal site of alcohol and drug detoxification, and these hepatocytes are likely to be more vulnerable to damage or destruction than those in zones 1 or 2.

MEDICAL CONSIDERATIONS

Type I (insulin-dependent) *diabetes mellitis* is marked by lack of insulin secretion and is an autoimmune reaction in which beta cells are destroyed by T lymphocytes. Type I diabetes frequently begins before adulthood. In *type II* (insulin-independent) *diabetes mellitis*, beta cells do secrete insulin, but the target cells lack insulin receptors in their membrane and therefore do not respond to insulin. Dietary control, weight reduction, and exercise may completely reverse the symptoms of type II diabetes.

LIVER FUNCTION DURING STARVATION

During initial stages of starvation (the first day), it is important to supply glucose to the brain and to preserve protein. Thus, instead of using glucose as a fuel, the body uses fatty acids and ketone bodies. Triacylglycerols are mobilized from adipose tissue, and gluconeogenesis occurs in the liver. The liver obtains energy by oxidizing fatty acids released from adipose tissue. Then, after approximately 3 days of starvation, the liver produces large amounts of 3-hydroxybutyrate (ketone bodies) and acetoacetate. The synthesis of these substances from acetyl coenzyme A increases because the citric acid cycle is unable to oxidize all acetyl units generated by the degradation of fatty acids. Thus, ketone bodies are formed from acetyl coenzyme A if fat breakdown predominates.

Stones or calculi that develop from cholesterol and a variety of bile components can block the passage of bile from the gallbladder.

Cirrhosis of the liver results from hepatitis or alcoholism. Effects on the liver include fatty infiltration, necrosis, fibrosis, and other forms of scarring. Hepatitis or inflammation of the liver may be due to a virus (hepatitis A, B, C, D, and E), which can be transmitted by such things as contaminated feces, water, food, sexual contact, and blood. Nonviral hepatitis is caused by toxins such as alcohol and drugs.

SELECTED BIBLIOGRAPHY

Adelson, J.W., and Miller, P.E. (1989). Heterogeneity of the exocrine pancreas. *Am. J. Physiol.* **256**, G817–G825.

Banfield, W.J. (1975). Physiology of the gallbladder. *Gastroenterology* **69**, 770–777.

Frizzell, R.A., and Heintze, K. (1980). Transport functions of the gallbladder. In *International Review of Physiology: Liver and Biliary Tract Physiology I*, Vol. 21, N.B. Javitt, ed. University Park Press, Baltimore.

Fushiki, T., and Iwai, K. (1989). Two hypotheses on the feedback regulation of pancreatic enzyme secretion. *FASEB J.* **3**, 121–126.

Gerber, M.A., and Swan, N.T. (1987). Histology of the liver. *Am. J. Surg. Pathol.* **11**, 709.

Kardon, R., and Kessel, R. (1980). Three-dimensional organization of the hepatic microcirculation in the rodent as observed by scanning electron microscopy of corrosion casts. *Gastroenterology* **79**, 72–81.

Mason, D.K., and Chisholm, D.M. (1975). *Salivary Glands in Health and Disease*. W.B. Saunders, Philadelphia.

Young, J.A., and Van Lennep, D.W. (1978). *The Morphology of Salivary Glands*. Academic Press, Orlando, FL.

The Endocrine System

The integration and harmonious coordination of all tissues and organ systems in the body are made possible largely by the nervous system and the endocrine system. The nervous system causes the release of chemical messengers (synaptic secretion) that profoundly affect the activity of resident cells of the body. The endocrine system synthesizes and exports a vast array of chemical messengers that circulate in the vascular system to affect target cells.

For the harmonious interaction of all cells in a complex multicellular organism, cell communication is a necessity. Cells can communicate locally by means of specific cell surface molecules, as well as by gap or communicating junctions. However, for communication over longer distances, it is necessary for chemical messengers to be synthesized and released to circulate to cells where interaction occurs with cell surface receptors. *Paracrine secretion* involves the secretion of chemical messengers that diffuse to act on nearby cells, providing for localized cell control. *Endocrine secretion* involves the release of chemical messengers into the bloodstream for distribution to act on specific target cells. The type of chemical messenger used in the endocrine system is called a *hormone*. The chemical nature of hormones can vary, with most of the common hormones falling into four categories: peptides, proteins, steroid derivatives, and tyrosine derivatives (Table 20.1). The hormones produced by endocrine gland cells typically exert their effects by interacting with specific receptor molecules in the plasma membrane, cytoplasm, or nucleus of the target cells. These events usually lead to stimulatory or inhibitory effects on the target cells. Positive and negative feedback loops commonly exist between the hormones and the specific target cells with which they interact; specific examples will be given.

The binding of a signaling molecule (e.g., hormone) to its receptor causes a cell to respond in a characteristic and programmed manner. Three major groups of cell surface receptors transduce extracellular signals in different ways and were discussed in Chapter 2. Enzyme-linked receptors may either be enzymes or are associated with enzymes, usually protein kinases, that phosphorylate specific proteins in responsive cells. Ion-channel-linked receptors are transmitter-gated ion channels that rapidly open and close after binding to a neurotransmitter. G-protein-linked receptors are the largest group of cell surface receptors. They cause the activation or inactivation of plasma membrane-bound enzymes or ion channels by means of *G proteins* (trimeric GTP-binding proteins). G-protein-linked receptors usually function by altering the concentration of small intracellular signaling molecules such as *cAMP* and *calcium* (Ca^{2+}).

G proteins couple receptors to adenylyl cyclase, thereby altering the level of cAMP in the cell. G proteins also couple receptors to the enzyme *phospholipase C*, which, after activation, results in the cleavage or splitting of *phosphatidylinositol-biphosphate* (PIP_2) into *inositol triphosphate* (IP_3) and *diacylglycerol*. IP_3 is rapidly dephosphorylated, and the calcium is pumped from the cell to limit the response. Diacylglycerol activates a calcium-dependent enzyme, *protein kinase C*, which phosphorylates selected proteins within the cells, leading to a response (see Chapter 2).

HYPOPHYSIS (PITUITARY)

ORIGIN AND ORGANIZATION

The hypophysis (pituitary gland) is structurally and functionally an endocrine extension of the hypothala-

Table 20.1 Chemical Nature of Common Hormones

Peptides (<20 Amino Acids)	Proteins (>20 Amino Acids)	Steroid Derivatives	Tyrosine Derivatives
Vasopressin	Glucagon	Estradiol	Dopamine
Oxytocin	Insulin	Progesterone	Thyroxine (tetra-iodothyronine)
Angiotensin	Prolactin	Testosterone	Triiodothyronine
Somatostatin	Calcitonin	Aldosterone	Epinephrine
Melanocyte-stimulating hormone	Adrenocorticotropic hormone	Cortisol	Norepinephrine
	Thyroid-stimulating hormone	Vitamin D	
	Follicle-stimulating hormone		
Gonadotropin-releasing hormone	Luteinizing hormone		
	Growth hormone		
	Corticotropin-releasing hormone		
Thyrotropin-releasing hormone	Growth hormone-releasing hormone		
	Chorionic gonadotropin		
	Chorionic somatomammotropin		
	Parathyroid hormone		

mus of the brain, to which it is attached (Fig. 20.1). The gland is surrounded by a connective tissue capsule, and lies within and is protected by the sella turcica (turkish saddle), a depression in the sphenoid bone. The hypophysis is attached superiorly by its infundibular stalk to the median eminence of the tuber cinereum, which is the basal portion of the hypothalamus.

The hypophysis has its embryonic origin from two different sources, neural and oral. This results in the pituitary's having two distinct parts that differ in both structure and function. The *adenohypophysis* arises from ectoderm in the roof of the embryonic oral cavity. The proliferation of ectoderm cells here results in a fold, called *Rathke's pouch*, that subsequently detaches from the

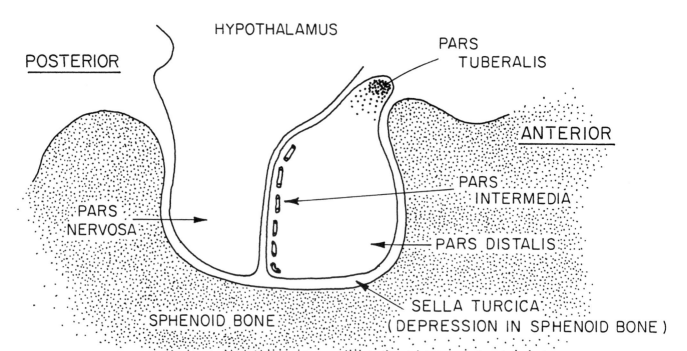

Figure 20.1. Diagram of a sagittal section of the pituitary gland with identification of parts. The pars nervosa is connected to the hypothalamus via the infundibulum.

oral cavity epithelium and migrates toward and fuses with a downgrowth from the floor of the embryonic diencephalon. This region of the embryonic diencephalon subsequently becomes the hypothalamus. The downgrowth of the embryonic diencephalon becomes the *neurohypophysis*. The neurohypophysis retains its connection to the hypothalamus and includes the *pars nervosa* and the *infundibulum*. That portion of the hypophysis that develops from oral ectoderm differentiates into a pars distalis, a pars tuberalis, and a pars intermedia.

The pars distalis is the principal glandular part of the hypophysis and contains different cell types that synthesize a broad spectrum of hormones with profound effects on their target cells (Plate 53A–D). The pars tuberalis is a collar-like upward extension of the pars distalis and partially surrounds the neural (infundibular) stalk. The pars intermedia is rudimentary in humans but more extensive in those vertebrates that exhibit marked changes in pigmentation or color. The pituitary is described as having two lobes, which relate to the neuro- and adenohypophysis, as shown in the following diagram.

$$\text{Neurohypophysis} \begin{cases} \text{infundibulum} \\ \text{pars nervosa} \end{cases}$$
$$\text{Adenohypophysis} \begin{cases} \text{pars intermedia} \\ \text{pars distalis} \\ \text{pars tuberalis} \end{cases}$$
posterior lobe

anterior lobe

The pars distalis is regulated by hypothalamic peptide hormones. These hormones are produced by neurosecretory cells and travel to the pars distalis via the hypophyseal-portal circulation. The hormones can then either stimulate or inhibit release of the pars distalis hormone. Distinct hypothalamic regulator hormones exist for all pars distalis hormones.

PORTAL CIRCULATORY SYSTEM

The pituitary is supplied by two sets of arteries: the right and left superior hypophyseal arteries and the right and left inferior hypophyseal arteries. The inferior hypophyseal arteries supply principally the pars nervosa. The anterior lobe has no direct arterial supply. The superior hypophyseal arteries supply the median eminence and neural stalk and terminate in a primary capillary plexus, which then join together as portal veins that travel into the pars distalis and end in a secondary capillary plexus. This *portal system* provides a route for neurosecretory substances released by neurons in the median eminence and infundibular stem to pass to cells in the pars distalis (Fig. 20.2). The capillaries of the portal system are fenestrated to facilitate rapid exchanges.

RELATIONSHIP BETWEEN HYPOTHALAMUS AND PARS DISTALIS

The secretion of hormones in the pars distalis is regulated by factors released from the hypothalamus. The hypothalamus has complete control over the pars distalis and pars tuberalis in determining whether or not the hormones will be released into the circulation. Both the anterior pituitary and the infundibular stalk have extensive plexuses of fenestrated endothelial capillaries that are connected by portal veins. Therefore, venous blood in the capillary plexuses in the hypothalamus and infundibulum flows to capillary plexuses in the pars distalis. This arrangement comprises the *hypophyseal-portal circulation*. It is now known that certain neurons in the hypothalamus can synthesize *releasing hormones* or factors and *release-inhibiting hormones* or factors that can be discharged into the portal circulatory system and travel to the pars distalis, causing secretory cells located in this region to either release or prevent release of their specific hormones. In every instance, a specific hypothalamic releasing hormone has been identified for each anterior pituitary hormone. However, recently, only three hypothalamic inhibiting hormones have been identified for three corresponding anterior pituitary hormones. The accompanying table indicates the specific hormones produced by cells in the pars distalis.

CELL TYPES IN THE ADENOHYPOPHYSIS

The cells in the adenohypophysis have long been classed on the basis of the staining properties of their secretory granules after exposure to various mixtures of acidic and basic dyes. *Chromophobes* (cells that "dislike" stain) are cells that have no granules and thus little affinity for dyes. In contrast, there are two populations of *chromophils*. Chromophils with granules that bind acid dyes are called *acidophils*, while those with granules that bind basic dyes are called *basophils* (Plate 53B,C). By immunocytochemistry it has been possible to identify the cells on the basis of the specific hormone they contain. In two cases, a single cell produces more than one hormone.

CELL TYPES IN THE PARS DISTALIS

There are two types of acidophils in the pars distalis based on their distinct hormone products (Fig. 20.3). The somatotropic cells (or *somatotrops*) are acidophilic chromophils that synthesize and release *growth hormone* (*GH*). Lactotropic cells (*lactotrops* or *mammotrops*) are acidopohilic chromophils that produce and secrete *prolactin*. There are three types of basophils. Gonadotropic cells or *gondadotrops* are basophilic chromophils that produce both *luteinizing hormone* (*LH*) and *follicle-stimulating*

Cell Type	Acidophil or Basophil	Hormone Produced: Chemical Nature	Physiologic Effects	Hypothalemic-Releasing (Humans) Hormone or Factor	Release-Inhibiting Hormone or Factor	Target
Somatotropic cell	Acidophil	Growth hormone (GH) Somatotropin or somatotropin hormone (STH) Protein	Promotes growth in mass and stimulates somatomedin production in liver; stimulates protein synthesis	Growth hormone-releasing hormone (GNRH), somatocrinin stimulates GH secretion	Somatotropin release-inhibiting factor (SRIF); somatostatin. Inhibits GH secretion	Most tissues
Mammotropic cell	Acidophil	Prolactin Protein	Promotes milk secretion	Prolactin-stimulating factor or PRL-releasing factor. Stimulates prolactin secretion	Prolactin inhibiting factor (PIF) Dopamine Inhibits prolactin secretion	Mammary glands
Gonadotropic cell	Basophil	Follicle-stimulating hormone (FSH) and luteinizing hormone (LH or ICSH) in same cell type	FSH promotes ovarian follicle development and estrogen secretion in female; stimulates spermatogenesis in male. LH stimulates ovulation of ripe ovarian follicle; corpus luteum formation; progesterone and estrogen secretion in female. LH stimulates Leydig cells to synthesize and secrete testosterone in male	Gonadotropin-releasing hormone (GnRH). Stimulates secretion of FSH and LH		Ovary / Testis
Thyrotropic cell	Basophil	Thyroid-stimulating hormone (TSH) or thyrotropin Glycoprotein	Stimulates synthesis and secretion of thyroid hormones	Thyrotropin-releasing hormone (TRH). Stimulates secretion of TSH and prolactin		Thyroid gland
Corticotropic cell	Basophil	Adrenocorticotropic hormone (ACTH) or corticotropin	Stimulates secretion of adrenal cortical hormones	Corticotropin-releasing hormone (CRH). Stimulates secretion of ACTH, β-LPH, and β-endorphin		Adrenal cortex
		Peptide α, β Melanocyte-stimulating hormone (MSH)	Pigment dispersion in melanocyte (some animals)	Melanocyte-stimulating hormone-releasing factor (MIF) Melanocyte-stimulating hormone-releasing factor (HRF).	Melanocyte-stimulating hormone-inhibiting factor	Melanocyte
		β, γ-Lipotropin (LPH)	Stimulates mobilization of lipids from adipose tissue. Role in human unknown			Adipocyte
		β-endorphin	Role unclear			General (?)

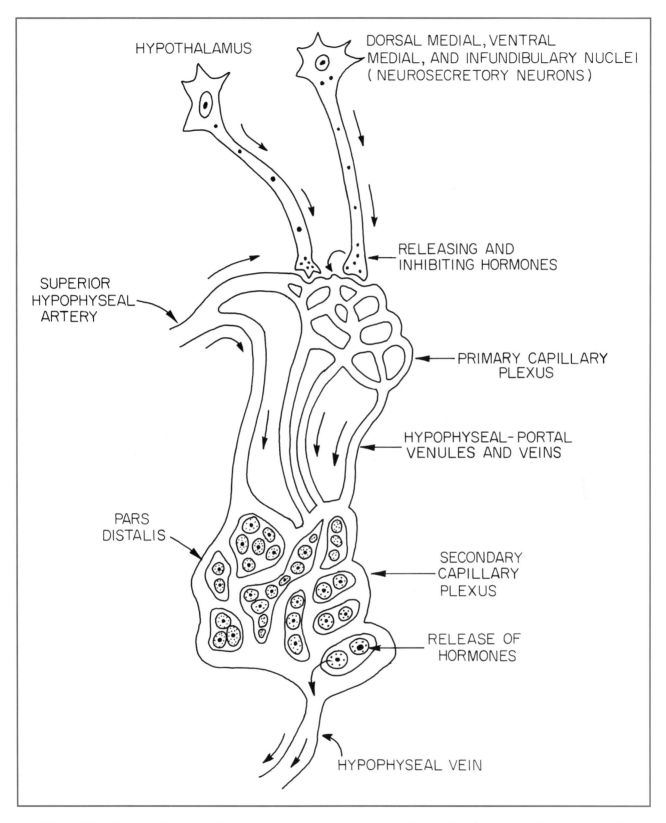

HYPOTHALAMUS

DORSAL MEDIAL, VENTRAL MEDIAL, AND INFUNDIBULARY NUCLEI (NEUROSECRETORY NEURONS)

RELEASING AND INHIBITING HORMONES

SUPERIOR HYPOPHYSEAL ARTERY

PRIMARY CAPILLARY PLEXUS

HYPOPHYSEAL-PORTAL VENULES AND VEINS

PARS DISTALIS

SECONDARY CAPILLARY PLEXUS

RELEASE OF HORMONES

HYPOPHYSEAL VEIN

Figure 20.2. Diagram of the hypophyseal-portal circulatory system. Neurons in the hypothalamus secrete releasing hormones or release-inhibiting hormones into the portal circulation and these hormones are carried to the pars distalis, where they determine whether the acidophils and basophils there will release their hormones into the circulation.

429

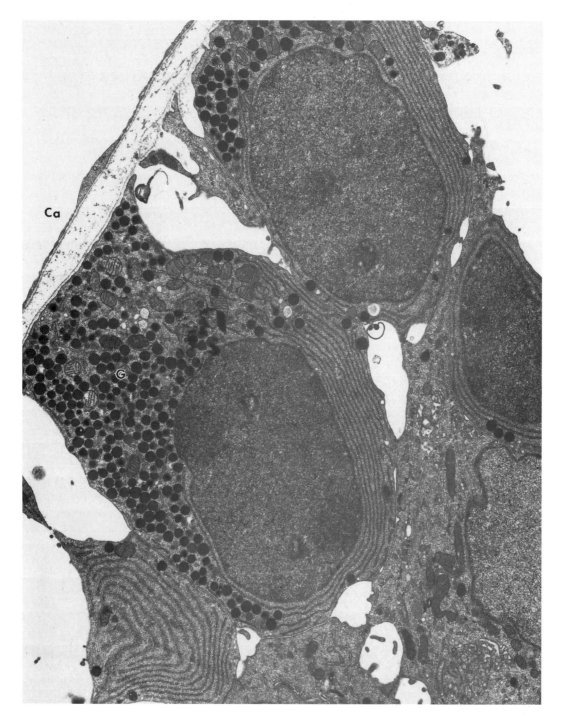

Figure 20.3. This group of chromophils in the pars distal terminates close to a fenestrated capillary (Ca). The secretory granules (G) are released toward the capillary side of the cell for easy and rapid movement into the adjacent fenestrated capillary. Cells contain abundant rER. ×9750.

hormone (FSH). Thyrotropic cells (or *thyrotrops*) are basophilic chromophils that produce and secrete *thyroid-stimulating hormone (TSH)*. Finally, corticotropic cells (also called adrenocorticolipotropic cells or *adrenocorticolipotrops*) are basophilic chromophils that synthesize and secrete *adrenocorticotropic hormone (ACTH)* and *lipotropic hormone (α, β lipotropin)* primarily. ACTH is also called *corticotropin* or *adrenocorticotropin* and consists of a family of peptides that also includes α- and β-

melanocyte-stimulating hormone (MSH), α- and β-*lipotropin*, and *β-endorphin*. In humans the physiologic role of these peptides, except ACTH, is unclear. MSH causes melanin pigment dispersion in melanocytes (i.e., darkening) in the skin of lower vertebrates but not in humans. In some animals, MSH is produced by the intermediate lobe, but this portion of the pituitary in humans is probably not functional except possibly in fetal life. The corticotrops secrete a prohormone that undergoes posttranslational cleavage to form ACTH, β-endorphin, and β-lipotropin.

Beta-lipotropin (β-LPH) stimulates lipid mobilization from adipose tissue in rabbits, but its role in humans is not known. Part of the β-LPH molecule contains a complete sequence of β-endorphin. Beta-endorphin reacts with the same receptors as those for morphine. All of these peptides result from the transcription and translation of a single gene. The gene product, called *pro-opiomelanocortin (POMC)*, is cleaved by trypsin-like endopeptidases, and this processing results in the final secretory products. Since the final processing of POMC appears to occur in secretory granules of the corticotropin cell, β-LPH and β-endorphin are released together with ACTH into the bloodstream.

NATURE AND FUNCTIONS OF PARS DISTALIS HORMONES

The secretory cells in the pars distalis, their products, the actions of these products, and the releasing and inhibiting hormones are listed in Table 20.2.

PITUITARY DYSFUNCTION

When GH is produced in excessive quantity, gigantism or acromegaly may result. Gigantism occurs when the growth of long bones continues past adolescence. Acromegaly results when hormone overproduction occurs later in life, resulting in overgrowth of some bones.

With insufficient production of GH the result may be dwarfism, in which there is insufficient growth of long bones, resulting in short stature.

Tumors of the hypophysis are frequently benign and involve cells that produce GH, prolactin, ACTH, and occasionally TSH. Lesions of the hypothalamus can sometimes occur, destroying the neurosecretory neurons and resulting in diabetes insipidus. Individuals with diabetes insipidus may excrete nearly 20 liters of urine per day and consume large quantities of liquids.

PARS INTERMEDIA AND PARS TUBERALIS

The *pars intermedia* is variable in structure among species. In humans, it is reduced to cystic cavities (follicles) and contains basophils and chromophobes. Its function in humans is unclear. In amphibians, the basophilic cells produce *MSH*, which causes pigment production in melanocytes. In humans, MSH may be a product of lipotrophic hormone (LPH) cleavage. The *pars tuberalis* is highly vascular and contains chromophil and chromophobe cells. Gonadotrophs are the most common functional cells present in this region.

NEUROHYPOPHYSIS

Organization

The posterior lobe is also known as the pars nervosa or neurohypophysis. It contains many unmyelinated axons of nerve cell bodies that are located in the paraventric-

Table 20.2 Anterior Pituitary Hormones

Cell Name	Acidophil/ Basophil	Hormone Produced	Chemical Nature	Major Physiologic Effects
Somatotrope	Acidophil	Growth hormone (GH or somatotropin)	Protein	Stimulates growth of long bones via somatomedins synthesized by liver
Mammotrope	Acidophil	Prolactin (PRL) or lactogenic hormone (LTH)	Glycoprotein	Promotes milk secretion
Thyrotrope	Basophil	Thyroid-stimulating hormone (TSH) or thyrotropin	Glycoprotein	Stimulates thyroid hormone— synthesis, storage, and discharge
Gonadotrope	Basophil	Follicle-stimulating hormone (FSH) *and* luteinizing hormone (LH)	Glycoprotein	FSH stimulates ovarian follicle development and estrogen secretion in females; stimulates Sertoli cells to secrete androgen binding protein. LH causes ovulation and corpus luteum formation in females; causes interstitial cells of Leydig to produce testosterone in males.
Corticotrope	Basophil	Corticotropin or adrenocorticotropic hormone (ACTH) and others	Peptide	Stimulates secretion of adrenal cortical hormones

ular and supraoptic nuclei of the hypothalamus. These neuronal fibers are unusual in that they terminate blindly on blood vessels of the rich capillary plexus in the pars nervosa rather than end in relation to other neurons or effector cells (Fig. 20.4). Resident cells in the pars nervosa resemble neuroglia found in the CNS, but are called *pituicytes* in the pars nervosa (Plate 53D). The functional role of these cells is unclear.

Hormones and actions

The neurons in the supraoptic and paraventricular nuclei produce two peptide hormones consisting of nine amino acids. Both vasopressin and oxytocin are synthesized and stored in nerve cells. Vasopressin and oxytocin differ chemically by only two amino acid residues. *Oxy-*

tocin is produced by neurons of supraoptic and paraventricular nuclei. Oxytocin causes contraction of myoepithelial cells of the mammary glands during nursing, causing milk to be ejected from secretory alveoli. During labor, oxytocin induces contraction of smooth muscle in the wall of the uterus. *Vasopressin* or *antidiuretic hormone* (*ADH*) is also produced by neurons in both supraoptic and paraventricular nuclei in the hypothalamus. Vasopressin promotes resorption of water from collecting tubules in the kidney. It also elevates blood pressure by causing contraction of smooth muscle in arterioles. The neurosecretion also contains ATP and a binding protein (neurophysin) that is specific for each hormone. The two hormones, in association with carrier proteins, travel along the axons as secretory granules to axon terminals in the pars nervosa. The secre-

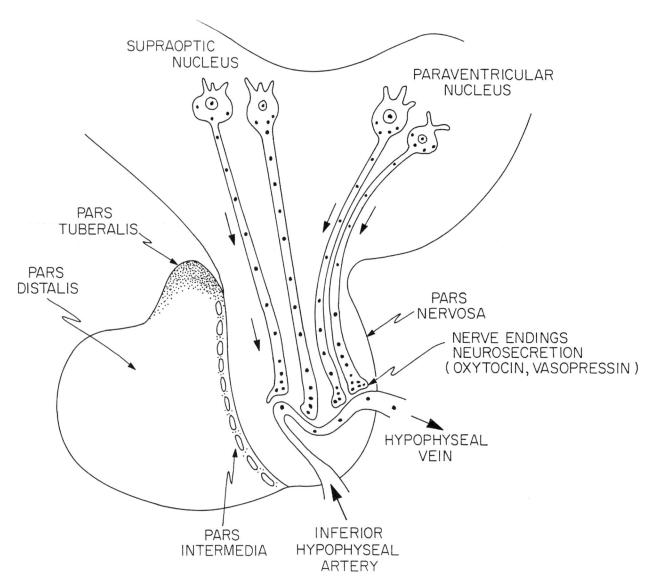

Figure 20.4. Diagram of neurosecretory neurons in supraoptic and paraventricular nuclei of hypothalamus. Axons of these neurons extend into the pars nervosa of the pituitary. The neurosecretion contains oxytocin and vaso- **pressin, which are released at the nerve endings into vessels in the pars nervosa to be distributed throughout the circulatory system.**

tion is stored in the ends of the axons and may be visible in LM preparations as small accumulations of secretion known as *Herring bodies* (Fig. 20.5). The secretion is then discharged by exocytosis in response to impulses in nerve fibers from the hypothalamus and enters nearby fenestrated capillaries.

Suckling stimulates nerve endings in the nipple and results in impulses in the CNS that stimulate neurosecretory cells to produce and release oxytocin. When the suckling stimulus ceases, negative feedback stops oxytocin release. In a positive feedback mechanism, the dilation of the uterine cervix late in pregnancy results in increased oxytocin release, which, in turn, causes enhanced uterine contraction (Table 20.3).

PINEAL GLAND

ORIGIN AND ORGANIZATION

The pineal gland or epiphysis cerebri is attached to the roof of a cavity, the third ventricle in the midbrain, and is covered by pia mater. The name *pineal* is derived from *pineus*, meaning "pine," and denotes the fact that the gland is shaped similarly to a pine cone. The gland arises as an outgrowth of the embryonic diencephalon and is thus derived from neural ectoderm. The major cell type is called the *pinealocyte*, which synthesizes melatonin

(Fig. 20.6). It is a secretory cell that somewhat resembles a neuron, for it has a large ovoid nucleus with a prominent nucleolus. A cytoplasmic process that extends from the cell body terminates in a club-shaped tip adjacent to capillaries. The gland is richly vascularized, and the capillaries lack fenestrations. *Glial cells*, which resemble astrocytes, are located among the pinealocytes. Glial cells are less numerous than pinealocytes and appear to have a supportive function.

Many sympathetic nerve fibers are present in the pineal gland. These nerve processes lose the myelin sheath upon entering the pineal, and some of the nerves appear to synapse in relation to the pinealocyte. The nerve terminals have synaptic vesicles containing norepinephrine. Postganglionic sympathetic fibers run to the pineal gland from the superior cervical ganglia of the sympathetic trunks. Impulses along sympathetic nerves, as well as the presence or absence of light entering the eyes, play important roles in regulating the secretory activity of the pinealocytes.

In addition to the pinealocytes, glial cells, and nerve process, calcified organic concretions appear within the organic matrix of the substance secreted by the pinealocytes. These concretions consist of calcium phosphates and calcium carbonates and are called *corpora arenacea, acervuli*, or *psammoma bodies* ("brain sand granules"). These calcified concretions may vary widely in size and shape; some may be so large that they fall

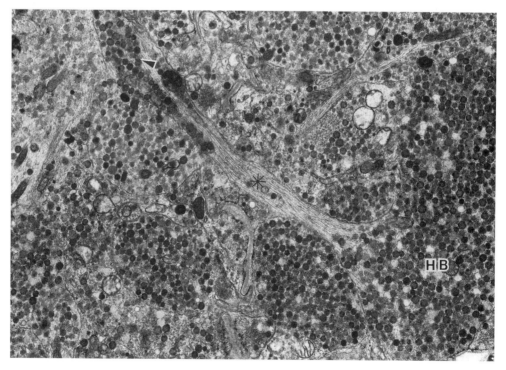

Figure 20.5. TEM of pars nervosa. The nerve process (*) in the center of the field contains neurosecretion (arrowhead). The neurosecretion (oxytocin and vasopressin) accumulates as Herring bodies (HB) at the nerve terminals prior to release into the circulatory system. ×8000. (From R. Roberts, R. Kessel, H. Tung. *Freeze Fracture Images of Cells and Tissues*, Oxford University Press, New York, 1991, with permission)

Table 20.3 Hormones Released from the Pars Nervosa

Parameter	Vasopressin or Antidiuretic Hormone (ADH)	Oxytocin
Chemical Nature	Peptide (nonapeptide)	Peptide (nonapeptide)
Source	Neurons in supraoptic and paraventricular nuclei of hypothalamus	Neurons in supraoptic and paraventricular nuclei of hypothalamus
Site of Action	Collecting ducts and ascending thick limb of Henle's loop (NaCl transport)	Uterus and cervix; myoepithelial cells of mammary gland
Stimulus (I) for Secretion	Increased osmolality of blood (also decreased blood volume; angiotensin II)	Increased dialtion of cervix; suckling (nerve impulses in nipple)
Function	Makes collecting ducts more permeable to water (increased water retention); also causes contraction of vascular smooth muscle (vasoconstriction)	Causes increased uterine muscle contraction; causes contraction of myoepithelial cells in mammary gland.
Rapidity of Response	Instantaneous	Rapid
Duration of Response	Minutes	Minutes
Mode of Action	cAMP	cAMP

out of sections of the gland (Plate 53D; Plate 54A). The concretions begin to form early in life and then increase in number with age. Their functional significance is unknown. They are visible in radiographic films and computed tomography scans.

MELATONIN SYNTHESIS

Melatonin synthesis is accomplished by the conversion of serotonin to n-acetyl serotonin, which, in turn, is converted to melatonin (an indolamine) (Fig. 20.6). The enzyme that catalyzes the conversion of serotonin to n-acetyl serotonin is n-acetyl transferase. Norepinephrine is released from the postganglionic sympathetic nerve endings in the pineal and binds to *β-adrenergic receptors* on the surface of the pinealocytes. The receptor binding activates the enzyme adenylate cyclase in the plasma membrane and catalyzes the conversion of ATP to *cAMP* inside the cell. Cyclic AMP stimulates the synthesis of n-acetyl transferase, which converts serotonin to *N*-acetyl serotonin. The enzyme *hydroxy indole-O-methyltransferase* (HIOMT) converts n-acetyl serotonin to melatonin. Because HIOMT can be made only in the dark, the same is true of melatonin.

Functional significance

Melatonin tends to cause rhythmic changes in the secretory activity of the gonads and hypophysis; it is thus a neuroendocrine transducer that can alter the function of other endocrine glands. Melatonin has a suppressive effect on gonadotropin secretion, inhibiting gonadal growth and function. The pineal hormone appears to suppress GnRH release. In humans, the pineal appears to play a role in preventing the onset of precocious gonadal function. Children with tumors that destroy the pineal parenchyma demonstrate precocious or early onset of puberty. While the pineal gland is comparatively large in infancy, involution begins just before puberty. It has been reported that when hamsters are maintained for a long time in the dark, they exhibit gonadal degeneration. Recent studies indicate that the pineal gland also produces a number of peptides or small polypeptides, but their functional role has not been defined.

ADRENAL (SUPRARENAL) GLANDS

The adrenal glands are paired, encapsulated endocrine glands that lie close (adrenal) to the superior pole of

Figure 20.6. Diagram illustrates how stimulation by postganglionic sympathetic nerve fibers can stimulate the pinealocyte to synthesize melatonin, which is then released into the bloodstream. Steps in the conversion of serotonin into melatonin are denoted.

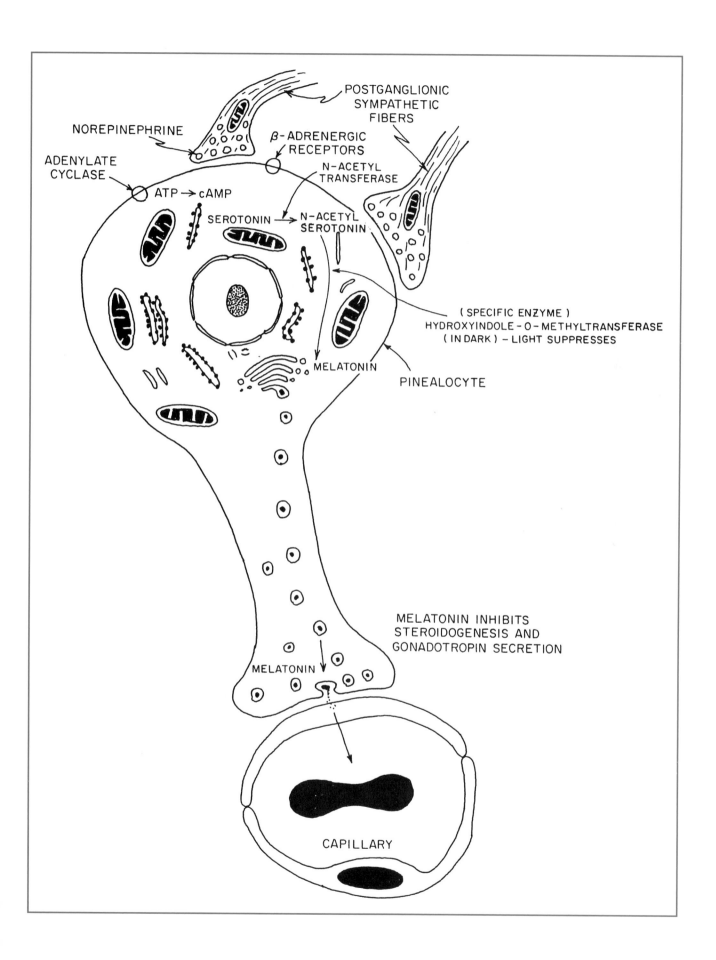

POSTGANGLIONIC
SYMPATHETIC
FIBERS

NOREPINEPHRINE

β-ADRENERGIC
RECEPTORS

ADENYLATE
CYCLASE

N-ACETYL
TRANSFERASE

ATP → cAMP

SEROTONIN → N-ACETYL
SEROTONIN

(SPECIFIC ENZYME)
HYDROXYINDOLE - O - METHYLTRANSFERASE
(IN DARK) - LIGHT SUPPRESSES

MELATONIN

PINEALOCYTE

MELATONIN INHIBITS
STEROIDOGENESIS AND
GONADOTROPIN SECRETION

MELATONIN

CAPILLARY

the kidneys or on top of (suprarenal) the kidneys. In humans the adrenal glands are somewhat flattened, and their maximum length is approximately 5 cm. If a fresh section of the adrenal gland is made, it consists of a yellowish peripheral layer (the adrenal cortex) and a reddish-brown central region (the adrenal medulla). The *adrenal cortex* and *medulla* have different embryologic origins and functions. The *provisional* or fetal adrenal cortex is formed from mesoderm. The provisional adrenal cortex develops in the fetus between the permanent cortex and the adrenal medulla but undergoes involution and disappears after birth, to be replaced by the permanent cortex. The fetal cortex synthesizes sulfated conjugates of androgens that can be transformed by the fetal placenta into active androgens and estrogens. A second, *permanent* adrenal cortex forms later from mesoderm. In contrast, *neural crest* cells migrate to form the coeliac ganglion (a prevertebral sympathetic ganglion), and some of these cells also migrate into the interior of the adrenal to form the medulla. The cells of the *adrenal medulla* produce and release the *catecholamine hormones epinephrine* and *norepinephrine*.

Branches of the superior, middle, and inferior suprarenal arteries branch to form a subcapsular plexus, from which arise branches to supply the capsule, cortex, and medulla. The capillaries are fenestrated for easy passage of hormones into the bloodstream. The medulla receives some blood that drains into it from the capillaries in the cortex. Thus, this blood contains hormones that have been released by the secretory cells in different layers of the cortex. The adrenal medulla is characterized by the presence of a large medullary vein.

ADRENAL CORTEX

The adrenal cortex consists of three layers that vary primarily in the arrangement of the secretory cells comprising each layer (Plate 54B–D). Cells in the adrenal cortex do not store secretion in granules, but rather synthesize and release low molecular weight, lipid-soluble cortical steriods when appropriately stimulated. The outermost layer, the *zona glomerulosa*, consists of somewhat spherical aggregations of cells (Figs. 20.7, 20.8). The middle and widest zone is called the *zona fasciculata*; here the cells are arranged in straight, radial cords of cells that are oriented at a right angle to the external capsule (Figs. 20.9, 20.10). The innermost layer of the cortex consists of cords of cells arranged into anastomosing networks. This layer is called the *zona reticularis*.

ZONA GLOMERULOSA

This region of the cortex comprises about 15% of the total volume of the adrenal. The zona glomerulosa secretes *mineralocorticoids*, and the primary one is *aldosterone*. With the use of differential centrifugation of cell fractions and biochemical analysis, the synthesis of aldosterone has been determined to involve the sER and mitochondria in these cells (Fig. 20.11).

Aldosterone production is stimulated by *angiotensin II*, which is produced in response to *renin* release from juxtaglomerular cells in the kidney. Aldosterone acts on the distal convoluted tubules and collecting ducts in the kidney, causing the reabsorption of sodium (see Fig. 21.33). Aldosterone may also act on cells of the gastric mucosa, as well as on the salivary glands and sweat glands to cause reabsorption of sodium.

ZONA FASCICULATA

The zona fasciculata contains cells that are arranged in straight cords oriented at a right angle to the capsule. Because of the large number of lipid droplets in these cells, they often appear vacuolated in routine histologic preparations since the lipid droplets are dissolved from the sections. The *sER* is unusually well developed and extensive in the cells of the zona fasciculata (Figs. 20.12, 20.13). The cells also have large quantities of *cholesterol* and abundant *mitochondria*. The cells produce *glucocorticoids* and to some extent, *sex steroids*. The glucocorticoids have a regulatory effect on carbohydrate and protein metabolism, as well as on lipid metabolism. The principal glucocorticoids are *cortisol* and *corticosterone*.

Glucorticoids stimulate the uptake and use of fatty acids, amino acids, and carbohydrates in the liver that are involved in *gluconeogenesis* and *glycogenesis*. In areas other than the liver, such as the muscle, skin, and adipose tissue, glucocorticoids tend to decrease synthetic activity and to promote degradation of protein and lipid.

Glucocorticoids also suppress the immune response and cause a marked reduction in the number of circulating lymphocytes. They tend to depress lymphocyte proliferation in lymphatic tissue and to stimulate increased destruction of existing lymphocytes. Glucocorticoids are therefore used to suppress the inflammatory response in some allergic reactions, to provide resistance to stress, and to raise the blood sugar level by producing carbohydrate from protein.

ZONA RETICULARIS

The cells of the zona reticularis produce *gonadocorticoids* or sex hormones that are involved to some extent in the development of sexual characteristics. The principal sex hormone secreted in significant quantity is *dehydroepiandrosterone*. This has a masculinizing and anabolic effect but is much less potent than testicular androgens.

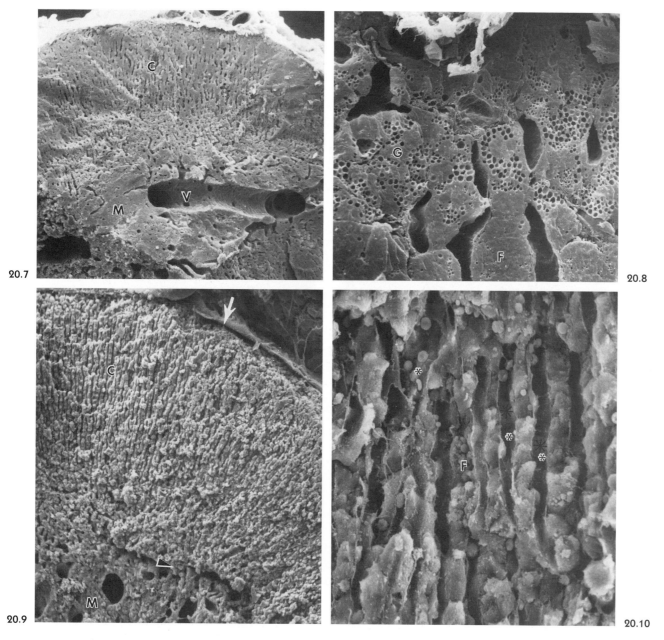

Figures 20.7–20.10. SEMs of rat adrenal gland. The cortex (C) and medulla (M) with a large collecting vein (V) are shown in Fig. 20.7. The zona glomerulosa (G) (vacuolated cells) and start of the zona fasciculata (F) are seen at the bottom in Figure 20.8 (×1485). Cut section of the adrenal in Figure 20.9 includes the capsule (arrow), cortex (C), and medulla (M) (junction denoted by arrowhead). ×150. The cords of cells and intervening sinusoids (*) of the zona fasciculata (F) are shown in Figure 20.10. ×75. (From R. Kessel and R.H. Kardon, *Tissues and Organs: A Text-Atlas of Scanning Electron Microscopy*. W.H. Freeman, New York, 1979, with permission)

CONTROL MECHANISM

Ultimate control of the adrenal cortex is provided by neurosecretory cells in the hypothalamus, which produce a releasing hormone for ACTH. This hormone circulates through the hypothalmo-hypophyseal portal system to the pars distalis and causes corticotrops to release ACTH. ACTH stimulates the synthesis and secretion of cortical hormones, especially the glucocorticoids. A feedback loop exists such that appropriate levels of glucocorticoids can inhibit cells in the hypothalamus and anterior pituitary that are involved in ACTH synthesis and release. ACTH seems to exert relatively little effect on the secretion of aldosterone, however.

ADRENAL MEDULLA

The adrenal medulla synthesizes and releases two catecholamines: *epinephrine* and *norepinephrine* (Fig. 20.14).

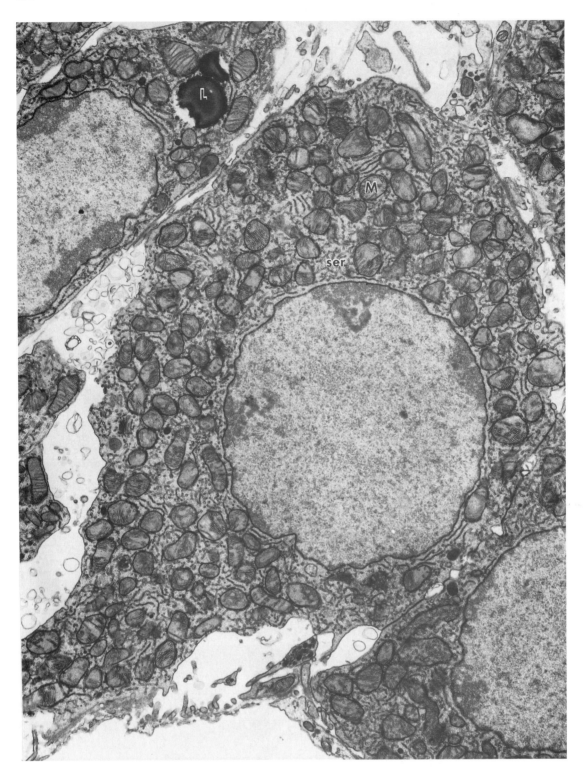

Figure 20.11. TEM of cells in the zona glomerulosa. Note the large number of mitochondria, occasional lipid (L) droplets, and elements of the sER (ser) among the mitochondria (M). ×10,000.

The adrenal medullary cells are also known as *chromaffin cells* or *pheochromocytes* because they stain yellowish-brown when treated with chromic acid or reducible chromium salts. Adrenal medullary cells are innervated by preganglionic sympathetic fibers. Thus, the cells of the medulla appear to be equivalent to sympathetic ganglion cells. Postganglionic sympathetic neurons may, in fact, also be scattered among the chromaffin cells.

Two different cell types are involved in the synthesis of adrenal medullary hormones, and the secretory granules in the two cells types are distinctive in ultrastructure. Epinephrine-secreting cells have smaller and

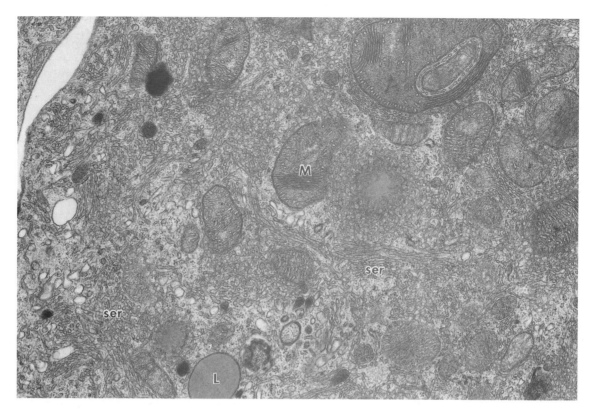

Figure 20.12. TEM of the adrenal cortex and zona fasciculata. Note the numerous mitochondria (M), lipid (L) droplets, and sER (ser). ×19,840.

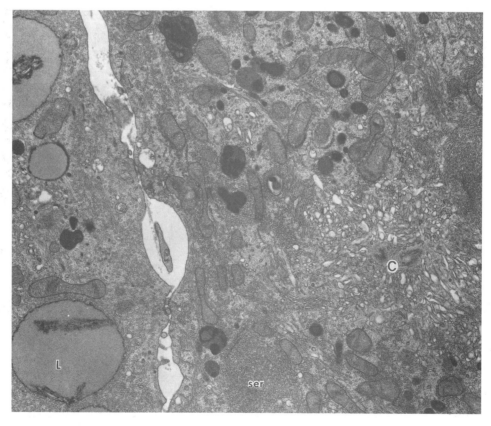

Figure 20.13. TEM of an adrenal cortical cell. The cell contains many electron-dense lysosomes and pigment granules and extensive sER (ser), which often surround lipid (L) droplets. A centriole (C) in the centrosome region is denoted. ×13,475.

Both synthesized from phenylalanine

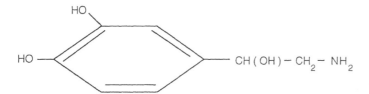

NORADRENALIN   (NOREPINEPHRINE)

INCREASES BLOOD PRESSURE
CONSTRICTS BLOOD VESSELS

ADRENALIN   (EPINEPHRINE)

Has extra methyl group

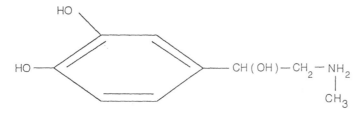

INCREASES HEARTBEAT
STIMULATES ACTH
MOBILIZES LIVER CARBOHYDRATE STORES

Figure 20.14. Structural formulas of the catecholamines, noradrenalin, and adrenalin (which has an extra methyl group) and their biological effects.

less electron-dense secretory granules than norepinephrine-secreting cells (Fig. 20.15). Furthermore, while the granules in epinephrine-secreting cells are completely filled, there is an electron-lucent layer at the periphery of the granules in norepinephrine-secreting cells. Both kinds of secretory cells can synthesize their product and store it in secretory granules until stimu-

lated to discharge. The secretory cells in the adrenal medulla are innervated by cholinergic endings of preganglionic sympathetic neurons. As described in the accompanying table, the two types of adrenal medullary cells differ with respect to their blood supply, and the source of their blood supply influences their secretory product. The secretory granules of the adrenal

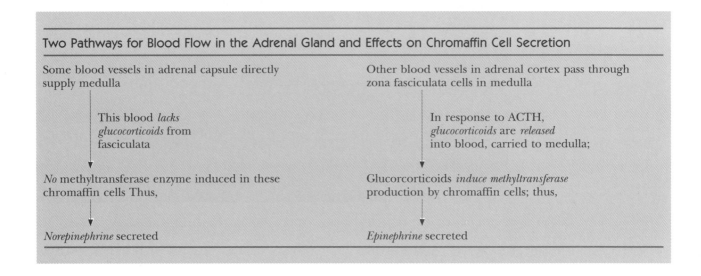

Two Pathways for Blood Flow in the Adrenal Gland and Effects on Chromaffin Cell Secretion

Some blood vessels in adrenal capsule directly supply medulla	Other blood vessels in adrenal cortex pass through zona fasciculata cells in medulla
This blood *lacks glucocorticoids* from fasciculata	In response to ACTH, *glucocorticoids* are *released* into blood, carried to medulla;
No methyltransferase enzyme induced in these chromaffin cells Thus,	Glucorticoids *induce methyltransferase* production by chromaffin cells; thus,
Norepinephrine secreted	*Epinephrine* secreted

medullary cells also contain ATP, the enzyme dopamine β-hydroxylase, substances resembling enkephalins, and proteins called chromogranins. Chromogranins appear to represent binding proteins for the catecholamines.

Synthesis of Norepinephrine and Epinephrine by Adrenal Chromaffin Cells

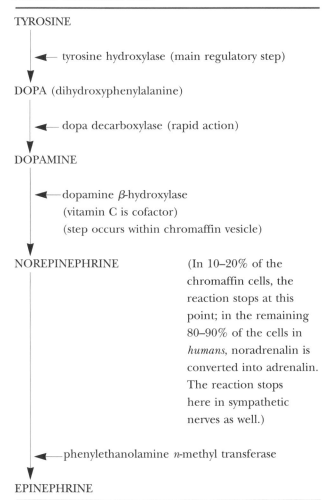

TYROSINE

→ tyrosine hydroxylase (main regulatory step)

DOPA (dihydroxyphenylalanine)

→ dopa decarboxylase (rapid action)

DOPAMINE

→ dopamine β-hydroxylase
(vitamin C is cofactor)
(step occurs within chromaffin vesicle)

NOREPINEPHRINE   (In 10–20% of the chromaffin cells, the reaction stops at this point; in the remaining 80–90% of the cells in *humans*, noradrenalin is converted into adrenalin. The reaction stops here in sympathetic nerves as well.)

→ phenylethanolamine *n*-methyl transferase

EPINEPHRINE

In the synthesis of epinephrine, tyrosine is taken into the cell and coverted to DOPA by the enzyme tyrosine hydroxylase; this is the main regulatory step. DOPA is rapidly converted by dopa decarboxylase to dopamine. Dopamine is converted to norepinephrine by dopamine β-hydroxylase; this step occurs within the chromaffin granules, but the previous steps occur in the cytosol. Vitamin C is a cofactor in the action of dopamine β-hydroxylase. In 10–20% of the chromaffin cells, the reaction stops at this point. In the remaining 80–90% of the cells in humans, norepinephrine is converted to epinephrine by the enzyme phenylethanolamine n-methyl transferase. Thus, epinephrine is produced by the methylation of norepinephrine.

When glucocorticoid secretion is stimulated by ACTH, the *glucocortocoids* are released into nearby cortical sinusoids that drain into the medulla. The glucocorticoids induce the secretion of *methyltransferase* enzyme in the chromaffin cells, which leads to the production of epinephrine. The medullary chromaffin cells supplied by a direct flow of blood from the capsule, which therefore lack glucocorticoids, do not produce methyltransferase and thus secrete norepinephrine.

Epinephrine and norepinephrine are released into the bloodstream by chromaffin cells in response to emotional reactions (fright, fight, or flight) as a result of impulses in sympathetic nerves. When ACh is released from nerve endings during neuronal stimulation, sodium ions enter the cells and depolarize the plasma membrane. This leads to an influx of calcium ions into the chromaffin cells; these ions are required for catecholamine secretion by chromaffin cells. The effects of catecholamines are produced within seconds and dissipate rapidly; they are thus suited for rapid, short-term behavior modifications. Most cells in the body have receptors for both epinephrine and norepinephrine; they are called *adrenergic receptors* and are subdivided into α_1, α_2, β_1, and β_2. Receptors β_1 and β_2 are identical except that β_2 receptors have low sensitivity to norepinephrine. The signal transduction mechanism of the receptor types is variable. Epinephrine interacts with receptors on various cells to increase the heartbeat rate, increase blood *pressure* (vasoconstriction, hypertension), and release additional sugar from hepatocytes for use by muscles in the fight-or-flight reaction. Epinephrine is more effective in raising blood glucose levels and in increasing cardiac output than norepinephrine, but norepinephrine is more effective in raising systolic and diastolic blood pressure.

ABNORMALITIES IN ADRENAL GLAND FUNCTION

Abnormalities in the functioning of the adrenal cortex can involve hyperfunction (overfunctioning) or hypofunction (underfunctioning). Tumors of the adrenal cortex can result in overproduction of glucocorticoids, a condition known as *Cushing's syndrome*. This condition is ususally due to a pituitary adenoma that results in overproduction of ACTH. Overproduction of aldosterone occurs in *Conn's syndrome*. Overproduction of adrenal androgens generally has little effect in males but can result in abnormal hair growth (hirsutism) and virilization in females and precocious puberty in males. *Addison's disease* usually results in failure to secrete glucocorticoids and mineralocorticoids and commonly is due to autoimmune destruction of the adrenal cortex. Tumors of the adrenal medulla, called *pheochromocytoma*, cause hyperglycemia and transiently elevated blood pressure.

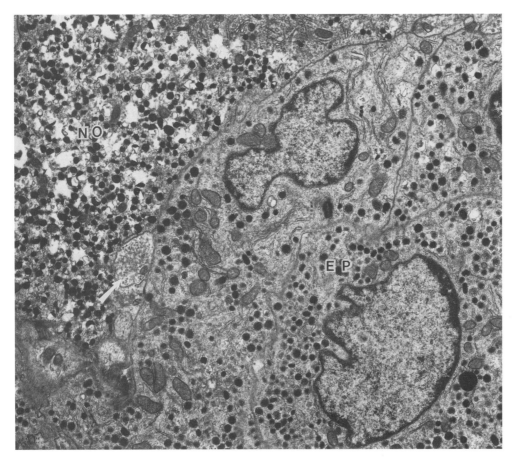

Figure 20.15. TEM of the adrenal medulla. Cells with characteristics of epinephrine (EP)- and norepinephrine (NO)-producing cells are identified. There are also sections of preganglionic sympathetic nerves (arrow) that terminate on the chromaffin cells. ×9750. (From R. Roberts, R. Kessel and H. Tung. *Freeze Fracture Images of Cells and Tissues.* Oxford University Press, New York, 1991, with permission)

THYROID GLAND

ORIGIN, ORGANIZATION, GENERAL FUNCTION

The thyroid develops early in embryonic life as an outgrowth of the embryonic pharynx. Its two lobes are located anterior to and on either side of the trachea and are connected by an isthmus. A rather thin connective tissue capsule extends as septae into the interior of the well-vascularized gland, dividing it into irregular lobules. The parenchyma of the thyroid contains a multitude of spherical glandular units called *follicles* (Plate 55A; Fig. 20.16). The follicles consist of roughly spherical compartments that contain stored colloid and are surrounded by follicular epithelial cells (Fig. 20.17).

The thyroid gland also contains scattered cells that originate from neural crest cells in the embryo. These neural crest cells migrate into the pharyngeal pouches during formation of the thyroid gland. The cells are called *parafollicular cells* (*C cells*), and they produce the hormone *calcitonin* (Plate 55C).

The thyroid begins to function at about the 10th week of fetal life. The gland plays an important role in regulating tissue metabolism and general growth and development. In addition to increasing the metabolic rate, thyroid hormone increases absorption of carbohydrates and regulates lipid metabolism. The thyroid follicle cells produce thyroid hormone. Two circulating forms of thyroid hormone exist: *thyroxine* (or *tetraiodothyronine*, T_4) and *triiodothyronine* (T_3).

The follicles vary markedly in diameter. The shapes of the epithelial cells comprising the follicles also vary from squamous to low columnar. Larger follicles that are filled with colloid have a squamous or cuboidal epithelium. Glands with follicles that have predominantly squamous epithelial cells are considered to be hypoactive. When the gland is stimulated to synthesize thyroid hormone, the follicular epithelial cells become columnar and the amount of colloid is reduced.

CONTROL OF THYROID ACTIVITY

The thyroid is controlled mainly by the thyroid-stimulating hormone (TSH or thyrotropin), which is released from a population of basophils in the pars distalis in re-

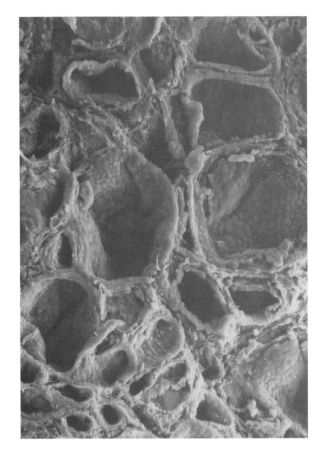

Figure 20.16. An SEM of thyroid follicles that were sectioned and colloid was removed. ×285. (From: R. Kessel and R. Kardon, *Tissues and Organs: A Text-Atlas of Scanning Electron Microscopy*. W.H. Freeman, New York 1979, with permission)

sponse to the thyrotropin-releasing hormone produced by neurons in the hypothalamus and released into the hypothalmo-hypophyseal portal circulatory system. The thyroid epithelium resides on a basement membrane, and the intervening connective tissue contains highly vascularized, fenestrated capillaries. Terminals of sympathetic and parasympathetic nerves end close to the basal regions of the follicle cells

SYNTHESIS OF THYROGLOBULIN: ULTRASTRUCTURE OF FOLLICLE CELLS

The synthesis of thyroglobulin involves the active uptake of iodide from the circulation. An iodide pump is located in the basal plasma membrane of the follicle cells and is sensitive to the level of TSH. The iodide is then oxidized by thyroid peroxidase to an intermediate that combines with the tyrosine residues in the colloid. The iodination of tyrosine in the thyroglobulin occurs in the colloid adjacent to the plasma membrane at the apical end of the cells. The apical membrane has short microvilli projecting into the colloid (Fig. 20.18).

The thyroid follicle cells contain an extensive system of rER that is located in the basal region of the cell. It is here that the protein thyroglobulin is synthesized. Mitochondria, a supranuclear Golgi complex, and a number of lysosomes and digestive vacuoles are also located in the cells. There are also secretory granules, apical vesicles, and phagosomes that vary in number, depending upon the physiologic state of activity.

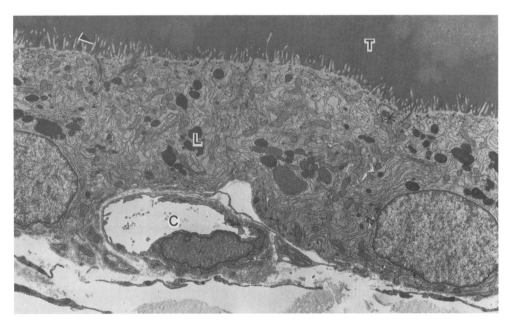

Figure 20.17. TEM of a thyroid follicle cell. Thyroglobulin (T) is present in the colloid and, under appropriate stimulus, is taken into the cell (*) and digested by means of lysosomes (L). Capillary (c). ×2500. (From R. Roberts, R. Kessel, H. Tung. *Freeze Fracture Images of Cells and Tissues*. Oxford University Press, New York, 1991, with permission)

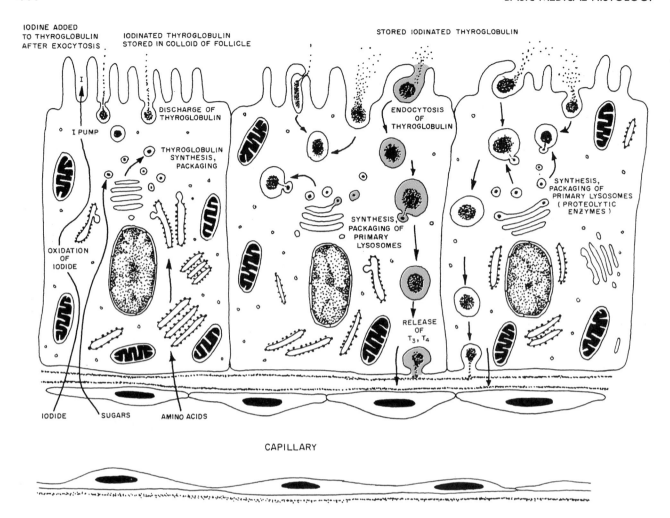

Figure 20.18. Diagram of stages in the synthesis of thyroglobulin (left cell). Cells in the center and on the right illustrate endocytosis of thyroglobulin and its degradation into thyroxine, which is released at the base of cell into capillaries.

PROCESSING OF COLLOID— SECRETION OF HORMONE

In response to TSH, the follicle cells internalize small packets of the stored thyroglobulin into pinocytotic vesicles at the apical end of the cells (Fig. 20.18). These pinocytotic vesicles then fuse with lysosomes; as a result, proteases in the lysosomes rupture the peptide bonds between iodinated residues. The resulting products include T_4, T_3, diiodotyrosine (DIT), and monoiodotyro-

sine (MIT), which enter the cytoplasm. As is apparent from the structural formulas of these substances, the condensation of two molecules of DIT (3,5, diiodotyrosine) with the elimination of an alanine residue results in the formation of tetraiodothyronine (T_4 or thyroxine). The condensation of one molecule of MIT (3-monoiodtyrosine) and one molecule of DIT, followed by the elimination of one alanine residue, results in the formation of triiodothyronine (T_3).

The T_4 and T_3 leave the cell and enter the capillaries (Fig. 20.19), but DIT and MIT do not leave the cell. DIT and MIT are converted by an enzymatic reaction to iodine and tyrosine, which can be reutilized by the follicle cells. T_3 is more potent than T_4 and acts more rapidly, but T_4 is the main form of the hormone that is secreted (about 95%).

THYROID DYSFUNCTION

When the diet is deficient in iodine, this interferes with iodination of thyroglobulin. As a result, there is increased TSH production resulting in an iodine deficiency goiter. When there is a deficiency of thyroid hormone from the time of birth, a dwarf child who is mentally retarded may result; such children suffer from cretinism. Overactivity of the thyroid (hyperthyroidism) may be due to a number of factors. In Graves' desease, the thyroid is overactive (hyperthyroidism), even with low levels of TSH, due to an immunologic disturbance in which an immunoglobulin has an effect similar to that of TSH. In Hashimoto's disease, there is an autoimmune reaction in which the body's lymphocytes destroy the thyroid gland, resulting in hypothyroidism.

PARAFOLLICULAR (C) CELLS AND CALCITONIN

The parafollicular cells are located between the follicles in the thyroid (Plate 55C). They are not part of the follicle and do not contact the colloid, but instead release their secretion into adjacent capillaries. Numerous secretory granules are present in the cells; these granules contain the polypeptide hormone *calcitonin* (Fig. 20.20). Calcitonin lowers the blood calcium level. Calcitonin acts on the ruffled borders of osteoclasts to decrease bone-resorbing activity. Calcitonin also promotes the excretion of calcium and phosphate ions from the kidneys.

PARATHYROID GLANDS

ORIGIN AND ORGANIZATION

There are usually four, but sometimes only two or as many as six, small parathyroid glands embedded in the connective tissue sheaths on the posterior surface of the two lobes of the thyroid gland. The parathyroids are derived from the endoderm of the embryonic third and fourth pharyngeal pouches. A thin connective tissue capsule extends into the glands as thin septae that incompletely divide the glands into lobules. The cells comprising the glandular parenchyma are supported by reticular fibers. There are two major cell types in the parathyroid. The *chief*, or *principal, cells* are the most nu-

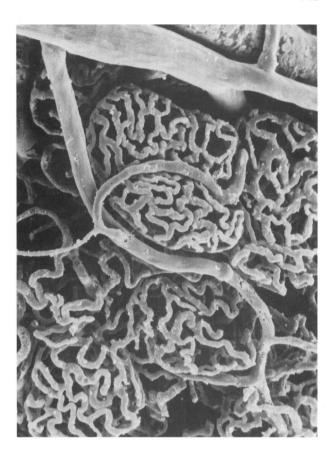

Figure 20.19. An SEM of a microvascular cast of the capillary plexuses associated with four thyroid follicles. ×210. (From: R. Kessel and R. Kardon. *Tissues and Organs: A Text-Atlas of Scanning Electron Microscopy.* W.H. Freeman, New York 1979, with permission)

merous and secrete *parathyroid hormone (PTH)*. Their cytoplasm contains a few electron-dense cytoplasmic granules. *Oxyphil cells* are larger than chief cells and have an intensely acidophilic-staining cytoplasm (Plate 55B). Oxyphil cells may exist singly and are widely distributed, but they are sometimes located in more extensive cell clusters. Oxyphil cells usually appear shortly before puberty, and their functional role is unknown. They are structurally unusual in that they have an extremely high concentration of mitochondria. Glycogen granules are also present in the cells. Structural variations observed in various cell types in the parathyroid suggest that the chief and oxyphil cells are transitions in only a single cell type.

FUNCTION OF PTH

As dicussed in Chapter 7, when the blood or plasma calcium level drops below normal, the parathyroid gland cells respond by synthesizing and releasing *PTH*. Due to the release of PTH, osteoclasts increase in number and are activiated to resorb bone, thus elevating the

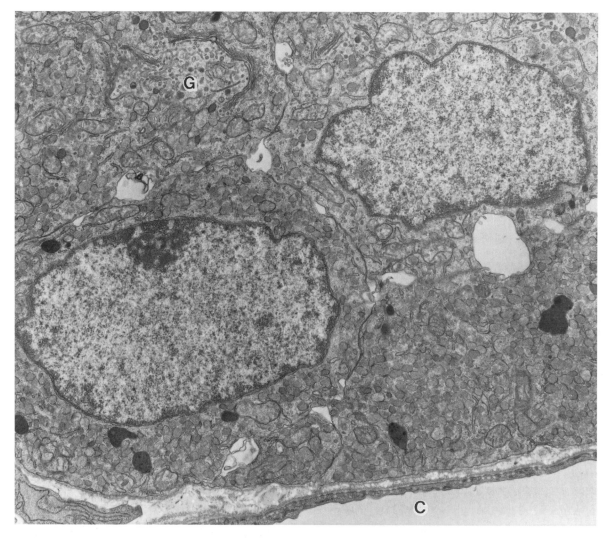

Figure 20.20.   TEM of parafollicular cells in the thyroid. Numerous secretory granules are present in these cells. The Golgi complex (G) is identified, and a fenestrated capillary (C) is present in the lower right of the field. ×12,500.

blood calcium level. The rising blood calcium level causes the chief cells to decrease or stop the release of PTH. Thus a feedback loop exists between the blood calcium level, parathyroid chief cells, and osteoclasts in regulating the blood calcium level. Recent evidence indicates that the action of PTH on osteoclasts is indirect.

ABNORMAL PARATHYROID FUNCTION

In cases of pronounced *hyperparathyroidism* (i.e., overactive parathyoids), there is a high concentration of calcium in the bloodstream but the blood phosphate level is low; this situation may result in pathological deposits of calcium in such locations as arteries and kidneys. *Hypoparathyroidism* (i.e., underactive parathyroids) is a condition in which the blood calcium level is quite low and the phosphate ion concentration is elevated. This con-

dition may lead to spastic contractions of skeletal muscle resulting in convulsions (tetany). These actions are due to increased excitability of the nervous system from the lack of sufficient blood calcium.

ISLETS OF LANGERHANS

The islets of Langerhans consist of highly vascularized, spherical aggregations of cells. The islets are separated from the exocrine pancreas by a thin aggregation of reticular fibers (Plate 55D). It has been estimated that the human pancreas contains 500,000 to 1 million islets of Langerhans that are more concentrated in the tail region. All cells in the islets are in contact with fenestrated capillaries and are supported by fine reticular fibers. The cells in the islets are coupled by intercellular junctions of the gap junction type. Different cell types have been identified in the islets based on specific staining techniques and, more recently, on immunologic cytochemical procedures.

CELL TYPES

The *beta cells* are the most numerous, comprising about 75% of all cells (Fig. 20.21). These cells produce *insulin*, which reduces the blood sugar level. An elevated blood glucose level causes insulin secretion, which, in turn, causes a reduction in blood sugar level. The reduction in sugar is accomplished by stimulating glucose transport into liver and muscle for storage in the form of glycogen. Insulin facilitates glucose transport by its action on glucose transporters. Glucose transporters are plasma membrane carriers involved in glucose transport into the cell in response to increased insulin secretion. When insulin secretion is reduced, glucose transporters are removed from the plasma membrane of responsive cells and become part of an intracellular pool of these transporters. The hormone insulin boosts protein synthesis and controls blood glucose levels. When beta cells in the pancreas detect a high glucose level, insulin is released into the blood and, by acting on insulin receptors in target cells, instructs adipocytes and skeletal muscle fibers to synthesize more of those enzymes that catalyze the synthesis of fats and/or muscle proteins. Early on, it was recognized that insulin can regulate the activities of a cell without actually entering the cell. Insulin interacts with an insulin receptor embedded in the plasma membrane.

Alpha cells comprise about 20% of the islets in humans (Fig. 20.22). These cells are more concentrated at the periphery of the islet and produce *glucagon*. Low blood glucose levels cause glucagon secretion, which stimulates the conversion of glycogen to glucose in liver cells and its release into the blood for energy between meals. Glucagon is antagonistic to insulin and has the effect of increasing the blood glucose concentration. Two major effects of glucagon on glucose metabolism are: *glycogenolysis*, the breakdown of liver glycogen, and *gluconeogenesis*, the formation of glucose from amino acids and the glycerol portion of fat.

The delta cells comprise about 5% of the islets. It has been suggested that the delta cells produce *somatostatin*, a peptide that in the pituitary inhibits the release of GH. However, somatostatin released from the delta cells may act in a paracrine manner to suppress secretion of insulin and glucagon by the islet cells. It has also been suggested that the gastrin secreted by the islets may be derived from alpha and delta cells. A PP cell has been described in the islets; the granules in this cell react immunocytochemically to *human pancreatic polypeptide* (hPP). In addition, *vasoactive intestinal polypeptide* (VIP) is secreted by a type of D cell, and serotonin is secreted by an enterochromaffin (EC) cell in the islet.

SECRETORY PRODUCTS OF ISLETS

The secretory products that have been described to originate from the islets of Langerhans and the cellular source of these secretory products are summarized in the accompanying table.

Islets of Langerhans

Cell Type	Substance Produced	Major Action	% of Cells
Beta	Insulin (polypeptide)	Reduces blood sugar (inhibits release of glucagon, paracrine)	75%
Alpha	Glucagon (polypeptide)	Elevates blood sugar (glycogenolysis = liver glycogen → glucose) (gluconeogenesis = amino acids + glycerol → glucose) (stimulates release of insulin and pancreatic somatostatin; paracrine)	20%
Delta (D)	Somatostatin (peptide)	Suppresses insulin and glucagon secretion (paracrine regulation) (inhibits release of hormone by neighboring cells)	5%
D1	Vasoactive intestinal peptide (VIP)	Unknown	?
G	Gastrin	Stimulates HCl production and release by parietal cells in stomach (presence in normal pancreas questionable)	<1%
EC	Serotonin (also motilin, substance P)	Dilation and increased permeability of blood vessels; neurotransmitter	<1%
PP	(Human) pancreatic polypeptide (hPP)	Inhibits release of exocrine secretions of pancreas	<1%

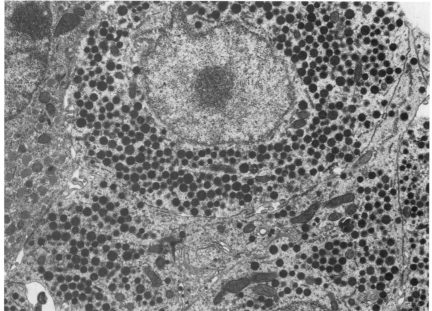

20.21

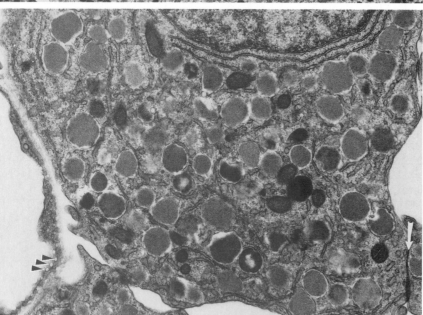

20.22

Figures 20.21, 20.22. TEM of an islet of Langerhans. Cells characteristic of α-glucagon cells are located in figure 20.21, while a portion of an insulin-producing beta cell is located in figure 20.22. Beta cells are coupled by gap junctions (arrow). Note the fenestrated endothelium (arrowheads) of capillary close to the beta cell in the lower figure. Figure 20.21, ×8000. Figure 20.22, ×9750. (Fig. 20.22 from: R. Roberts, R. Kessel, H. Tung. Freeze Fracture Images of Cells and Tissues. Oxford University Press, New York, 1991, with permission.)

TYPE I AND TYPE II DIABETES

Type I (insulin-dependent) diabetes mellitus, which is marked by lack of insulin secretion, is an autoimmune reaction in which beta cells are destroyed by appropriately activated T lymphocytes. Type I diabetes frequently begins before adulthood. In Type II (insulin-independent) diabetes, beta cells do secrete insulin, but the target cells of insulin lack (down regulation) insulin receptors in the membrane and therefore do not respond to insulin. Dietary control, weight reduction, and exercise may completely reverse the symptoms of type II diabetes.

A summary of the principal endocrine glands, their hormones, targets and functions is presented in Table 20.4

Table 20.4 The Principal Endocrine Glands: Hormones, Targets, and Functions

Gland	Hormones	Target Cells, Tissues Organs	Chief Functions
Hypothalamus	Releasing hormones	Anterior pituitary	Stimulates anterior pituitary to release specific hormones
	Inhibiting hormones	Anterior pituitary	Inhibits anterior pituitary from releasing specific hormones
Anterior pituitary	Thyroid-stimulating hormone (TSH)	Thyroid gland	Stimulates secretion of thyroid hormones
	Prolactin (PRL)	Mammary glands	Causes milk synthesis, secretion
	Growth hormone (GH, somatotropin)	Bones, other tissues	Promotes growth; protein synthesis, maintenance of adult size
	Adrenocorticotropin (ACTH)	Adrenal cortex	Stimulates adrenal cortex; mainly glucocorticoids
	Gonadotropic hormones	Ovary	Stimulates gonads; folliculogenesis, germ cell differentiation
	FSH (follicle-stimulating hormone)	Testis	Secretion of androgen-binding protein (ABP) by Sertoli cells
	LH (luteinizing hormone)	Ovary	Release of oocyte at ovulation; formation of corpus luteum
		Testis	Testosterone secretion by Leydig cells
Hypothalamus (Supraoptic and paraventricular nuclei) Hormones released from posterior pituitary	ADH (antidiuretic hormone, vasopressin)	Kidneys (collecting ducts)	Causes water reabsorption by kidneys
	Oxytocin	Smooth muscle of uterus, myoepithelial cells of mammary gland	Causes smooth muscle contraction (labor); stimulates milk ejection into ducts
Pineal	Melatonin	Brain, gonads	"Time-keeping gland"; inhibits gonadal growth and function; suppresses gonadotropin-releasing hormone (GnRH)
Thyroid	Thyroxine (tetraiodothyronine and triiodothyronine)	All cells, tissues	Increases general metabolic rate ($\uparrow O_2$ consumption); increases body temperature and nutrient utilization
	Calcitonin	Bones, kidneys, digestive tract	Decreases plasma calcium; calcium enters bones; excretion of calcium in kidneys, digestive tract
Parathyroid	Parathormone (PTH)	Bones, kidneys, digestive tract	Increases plasma calcium and phosphorus levels; stimulates bone
Adrenal cortex	Mineralocorticoids (aldosterone)	Kidneys (distal nephron)	Causes sodium retention and postassium excretion by distal nephrone
	Glucocorticoids (cortisol)	Most tissues, liver	Causes gluconeogenesis; breakdown of protein, fat; anti-inflammatory; adaptation to stress
	Androgens	Male fetus	Masculinization resorption; conservation of calcium by reabsorption in kidneys

Table 20.4 The Principal Endocrine Glands: Hormones, Targets, and Functions continued

Gland	Hormones	Target Cells, Tissues Organs	Chief Functions
Adrenal medulla	Norepinephrine	Cardiac, skeletal muscle, glands	Promotes "fight or flight"; blood vessels constrict; increased blood pressure
	Epinephrine	Cardiac, skeletal muscle, glands	Elevates heartbeat; mobilizes liver carbohydrate stores
Pancreas (islets of Langerhans)	Insulin	Liver, muscles, adipose tissue, blood glucose	Decreases blood sugar; promotes entry of glucose into cells; stimulates glycogenesis, fat storage, and protein synthesis
	Glucagon	Liver, muscles, adipose tissue, blood glucose	Elevates blood sugar level by stimulating glycogenolysis and gluconeogenesis; mobilizes fat
Thymus	Thymulin, thymopoietin and thymosin α1	T lymphocytes	Promotes division, differentiation, and maturation of T lymphocytes
Testes	Testosterone	Sex organs, bones, muscle, integument	Growth and development of secondary male sex characteristics; promotes spermatogenesis
Ovaries	Estrogen	Sex organs, bones, muscle, integument	Ovarian development, development of uterine endometrium, secondary female sex characteristics
	Progesterone (corpus luteum)	Uterus, ovary	Prepares body for implantation; maintain secretory uterine endometrium; prevent follicle development
	Relaxin	Pubic symphysis	Softening of ligaments at parturition
Fetal placenta	Human chorionic gonadotropin (hCG)	Corpus luteum	Maintains functional corpus luteum during initial stages of implantation
	Human chorionic somatomammotropin	Mother, fetus	Lactogenic and growth-stimulating effects
	Relaxin	Uterus, symphysis pubis	Quiets uterine muscle; soften symphysis pubis late in pregnancy
	Progesterone	Uterine endometrium	Maintains uterine endometrium during most of pregnancy
	Estrogen	Hypothalamus—pituitary	Prevents FSH release during pregnancy
	Chorionic thyrotropin	Thyroid	Stimulates thyroid
	Chorionic corticotropin	Adrenal cortex	Stimulates activity
Kidney	Renin	Elevates blood pressure	Secreted in response to blood ↓ Na$^+$ or ↓ blood pressure
	Erythropoietin	Bone marrow	Acts on early stages of erythroid proliferation to promote erythrocyte differentiation
Digestive tract	Gastrin	Stomach	Stimulates HCL secretion
	Secretin	Ducts of exocrine pancreas	Concentration of pancreatic digestive enzymes
	Cholecystokinin/ pancreozymin (CCK)	Gallbladder	Gallbladder contraction
		Exocrine pancreas	Stimulates secretion of pancreatic digestive enzymes

SELECTED BIBLIOGRAPHY

Brinkley, S. (1988). *The Pineal: Endocrine and Nonendocrine Function.* Prentice Hall, Englewood Cliffs, NJ.

Burrow, G., Oppenheimer, J., and Volpe, R. (1989). *Thyroid Function and Disease.* W.B. Saunders, Philadelphia.

Carey, R.M., and Sen, S. (1986). Recent progress in the control of aldosterone secretion. *Rec. Progr. Horm. Res.* **42**, 251–289.

Carmichael, S.W., and Winkler, H. (1985). The adrenal chromaffin cell. *Sci. Am.* **253**, 40–49.

Cohn, D.V., Kumarasamy, R., and Ramp, W.K. (1986). Intracellular processing and secretion of parathyroid gland proteins. *Vitamins Horm.* **43**, 285–315.

Cooperstein, S.J., and Watkins, D., Eds. (1981). *The Islets of Langerhans: Biochemistry, Physiology, Pathology.* Academic Press, New York.

Falke, N. (1991). Modulation of oxytocin and vasopressin release at the level of the neurophypophysis. *Prog. Neurobiol.* **36**, 465–484.

Goodman, H.M. (1988). *Basic Medical Endocrinology.* Raven Press, New York.

Habener, J., Roseblatt, M., and Potts, J.T., Jr. (1984). Parathryoid hormone: biochemical aspects of biosynthesis, secretion, action, and metabolism. *Physiol. Rev.* **64**, 985–1054.

Kannan, C.R. (1987). *The Pituitary Gland.* Plenum, New York.

Kannan, C.R. (1988). *The Adrenal Gland.* Plenum, New York.

Marx, J. (1991). How peptide hormones get ready for work. *Science* **252**, 779–780.

Nussdorfer, G.C. (1986). Cytophysiology of the adrenal cortex. *Int. Rev. Cytol.,* **98**, 1–394.

Petersen, O.H. (1990). Control of insulin secretion in pancreatic b-cells. *NIPS* **5**, 254–258.

Reichlin, S., ed. (1984). *The Neurohypophysis: Physiological and Clinical Aspects.* Plenum, New York.

Reiter, R.J. (1987). Mechanisms of control of reproductive physiology by the pineal gland and its hormones. *Adv. Pineal Res.* **2**, 109–125.

Reiter, R.J. (1991). Melatonin: that ubiquitously acting pineal hormone. *NIPS,* **6**, 223–227.

Schatzberg, A.F., and Nemeroff, C.B., eds. (1988). *The Hypothalamic-Pituitary-Adrenal Axis.* Raven Press, New York.

Steiner, D.F., and James, D.E. (1992). Cellular and molecular biology of the beta cell. *Diabetologia* **35**, S41–S48.

Ungar, A., and Phillips, J.J. (1983). Regulation of the adrenal medulla. *Physiol. Rev.* **63**, 787–843.

Wilson, J.D., and Foster, D.W. (1985). *Williams Textbook of Endocrinology,* 7th ed., W.B. Saunders, Philadelphia.

CHAPTER 21

The Urinary (Excretory) System

GENERAL FUNCTIONS

The excretory system consists of paired kidneys, ureters, and a single urinary bladder and urethra. The regulatory activity of the kidney involves a variety of physiologic processes including filtration, active transport (absorption), passive absorption, and secretion. The kidneys perform an important function in eliminating the waste products of protein catabolism. These nitrogenous and other waste products are filtered from the blood by over 1 million filters called *renal corpuscles* that are present in each kidney. The kidneys maintain fluid balance and function to conserve water. Since the kidneys also regulate the loss of electrolytes in the urine, they are exceedingly important in the maintenance of blood homeostasis. Thus, the process of reabsorption of molecules (such as amino acids, glucose, and small proteins), as well as ions (Na^+, Cl^-, Ca^{2+}, PO_4^{3-}) and water, are as important as the excretory role of the urinary system. The kidneys also produce an enzyme called *renin*, which is important in stabilizing blood pressure and maintaining the proper oxygen level in the blood. In addition, the kidney produces a hormone, *erythropoietin*, that is involved in regulating erythrocyte production.

GENERAL ORGANIZATION

The human kidneys are paired bean-shaped structures about 10–12 cm in length and are retroperitoneal (i.e., outside the peritoneal cavity). The superior pole of each kidney is capped by a suprarenal gland. The hilum is a concavity in which the renal artery, renal vein, renal pelvis, nerves, and lymph vessels are located (Fig. 21.1).

The kidneys are compound tubular glands consisting of many tubular units called *uriniferous renal tubules* (Fig. 21.2). Each uriniferous tubule consists of a nephron and a collecting duct, which are positioned such that when a medial sagittal section of the kidney is viewed grossly, an inner portion called the *medulla* appears to be somewhat striated in appearance, but an outer *cortex* appears to be finely granular and homogeneous (Fig. 21.1). Each nephron consists of a renal corpuscle and a recurrent tubular portion.

The renal corpuscles, which are located only in the cortex, give this region its finely granular appearance. The kidney is both an exocrine (urine) gland and an endocrine (erythropoietin) gland. The kidney differs significantly in microscopic anatomy from other glands in that no connective tissue septa extend from the capsule into the parenchyma of the kidney. Therefore, the kidney cannot be divided into distinct lobes based on the presence of connective tissue septae, as is typical of salivary glands, for example.

The rat kidney consists of but one lobe and is called a *unilobar kidney*. In a unilobar kidney there is one medullary pyramid with associated overlying cortical tissue. The human kidney, however, is *multilobar* and may contain as many as 18 lobes. Each lobe in the human kidney consists of a pyramid, located in the medulla, together with the overlying cortical tissue (Fig. 21.1).

In the human kidney, groups of closely packed straight tubules, called a *medullary ray*, extend from the base of a pyramid into the cortex. These groups of straight tubules are oriented at a right angle to the overlying capsule. Each medullary ray consists of collecting ducts and the straight portions of a number of nephrons and blood vessels. The filtrate drains through a branching system of collecting ducts into the renal pelvis, which

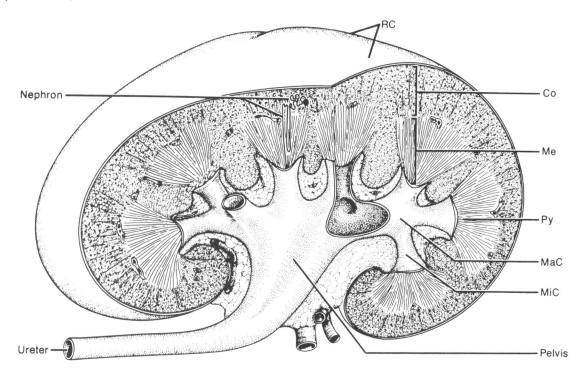

Figure 21.1. Drawing of the mid-sagittal section of a multilobar kidney. Renal capsule (RC), cortex of the kidney (Co), medulla of the kidney (Me), pyramid (Py), major calyx (MaC), minor calyx (MiC), pelvis, and ureter are identified. The position of a single nephron is denoted. (From R. G. Kessel and R. H. Kardon, *Tissues and Organs: A Text-Atlas of Scanning Electron Microscopy*. W.H. Freeman, New York, 1979, with permission)

is the funnel-like proximal end of the ureter. By means of muscular contractions (peristalsis) of the tubular ureters, urine passes to the urinary bladder, where it may be stored before elimination through the urethra. The *renal pelvis* is divided into *major calyces* and *minor calyces* (Fig. 21.1)

CIRCULATORY SYSTEM

The kidneys are strategically located to filter blood. Each kidney is supplied by either the large left or right renal arteries, which branch directly from the descending aorta. As a result, the kidneys receive approximately 20% of the cardiac output per minute. In a 24-hour period, an average human produces ~180 liters of fluid ultrafiltrate, which passes through the kidney tubules. Of this amount, however, only about 1.5 liters is excreted as urine; the remaining ~178.5 liters is reabsorbed by the tubule cells and reenters the blood vascular system.

Another way of emphasizing the importance of the blood in kidney function is the fact that the kidneys filter about 1.25 liters of blood per minute. This means that all the blood in the body flows through the kidneys every 5 minutes or less. From this, the two kidneys produce about 125 ml of filtrate per minute, but 124 ml of this amount is reabsorbed. Thus, in a 24-hour period, approximately 1.5 liters of urine is produced.

The renal artery branches inside the kidney into several *interlobar* arteries that traverse the medulla to the junction of the medulla and cortex, where they branch at right angles into *arcuate* arteries that then run parallel to the cortical-medullary junction (Fig. 21.3). A number of *interlobular* arteries arise by branching at right angles from each arcuate artery and then extend through the cortex to the capsule. *Intralobular* arteries may branch from the interlobular arteries to become afferent arterioles, which form the glomeruli and supply each Bowman's capsule. However, interlobular arteries may also branch directly into *afferent arterioles*. The afferent arterioles then narrow and subdivide to form a capillary tuft called the renal *glomerulus* (Fig. 21.4). The capillaries of the glomerulus coalesce into an efferent arteriole that exits the renal corpuscle (Fig. 21.4). The placement of a capillary tuft interposed between two arterioles is unique and serves to maintain a high filtration pressure in the renal corpuscle. The *efferent arterioles* of more superficially located glomeruli in the cortex break down into another capillary plexus called the *peritubular plexus*, which closely surrounds and invests the tubular portion of these nephrons (Fig. 21.4). In more deeply located glomeruli, thin, straight loops of vessels arise from the efferent arteriole of these juxtamedullary glomeruli and are called *arteriolae rectae spuriae*. These vessels travel parallel to the loops of Henle and extend deep into the medulla (Fig. 21.3).

Depending upon the location of the renal corpus-

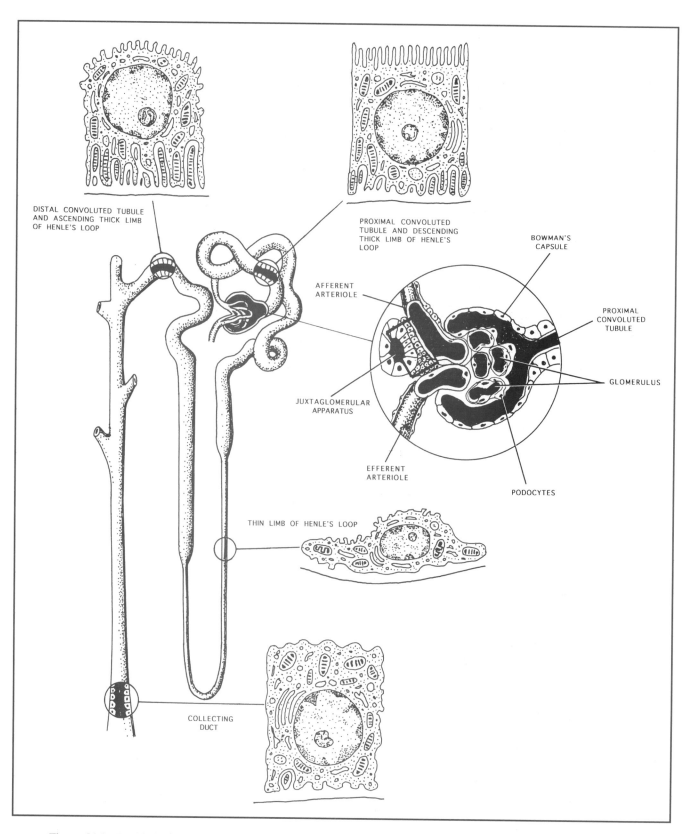

Figure 21.2. Drawing of parts of a uriniferous tubule and the ultrastructural organization of cells in different parts of the tubule.

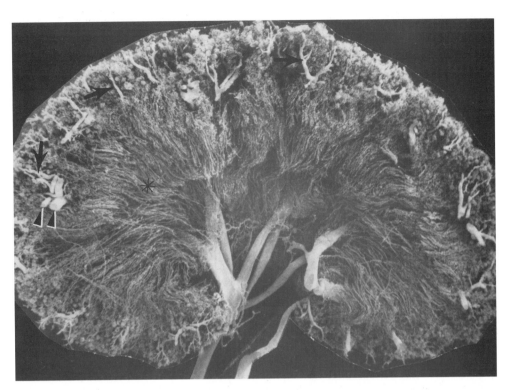

Figure 21.3. Microvascular cast of the entire rat kidney. The arcuate artery and vein (arrowheads) are located at the cortical-medullary junction. Interlobular vessels are denoted by arrows. Vasa rectae (*). ×7. (From R. Kessel and R. Kardon, *Tissues and Organs: A Text-Atlas of Scanning Electron Microscopy*, W.H. Freeman, New York, 1979, with permission)

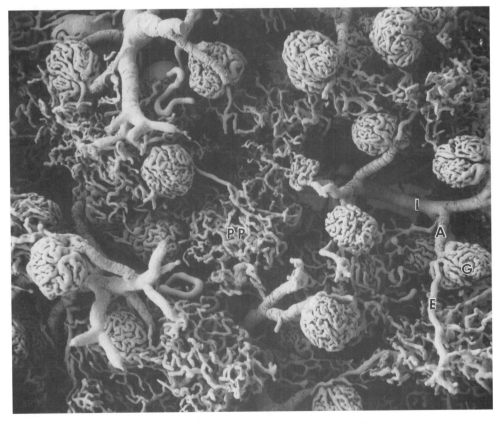

Figure 21.4. Microvascular cast of the renal cortex illustrates an intralobular vessel (I), afferent arteriole (A), glomerulus (G), efferent arteriole (E), and peritubular capillary plexus (PP). ×100. (From R. Kessel and R. Kardon, *Tissues and Organs: A Text-Atlas of Scanning Electron Microscopy*, W.H. Freeman, New York, 1979, with permission)

cle, it is possible to distinguish cortical, midcortical, and juxtamedullary glomeruli or nephrons (Fig. 21.5). Cortical nephrons have short loops of Henle. The afferent arterioles subdivide into a glomerulus, or capillary plexus, that exits the renal corpuscle as an efferent arteriole (Fig. 21.4). Since the afferent and efferent arterioles are similar in diameter, there is very little pressure drop in the glomerulus. In the case of cortical and subcortical glomeruli, the efferent arteriole once again breaks down into a *peritubular capillary plexus* (Figs. 21.4,

21.5). This arrangement actually represents an *arterial portal system* that closely invests much of the tubular portion of the nephron. These capillaries have a relatively high colloidal osmotic pressure because they are postglomerular capillaries, and much of the fluid and crystalloids pass out of the blood in the glomerular capillaries. However, most of the proteins are retained; thus the blood in this region has a *high colloidal osmotic pressure*. As a result, the peritubular capillaries are suited to reabsorb substances from the collecting ducts because

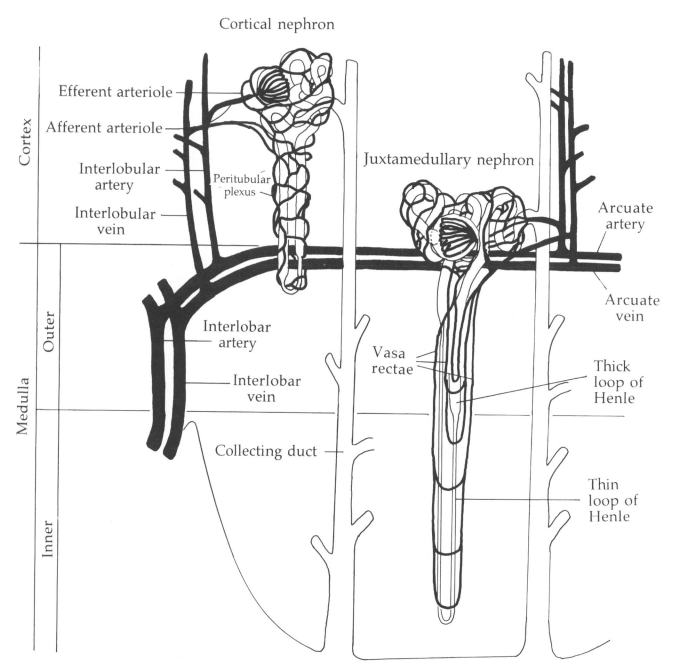

Figure 21.5. Drawing of cortical and juxtamedullary (lower) nephrons and their blood supply. The cortical nephrons are surrounded by a peritubular capillary plexus into which certain substances are reabsorbed from the tubules. The tubules of juxtamedullary nephrons, however, are invested by "straight" vessels called *vasa rectae*.

of the high colloidal osmotic pressure in the peritubular capillaries.

Most of the efferent arterioles from juxtamedullary nephrons divide several times to form several long, straight, hairpin-like loops that extend into the medulla. These vessels are collectively called *vasae rectae* ("straight vessels"), but those that extend from the efferent arterioles into the medulla are called *arteriolae rectae spuriae* (Fig. 21.5). In the inner medulla, the arteriolae rectae spuriae make a hairpin turn, and ascend again as recurrent venules in the region adjacent to the descending limb, and form a vascular countercurrent exchanger (Fig. 21.5). After the hairpin turn in the vessels, the *venous branches* of the *vasae rectae* empty into the *arcuate* or *interlobular veins*. The vasae rectae collectively comprise the *rete mirabile* or "marvelous network" and function in countercurrent exchange.

URINIFEROUS TUBULE

Each uriniferous tubule is about 6.5 cm long and consists of a *nephron* and a *collecting duct* (Fig. 21.2, 21.6) There are approximately 1.3 million nephrons in each kidney, and each nephron is composed of a *renal corpuscle* (or *Malpighian corpuscle*) and a long tubular portion consisting of several regions, including a *proximal convoluted tubule*, a *thick descending limb* of *Henle*, a *thin descending limb* of the loop of Henle, *a thin ascending limb* of *Henle*, an *ascending thick limb* of *Henle*, and a *distal convoluted tubule* that empties into a *collecting tubule* (Fig. 21.2).

Each renal corpuscle consists of a capillary tuft called a *glomerulus* and an investing epithelial structure called *Bowman's capsule* that has two layers (Figs. 21.7–21.9). The cortical corpuscles produce an ultrafiltrate of the blood, while the tubular portion, which extends from the cortex into the medulla and back into the cortex again, modifies the ultrafiltrate as it passes through the tubule.

THE NEPHRON

STRUCTURE

The *nephron* consists of a rounded *renal corpuscle* (Figs. 21.10–21.13) or Malpighian corpuscle that is about 200–300 μm in diameter and a recurrent *tubular portion* that is some 50–77 mm long. The tubule consists of a simple epithelium that varies from squamous to cuboidal to columnar. The relationship of the renal corpuscle and the tubular portion is erroneously represented in most textbooks by necessity. For if the renal corpuscle in a drawing were the size of a penny, then the loop of Henle (descending limb, thin segment, and ascending limb) would require a distance of ~7.5 m to

accurately convey the size relationships. In addition, the components of the nephron and uriniferous tubule are much more compact than those usually depicted by drawings.

The descending and ascending limbs and collecting ducts are very closely aggregated in groups, and these collections of straight tubules that extend into the kidney cortex are called *medullary rays* (*of Ferrein*) (Fig. 21.6). The region of the cortex located between medullary rays contains renal corpuscles, proximal and distal convoluted tubules, and blood vessels (Plate 56A; Figs. 21.6–21.9). A kidney *lobule* is defined as a single collecting duct of Bellini and the surrounding nephrons that drain into it. The extensive U shape of the nephron is directly related to water conservation or water recovery. In addition, the U shape of the nephron is associated with the development of high osmolarity ("saltiness") in the interstitial fluid that bathes the outer surface of the tubules and ducts.

The parietal layer of Bowman's capsule is continuous with the proximal convoluted tubule, which is the longest portion of the tubule in the cortex (~15 mm long and ~60 μm in diameter). Therefore, the proximal convoluted portion of the tubule is most frequently observed in a random section of the cortex. The proximal convoluted tubule extends in a straight fashion toward the medulla and is called the *pars recta* of the proximal convoluted tubule or, more commonly, the *thick descending limb of the loop of Henle* (~30 μm). It begins in the medullary ray and extends for varying depths toward and into the medulla, depending upon the position of the nephron. Near the border between the outer and inner stripes of the medulla, the tubule becomes thinner (~20 μm) and is called the *descending thin limb of Henle's loop*. After making an abrupt hairpin loop, the thin segment is called the *ascending thin limb of Henle's loop*. Near the border of the inner and outer medullas, the thin ascending portion of Henle's loop once again becomes larger in diameter (~40 μm) and is usually called the *thick ascending limb of Henle's loop* (or the *pars recta of the distal tubule*) (Fig. 21.2). This tubule extends through the outer medulla in the medullary ray toward the vascular pole of the renal corpuscle in the cortex. The distal convoluted tubule begins at the vascular pole of the renal corpuscle and is approximately 5 mm long and ~40–50 μm in diameter. The distal convoluted tubule empties into a collecting duct.

RENAL CORPUSCLE

POLES

Each renal corpuscle has a *vascular pole* (Fig. 21.9) where the afferent arteriole enters and the efferent arteriole exits the renal corpuscle. Each renal corpuscle has an

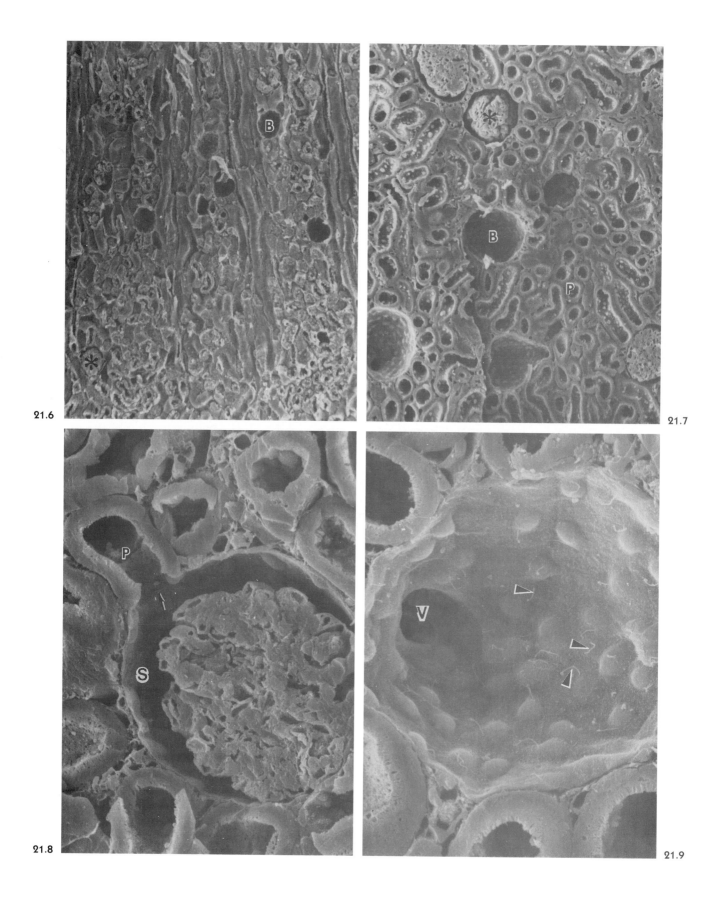

21.6

21.7

21.8

21.9

458

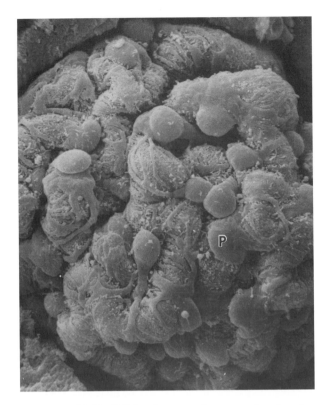

Figure 21.10. SEM of a renal corpuscle showing podocytes (P) comprising the visceral layer of Bowman's capsule. ×1230. (From R. Kessel and R. Kardon, *Tissues and Organs: A Text-Atlas of Scanning Electron Microscopy*, W.H. Freeman, New York, 1979, with permission)

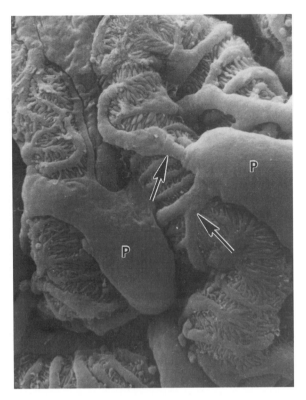

Figure 21.11. Podocytes (P) have many processes (primary, secondary, and tertiary) extending from the cell bodies (arrows). These podocytes surround the glomerular capillary. ×3640. (From R. Kessel and R. Kardon, *Tissues and Organs: A Text-Atlas of Scanning Electron Microscopy*, W.H. Freeman, New York, 1979, with permission)

opposite pole, called the *urinary pole* (Fig. 21.8), which is continuous with the proximal convoluted tubule.

BOWMAN'S CAPSULE: PARIETAL LAYER

The glomerular capillary is surrounded by a double-walled cup called *Bowman's capsule* (Figs. 21.8, 21.9). It consists of an inner *visceral layer* made up of highly branched cells called *podocytes* that completely invest the glomerular capillary (Figs. 21.10–21.13). The outer layer is called the *parietal layer of Bowman's capsule* and consists of simple squamous epithelium that is continuous at the *urinary pole* of the renal corpuscle with the proximal convoluted tubule (Fig. 21.8). The space between the visceral and parietal layers of Bowman's capsule is called the *urinary space* (*capsular space* or *Bowman's space*) (Fig. 21.8). The primitive urinary filtrate passes

into the urinary space and then into the proximal convoluted tubule. The glomerulus is suspended from a *vascular pole* of the renal corpuscle by *mesangial cells*. The *macula densa* is a region of the distal convoluted tubule that adheres to the Bowman's capsule between the afferent and efferent arterioles.

BOWMAN'S CAPSULE: VISCERAL LAYER

The fenestrated glomerular capillary is completely covered by the visceral epithelial layer of Bowman's capsule; these cells are called *podocytes* (Figs. 21.10–21.13). The podocytes are highly branched or dendritic and extend primary and secondary branches (Fig. 21.12). The primary branches tend to extend parallel with the capillary. The secondary branches come off at right angles

Figures 21.6–21.9. SEMs of renal corpuscles (*), some of which have had the glomerulus removed so that only Bowman's capsule (B) is present. Proximal (P) tubules and other tubules are numerous; the continuity between the urinary space and proximal (P) tubule at the urinary pole is shown in Figure 21.8 (arrow); urinary space (S). Note the cilia (arrowheads) extending from cells of the parietal layer of Bowman's capsule (Fig. 21.9); vascular pole (V). Figure 21.6, ×75; Figure 21.7, ×145; Figure 21.8, ×600; Figure 21.9, ×910. (From R. Kessel and R. Kardon, *Tissues and Organs: A Text-Atlas of Scanning Electron Microscopy*, W.H. Freeman, New York, 1979, with permission)

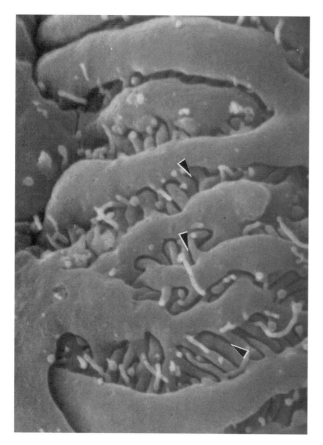

Figure 21.12. SEM of podocyte pedicels. Pedicels of one podocyte interdigitate with those of another podocyte; thin spaces between adjacent pedicels are the filtration slits (arrowheads). ×15,600. (From R. Kessel and R. Kardon, *Tissues and Organs: A Text-Atlas of Scanning Electron Microscopy*, W.H. Freeman, New York, 1979, with permission)

to the primary branches and are annular in orientation with respect to the fenestrated capillary (Figs. 21.14–21.17). Smaller divisions, called *pedicels*, branch at right angles to the secondary branches. As a result, the glomerular capillary is covered with a multitude of finger-shaped *pedicels* that interdigitate like the fingers of two hands. That is, a pedicel always interdigitates with one from another podocyte, never with the same podocyte (Fig. 21.12). The narrow slits (20–30 nm) between adjacent pedicels are called *filtration slits* (Figs. 21.12, 21.13). The filtration slits are spanned by a *filtration slit diaphragm* that consists of a lattice with openings measuring approximately *6 by 14 nm.* The functional role of the filtration slit diaphragm is unclear.

GLOMERULAR CAPILLARIES

At the renal corpuscle, the afferent arteriole breaks down into a tuft of anastomosing capillaries called the *glomerulus.* The five to seven glomerular branches have an endothelium that is fenestrated; that is, it is pierced

ly 50- to 100-nm-diameter pores (Figs. 21.13–21.17). Unlike most fenestrated capillaries, these have no occluding diaphragms; they are completely open, and this feature facilitates formation of ultrafiltrate (Fig. 21.13). The fenestrated endothelium retains primarily platelets and blood cells. Since the glomerular capillaries are interposed between two arterioles, there is little pressure drop compared to those capillaries drained by veins. This arrangement is suited for the production of abundant quantities of glomerular filtrate.

GLOMERULAR BASEMENT MEMBRANE

A relatively thick, highly differentiated basement membrane is located between the glomerular capillaries and the overlying podocytes (Figs. 21.11, 21.18, 21.19). It acts as a molecular sieve, permitting the passage of only small molecules. The glomerular basement membrane (which lacks a fibroreticularis layer) is the main filtration barrier. It represents the fused basal laminae of an

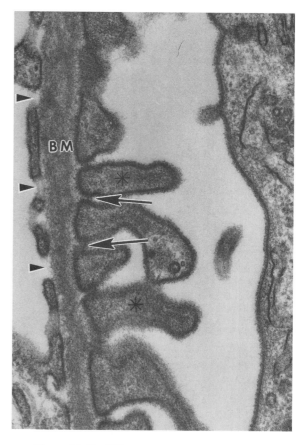

Figure 21.13. TEM of pedicels (*) with filtration slit diaphragms (arrows) between adjacent pedicels; fenestrated (arrowheads), glomerular capillary endothelium, and basement membrane (BM) are shown. ×48,825. (From R. Kessel and R. Kardon, *Tissues and Organs: A Text-Atlas of Scanning Electron Microscopy*, W.H. Freeman, New York, 1979, with permission)

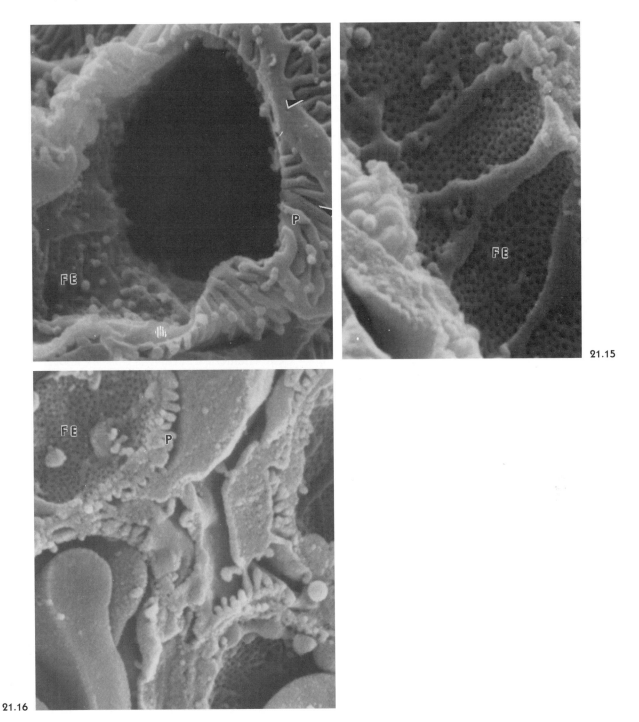

Figures 21.14–21.16. SEMs of the glomerular capillary. Podocyte pedicels (P), filtration slits (arrowheads), and fenestrated endothelium (FE) are identified. Figure 21.14, ×16,900; Figure 21.15, ×22,750; Figure 21.16, ×16,250.

(From R. Kessel and R. Kardon, *Tissues and Organs: A Text-Atlas of Scanning Electron Microscopy*, W.H. Freeman, New York, 1979, with permission)

epithelium (podocytes) and an endothelium (glomerulus). With TEM, the basement membrane has three layers (Fig. 21.20). The layer adjacent to the endothelium is called the *lamina lucida (rara) interna*. The middle layer is the thickest and is called the *lamina densa*. A third layer, called the *lamina lucida (rara) externa*, is lo-

cated adjacent to the glomerular epithelium (pedicels of the podocytes).

The glomerular basement membrane is approximately 0.1 nm wide or thick, and contains *type IV collagen* and a *GAG* that is rich in *heparan sulfate*. Evidence indicates that new glomerular basal lamina material is

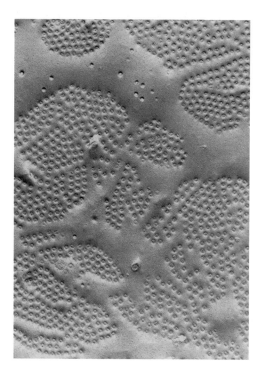

Figure 21.17. Freeze fracture replica of glomerular capillary endothelium showing en face views of the fenestrations. ×15,500. (From R. Roberts, R. Kessel and H. Tung. *Freeze Fracture Images of Cells and Tissues.* Oxford University Press, New York, 1991, with permission)

continually added by glomerular *epithelial cells* (*podocytes*). *Mesangial cells* appear to dispose of old basement membrane material or that which has become clogged with protein and other substances. With the use of tracer studies, it has been determined that the basement membrane acts as a barrier to substances more than about *69 kD* in size. Useful substances of lower molecular weight that escape the basement membrane are reabsorbed by the proximal convoluted tubule cells. Also, substances with a high net negative charge (polyanionic molecules) do not normally transverse the basement membrane. The half-life of the basement membrane is about 6 months. The heparan sulfate proteoglycan appears to be chiefly responsible for preventing proteins such as plasma albumin from traversing the basement membrane and entering the urinary filtrate because enzymatic removal of the heparan sulfate proteoglycan from the basement membrane causes a marked increase in its permeability to negatively charged substances. Thus, the basement membrane acts as a physical filter, primarily due to the type IV collagen in the lamina densa. Heparan sulfate has been localized in the laminae lucidae (laminae rarae), and this polyanionic molecule provides a charge barrier in the basement membrane.

There are two types of mesangial cells. The first type is located in the glomerulus. These *intraglomerular*

mesangial cells have long processes that intercalate among the podocyte pedicels and end in close proximity to the basement membrane (Figs. 21.18, 21.19). The mesangial cell is a specialized pericyte that has characteristics of a smooth muscle cell. The mesangial cell contracts or relaxes in response to a number of vasoactive agents; thus, this cell can locally modify glomerular filtration. Mesangial cells reportedly contract when stimulated by angiotensin to decrease capillary blood flow. Mesangial cells also produce vasoactive agents including renin, prostaglandin, and platelet-activating factor. In addition, mesangial cells play a role in basement membrane remodeling in the glomerulus, and the cells can produce IL-1. There is evidence that the intraglomerular mesangial cells are phagocytic, and act as a macrophage to *phagocytose* larger protein molecules that might pass through the fenestrated endothelium and become lodged in the glomerular basement membrane. The second type of mesangial cells, called *extraglomerular mesangial cells*, are located between the macula densa and the afferent and efferent arterioles (Fig. 21.18). The extraglomerular mesangial cells are known as *lacis cells* and may be continuous with the intraglomerular mesangial cells. Gap junctions are prevalent between lacis cells and between lacis cells and juxtaglomerular (JG) cells.

JUXTAGLOMERULAR APPARATUS

Juxtaglomerular (JG) cells are modified smooth muscle cells in the tunica media of the afferent arteriole close to the renal corpuscle (Fig. 21.18). Acidophilic-staining granules that contain *renin* and *erythropoietin* are present in the JG cells (Plate 56C,D). Erythropoietin is a hormone that stimulates maturation of red blood cells in the bone marrow in response to reduced oxygen tension. Renin, an aspartyl peptidase enzyme, plays an important role in water conservation and regulation of blood pressure.

The JG cells are located close to the macula densa of the distal convoluted tubule. In the macula densa region, the tubule cells are much taller and narrower than the remaining cells. Therefore, the nuclei are much closer together in these cells than in the remainder of the distal convoluted tubule wall. In addition, the Golgi apparatus is located basally in the macula densa cells. Evidence suggests that the composition of the tubule fluid in the region of the macula densa influences renin release. The cells of the macula densa appear to be sensitive to changes in NaCl concentration. When the NaCl concentration or blood pressure falls, renin is released from JG cells. There is also a cluster of cells close to the vascular pole of the renal corpuscle between the afferent and efferent arterioles. These cells are variously called the *polkissen, lacis cells,* or *extraglomerular mesangial cells.* The macula densa, JG cells, and polkissen comprise the *juxtaglomerular apparatus.* Intraglomerular mesangial

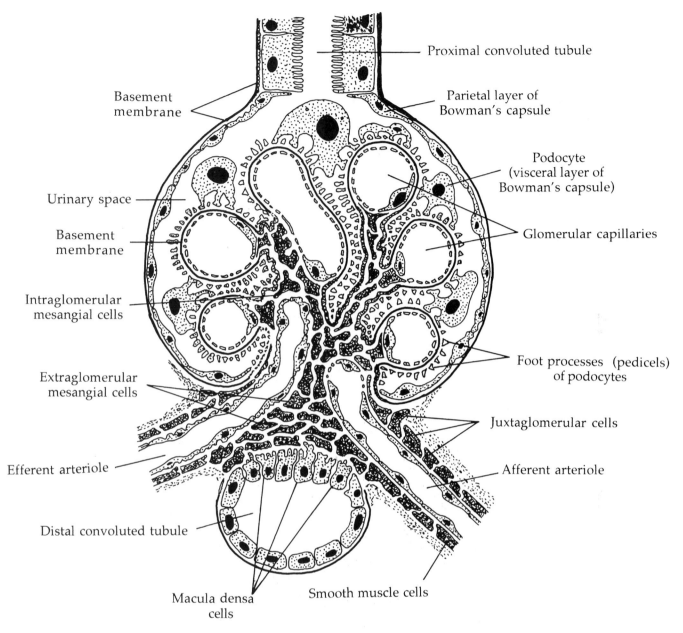

Figure 21.18. Diagram of the renal corpuscle and its relationship to the proximal convoluted tubule and renal pole and the afferent and efferent arterioles at the vascular pole. The positions of the macula densa and, intraglomerular and extraglomerular mesangial cells are also denoted. (Re-printed from Nephrology: Proceedings of the Tenth Intern. Congress of Nephrology, W. Kriz and T. Sakai. Morphological aspects of glomerular function. 1987. By permission of publisher Bailliere Tindall, London, with permission)

cells are located within the renal corpuscle and were described previously.

PROXIMAL CONVOLUTED TUBULE

The proximal convoluted tubule is the widest segment of the nephron and stains acidophilic (Plate 56A,B). The cells have a well-developed brush border (microvilli) that is quite susceptible to postmortem degenerative changes. The cuboidal or columnar cells have extensive lateral and basal interdigitations and many basal plasma membrane infoldings (Figs. 21.22–21.25). Long *mitochondria* with a basal-apical orientation are located between the plasma membrane infoldings. The cells contain lysosomes and digestive vacuoles and may contain many spherical or tubular pinocytotic vesicles at the base of the microvilli. Peroxisomes and a prominent Golgi apparatus are also located in the cells.

The proximal convoluted tubule is responsible for

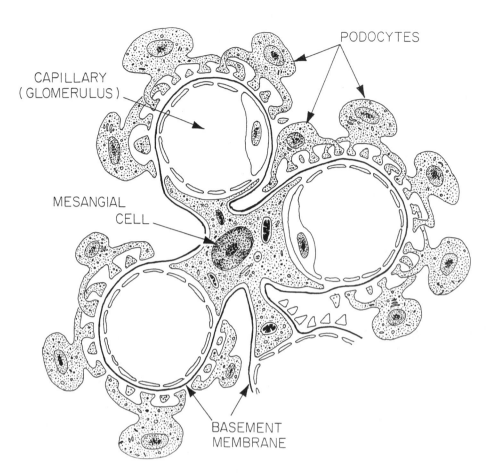

CAPILLARY
(GLOMERULUS)

PODOCYTES

MESANGIAL
CELL

BASEMENT
MEMBRANE

Figure 21.19. Diagram of the relationships of the renal glomerular capillary, podocyte, mesangial cells, and basement membrane.

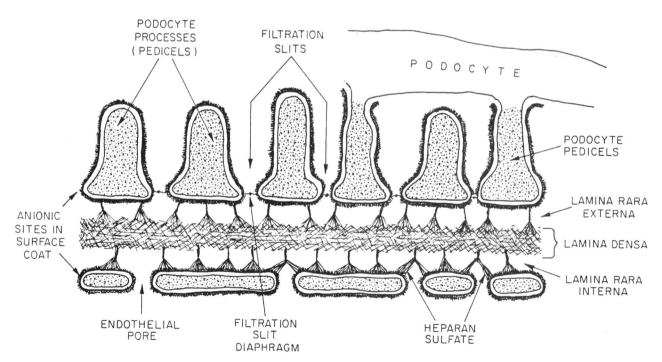

PODOCYTE
PROCESSES
(PEDICELS)

FILTRATION
SLITS

PODOCYTE

PODOCYTE
PEDICELS

ANIONIC
SITES IN
SURFACE
COAT

LAMINA RARA
EXTERNA

LAMINA DENSA

LAMINA RARA
INTERNA

ENDOTHELIAL
PORE

FILTRATION
SLIT
DIAPHRAGM

HEPARAN
SULFATE

Figure 21.20. The filter in the renal corpuscle consists of podocyte pedicels and filtration slit diaphragms. The basement membrane and the fenestrated endothelium and their relationships are illustrated. (Redrawn from M. Farquhar, 1979. *J. Cell Biol.* 81, 137 by copyright permission of Rockefeller Univ. Press)

464

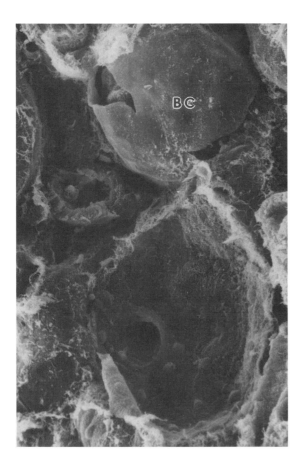

Figure 21.21. SEM of the parietal layer of Bowman's capsule from the outside (BC) and from the inside (lower part of the figure). ×615. (From R. Kessel and R. Kardon, *Tissues and Organs: A Text-Atlas of Scanning Electron Microscopy*, W.H. Freeman, New York, 1979, with permission)

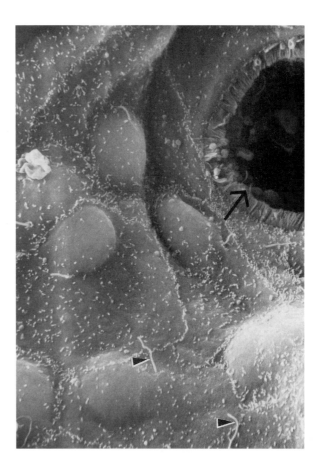

Figure 21.22. SEM of the inner surface of the parietal layer of Bowman's capsule at the urinary pole; entrance to the proximal convoluted tubule (arrow). The bulge in the cells is due to the inner location of the nucleus; note the cilia (arrowheads) extending from each cell. ×925. (From R. Kessel and R. Kardon, *Tissues and Organs: A Text-Atlas of Scanning Electron Microscopy*, W.H. Freeman, New York, 1979, with permission)

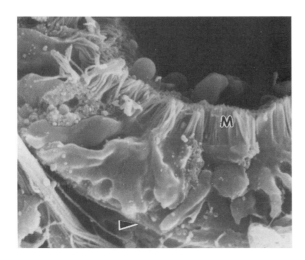

Figure 21.23. SEM of cells in the proximal convoluted tubule. Microvilli (M) and basement membrane (arrowhead) are identified. ×4860. (From R. Kessel and R. Kardon, *Tissues and Organs: A Text-Atlas of Scanning Electron Microscopy*, W.H. Freeman, New York, 1979, with permission)

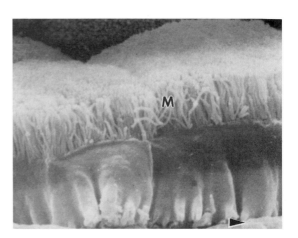

Figure 21.24. Kidney tubule cells with microvilli (M), and basement membrane (arrowhead). (From R. Kessel and R. Kardon, *Tissues and Organs: A Text-Atlas of Scanning Electron Microscopy*, W.H. Freeman, New York, 1979, with permission)

465

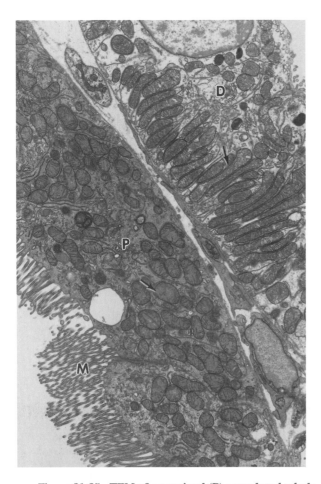

Figure 21.25. TEM of a proximal (P) convoluted tubule with extensive microvilli (M) and a distal (D) convoluted tubule with few microvilli, but with basal plasma membrane infoldings and numerous mitochondria (arrows). ×5135. (From R. Kessel and R. Kardon, *Tissues and Organs: A Text-Atlas of Scanning Electron Microscopy,* **W.H. Freeman, New York, 1979, with permission)**

convoluted tubule reabsorbs sodium and chloride at the same rate as water, the filtrate that enters the loop of Henle has the same osmotic pressure as that which entered the proximal convoluted tubule from the urinary space. Those substances resorbed from the proximal convoluted tubules enter the peritublar capillaries. A number of organic acids and bases are actively secreted into the lumen of the proximal convoluted tubule. The proximal convoluted tubule cells reabsorb bicarbonate ions. A small amount of plasma protein in the filtrate is taken into the cells by micropinocytosis and degraded within lysosomes to amino acids, which enter the bloodstream. Certain dyes, drugs, and penicillin are secreted into the proximal convoluted tubule lumen. When transverse sections of proximal and distal convoluted tubules are compared, the proximal convoluted tubules are found to be wider (larger), have a more pronounced brush border, are more acidophilic in staining, and have a smaller lumen than that of the distal convoluted tubule.

LOOP OF HENLE

The thick descending limb (also called the *pars recta of the proximal convoluted tubule*) of the loop of Henle contains cells organized much like those in the proximal convoluted tubule, but the cells are more cuboidal and the brush border is less well developed (Figs. 21.25, 21.27). The functions of the thick descending limb are greatly reduced, and this region is permeable to diffusion of water and ions in either direction. In those regions of the kidney interstitium with a high osmolality (osmotic concentration), both Na^+ and Cl^- ions enter the tubule from the interstitium (Figs. 21.31, 21.32).

The thin segment (thin descending, thin ascending) is variable in length (Plate 57A,B). The cells are squamous and offer little resistance to the passive flow of ions and water in either direction (Fig. 21.26).

The thick ascending segment (limb) of the loop of Henle (or *pars recta of the distal convoluted tubule*) actively pumps ions from the lumen fluid through the cells to the interstitium (Plate 57A,B). The cells have basal and lateral infoldings of the plasma membrane, as well as numerous mitochondria that provide energy for active transport. There is a strong Cl^- pump in these cells that moves chloride ions from the lumen to the interstitium surrounding the cells (Fig. 21.31). Sodium ions also may be pumped or follow into the interstitium. Water does not move from the filtrate to the interstitium because the cells are impermeable to water. Because of the strong pumps and different positions of ascending thick limbs in the kidney, a gradient of osmotic pressure is created in the kidney interstitium (i.e., the region surrounding the tubules) (Fig. 21.32). In humans, the osmotic pressure in the outer cortex is approximately *300 mOsm*, while that of the inner medulla is about *1400 mOsm*.

the reabsorption of approximately *seven-eighths (80%)* of all the proteins, amino acids, glucose, water, and most ions and electrolytes (sodium, chloride, calcium, phosphates) from the tubular filtrate. There is an active transport of Na^+ ions through the base of the cells into the interstitium; these ions then enter the peritubular capillaries. The many mitochondria operate an *Mg^{2+}-dependent Na^+, K^+ activated ATPase pump* located in the basal part of the cell membrane. Chloride ions passively follow the actively transported Na^+ ions. By the active transport of Na^+ ions from the glomerular filtrate into the peritubular capillaries, an electrochemical gradient is created that allows Cl^- ions to follow the sodium ions by passive transport in all regions of the tubule except the thick ascending limb of Henle's loop. The accumulation of ions outside the base of the cell causes water to move passively out of the tubule lumen; this water is called *obligatory water*. Because the proximal

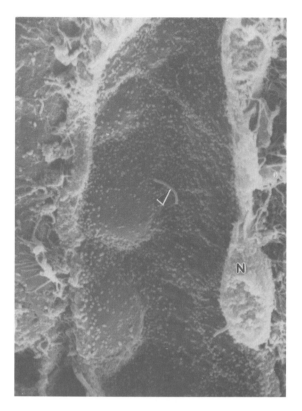

Figure 21.26. SEM of a longitudinal section of a thin loop of Henle. The nucleus (N) and a single cilium (arrowhead) of these simple squamous cells are denoted. ×3900. (From R. Kessel and R. Kardon, *Tissues and Organs: A Text-Atlas of Scanning Electron Microscopy*, W.H. Freeman, New York, 1979, with permission)

DISTAL CONVOLUTED TUBULE

The cuboidal cells of the distal convoluted tubule are shorter than those of the proximal convoluted tubule and do not have a prominent brush (microvillous) border (Plate 56A,B). The basal plasma membrane of the cells is infolded, and these infoldings interdigitate with those of neighboring cells. Mitochondria are numerous and concentrated in the base of the cells. Sodium ions are actively transported from the tubular filtrate into the interstitium. NH_3^+ ions are secreted into the lumen in this region. In the lumen, ammonia ions combine with H^+ ions to form *urea*.

In the region of the macula densa, the cells in the distal tubule have a reversed polarity. That is, the Golgi apparatus is located between the nucleus and the basal portion of the cell. In this region, only a thin basement membrane separates the macula densa cells from the nearby JG cells of the afferent arteriole. The macula densa is thought to be sensitive to the sodium concentration in the distal tubule fluid. The cells of the macula densa thus represent sodium receptors.

DISTAL PORTION OF THE DISTAL CONVOLUTED TUBULE AND CORTICAL COLLECTING DUCT SYSTEM

The distal portion of the distal convoluted tubule and the cortical collecting ducts (Figs. 21.28, 21.29) have similarities in structure and function. Both segments reabsorb sodium ions (controlled primarily by aldosterone) (Fig. 21.33). With the transport of sodium out of the tubular lumen, potassium ions are transported into the tubular lumen. The potassium ions are actively secreted by the distal tubule and cortical collecting ducts and play an important regulatory role, controlling the K^+ ion concentration in the extracellular fluids of the body. The dark cells (sometimes referred to as *brown cells*) appear to be involved in the active secretion of H^+ ions against a strong concentration gradient (Fig. 21.30). These cells are thus important in producing acidification of the urine. The extremely distal portion of the distal convoluted tubule and the cortical collecting duct system are also permeable to water in the presence of antidiuretic hormone, but these cells are impermeable to water in the absence of antidiuretic hormone.

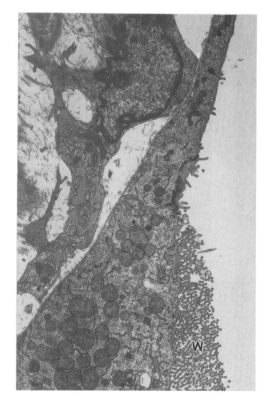

Figure 21.27. TEM of the junction between a thin limb of loop of Henle and a thick ascending portion, which acquires microvilli (M) and numerous mitochondria. ×5425.

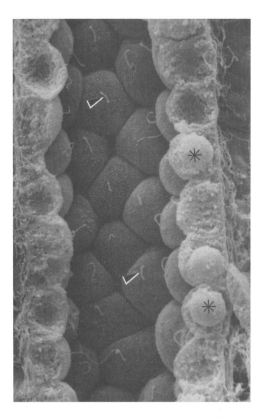

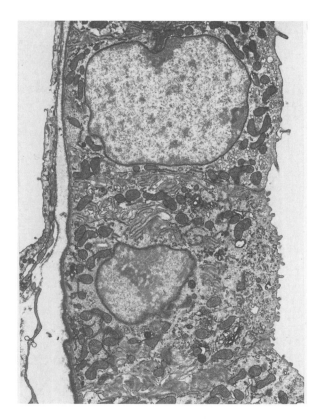

Figure 21.28. SEM of a section through a collecting duct. Note that the apical surface of each duct cell has a single cilium (arrowheads). Cells have been cut open so that the nucleus (*) is exposed in some cells. ×730.

Figure 21.29. TEM of a collecting tubule. Plasma membrane infoldings and mitochondria are present in the basal region of the cells. ×5000 (From R. Kessel and R. Kardon, *Tissues and Organs: A Text-Atlas of Scanning Electron Microscopy*, W.H. Freeman, New York, 1979, with permission)

COLLECTING DUCTS

The collecting ducts vary somewhat in size, and the shape of the cell can vary from cuboidal to columnar (Plate 57C). Two cell types have been described as making up the wall of the collecting tubule. On the basis of TEM observations, they have been described as light and dark cells. By SEM, the luminal surface of the more numerous light cell is characterized by the presence of one or two central cilia. The apical surface of the dark cell, in contrast, contains microfolds and broader projections (Fig. 21.30). The number of dark cells increases during respiratory acidosis, which suggests that these cells, in conjunction with cells in the distal convoluted tubule, may play a role in acid-base balance.

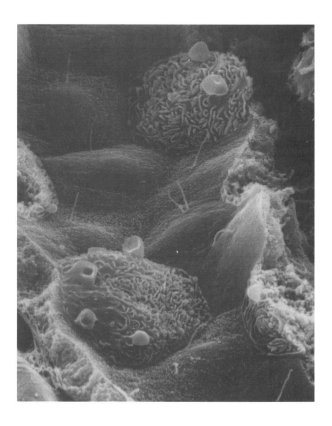

Figure 21.30. SEM of a collecting tubule. Light cells contain one or two cilia, while dark cells possess folds (microplicae). Dark cells may play a role in acid-base balance. ×3055. (From R. Kessel and R. Kardon, *Tissues and Organs: A Text-Atlas of Scanning Electron Microscopy*, W.H. Freeman, New York, 1979, with permission)

A number of *collecting tubules* may join to form several large, straight collecting ducts called *papillary ducts* or *ducts of Bellini*. They empty into the renal calyx through several apertures in a region that comprises the *area cribrosa* of the kidney papilla.

The permeability of the collecting duct cells to water is affected by the *antidiuretic hormone* (ADH) (vasopressin), which is released from the posterior lobe of the pituitary gland. When blood levels of ADH are high, the permeability of the collecting duct cells to water is increased (Fig. 21.33). As a result, the hypertonic interstitium causes more water to move from the tubule lumen to the capillaries in the interstitium, resulting in a more concentrated urine. When the osmolarity (salt concentration or tonicity) of the blood is abnormally elevated, the posterior lobe releases ADH (Fig. 21.33). The additional water resorbed from the tubules causes a lowering of the blood osmolarity. Under certain conditions, ADH is not produced. This results in *diabetes insipidus*, in which large amounts of dilute urine are produced.

The collecting ducts thus provide the last place in the tubule for water conservation. This is important because the extent of water conservation is under physiologic control, being regulated by ADH according to the varying needs of the body.

WATER CONSERVATION

Water conservation is an important homeostatic mechanism, especially for land-dwelling animals, who have to cope with the constant problem of dessication. It should be emphasized that nearly 80% of the water filtered into the nephron at Bowman's capsule by glomerular filtration is reabsorbed in the proximal convoluted tubule by a mechanism that involves active transport of sodium chloride with water following from the filtrate by passive diffusion (Fig. 21.31). Water conservation in the remainder of the tubule (i.e., the loop of Henle's countercurrent multiplier effect) is a way of concentrating urine and conserving the last remaining water by means that can be regulated.

The loop of Henle creates an environment for retention of water by producing a hypertonic urine and conserving body water. The loop of Henle creates a gradient of increasing hypertonicity or concentration that is lowest in the cortex and highest in the inner medulla.

Figure 21.30 Major Transport Events in the Uriniferous Tubule

Nephron Segment	Interstitium to Lumen	Lumen to Cell or Interstitium
Proximal convoluted tubule	Organic acids, bases Dyes, drugs, penicillin	Active transport (Na^+, Mg^{2+}-dependent Na^+,K^+-activated ATPase)
		Obligatory water
		~75% glucose, amino acids resorbed
		Small proteins (micropinocytosis)— degraded by lysosomes
		Reabsorb HCO_3^- ions
		Reabsorb Ca^{2+}, PO_4^{3-}
Thick descending limb (loop of Henle) (freely permeable to diffusion of water and ions)	Na^+ and Cl^- ions enter when osmolality in intersitium is high	
Thick ascending limb (loop of Henle)		Strong Cl^- pump moves Cl^- ions to interstitium; Na^+ follows
		Impermeable to water
Distal convoluted tubule	Active secretion of H^+ ions	Sodium actively pumped to interstitium
	$NH_3^+ + H^+ \rightarrow NH_4$ (urea)	Distal portion permeable to water in presence of ADH
	Active K^+ ion transport	
	Reabsorbs Na^+ (aldosterone)	
Collecting tubules	Active secretion of H^+ ions	Reabsorbs water osmotically (ADH increases permeability of cells to water)
	Active K^+ ion transport	
	Reabsorbs Na^+ (aldosterone)	

This hypertonic interstitium concentrates the urine as it flows through the collecting ducts that pass through the hyperosomotic kidney medulla. Sodium and chloride can enter the descending thick limb from the interstitium and are thereby available to pass once again into the thick ascending limb, to be repumped into the interstitium, thereby concentrating the interstitium and increasing the osmolarity of this region, as achieved by the countercurrent multiplier mechanism. The loop of Henle thus establishes a hyperosmotic interstitium that is a concentrated region surrounding the tubules. Because of this hyperosmotic medulla, water is reabsorbed into the collecting tubules as they pass through the medulla. Because of the osmotic pressure, the water from the tubule lumen passes into the capillaries in the medullary interstitium and is conserved.

The thin ascending limb, the thick ascending limb, and the initial part of the distal convoluted tubule are impermeable to water. The thick ascending limb actively transports chloride ions to the interstitium; there is a also a passive reabsorption of sodium ions into the interstitium (Fig. 21.31). This causes the tubule fluid in this location to be diluted but concentrates the interstitium, making it more hyperosomotic (Fig. 21.32). Water is reabsorbed down its osmotic gradient in the distal portion of the distal convoluted tubule, as well as in the collecting tubule and ducts.

Water and some urea are reabsorbed from the collecting duct in the inner medulla region (Fig. 21.31), and some of the urea reenters the loop of Henle. Urea recycling tends to cause the urea to accumulate in the medullary interstitium, where it plays a role in extract-

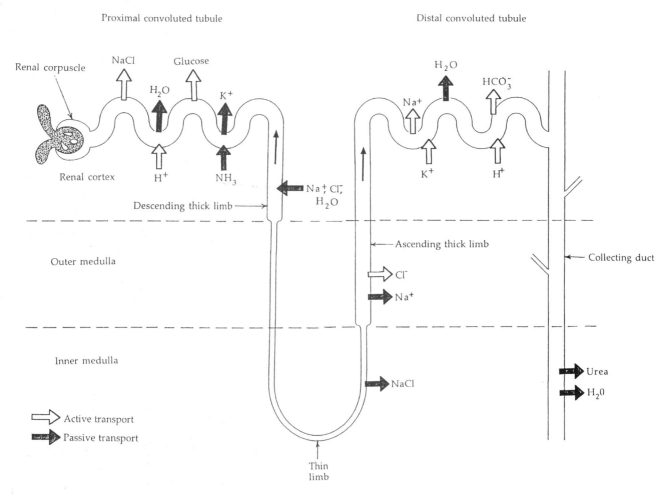

Figure 21.31. The diagram summarizes the major transport events in the uriniferous tubule. The direction of movement is indicated by the arrows from the tubule to the interstitium (and blood vessels) or from the interstitium to the tubule. Active and passive transport are denoted by the open and solid arrows. The descending limb (of Henle) is freely permeable to water, Na^+, and Cl^- ions, and these pass into the tubule lumen from the outside (interstitium). The ascending limb actively pumps Cl^- ions from the tubule lu-men to the interstitium (outside); Na^+ ions follow the Cl^- ions to maintain ionic neutrality. The ascending limb is impermeable to water, so it remains in the tubule lumen. Na^+ and Cl^- ions in the interstitium can reenter the descending limb and circulate to the ascending limb once again, to be pumped into the interstitium. This produces a multiplier effect and leads to increasing hypertonicity (saltiness) of the interstitium compared to the fluid in the tubule lumen.

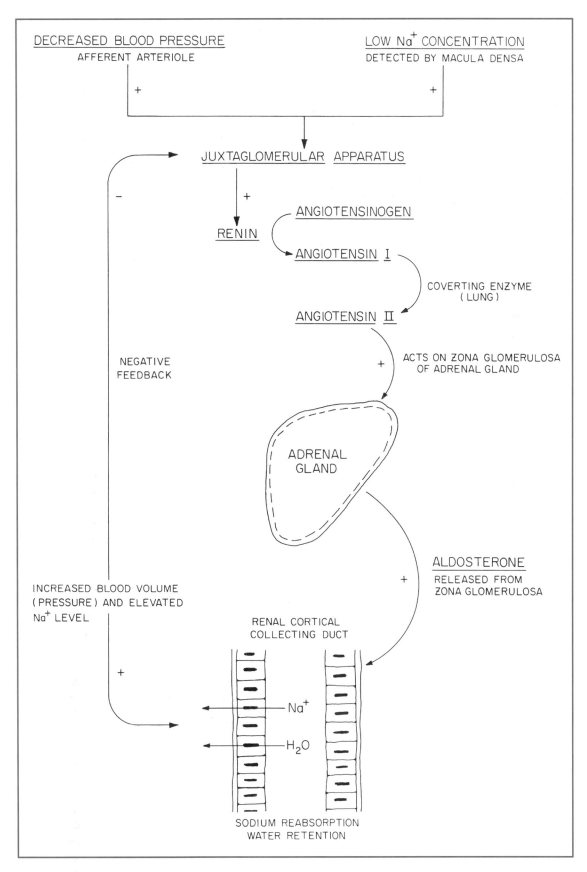

Figure 21.32. The diagram summarizes the events leading to the release of aldosterone from the adrenal cortex and its effect on uptake of sodium and water from the renal collecting ducts. See text for additional description.

ing water from the descending limb so as to concentrate sodium chloride in the descending limb.

Since nephrons in different regions of the cortex have tubules in different parts of the medulla, they can produce different concentrations of urine. Cortical nephrons produce a more dilute urine, while juxtamedullary nephrons produce a more concentrated urine. Sympathetic nerve stimulation causes contraction of sphincters in the afferent arterioles by shunting blood to predominantly juxtamedullary or cortical nephrons. The major transport events in the uriniferous tubule are summarized in the accompanying table.

RENIN FUNCTION

In response to a decreased rate of blood flow in the kidney, as in cases of severe blood loss, or a lowered sodium or chloride concentration in the blood (sodium depletion), or a decrease in extracellular fluid volume (dehydration), renin is released from the JG cells. Renin causes increased blood pressure as well as sodium and water retention by the distal nephron, but it does this in an indirect way. *Renin* acts on a substance (globulin) in the blood plasma called *angiotensinogen*, causing it to be converted to an inactive decapeptide called *angiotensin I* (Fig. 21.32). Angiotensin I loses two amino acids and is converted to *angiotensin II*, an octapeptide, by a *converting enzyme* called *peptidyl dipeptidase* that is produced by *endothelial cells*, especially those in the lung. *Angiotensin II* is a *potent vasoconstrictor* of arterioles, and this elevates blood pressure. In addition, angiotensin II acts on cells in the *zona glomerulosa of the adrenal cortex*, causing the cells to release *aldosterone* (Fig. 21.32). Aldosterone stimulates the distal nephron to reabsorb more sodium and chloride ions in exchange for hydrogen or potassium ions. This causes an increase in fluid volume in the circulatory system, thus raising the blood pressure. *JG cells* respond by sensing the degree of stretching in the afferent arteriole. The JG cells can also participate in the regulation of the Cl^- concentration in the filtrate reaching the distal convoluted tubule. Chloride ions fall in concentration when there is a decrease in blood pressure.

Although much of the urinary filtrate is reabsorbed in the proximal convoluted tubule, far too much water would be lost were it not for the loop of Henle. The loop of Henle acts as a *countercurrent multiplier*, increasing the tonicity or osmotic pressure of the renal interstitium. Further, there are two countercurrent exchangers represented by the descending and ascending vasae rectae, as well as the large collecting ducts that pass through the medulla. The thick ascending segment of the loop of Henle concentrates the interstitium by pumping chloride ions from the lumen to the interstitium; sodium is transported as well. However, the cells in this region are impermeable to water, which remains

in the tubule lumen. The chloride and sodium ions can move into the thick descending limb, with water following, to be recirculated to the thick ascending limb, where it can once again be pumped into the interstitium. This is sometimes referred to as the *hairpin countercurrent osmotic multiplier*, and is the mechanism for producing a hypertonic interstitium through which the collecting ducts and tubules pass. As a result of their permeability, the water is removed by osmosis from the collecting ducts and enters the capillaries in the interstitium.

The straight vessels or vasae rectae in the medulla do not alter the osmolality of the interstitium or the functioning of the loops of Henle. The arterial and venous divisions of the vasae rectae run together through the medulla. As the arterial divisions of the vasae rectae extend to the inner medulla, they gain sodium and lose water since the interstitium becomes more and more hyperosmotic. However, the venous division loses sodium and gains water as these vessels pass back to the inner medulla, where the interstitium is less hypertonic. Thus, water lost from the descending vessel is gained by the ascending vessel, while the sodium that enters the descending vessel leaves the ascending one. While the countercurrent flow does not alter the osmolarity, it does permit some recirculation of water and ions in the renal medullary interstitium.

ACID-BASE BALANCE

Kidneys play an important role in maintaining the acid-base balance of the blood. The blood is maintained at a pH of approximately 7.4 by a buffering system that involves carbonic acid (H_2CO_3) and bicarbonate ions (HCO_3^-). If the blood becomes more acid (less alkaline), carbonic acid dissociates to hydrogen and bicarbonate ions.

$$H_2CO_3 \xrightleftharpoons[\text{basic}]{\text{acidic}} H^+ + HCO_3^-$$

If the blood becomes less acid (more alkaline), the bicarbonate ions combine with the H^+ ions to produce H_2CO_3. The secretion of H^+ and NH_3 and the reabsorption of Na^+ and HCO_3^- are adjusted to maintain the pH within a normal range. If blood is acidic, H^+ is excreted along with ammonia, while Na^+ and HCO_3^- are reabsorbed (Fig. 21.33). If blood is basic, fewer H^+ ions are excreted and fewer Na^+ and HCO_3^- ions are reabsorbed (Fig. 21.33).

URETER, URINARY BLADDER, URETHRA

Urine is released into the major calyces, from which it travels to the renal pelvis, ureter, urinary bladder, and

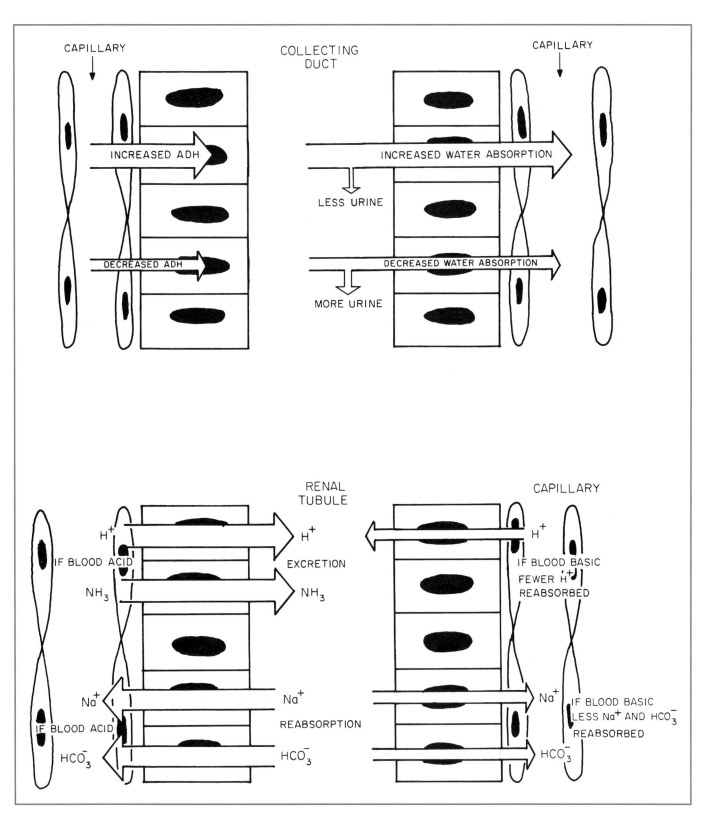

Figure 21.33. Upper portion of the drawing illustrates the effects of increased or decreased ADH release on increased or decreased water absorption form the renal collecting ducts. In the lower figure, when blood is acid, NH_3^+ and H^+ are excreted into the renal tubule, but if blood is basic, fewer H^+ ions are reabsorbed. If blood is acid, Na^+ and NCO_3^- are reabsorbed into the blood. If blood is basic, fewer of these ions are reabsorbed.

urethra. Transitional epithelium lines the lumen of the major calyces, renal pelvis, ureters, and urinary bladder. Transitional epithelium is unique to the urinary system and is designed for stretch. The ureter and urinary bladder have a mucosa consisting of transitional epithelium and loose connective tissue lamina propria. The superficial cells may be large and rounded when empty or flattened when the epithelium is stretched (Fig. 21.34).

Large polyploid nuclei or binucleate cells may be present. The exposed plasma membrane of the most superficial layer of epithelial cells is somewhat thicker and serves as an *osmotic barrier* between the urine and the tissue fluid and blood vessels in the lamina propria. Between the thickened plasma membrane plaques are thinner but much shorter regions of plasma membrane that appear to represent "hinges" permitting the plasma

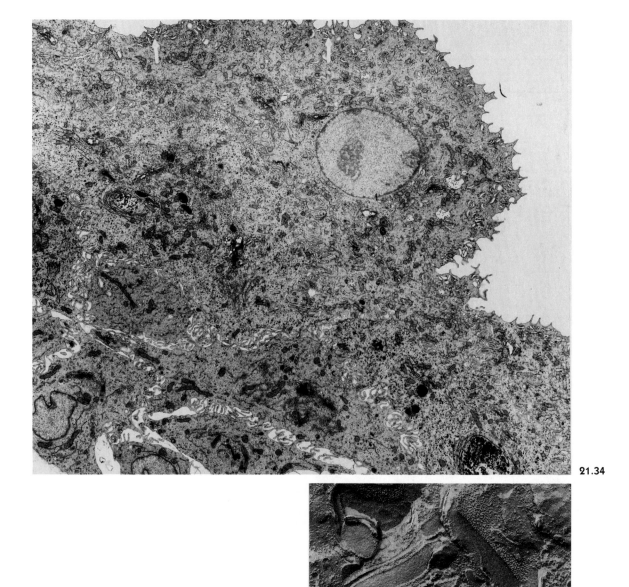

21.34

21.35

Figures 21.34, 21.35. TEM of urinary bladder epithelium. Apical ends of the cells contain variable numbers of discoid vesicles (arrows), which are enlarged in Figure 21.35. Discoid vesicles are believed to represent additional plasma membrane when cells expand due to filling of the bladder.

Figure 21.34, ×705 ; Figure 21.35, ×1670. (From R. Kessel and R. Kardon, *Tissues and Organs: A Text-Atlas of Scanning Electron Microscopy*, W.H. Freeman, New York, 1979, with permission)

membrane to fold when the bladder is empty. The excess plasma membrane appears as discoid vesicles in the apical cytoplasm of these epithelial cells when examined with the EM (Figs. 21.34–21.37). As the bladder expands from within, the discoid vesicles unfold and become incorporated once again into the superficial plasma membrane.

The muscularis externa of the ureter usually consists of two layers of smooth muscle. The *inner* layer is predominantly longitudinal in orientation, while the outer layer is largely circular. In the lower portion of the ureters, an additional outer layer of smooth muscle, predominantly longitudinal in orientation, appears. The urinary bladder has a thick muscularis externa layer containing smooth muscle with varied orientations. The upper part of the urinary bladder is covered with serosa (peritoneum), but the remainder of the urinary bladder and the ureters are covered externally by an adventitia layer.

The male urethra has several regions. The *prostatic urethra* passes through the prostate gland upon leaving the bladder and is lined with transitional epithelium. The prostatic urethra is continuous with a very short (approximately 1 cm), *membranous urethra* that is lined by stratified or pseudostratified columnar epithelium.

An *external sphincter* of *striated muscle* surrounds this portion of the urethra. Both the bulbous and pendulous components of the urethra extend through the *corpus spongiosum* of the penis. The epithelium in these regions may be pseudostratified columnar or stratified columnar. Mucus-secreting *glands* of *Littré* are located throughout the male urethra but are particularly numerous in the penile urethra. The glands may be present within the stratified epithelium or in the connective tissue and are connected by means of ducts to the urethral lumen.

The female urethra is tubular and only 4–5 cm long. It is lined by stratified squamous epithelium, although pseudostratified columnar epithelium may also be present. An external striated (voluntary) *muscle* is located in the wall of the female urethra about midway along its length.

MEDICAL CONSIDERATIONS

Acute renal failure involves a sudden loss of kidney function because of a deficiency of blood flowing through the kidneys, which can be the result of dehydration, shock, toxins, obstruction, or cardiovascular or renal disease. *Acute poststreptococcal glomerulonephritis* is an im-

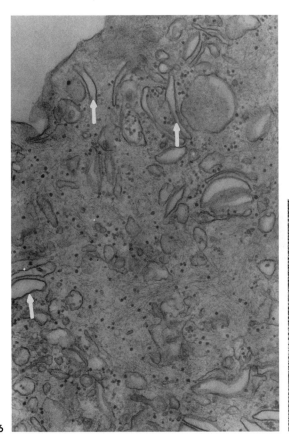

21.36

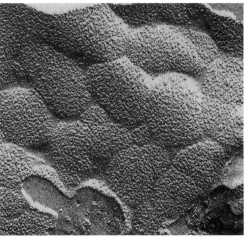

21.37

Figures 21.36, 21.37. **Freeze fracture images of the discoid vesicles in section and surface views (Fig. 21.37). Figure 21.36, ×38,595; Figure 21.37, ×40,000.**

munologic reaction in which antigen-antibody complexes trapped in the glomerulus cause inflammation and glomerular dysfunction and may follow a streptococcal infection in other regions. *Hydronephrosis* refers to the accumulation of fluid in the renal pelvis caused by an obstruction such as a tumor, calculus, or stenosis. *Pyelonephritis* is an inflammation of the kidney and renal pelvis due to bacterial infection. *Cystitis* is an inflammation of the urinary bladder, usually caused by bacterial infection, that travels from the outside. It is more common in women because of the shorter urethra in women. Degeneration of glomerular function (*diabetic nephropathy*) may occur after long-term diabetes mellitus.

Some Abnormal Conditions of the Urinary System

Albuminuria	Albumin in urine
Anuria	Absence of urine production
Bacteriuria	Bacteria in urine
Dysuria	Painful urination
Enuresis	Involuntary bedwetting
Hematuria	Blood in urine
Pyuria	Pus in urine
Uremia	Waste products accumulate in blood due to loss of renal function

SELECTED BIBLIOGRAPHY

Andrews, P.M. (1989). Shape changes in kidney glomerular podocytes: mechanisms and possible functional significance. In *Cells and Tissues: A Three-Dimensional Approach by Modern Techniques in Microscopy*. Alan R. Liss, New York.

Baylis, C., and Blantz, R. (1986). Glomerular hemodynamics. *NIPS* **1**, 86–89.

Brenner, B., and Rector, F., eds. (1992). *The Kidney*, Vol. 1. W.B. Saunders, Philadelphia.

Briggs, J.P., Skott, O., and Schnermann, J. (1990). Cellular mechanisms within the juxtaglomerular apparatus. *Am. J. Hypertension* **3**, 76–80.

Bulger, R.E., and Dobyan, D.C. (1982). Recent advances in renal morphology. *Annu. Rev. Physiol.* **44**, 147–158.

Dirks, J.H., and Sutton, R.A. (1986). *Diuretics: Physiology, Pharmacology and Clinical Use*. W.B. Saunders, Philadelphia.

Ganong, W.F. (1989). Formation and excretion of urine. In *Review of Medical Physiology*, 14th ed. Appleton & Lange, Norwalk, CT.

Gibbons, G.H., Dzau, V.J., Farhi, E.R., and Barger, A.C. (1984). Interaction of signals influencing renin release. *Annu. Rev. Physiol.* **46**, 291–308.

Greger, R. (1988). Chloride transport in thick ascending limb, distal convoluted, and collecting duct. *Annu. Rev. Physiol.* **50**, 111–123.

Kriz, W., Elger, M., Lemley, K., and Sakai, T. (1990). Structure of the glomerular mesangium: a biomechanical interpretation. *Kidney Int.* **38**(suppl 30), S2.

Kriz, W., and Lever, R. (1969). Renal countercurrent mechanisms: structure and function. *Am. Heart J.* **78**, 101–118.

Lewis, S. (1986). The mammalian urinary bladder: it's more than accommodating. *NIPS* **1**, 61–64.

Maunsbach, A., Olsen, T., and Christensen, E., eds. (1981). *Functional Ultrastructure of the Kidney*. Academic Press, New York.

Quinn, S.J., and William, G.H. (1988). Regulation of aldosterone secretion. *Annu. Rev. Physiol.* **50**, 409–426.

Sasaki, S., and Marumo, F. (1989). Mechanisms of transcellular Cl^- transport in mammalian renal proximal tubules. *NIPS* **4**, 18–22.

Schlondorff, D. (1987). The glomerular mesangial cell: an expanding role for a specialized cell. *FASEB J.* **1**, 272–281.

Seldin, D.W, and Giebisch, G. (1989). *The Regulation of Acid-Base Balance*. Raven Press, New York.

Silbernagl, S. (1986). Tubular reabsorption of amino acids in the kidney. *NIPS* **1**, 167–171.

Female Reproductive System

T he female reproductive system consists of paired ovaries, paired oviducts, mammary glands, a single uterus, a vagina, and external genitalia. The ovaries, oviducts, uterus, and mammary glands undergo cyclic changes in structure and function in response to changing concentrations of hormone during the menstrual cycle between menarche and menopause. The relationships of the ovary, oviduct, uterus, and vagina are illustrated in Figure 22.1.

OVARY

The human ovary is a bean-shaped structure that is variable in size, usually ranging from 2.5 to 5.0 cm in length, 1.5 to 3.0 cm in width, and 0.6 to 1.5 cm in thickness. One edge of the ovary, the hilus, is attached by the mesovarium to the broad ligament. The ovary is illustrated in section in Figure 22.2. The ovary is both an exocrine and an endocrine gland; the *exocrine* product is the female gamete, or *oocyte*, and its cyclic release begins at puberty and continues until menopause. The ovary is also an endocrine gland since it synthesizes and secretes a number of hormones into the bloodstream; two of the more important ones are *estradiol* (estrogen) and *progesterone*. Estradiol affects various target tissues, such as the oviduct and uterus, because these cells have estradiol receptors. In addition, after stimulation by estradiol, the target tissues may produce receptors for progesterone. The hypothalamic-pituitary complex plays an important role in the regulation of the female reproductive system, especially the cyclic nature of its transformations and transitions.

The ovary consists of a central *medulla* and an outer *cortex*. The boundary between the cortex and medulla is not pronounced. The ovary is surrounded by a layer of simple cuboidal epithelium (simple squamous epithelium in older females) called the *ovarian epithelium*, although in the past it was referred to erroneously as the germinal epithelium. The cortex is typically filled with numerous *germ cells* in different stages of development. The *ovarian stroma* refers to all the connective tissue in the ovary. However, the ovarian stroma differs in different parts of the ovary. The stroma consists of many spindle-shaped fibroblasts and many fine collagen fibers. Immediately adjacent to the ovarian epithelium, the stroma consists of densely arranged connective tissue; this portion is called the *tunica albuginea*. The connective tissue fibers in this region are oriented parallel to the overlying ovarian epithelium. Collagenic and reticular fibers are abundant in the tunica albuginea, and this region has a high concentration of amorphous intercellular substances. In deeper regions of the cortex, the ovarian stroma contains relatively more cells and fewer fibers than the tunica albuginea region. Thus, the inner portion of the ovarian cortex appears to be somewhat more loosely organized than the outer portion.

The medulla contains extensively vascularized connective tissue. Because the vessels are so prominent in this region, it is sometimes called the *zona vasculosa*. The medulla contains loose connective tissue in which numerous elastic fibers are present, as well as arteries, convoluted veins, and smooth muscle.

EARLY GERM CELL FORMATION

The ovaries develop from genital (or gonadal) ridges in the embryo. The mesoderm cells of the genital ridge develop into the epithelium that surrounds the ovary. The primordial *germ cells* develop from *yolk sac endoderm*

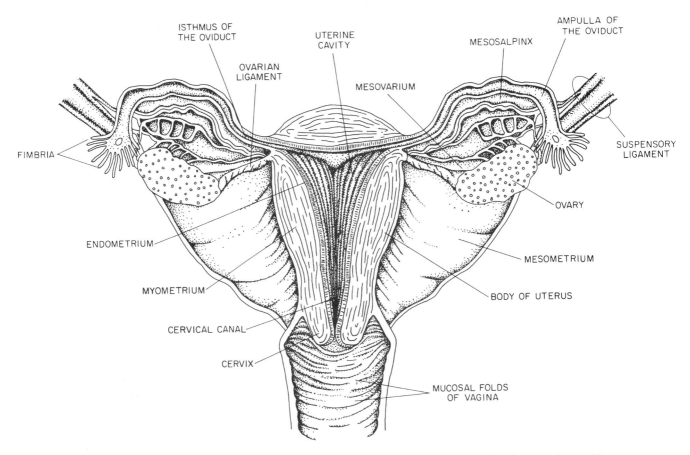

Figure 22.1. Diagram of the female reproductive system showing the relationships of paired ovaries, oviducts, uterus, and vagina.

as early as 1 month of fetal life and can divide several times as they migrate from the yolk sac into the forming genital ridges. The primordial germ cells in the female give rise to oogonia. As the germ cells migrate into the primitive gonad, they become surrounded by a single layer of squamous ovarian epithelial cells (Plate 58A); Fig. 22.3). Nests of closely packed *primordial germ cells* become concentrated in the ovarian cortex. Mitotic division of the germ cells in the ovarian cortex continues until about the fifth month of fetal development, at which time there are 1–3 million oogonia in each ovary. By the seventh month of fetal development, all of the oogonia have entered meiotic prophase and are called *primary oocytes*. However, many of the primary oocytes degenerate during this period in a process called *atresia*.

FOLLICULOGENESIS

In the adult human, only primary oocytes are present in ovarian follicles. Human primary oocytes do not complete meiosis I until ovulation. Thus, secondary oocytes are found only after ovulation. A true mature female gamete, or ovum, is not usually found in a human cycle because the second meiotic division is completed only if fertilization occurs.

The primary oocyte is contained within a follicle. During the period in which the oocyte progresses from meiotic prophase to ovulation, the follicle undergoes progressive changes to prepare it for ovulation. This sequence of stages in follicle development, called *folliculogenesis*, will be discussed prior to a description of hormonal interactions that influence ovarian activity. A *primordial follicle* consists of a primary oocyte arrested in the dictyate stage of meiotic prophase and a surrounding layer of simple squamous epithelial cells (granulosa cells). A prominent basal lamina invests the follicle. The oocyte is spherical and about 25 μm in diameter, with a large nucleus and a prominent nucleolus. The oocyte contains numerous mitochondria, Golgi complexes, ER, and annulate lamellae, which are initially all concentrated at one pole of the nucleus. The follicle cells have spot desmosomes and are surrounded by a basement membrane that separates the follicle from the vascular stroma. Typically, only a single germ cell is released by the ovaries in each menstrual cycle. The average duration of the menstrual cycle is 28 days in the human female.

MORPHOLOGIC STAGES

The initial sign that a primordial follicle has become activated is a change in the shape of follicle cells from squamous to cuboidal to columnar (Plate 58B; Figs. 22.3, 22.4). This *primary unilaminar follicle* contains only a single layer of follicle (granulosa) cells, although hyperplasia in follicle cells now follows. As a consequence of the proliferation of granulosa cells, the follicle becomes multilayered and is called a *multilaminar follicle* (Plate 58B). During this time, a homogeneous extracellular layer of glycoproteins appears around the surface of the oocyte, separating it from the granulosa cells. This layer is called the *zona pellucida*. Microvilli from the oocyte and microvilli from the innermost layer of granulosa cells extend into and interdigitate in the zona pellucida, which appears to be produced primarily by the oocyte (Plate 58C,D). A condensation of ovarian stroma, called the *theca follicluli*, is present around the follicle and will shortly differentiate into a *theca interna* and a *theca externa* layer. As the number of granulosa cell layers increases through proliferation, pools of fluid called the *vacuoles of Call-Exner* appear among the granulosa cells (Plate 58C,D). These vacuoles contain *follicular*

fluid, and this marks the beginning of the *secondary follicle stage* (Fig. 22.3).

As the proliferation of granulosa cells proceeds and as follicular fluid continues to accumulate in intercellular spaces within the follicle, the pools of fluid coalesce into a larger fluid-filled space called an *antrum* (Plate 59A–D). Such follicles are called *secondary (vesicular or antral) follicles*. The follicular fluid (called *liquor folliculi* or *follicular liquor*) contains transudates of plasma and substances secreted by granulosa cells. With further granulosa cell proliferation and an increase in antral size, a *Graafian follicle* stage is reached, which is ready for ovulation (Plate 59B,C; Figs. 22.3, 22.5).

The growth and development of the follicle involve the differentiation of the *theca folliculi* into a theca interna and a theca externa. The cells of the theca interna contain mitochondria, many lipid droplets, and extensive sER. The theca interna is richly vascularized and produces follicular fluid.

The granulosa cells become organized into a group that encloses and suspends the oocyte into the antrum; collectively, these cells are called the *discus proligerus* or *cumulus oophorus*. The single layer of granulosa cells immediately surrounding the germ cell is referred to as

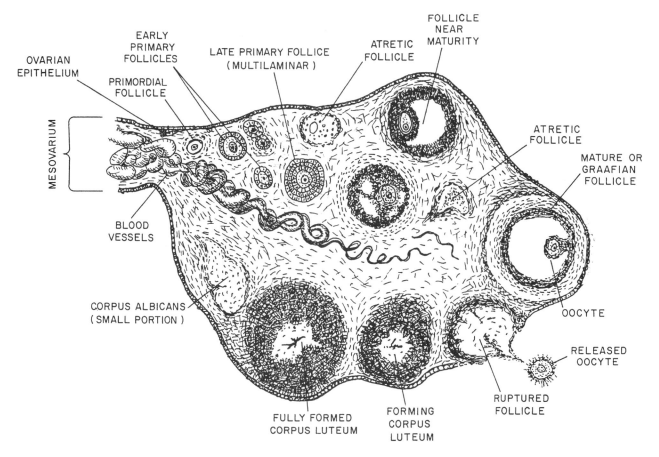

Figure 22.2. Diagram of the section of an ovary. Stages in follicle development are illustrated in the upper portion of the ovary; ovulated oocytes, stages in corpus luteum development, and a small portion of the corpus albicans are shown in the lower portion of the ovarian cortex.

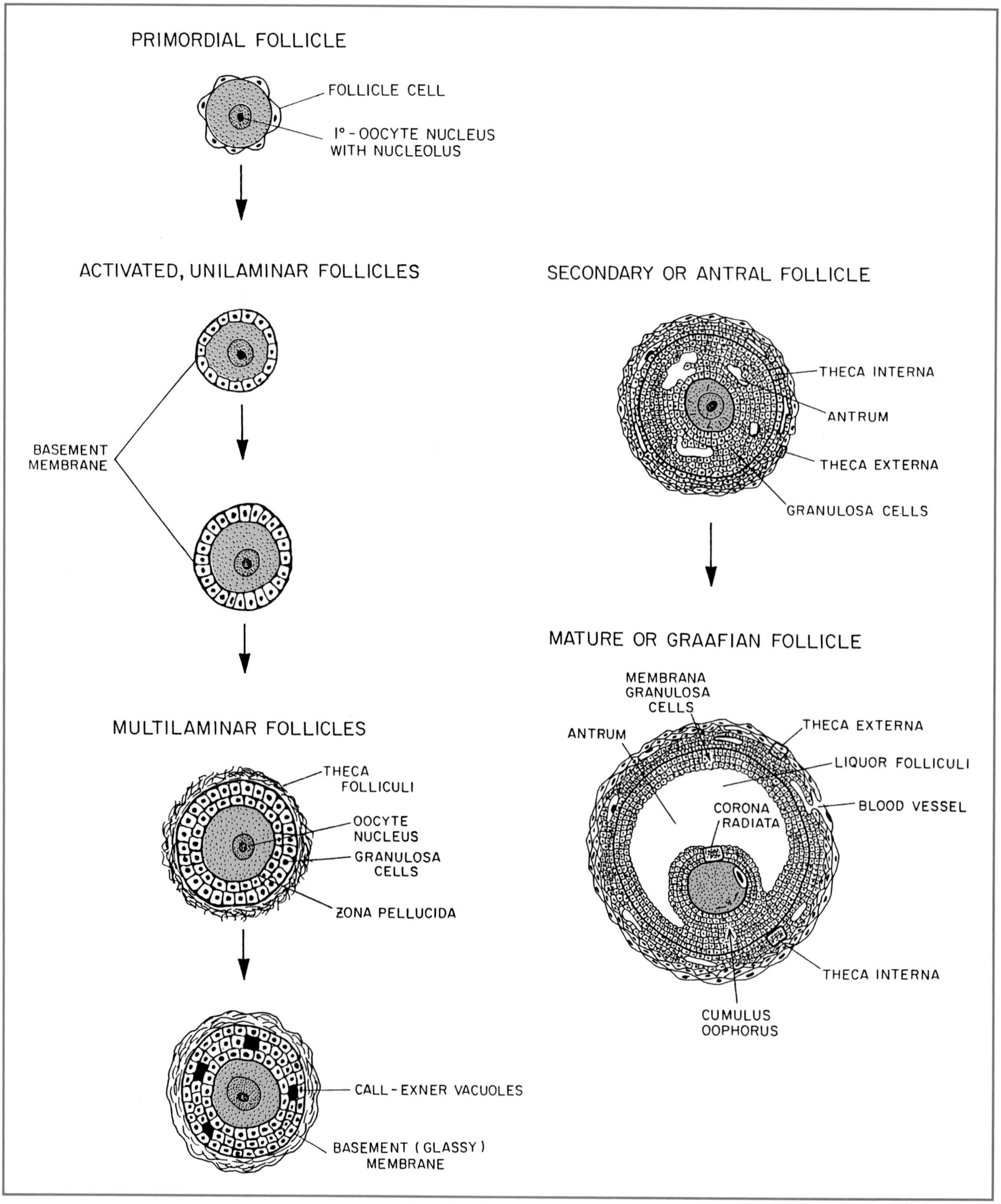

Figure 22.3. Diagrams of the stages in folliculogenesis that occur during the first 10–12 days of the menstrual cy- cle under the influence of FSH. All major structures are identified.

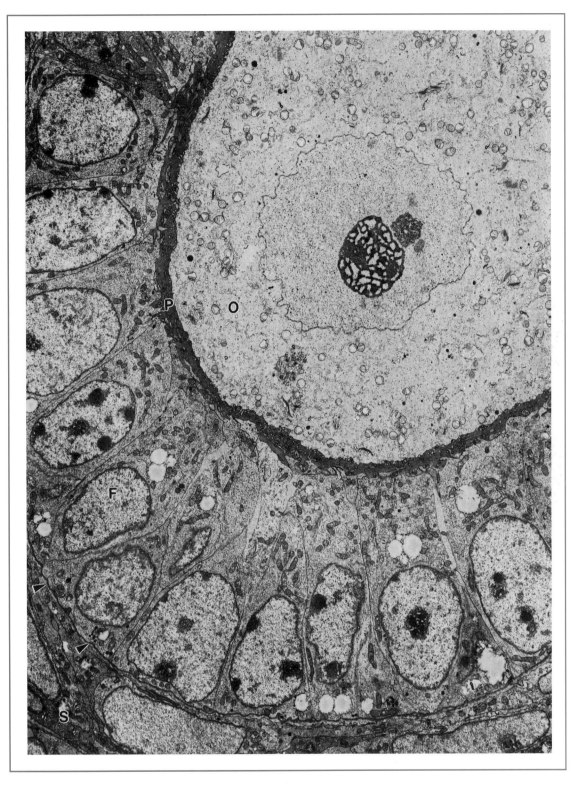

Figure 22.4. TEM of activated follicle shows oocyte (O) and columnar follicle (F) cells. The basement membrane (arrowheads), ovarian stroma (S), and zona pellucida (P) are identified. A nucleolus is present in the oocyte nucleus. ×4500. (From R. Roberts, R. Kessel and H. Tung. *Freeze Fracture Images of Cells and Tissue.* Oxford University Press, New York, 1991, with permission)

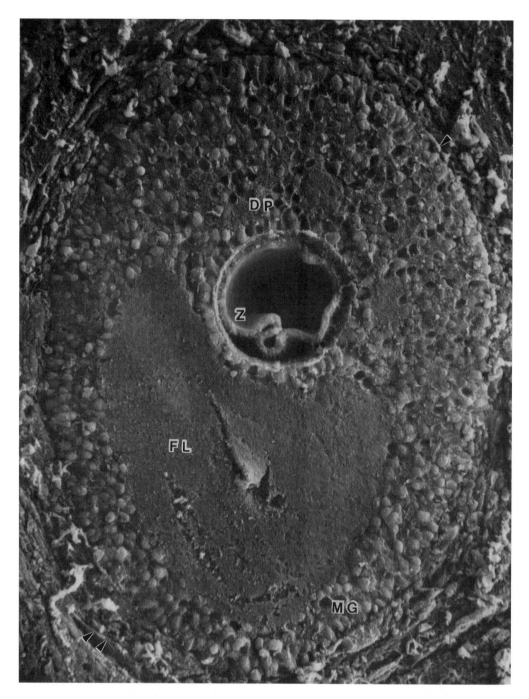

Figure 22.5. SEM of a section through a Graafian follicle. The oocyte was removed in making the section, but the zona pellucida (Z) remained. The follicle cells include those comprising the discus proligerus (DP) and the membrana granulosa (MG) surrounding the antrum, which in this preparation contains the coagulated follicular liquor (FL). The basement membrane is denoted by arrowheads. ×740. (From R. Kessel and R. Kardon, *Tissues and Organs: A Text-Atlas of Scanning Electron Microscopy*, W.H. Freeman, New York, 1979, with permission)

the *corona radiata.* The remainder of the granulosa cells surrounding the follicular antrum are collectively called the *membrana granulosa.* The mature (*tertiary*) *follicle* (*Graafian follicle*) is about 2.5 cm long and bulges from the surface of the ovary. The follicular cavity enlarges with increased liquor folliculi.

HORMONAL RELATIONS DURING FOLLICULOGENESIS

Puberty commences with the rhythmic secretion of *gonadotrophin-releasing hormone* (*GnRH*) from the hypothalamus, which permits the cyclic secretion of follicle-stimulating hormone (FSH), luteinizing hormone

(LH), and estrogen (Fig. 22.6). The physical changes that characterize puberty are the direct consequence of *estrogen* (estradiol). Estrogen is responsible for the acquisition of the secondary female characteristics, such as development of subcutaneous and mammary gland fat, growth of the pelvic girdle, and broadening of the hips. The cyclic secretion of FSH by gonadotropes causes the follicle to mature and produce progressively higher concentrations of estrogen (estradiol). Estrogen is thus produced as a consequence of the development of an ovarian follicle in the ovary beginning at puberty. The development of the follicle is a result of the production and release of FSH. The cyclic secretion of FSH by gonadotropes begins at puberty, causing the follicle to mature and produce higher concentrations of estrogen (estradiol). The squamous follicle cells develop FSH receptors and change shape from squamous to cuboidal to columnar. Estradiol promotes proliferation of granulosa cells, which then become more responsive to FSH. Estradiol also appears to stimulate proliferation of theca interna cells. Both estradiol and FSH induce the formation of LH receptors by granulosa cells, which are most numerous in preovulatory follicles.

The granulosa cells are the only cells in the ovary to have FSH receptors. LH receptors are found on cells of the theca interna and ovarian stroma prior to antrum formation, and LH stimulates the cells to synthesize and secrete steroid hormones. A marked increase in receptor density for LH occurs in theca cells of the dominant follicle.

FSH and LH hormones bind to specific receptors on granulosa and theca cells. This event activates adenylate cyclase, resulting in increased cytoplasmic concentrations of cAMP. This, in turn, activates a number of protein kinases that phosphorylate several proteins necessary for steroidogenesis. The rate-limiting step is the conversion of cholesterol to pregnenolone in the theca and granulosa cells. Both theca and granulosa cells can synthesize estrogen, but optimum estrogen production requires the cooperation of both cell types. In response to LH, theca interna cells produce quantities of androstenedione and testosterone, which are precursors of estrogens. Because of variations in chemical reactions that can occur in the theca and granulosa cells, granulosa cells can transform androgens produced by theca interna cells into estrogen when stimulated by FSH. Also, 21–carbon steroids produced by granulosa cells can be converted to androgens by cells in the theca interna. Therefore, for proper estrogen production, the participation of both theca interna and granulosa cells, each one responsive to different hormones (LH and FSH, respectively), is necessary.

The spindle-shaped theca interna cells secrete substantial androgen substrates including *estradiol*. There is evidence that the theca interna cells synthesize and release *androstenedione*, which is converted to *estradiol* by granulosa follicle cells. Granulosa follicle cells contain

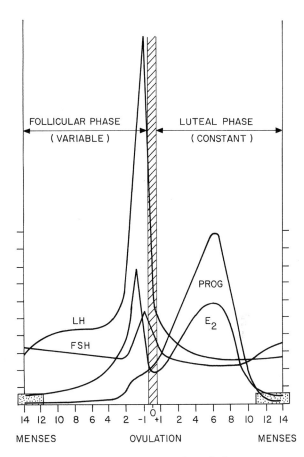

Figure 22.6. Graphs illustrate the relative concentrations of hormones in the menstrual cycle during the follicular, ovulatory, and luteal phases of ovarian development. E$_2$, estrogen.

cholesterol. All enzymes necessary for the synthesis of *estradiol-17β* are present in the granulosa cells.

Granulosa cells appear to produce a substance, *oocyte maturation inhibitor*, which is released into the follicular liquor and prevents the oocyte from completing meiotic division prior to ovulation. LH is thought to block the production of the oocyte maturation inhibitor at the time of ovulation. Other substances in the follicular liquor includes *GAGs*, several proteins (including *steroid-binding proteins*), and high concentrations of *progesterone, androgens,* and *estrogens,* as well as most inorganic ions.

The relative concentration of hormones of the menstrual cycle are illustrated in Figure 22.6.

ATRESIA

Because of the extensive degeneration (atresia) of primordial follicles, there are only approximately 400,000 germ cells in both ovaries at puberty. Only about 450 of the germ cells will be ovulated during the 30–40 years comprising the normal fertile life span of a human female. During the process of atresia, which can occur at any stage of follicular development, division of granulosa cells stops and the cells may become detached from the remainder of the follicle to float in the follicular liquor. The nuclei of the granulosa cells become pyknotic. The membrana granulosa may also detach from the surrounding basement membrane (Plate 60A,B). Macrophages usually invade the oocyte and other parts of the follicle. Deposition of some connective tissue may occur in the atretic follicle. It has been noted that atresia seems to occur when cells in the follicle have a maximal number of receptors for FSH and LH, but the hormonal levels are low at this time. Follicular atresia is particularly prevalent shortly after birth, when maternal hormones no longer have an influence. Atresia is also prevalent at puberty and during pregnancy. Although the granulosa cells and oocytes degenerate during atresia, theca interna cells persist and continue to secrete steroids. These cells are called *interstitial cells* or *interstitial glands* and produce ovarian androgens.

OVULATION

The concentration of LH rises to a peak approximately 16 hours prior to ovulation (Fig. 22.6). Ovulation is triggered by a surge in LH, and both theca and granulosa cells have receptors for this hormone (Fig. 22.7). In fact, the acquisition of LH receptors by granulosa cells is induced by both FSH and estrogen. LH is the physiologic switch for ovulation. Blood levels of FSH also peak at this time. In sufficient concentration, estrogen inhibits FSH release via a release-inhibiting hormone produced

and released by neurons in the hypothalamus. High concentrations of estrogen also stimulate GnRH for LH to be released by neurons in the hypothalamus. A substance called *follicular inhibin* (or *folliculostatin*) is also produced by follicle cells. Follicular inhibin is also thought to inhibit the release of FSH, probably by acting at the hypothalamus and pituitary levels.

Ovulation occurs approximately midway (day 14) during a 28-day menstrual cycle. Shortly before ovulation, meiosis I is completed and the secondary oocyte is blocked in metaphase of the second maturation division (meiosis II), which is completed only if fertilization occurs. Prior to ovulation, the oocyte and surrounding cells comprising the cumulus mass separate from the remainder of the follicle in anticipation of ovulation. Preovulatory changes in the ovary begin about 36 hours prior to release of the ovum and associated cumulus mass (follicle cells of the cumulus oophorus). The antral fluid or follicular liquor increases in amount and becomes less homogeneous, and there is an increase in hyaluronic acid content. The basement membrane, or glassy membrane, breaks down and the follicle bulges from the ovarian surface. This region of the ovarian surface becomes thinner and blanches due to reduced blood flow. In addition, there is a rupture with the loss of a small drop of blood (a corpus hemorrhagicum). A marked increase in proteases, such as collagenase and plasmin, appears to be important in dissolving the cortical ovarian stroma. Prior to ovulation, hydrolytic enzymes, including those that can digest the collagen of

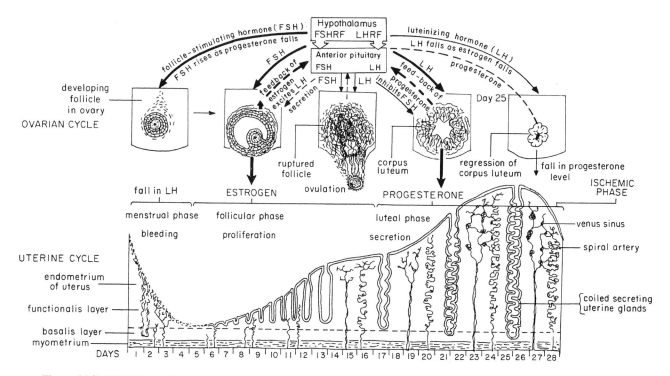

Figure 22.7. This illustration shows the changes that occur in the ovary and in the uterus (endometrium) at differ-

ent times during the menstrual cycle in response to specific hormones.

the ovarian stroma, increase in activity. Plasminogen activator is secreted by granulosa cells and releases the active proteolytic enzyme from plasminogen that is present in the follicular liquor.

The final steps in maturation of the tertiary or Graafian follicle is caused by LH. The surge of LH stimulates receptors for LH on the granulosa and theca cells; these LH receptors are induced by a combination of FSH and estrogen. GnRH produced by neurons in the hypothalamus causes the gonadotrophs to synthesize and release gonadotropins. When released, FSH causes follicular growth and differentiation and a consequent production of estrogen. The rising estrogen level in the blood depresses the synthesis and the release of FSH by gonadotrophs. The estrogen level peaks approximately 1 day prior to the midcycle surge in LH, which, in turn, is caused by the high estrogen level.

In addition to ovulation, LH causes luteinization of the ruptured follicle. In response to LH, the remaining granulosa and theca cells transform into a corpus luteum (yellow body) with large *granulosa lutein cells* and smaller, flattened *theca lutein cells*. Unless fertilization occurs, the corpus luteum has a life span of only about 14 days. This endocrine gland becomes richly vascularized, and the cells produce both *progesterone* and *estrogen*. The granulosa lutein cells produce most of the progesterone. Both theca cells and interstitial cells can also synthesize some progesterone. Progesterone is responsible for ensuring that the uterine endometrium is suitably prepared for implantation of a fertilized ovum (Fig. 22.7).

CORPUS LUTEUM

In addition to ovulation, the second major effect of LH is luteinization of the ruptured follicle which involves the formation of the corpus luteum (Plate 60C). In the living, this body has a yellow color due to the presence of a yellow pigment. The corpus luteum functions for about 12 days following ovulation under the influence of LH. Two cell types are present in the corpus luteum; these are the large, rounded granulosa lutein cells, the more numerous cell type, and the less numerous but flattened theca lutein cells. The granulosa lutein cells are derived from the membrana granulosa cells that remain in the ovulated follicle. The theca lutein cells are derived from the cells in the theca interna. Unless fertilization occurs, the corpus luteum undergoes involution and becomes scar tissue (Plate 60D). Following follicular rupture, the theca and granulosa cells become a compact mass of cells that are richly vascularized. Following ovulation, the blood vessels in the theca interna grow into the mass of remaining granulosa cells to vascularize the forming corpus luteum.

Both *progesterone* and *estrogen* are produced by the *corpus luteum*. The granulosa lutein cells appear to produce the major quantity of progesterone, but theca cells and interstitial cells can also synthesize progesterone. Progesterone plays an important role in causing major changes in the endometrium of the uterus to prepare for implantation of an early embryo. The estrogen that is produced following ovulation is produced by granulosa lutein cells, theca lutein cells, and interstitial cells of atretic follicles.

The high concentration of progesterone and estrogen produced by the active corpus luteum has a negative feedback on GnRH for LH. The combination of *progesterone* and *estrogen* is so effective in *inhibiting* the secretion of *GnRH* that pharmacologic doses of these two steroids are employed in *birth control pills* to *suppress ovulation*. The decline in blood progesterone and estrogen levels that results from the death of the corpus luteum leads to menstruation or shedding of a major part of the uterine endometrium. As a result, the corpus luteum involutes and transforms into scar tissue, which is then called the *corpus albicans* since it has a whitish color in the fresh state (Plate 60D). If fertilization and implantation occur, the corpus luteum does not undergo involution. It continues to produce progesterone and estrogen in sufficient quantity to maintain a secretory uterine endometrium until the 9th or 10th week of pregnancy. At this time, the fetal placenta produces progesterone directly in cooperation with the fetal adrenal cortex and liver.

Continued activity and functioning of the corpus luteum after fertilization and implantation is due to the production of a glycoprotein hormone called *human chorionic gonadotrophin* (hCG), which is produced by cells of the fetal placenta, specifically the *syncytiotrophoblast* cells of the chorionic villi. HCG replaces LH to maintain the corpus luteum of pregnancy until about 9–10 weeks of gestation. At this time, the corpus luteum of pregnancy begins an involution and is eventually converted into the scar tissue characteristic of a corpus albicans.

FALLOPIAN TUBES (OVIDUCTS)

The fallopian tubes (uterine tubes or oviducts) have a length of approximately 12 cm. At one end, the oviduct is continuous with the uterus; at the other end, the oviduct opens into the peritoneal cavity near the ovary. At the proximal end near the ovary, there is a flared region containing a number of processes or fimbriae that extend from a region called the *infundibulum*. The opening into the infundibulum is called the *ostium*. The infundibulum is continuous with a long *ampulla*. The ampulla is continuous with a thicker-walled *isthmus*. Finally, a short *intramural* or *interstitial* portion (pars interstitialis) traverses the wall of the uterus to communicate with the uterine lumen. At ovulation, the fimbriae become engorged with blood and the fimbriated lips of the infundibulum actively sweep over the ovarian surface. The ovulated oocyte and cumulus mass is sticky and adheres to the folded fimbriae. In addition, the surface cells of the fimbriae are heavily ciliated and the cilia beat, propelling the cumulus mass into the ostium of the oviduct. Fertilization usually occurs in the upper portion of the ampulla, and early cleavage of the ovum occurs as the zygote enters the uterus some 3–4 days following ovulation.

The wall of the oviduct consists of three layers. Internally, the *mucous membrane* or mucosa consists of simple columnar epithelial cells that overlie a connective tissue lamina propria. Both ciliated and nonciliated (secretory) columnar cells are present (Figs. 22.8, 22.9). The *muscularis layer* consists of circular and longitudinal smooth muscle layers that undergo peristalsis, which helps to propel the oocyte or zygote through the oviduct. A thin outer *serosa* covering the oviduct consists of a layer of simple squamous epithelium and a small amount of loose connective tissue.

The oviduct varies regionally in the extent to which the mucosa is folded. In the ampulla there are elaborate folds of mucous membrane such that the lumen is greatly reduced. The highly folded mucosa is very important in protecting against both physiologic and mechanical damage to the ovum and in ensuring that it is kept moist and closely applied to the mucosal epithelial surface. The cilia that develop on many of the colum-

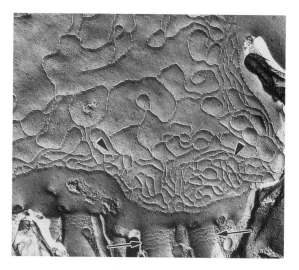

Figure 22.9. Freeze fracture replica of the apical end of ciliated oviduct epithelial cells. A complicated network of sealing strands (arrowheads) reflects the prominent circumferential tight junctions between epithelial cells and comprises a barrier to intercellular traffic. Also, note that at the base of the cilia there are four or five rows of intramembraneous particles that form "necklaces" in this region (arrows). ×30,000 (From: R. Roberts, R. Kessel, and H. Tung. *Freeze Fracture Images of Cells and Tissues.* Oxford University Press, New York, 1991, with permission)

nar epithelial cells during the follicular phase of the menstrual cycle do so under the influence of estrogen. The cilia are maximally developed at ovulation, and the secretory cells are then prepared to discharge their secretory product. While progesterone may initially increase the speed of ciliary beating, longer exposure to the hormone causes eventual degeneration or loss of cilia on the epithelial cells of the oviduct mucosa. Since fertilization usually occurs in the upper part of the ampulla, movement of the ovum is accomplished by both peristaltic contractions of the smooth muscle and the beat of cilia toward the uterus. The secretion produced by the secretory cells is rich in glycoproteins that help prevent dessication of the ovum and perhaps have a nutritive function. In addition, the secretion is important in activation or capacitation of sperm.

In certain limited cases, it is possible for the embryo to implant in the mucosa of the fallopian tube rather than the uterus. In such an *ectopic pregnancy*, the lamina propria behaves somewhat like the endometrium to the extent of forming decidual cells. Since the oviduct is easily ruptured during an ectopic pregnancy, extensive hemorrhage can be fatal if not dealt with promptly.

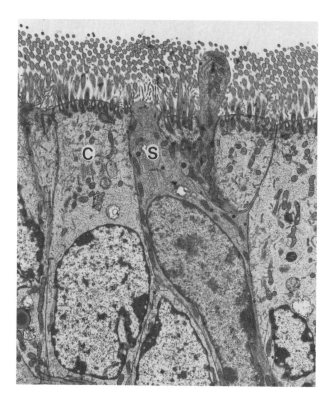

Figure 22.8. TEM of epithelium lining the oviduct. Both ciliated (C) and nonciliated (secretory) cells (S) are present. ×3875.

UTERUS

The uterus is an extremely important organ in the reproductive process, and it must prepare monthly for the implantation of a fertilized ovum, whether an oocyte is fertilized or not. The uterus must participate in the implantation process of the fertilized ovum, and it forms the maternal component of the placenta when pregnancy occurs.

The major portion of the uterus is called the body or *corpus* and contains a large *uterine cavity* (Fig. 22.1). The portion of the uterus above the points of entry of the oviducts is called the *fundus*. The uterine cavity narrows to a *cervical canal* within the narrower *cervix*. The cervix is the lower portion of the uterus and projects into the vagina as the *portio vaginalis*. The upper extension of the vagina around the portio vaginalis is called the *fornix*.

There are three layers to the uterus. The outer layer is either a *serosa* or an *adventitia*, depending upon the particular location. The middle *myometrium* is a thick layer of smooth muscle with various orientations. The inner layer, the *endometrium*, is the mucosa or mucous membrane of the uterus. The endometrium consists of simple columnar epithelial cells; a large population of these cells is secretory, and another population of cells is ciliated. Ciliated cells are generally confined to the surface epithelial layer. The uterine wall varies markedly in thickness during the menstrual cycle.

The myometrium consists of three or four ill-defined layers of smooth muscle surrounded by connective tissue. The middle layer is called the *stratum vasculare* because of the many large blood vessels present there. It is estimated that the mass of the uterus increases over 20 times during pregnancy. The smooth muscle cells may be 50 μm in length, but they can also enlarge markedly during pregnancy to nearly 500 μm. Smooth muscle cells thus hypertrophy, and there is also evidence that these cells can divide (hyperplasia). In addition, there is a marked increase in connective tissue elements during pregnancy, including a fivefold increase in collagen, which is produced by smooth muscle cells. After pregnancy, enzymatic degradation of collagen occurs; some of the smooth muscle cells are destroyed, and others decrease in size.

To a considerable degree, the normal size and state of differentiation of uterine smooth muscle are due to estrogen because, in the absence of estrogen, uterine smooth muscles tend to atrophy and lose their capacity to generate action potentials. In the nonpregnant uterus, the musculature undergoes shallow, intermittent contractions that may become exaggerated during sexual stimulation or menstruation, resulting in cramp-like pain. *Increased contractions* of the smooth muscle of the uterine myometrium can occur in response to *oxytocin* as well as *prostaglandins*. As a result, these substances have been used as *abortifacients*. Both *relaxin* and *progesterone decrease contractions* of the uterine smooth muscle and tend to quiet this muscle during pregnancy. Relaxin is a polypeptide produced by theca lutein cells in the corpus luteum of pregnancy and by the fetal placenta. Relaxin appears to play the major role in quieting the uterine smooth muscle during pregnancy. Some relaxin is also produced by *decidua cells* in the pregnant uterus and softens the *pubic symphysis* to facilitate *parturition*.

The layer of ciliated and secretory cells comprising the columnar epithelium of the uterine mucosa or mucous membrane (endometrium) is invaginated many times to form many simple tubular or branched tubular glands called *uterine glands*. The loose connective tissue of the lamina propria, called *endometrial stroma*, forms a thin packing among the many uterine glands. The endometrium (mucosa) has two layers (functionalis and basalis), one of which is a wide, superficial layer that contains most of the uterine glands and is called the *stratum functionalis* or functionalis layer of the endometrium (Fig. 22.7). The functionalis layer undergoes marked cytologic changes during the menstrual cycle. The second layer, which is much thinner and does not undergo marked changes during the menstrual cycle, is called the *basalis layer* or *stratum basalis* (Fig. 22.7). Beginning at puberty and terminating at menopause, the functionalis layer of the uterine mucosa undergoes marked cyclic changes in response to changing levels of hormone in the bloodstream. At the end of the menstrual cycle, the entire functionalis layer of the endometrium degenerates and is shed or sloughed during menstrual flow, which normally continues for approximately 2–4 days.

HORMONES AFFECTING THE UTERUS

Estrogen is primarily responsible for the repair or regeneration of the functionalis layer of the endometrium after it is lost during menstruation. The regeneration of this layer occurs at the same time that a follicle develops in the ovary. Estrogen not only stimulates cell proliferation of connective tissue and uterine gland cells, but also causes increased blood flow in the endometrium and a generalized increase in metabolic activity in this layer. After ovulation, progesterone is produced in the corpus luteum (and later in the fetal placenta if a pregnancy occurs), and progesterone stimulates the regenerated uterine glands to become highly coiled and secretory (Plate 61B).

Specific changes in the uterus, especially in the endometrium, in response to hormones of the menstrual cycle are characterized by four distinct stages or phases.

1. *Menstrual Phase.* This phase of the uterine endometrium is the period in which the entire functionalis layer is shed from the remainder of the endometrium—the basalis. This phase is a time of menstrual flow and, although variable, occurs during approximately days 1 through 4 of the menstrual cycle.

2. *Proliferative Phase*. This phase begins with the end of menstrual flow and extends to the time of ovulation, which in a relatively normal menstrual cycle is considered to be day 14 (Fig. 22.7). However, this is the most variable in duration of all the phases. This phase is called the *proliferative* or *reparative phase* because it is characterized by the rapid regeneration of the entire functionalis layer from the narrow basalis layer of endometrium remaining after menstruation (Plate 61A). Since the regeneration of the functionalis is caused by estrogen, it is also known as the *estrogenic phase*. Since folliculogenesis occurs in the ovary during this time, it is also known as the *follicular phase*.

During this phase, epithelial cells at the base of uterine glands and connective tissue cells of the stroma proliferate markedly, and cell migration occurs to reconstitute the entire functionalis layer. The uterine glands eventually become tall, straight, and closely packed. In addition, blood vessels consisting of many *coiled arteries* grow into the functionalis layer. The coiled arteries develop from basal arteries that persist in the basalis layer of the endometrium at the end of menstruation. During this phase, the endometrium increases from approximately 0.5–1 mm to approximately 2–3 mm in thickness. Ovulation normally occurs at the end of this phase.

3. *Secretory Phase*. This secretory phase is always associated with the formation of a functional corpus luteum in the ovary; the changes are caused primarily by *progesterone* (Fig. 22.7). The phase thus begins after ovulation and continues for about 10–12 days. Under the influence of progesterone the uterine glands initiate an intense secretory activity; consequently, the phase is sometimes called either the *progestational phase* or the *secretory phase* (Plate 61B). The glands become so active that the formerly straight, tubular uterine glands become more extensively coiled and secretion appears in their lumens. The glandular lumen may also become dilated. As a consequence of these activities, when the uterine glands are observed in longitudinal sections, they are described as having a corkscrew configuration. The secretory products of the uterine gland cells consist of *glycogen, mucin,* and *fat*. Because a pregnancy, if it occurs, does so during this phase, it is also called the *progravid phase*. The width or thickness of the endometrium increases to approximately 4 or 5 mm, primarily due to hypertrophy of gland cells and increased vascularity of the functionalis.

4. *Ischemic or Premenstrual Phase*. The last couple of days of the secretory or progestational phase of the uterus are sometimes identified as the *ischemic* or *premenstrual phase*. During this time, changes occur in the circulatory pattern of the coiled arteries that herald or mark vascular changes that will ultimately lead to the complete sloughing of the entire functionalis during the menstrual phase.

MENSTRUATION

The blood vessels of the endometrium are derived from circumferentially arranged arcuate arteries in the stratum vasculare of the myometrium. Two sets of arteries extend from the arcuate arteries: the straight arteries that supply only the basalis layer of the endometrium and *coiled arteries* that supply blood to the functionalis layer of the endometrium.

Progesterone production by the corpus luteum occurs for only about 10–12 days because of decreasing LH production and release. The corpus luteum then undergoes involution and ceases production of the progesterone necessary to maintain the functionalis layer of the endometrium in a thick, vascular, and highly secretory state. If no fertilization occurs, the entire functionalis layer of the endometrium will be shed.

Near the end of the secretory or progestational phase, in response to slightly lowering levels of progesterone, the coiled arteries in the functionalis layer of the endometrium tend to contract and relax in a somewhat rhythmic sequence. Because of the orientation of the coiled arteries, with contraction of the smooth muscle in the arterial wall, they tend to withdraw somewhat from the most superficial region of the functionalis, so that this region may become blanched for a time by being deprived of blood. The constriction of the coiled arteries becomes more pronounced and longer in duration such that an initial softening of the uterine stroma occurs immediately prior to initiation of incipient necrosis. As the concentration of progesterone and estrogen in the blood continues to decrease as the corpus luteum becomes more dysfunctional, the coiled arteries contract for longer periods of time, so that the surrounding uterine stroma and glands, as well as the tips of the arteries themselves, may become necrotic. As parts of arteries superficial to the constriction rupture, the initial blood loss (menstruation) begins. Initially, pools or lacunae of blood may accumulate in intercellular spaces in the degenerating functionalis tissue. As necrosis continues, these pools of blood may rupture and enter the uterine cavity. Further, since necrosis involves the smooth muscle of coiled arteries themselves, if and when these arteries relax, some bleeding from the ends of these necrotic vessels may occur directly into the uterine cavity. The coiled arteries become increasingly coiled to accommodate to the thinning functionalis layer. Increasingly deep layers of the functionalis become deprived of blood so that necrosis proceeds to involve progressively more of the stroma, glands, and blood vessels in the functionalis. The necrosis and sloughing of the endometrium continue until the entire functionalis layer is lost and only the basalis layer remains. The basalis layer escapes the menstrual process because its blood supply is derived from uncoiled basal arteries.

Regression of the functionalis in the ischemic and menstrual phases is due to pronounced vasoconstriction of the coiled arteries for progressively longer periods of time. The vasoconstriction is believed to be due to the falling levels of progesterone and estrogen in the blood as the corpus luteum fails. During menstruation approximately 35 ml of blood is lost, although this amount is highly variable. Menstrual fluid contains blood, glandular secretion, degenerative gland cells, and degenerating uterine stroma and blood vessels.

If fertilization and implantation occur, the hormone *human chorionic gonadotrophin* (hCG) is synthesized by cells in the developing embryo very soon after its implantation into the uterine endometrium. The hCG has an effect very similar to that of LH and maintains a functional corpus luteum even while LH levels are falling, thereby maintaining the endometrium.

EARLY EMBRYONIC DEVELOPMENT AND IMPLANTATION

As previously noted, the oocyte is usually fertilized in the ampulla or at the ampulla-isthmus junction of the oviduct. When ovulated, the oocyte is blocked at metaphase of the second meiotic division and is surrounded by the zona pellucida and a mass of cumulus (granulosa) follicle cells. The oocyte-cumulus mass does not remain viable for more than approximately 2 days. During fertilization, many sperm cause the dispersal of the cumulus mass and the fertilizing spermatozoon traverses the zona pellucida to fuse with and enter the oocyte. Fertilization results in the completion of meiosis II, with consequent formation of the second polar body (Fig. 22.10). The *zona pellucida* is important in the recognition of homologous sperm, in blocking polyspermy, and in keeping the blastomeres in a restrained and compacted cluster. The zona pellucida surrounds the egg until it reaches the uterus and may prevent the cleaving cells from sticking to the oviduct rather than traveling to the uterus. In humans, when the blastocyst adheres to the oviduct, a tubal or ectopic pregnancy can result, which has the potential to cause a severe hemorrhage. The blastocyst hatches from the zona by lysing a small hole through which the blastocyst emerges.

The fertilized egg or zygote initiates *holoblastic cleav-*

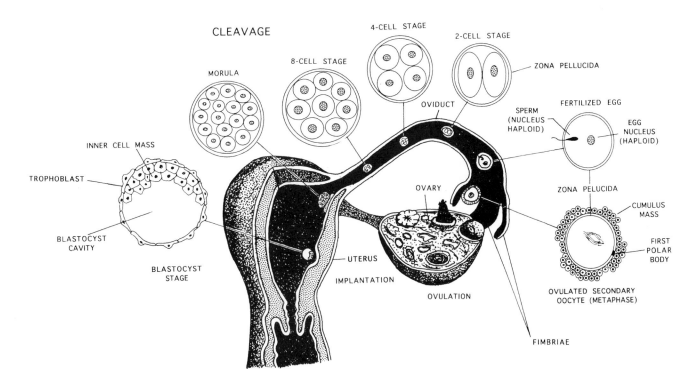

Figure 22.10. Diagrams of ovulation, fertilization, and early embryonic development during oviduct transport to the uterus.

age as it travels through the oviduct to the uterine cavity (Fig. 22.10). Some 3 to 4 days following ovulation and fertilization, the *morula stage embryo* enters the uterine cavity and becomes a *blastocyst stage*. By this time, a number of blastomeres have formed an inner cell mass (from which the embryo will form) and a single layer of *trophoblast* cells that surrounds a *blastocyst cavity*. The trophoblast layer represents the precursor of the fetal component of the placenta. By this time, a fluid that initially accumulated among the blastomeres now fills the blastocyst cavity. The blastocyst may remain in the uterine cavity for perhaps as long as 3 days before the zona pellucida is finally shed and implantation into the functionalis layer of the uterine endometrium occurs. The youngest blastocyst recovered from the uterine cavity was estimated to be approximately 7.5 days old and had the structural characteristics depicted in Figure 22.10. After the zona pellucida is shed, the blastocyst begins an invasive attack on the highly glandular endometrium on about day 21 or 22 of the menstrual cycle. As the cells begin to erode through the endometrial epithelium, they become highly proliferative (Fig. 22.11). As the trophoblast cells divide and invade the endometrium, they begin to form an outer syncytial layer and an inner cellular layer (Figs. 22.11). These layers become progressively more extensively folded and are called fetal *chorionic villi* (Plate 61C). The finger-like villi are surrounded on the outside by a syncytial layer called the *syncytiotrophoblast* (Plate 62B). The inner cellular layer, with distinct cell boundaries, is called the *cytotrophoblast layer* or *Langhans layer*, and it is this layer that forms the outer syncytial layer (Plate 61D). This differentiation occurs some 9–11 days following ovulation.

The complex interactions associated with the invasion of the fetal trophoblast into the maternal uterine functionalis are not completely understood (Fig. 22.11). It appears, however, that the invasion through the uterine epithelium involves proteases perhaps bound to the trophoblast cell surface. Once the invasion is initiated, it must be precisely regulated. The uterine decidua plays an important role in delimiting the boundaries of the invasion. One substance believed to be produced in the uterine decidua to regulate implantation is transforming growth factor.

The nuclei of cytotrophoblast cells are larger and lighter stained than the smaller, dark-staining nuclei in the syncytiotrophoblast layer (Plate 61D; Plate 62C). The cytotrophoblast cells contain many free polyribosomes, mitochondria, and glycogen but little rER. The syncytiotrophoblast cells contain extensive rER and sER, a well-developed Golgi apparatus, many mitochondria, lipid droplets, and cholesterol. It is thought that the syncytiotrophoblast is the principal synthetic cell and produces the glycoprotein *hCG*, as well as other hormones. The important hormones produced by the syncytiotrophoblast are summarized in Table 22.1. The exposed surface of the syncytiotrophoblast has folds in the form of microvilli and extensive micropinocytotic vesicles. The lytic activity of the syncytiotrophoblast causes the rupture of maternal arterial and venous blood vessels in the establishment of the maternal component of the placenta (Fig. 22.11). Blood vessels develop in the cores of the many fetal chorionic villi (Plate 62B,C). Spot desmosomes and circumferential tight junctions (zonule occludentes) are present between *Langhans cells*, as well as between *Langhans cells* and the *syncytiotrophoblast* layer. Since the placental syncytium or *syncytiotrophoblast* is a complete layer and there are no intercellular spaces, this condition establishes a very effective *maternal blood–fetal blood barrier*. The blood vessels in the fetal chorionic villi are thus separated from maternal blood by the syncytiotrophoclast cell layer, an adjacent cytotrophoblast cell layer (which may later be incomplete), the trophoblast basement membrane, the loose connective tissue in the core of the villus, and the endothelium and its basal lamina.

The chorion becomes so highly folded that the resulting chorionic villi are related to the maternal decidua in a manner similar to a hand-and-glove arrangement. The Langhans cells begin to disappear during the second month of pregnancy and no longer form a complete layer. Most of the Langhans cells are gone at about the fifth month of pregnancy.

The placenta consists of a fetal portion called the *chorion* and the maternal part, the *decidua basalis*. After implantation the endometrial stroma cells enlarge and are called *decidua cells* (Plate 62A). The decidual cells, which develop in response to progesterone, have been considered to be transformed uterine stroma cells by some, but others believe them to be derived from precursor periarteriolar cells. The *decidua* has an endocrine function and produces *prolactin, relaxin,* and *prostaglandins*. The binding of oxytocin to receptors on the decidua cells appears to result in the production of prostaglandins. *Prolactin* tends to increase spontaneous contractions of smooth muscle; however, relaxin decreases contractions of smooth muscle. Some decidua cells have been described to produce vitamin D.

A layer of extracellular material called *fibrinoid* is located between the maternal decidua and fetal chorionic villi (Plate 62A). This material contains *sulfated proteoglycans* that exhibit a strong negative charge. It has been suggested that the fibrinoid might form an *immunologic barrier* between the fetus and mother, perhaps by hiding the genetically foreign fetal tissues.

The syncytiotrophoblast cells synthesize *hCG* (a glycoprotein), *placental lactogen* (a protein), which has lactogenic and growth-stimulating activity, *estrogen* (steroid), *progesterone* (steroid), *chorionic corticotropin*, and *chorionic thyrotropin*. The hCG and human chorionic sommatomammotropin (hCS) have lactogenic and growth-promoting effects, and also affect fat and carbohydrate metabolism. The hCS is also called *human placental lactogen* (*hPL*).

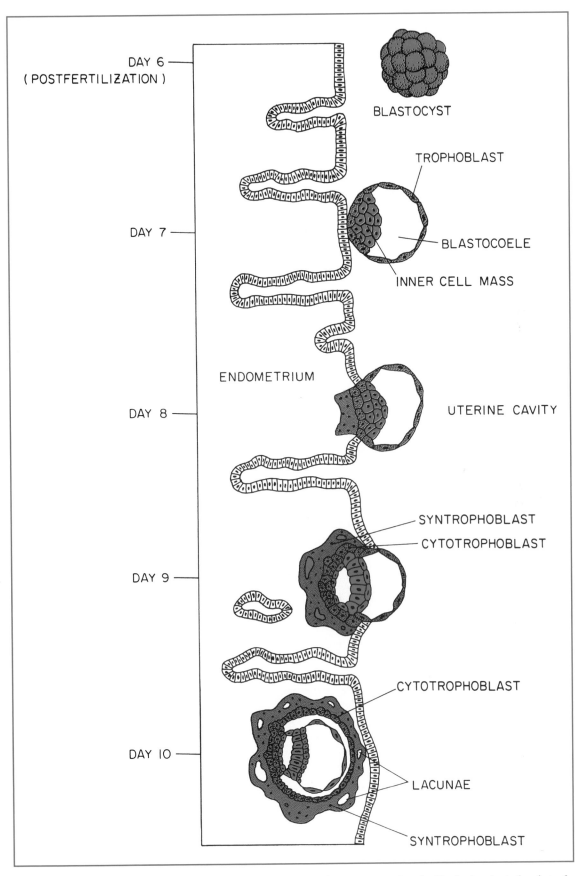

DAY 6
(POSTFERTILIZATION)

BLASTOCYST

TROPHOBLAST

DAY 7

BLASTOCOELE

INNER CELL MASS

ENDOMETRIUM

DAY 8

UTERINE CAVITY

SYNTROPHOBLAST

CYTOTROPHOBLAST

DAY 9

CYTOTROPHOBLAST

DAY 10

LACUNAE

SYNTROPHOBLAST

Figure 22.11. Diagrams of the organization of a blastocyst and the early events associated with the implantation into the uterine endometrium.

Table 22.1 Hormones of the Reproductive System and Placenta

Hormone	Source	Regulation	Action (Effects)
Reproductive System			
GnRF (gonadotropin-releasing hormone)	Hypothalamus	Female: inhibited by estrogens, progestins	Stimulates LH synthesis, FSH secretion
		Male: inhibited by testosterone	
FSH (follicle-stimulating hormone)	Anterior pituitary	Female: stimulated by GnRF; inhibited by estrogens and/or progestins	Female: stimulates follicle development, estrogen production, oocyte maturation
		Male: stimulated by GnRF, inhibited by inhibin	Male: stimulates spermatogenesis
Estrogens (primarily estradiol)	Follicle and interstitial cells in ovaries	Stimulated by FSH	Stimulates LH secretion, maintains secondary sex characteristics, stimulates endometrial repair, inhibits GnRF secretion
Inhibin	Sustentacular (Sertoli) cells in testes	Stimulated by FSH	Inhibits GnRF and FSH secretion in male
LH (luteinizing hormone)/ICSH (interstitial cell hormone)	Anterior pituitary	Female: production stimulated by GnRF, secretion by estrogens	Female: stimulates follicle and interstitial cells
		Male: stimulated by GnRF	Male: stimulates interstitial (Leydig) cells
Progestins (mainly progesterone)	Corpus luteum	Stimulated by LH	Stimulates endometrial growth, glandular secretions, inhibits GnRF secretion
Androgens (mainly testosterone)	Interstital (Leydig) cells in testes	Stimulated by ICSH	Maintains secondary sex characteristics, sexual behaviors; promotes maturation of spermatozoa; inhibits GnRF secretion
Prolactin (or lactaogenic hormone)	Anterior pituitary	Neurohormonal reflexes	Promotes mammary gland development and lactation during and after pregnancy
HCG (human chorionic gonadotropin)	Fetal placenta		Maintains corpus luteum early in pregnancy (mimics action of LH)
Relaxin	Fetal placenta		Dilates cervix; increases flexibility of pubic symphysis
HPL (human placental lactogen) (or sommato-mammotropin	Fetal placenta		Cooperates with prolactin to prepare mammary glands for milk production
Progesterone (~day 23 of pregnancy)	Fetal placenta		Maintains endometrium during pregnancy
Estrogen	Fetal placenta		Inhibits GnRH and FSH release (formation by placenta requires cooperation of fetal adrenal cortex and fetal liver)
Chorionic corticotropin	Fetal placenta		Stimulates adrenal cortex
Chorionic thyrotropin	Fetal placenta		Stimulates thyroid gland

The hCG is a glycoprotein that contains hexosamine and galactose and has a molecular weight of about 100,000. This hormone can be detected in the maternal blood in 11–day implantation stages. *Chorionic gonadotropin* has *LH activity* and it has also been suggested to have a capacity for *maternal lymphocyte suppression*, perhaps by blocking trophoblastic surface antigens from maternal lymphocytes. Direct production of *progesterone* from the *syncytiotrophoblast* has been detected at about the *23rd day* of *pregnancy*; hence hCG is no longer required to maintain the corpus luteum of pregnancy.

Maternal blood is directly exposed to the syncytiotrophoblast (Plate 62B). Since embryonic blood vessels develop from mesenchyme cells in the cores of the chorionic villi, the blood diffusion distance between maternal and fetal blood is quite short and involves the syncytiotrophoblast layer, perhaps some cytotrophoblast cells, basement membranes, and fetal endothelial cells. Substances with a molecular weight between *600* to *1000* tend to easily cross the placental barrier.

VAGINA

The vagina consists of an inner mucosa, a middle muscular layer, and an outer adventitia layer. The vagina has no glands in its wall, but *mucus* from *cervical glands* may enter the vagina. The mucosa is lined by stratified squamous epithelium, and these cells may synthesize *glycogen* in response to the hormone *estrogen*. The glycogen enters the vaginal lumen when surface epithelial cells desquamate. *Bacteria* located in the vaginal lumen metabolize the glycogen to lactic acid, and this results in an acid pH. Considerable amounts of elastic fibers are present in the lamina propria. Neutrophils and lymphocytes can migrate through the vaginal epithelium and into the vaginal lumen.

EXTERNAL GENITALIA

The external genitalia include the clitoris, labia minora, and labia majora. The labia majora enclose a small cavity called the *vestibulum*. The glands of Bartholin are located on either side of the vestibule and secrete mucus. The urethra opens into the vestibulum. The clitoris consists of erectile tissue and is covered by stratified squamous epithelium. The external genitalia are abundantly supplied with nerve endings, Meissner's plexuses, and Vater-Pacini corpuscles.

MAMMARY GLAND

The mammary gland is a *compound alveolar gland* that consists of approximately 20 lobes. Each lobe is surrounded by connective tissue and is linked to the nipple by means of a *lactiferous duct*. The "resting" mammary gland has no secretory alveoli and consists principally of ducts. An "active" or lactating mammary gland develops secretory alveoli at the ends of the ducts. *Myoepithelial cells* surround the secretory alveoli. Large quantities of adipose connective tissue are often present in the connective tissue septae of the gland. *Ligaments of Cooper* are elastic fibers that attach the breast to the integument. The *areolar glands* of *Montgomery*, once thought to be modified sebaceous glands that open onto the surface of the mammary gland, have been described as modified mammary gland alveoli.

Estrogen has an important role at puberty on breast development, including the accumulation of adipose connective tissue and collagenic fibers. The proliferation of the lactiferous ducts is also influenced by estrogen. *Lactogenic hormone* (*LTH*) and *prolactin* are involved in growth and development of the mammary glands. *Oxytocin* is involved in *milk ejection* and acts on the *myoepthelial cells*. Lactiferous ducts are lined by stratified cuboidal or stratified columnar epithelium. Myoepithelial cells closely surround the duct cells. Plasma cells and lymphocytes are located in the intralobular connective tissue. The plasma cells deliver *secretory IgA* into the milk at the end of pregnancy to provide *passive immunity* for the newborn.

During pregnancy there is marked growth and proliferation of secretory alveoli at the ends of terminal interlobular ducts. The alveoli contain milk-secreting cells (Plate 62D). The apical end of the cells contains membrane-bound secretory granules that contain *caseins*, α-lactalbumin, and *IgA*. *Lipid* droplets containing *neutral lipids* are also present in the cytoplasm. *Lactose* or milk sugar is synthesized from *glucose* and *galactose*. The milk contains 7% lactose, 4% lipids, and approximately 1.5% protein. The first secretion of the mammary gland after birth is *colostrum*, which contains more proteins and secretory IgA and less fat than regular milk.

SELECTED BIBLIOGRAPHY

Armstrong, D.T., Zhang, X., Banderhyden, B.C., and Khamsi, F. (1991). Hormonal actions during oocyte maturation influence fertilization and early embryonic development. *Ann. N.Y. Acad. Sci.* **626**, 127–158.

Austin, C.R., and Short, R.V., eds. (1982). *Reproduction in Mammals: I. Germ Cells and Fertilization.* Cambridge University Press, Cambridge.

Beaconsfield, P., Birdwood, G., and Beaconsfield, R. (1980). The placenta. *Sci. Am.* **243**, 94–109.

Blandau, R.J. (1971). *The Biology of the Blastocyst.* University of Chicago Press, Chicago.

Conley, A.J., and Mason, J.I. (1990). Placental steroid hormones. *Bailliere's Clin. Endocrinol. Metab.* **4**, 249–272.

Crowley, W.F., Jr., Filicori, M., Spratt, D.I., and Santoro, N.F. (1985). The physiology of gonadotropin-releasing hormone (GnRH) in men and women. *Rec. Prog. Horm. Res.* **41**, 473–526.

Davis, O.K., and Rosenwaks, Z. (1992). Current status of in vitro fertilization and the new reproductive technologies. *Curr. Opin. Obstet. Gynecol.* **4**, 354–358.

George, F.W., and Wilson, J.D. (1986). Hormonal control of sexual development. *Vitamins Horm.* **43**, 143–196.

Gruhn, J.G., and Kazer, R.R. (1989). *Hormonal Regulation of the Menstrual Cycle.* Plenum, New York.

Hanson, L.A. (1988). *Biology of Human Milk.* Raven Press, New York.

Hendrick, J.L. (1986). *The Molecular and Cellular Biology of Fertilization.* Plenum, New York.

Hodgen, G.D. (1986). Hormonal regulation in in vitro fertilization. *Vitamins Horm.* **43**, 251–282.

Irianni, F., and Hodgen, G.D. (1992). Mechanism of ovulation. *Endocrinol. Metab. Clin. North Am.* **21**, 19–38.

Jaffe, R.B. (1986). Endocrine physiology of the fetus and fetoplacental unit. In *Reproductive Physiology*, 2nd ed., S.S.C. Yen and R.B. Jaffe, eds. W.B. Saunders, Philadelphia.

Kaufmann, P., and Miller, R.K., eds. (1988). *Placental Vascularization and Blood Flow.* Plenum, New York.

Longo, F.J. (1987). *Fertilization.* Chapman and Hall, London.

Richards, J.S., and Hedin, L. (1988). Molecular aspects of hormone action in ovarian follicular development, ovulation, and luteinization. *Annu. Rev. Physiol.* **50**, 441–446.

Richards, J.S., Jahnsen, T., Hedin, L., Lifka, J., Ratoosh, S., Durica, J.M., and Goldring, N.B. (1987). Ovarian follicular development: from physiology to molecular biology. *Rec. Prog. Horm. Res.* **43**, 231–270.

Roberts, A.J., and Skinner, M.K. (1990). Estrogen regulation of theca cell steroidogenesis and differentiation: thecal cell-granulosa cell interactions. *Endocrinology* **127**, 2918–2929.

Strickland, S., and Richards, W.G. (1992). Invasion of the trophoblasts. *Cell* **71**, 355–357.

Tabibzadeh, S. (1991). Human endometrium: an active site of cytokine production and action. *Endocrine Rev.* **12**, 272–290.

Wassarman, P. (1988). Fertilization in mammals. *Sci. Am.* **256**, 78–84.

Wynn, R.M., and Jollie, W., eds. (1989). *The Biology of the Uterus.* Plenum, New York.

Yen, S.S.C., and Jaffe, R.B. (1986). *Reproductive Endocrinology*, 2nd ed. W.B. Saunders, Philadelphia.

Male Reproductive System

GENERAL ORGANIZATION AND FUNCTION

The male reproductive system consists of paired testes, excurrent ducts, accessory glands, and a copulatory organ (Figs. 23.1, 23.2). The system functions to produce male germ cells or spermatozoa, to produce the male hormone testosterone, and to facilitate fertilization by depositing sperm in close proximity to the female gamete in the female reproductive tract. The testes or gonads produce the spermatozoa in an extensive process of cellular differentiation called *spermatogenesis*. The testes also produce *androgens*, primarily *testosterone*. The sperm produced in the testis are transported through a series of excurrent ducts including the epididymis, ductus deferens, and ejaculatory duct. The *accessory glands* provide a nutritive vehicle for the spermatozoa. The spermatozoa and the glandular secretions are referred to as *semen*. The penis is the copulatory organ that permits internal fertilization. The ejaculatory duct and vas deferens serve primarily a conducting function to rapidly propel the semen.

TESTES

The testes develop in the abdomen but descend into a sac-like structure called the *scrotum* during fetal life. The testes are located outside the body because a temperature slightly lower than body temperature is necessary for differentiation of the male germ cells. In those cases where the testes fail to descend into the scrotum, sterility can result. Vitamin E, FSH, and LH are also required for spermatogenesis. Each testis is suspended in the scrotum at the end of a spermatic cord. The *spermatic cord* consists of the major excretory duct of the testis called the *vas deferens*, the *cremaster skeletal muscle*, *arteries*, *nerves*, and a plexus of veins called the *pampaniform*

plexus. Each testis is surrounded anteriorly and laterally by a *tunica vaginalis* (Fig. 23.1). The tunica vaginalis has parietal and visceral layers that enclose a small cavity; this condition results when the testes descend into the scrotum and carry peritoneum with them. Each testis is surrounded by a thick, dense, regularly arranged connective tissue capsule called the *tunica albuginea* (Figs. 23.1, 23.2). Some of this connective tissue extends into the interior of the testis as the *septuli testis* and, in doing so, forms some 250 compartments called the *lobuli testis*. Therefore, the connective tissue of the septuli testis separates the testis into *lobules*.

Each lobule consists of one to four highly folded or convoluted tubules called *seminiferous tubules* (Fig. 23.2). In a section of the testis, numerous section planes of seminiferous tubules are apparent (Figs. 23.3). These seminiferous tubules actually represent the exocrine portion of the testis, and it is here that spermatogenesis occurs (Fig. 23.4). There are about 500 seminiferous tubules per testis, representing a length of some 275 yards! At the apex of each lobule, the seminiferous tubules are continuous with short, straight, thin-walled tubules called the *tubuli recti*. The tubuli recti, in turn, are continuous with a system of thin-walled epithelium-lined spaces called the *rete testis* (Fig. 23.2). The connective tissue surrounding the rete testis is called the *mediastinum testis*. Extending from the rete testis are approximately 15–20 tubules called the *ductuli efferentes*, which extend from the testis to the nearby head of the epididymis. The highly coiled *epididymis* continues as the *ductus deferens*.

ORIGIN OF GERM CELLS: SPERMATOGENESIS

Spermatogenesis is the term used to denote all the sequences involved in the transformation of a spermatogonium into spermatozoa. In males, the primordial

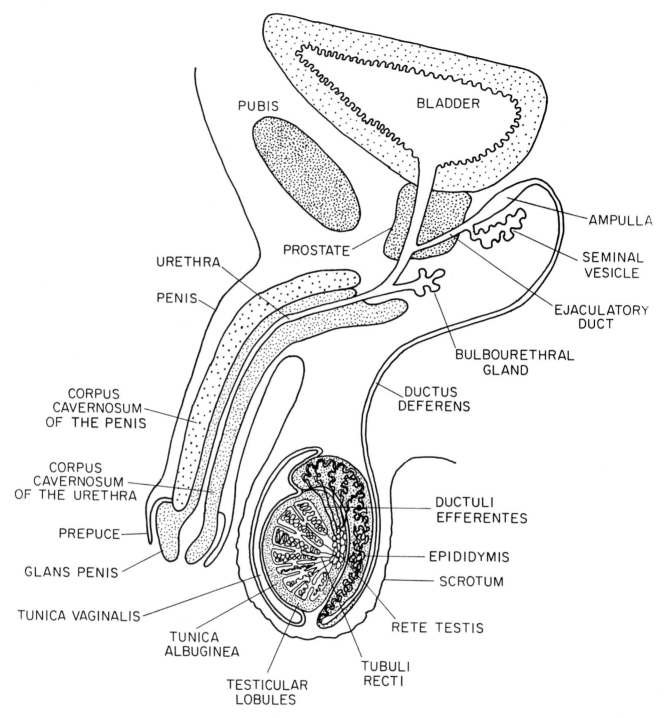

Figure 23.1. Diagram of the parts of the male reproductive tract in a lateral view. (Redrawn from L.C. Jun- queira, J. Carneiro, and R.O. Kelley. *Basic Histology.* 7th ed., Appleton and Lange, Norwalk, CT, 1992)

germ cells originate from *yolk sac endoderm* cells that migrate to and into the developing testis. These germ cells become located in epithelial cords that subsequently develop into seminiferous tubules. The diploid spermatogonia are derived from primordial male germ cells, spermatogonia that remain quiescent until near adolescence, when they proliferate by mitosis. Some of the resulting cells serve as a reserve source of proliferating cells, while others begin spermatogenesis at puberty. Following *meiotic prophase I,* the primary spermatocytes

complete meiosis (reduction-division) and *two haploid secondary spermatocytes* result. The *secondary spermatocytes quickly* undergo an *equational* (mitotic) *division* resulting in *four haploid spermatids* (Figs. 23.5, 23.6A,B), each of which undergoes cellular changes but no division, to produce a mature spermatozoon. The final step, which involves the morphologic transformation of a spermatid into a spermatozoon, is called *spermiogenesis.*

During spermatogenesis, a single spermatogonium develops into four spermatozoa. During oogenesis, how-

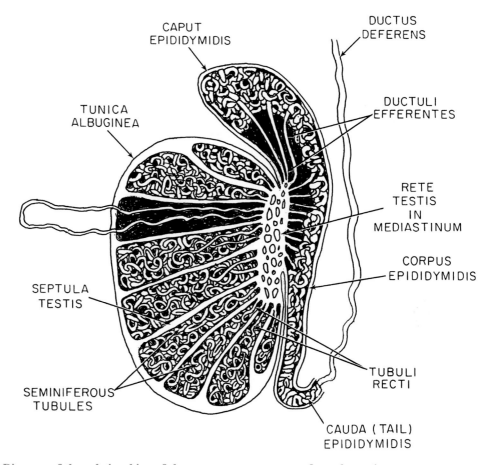

Figure 23.2. Diagram of the relationships of the excurrent passageways from the testis.

ever, a single oogonium develops into a single egg precursor (oocyte). During oogenesis, in contrast, the divisions of the oocyte are highly unequal, such that only one egg precursor is formed and the smaller polar bodies degenerate. Spermatogonia usually remain active throughout life, constantly proliferating to yield new primary spermatocytes and to continually replenish the supply of spermatogonia. This situation is unlike that in the human female, where all oogonia are produced by the time of birth and are arrested in meiosis.

HORMONAL RELATIONSHIPS DURING PUBERTY

The interstitial cells, which are located in the connective tissue surrounding the seminiferous tubules (Fig. 23.6A), secrete androgens in fetal life, but this occurs at a reduced rate during childhood. At about the time of puberty, approximately age 14, the anterior pituitary secretes *LH*, causing an increase in androgen production by Leydig cells (Fig. 23.6A). The elevated androgen level, as well as the action of FSH, stimulates spermatogenesis. At this time, the groups of interstitial cells of Leydig become more apparent and a distinct lumen appears in the seminiferous tubules. These processes are summarized in the accompanying diagrams.

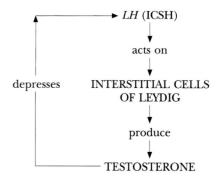

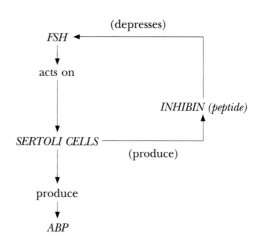

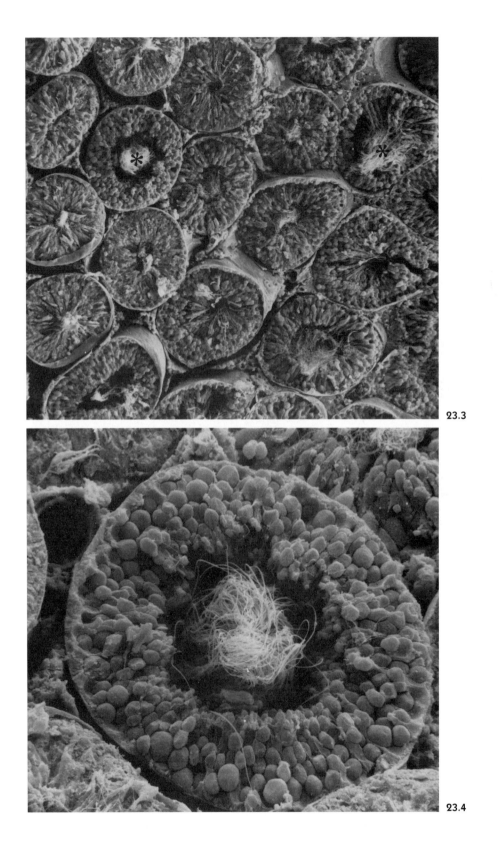

23.3

23.4

Figures 23.3, 23.4. Transverse sections of seminiferous tubules of the testis are illustrated in this SEM. Some of the tubules have sperm flagella in the lumen (*). Fig. 23.3, ×135; Fig. 23.4, ×510. (From R. Kessel and R. Kardon, *Tissues and Organs: A Text-Atlas of Scanning Electron Microscopy*, W.H. Freeman, New York, 1979, with permission)

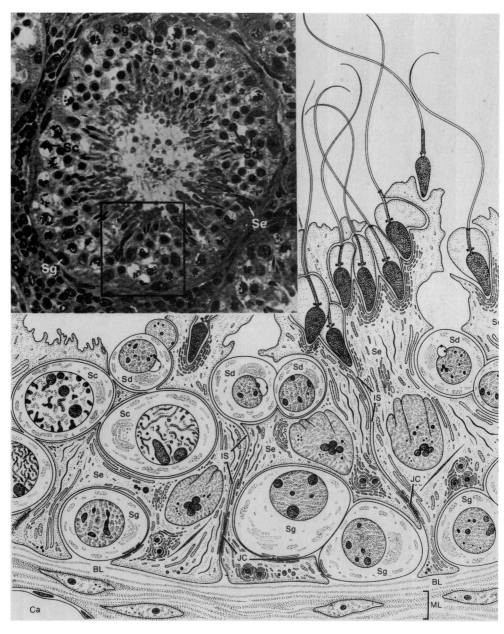

Figure 23.5. Diagram depicts a portion of the wall of the seminiferous tubule. The Myoid cell layer (ML), basal lamina (BL), capillary (Ca), spermatogonia (Sg), spermatocyte (Sc), spermatid (Sd), Sertoli cell (Se), intercellular spaces between Sertoli cells, and region of junctional complexes (circumferential tight junctions) (JC) are identified.

The inset is a low-magnification view of the seminiferous tubule, with a Sertoli (Se) cell, spermatogonium (Sg), spermatocytes (Sc), and spermatid (Sd) identified. From: R. Kessel and R. Kardon, *Tissues and Organs: A Text-Atlas of Scanning Electron MIcroscopy*, W.H. Freeman, New York, 1979, with permission)

HORMONAL RELATIONSHIPS IN GENERAL

Sufficient quantities of both LH and FSH are required for normal levels of spermatogenic activity. FSH seems to be particularly important for spermatid differentiation or maturation. LH production stimulates testosterone production by interstitial cells. Testosterone that is produced in response to LH is critical for spermatogenesis. In *negative feedback*, the rising testosterone level suppresses the further release of LH. FSH release by the gonadotrops in the anterior pituitary stimulates *Sertoli cells*, which are present in the seminiferous tubules, to release an *androgen-binding protein (ABP)*. The ABP passes into the lumen of the seminiferous tubules to bind testosterone and thereby maintain high levels of hormone in the tubules. The negative feedback regulation of FSH release appears to occur by a polypeptide called *inhibin*, which is produced by Sertoli cells in response to FSH. The release of FSH is thus reduced in response to the rising level of inhibin.

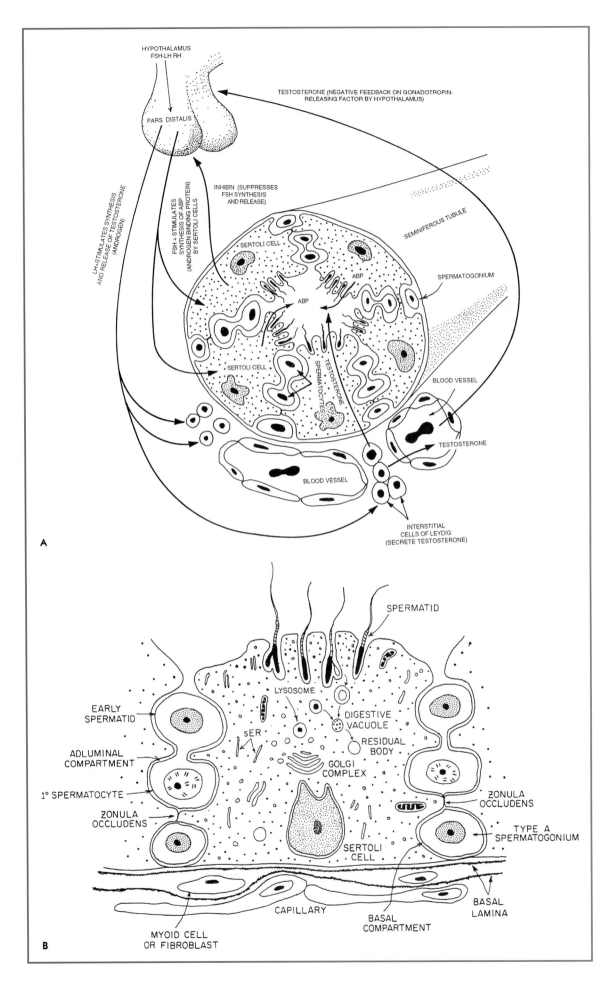

A

HYPOTHALAMUS
FSH-LH RH

PARS DISTALIS

TESTOSTERONE (NEGATIVE FEEDBACK ON GONADOTROPIN-
RELEASING FACTOR BY HYPOTHALAMUS)

LH→STIMULATES SYNTHESIS
AND RELEASE OF TESTOSTERONE
(ANDROGEN)

FSH + STIMULATES
SYNTHESIS OF ABP
(ANDROGEN BINDING PROTEIN)
BY SERTOLI CELLS

INHIBIN (SUPPRESSES
FSH SYNTHESIS
AND RELEASE)

SEMINIFEROUS TUBULE

SERTOLI CELL

ABP

ABP

SPERMATOGONIUM

SERTOLI CELL

SPERMATOCYTES

TESTOSTERONE

BLOOD VESSEL

BLOOD VESSEL

TESTOSTERONE

INTERSTITIAL
CELLS OF LEYDIG
(SECRETE TESTOSTERONE)

SPERMATID

EARLY
SPERMATID

ADLUMINAL
COMPARTMENT

1° SPERMATOCYTE

ZONULA
OCCLUDENS

LYSOSOME

DIGESTIVE
VACUOLE

RESIDUAL
BODY

SER

GOLGI
COMPLEX

ZONULA
OCCLUDENS

TYPE A
SPERMATOGONIUM

SERTOLI
CELL

BASAL
LAMINA

MYOID CELL
OR FIBROBLAST

CAPILLARY

BASAL
COMPARTMENT

B

Figure 23.7. SEM of a rat seminiferous tubule in transverse section.
Note the stratified germinal epithelium and the spermatids, which are
closely associated with the Sertoli
cells (arrows). Sperm flagella (*).
×390.

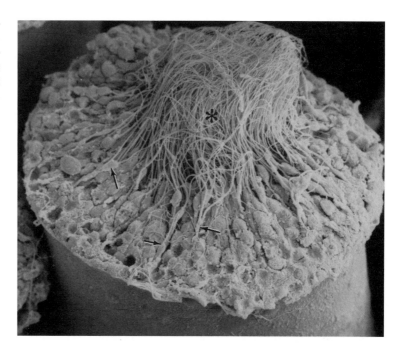

The accompanying table summarizes the actions of these hormones.

SEMINIFEROUS TUBULES

The highly coiled seminiferous tubules are the site of spermatogenesis. These tubules therefore contain all the cells of the spermatogenic series, as well as Sertoli cells (Plate 63A,B). One or more layers of *myoid cells* and loose connective tissue are associated with the outer surface of the highly folded seminiferous tubules external to the basement membrane. Interstitial cells (of Leydig) are present in the connective tissue (Septuli testis). The flattened myoid cells are also called *peritubular contractile cells.* The cells appear to cause rhythmic but shallow contractile waves in the seminiferous tubules. The principal cellular elements in the wall of the seminiferous tubules include *sustentacular cells of Sertoli* and *germ cells* in various stages of differentiation (spermatogenesis) (Figs. 23.7, 23.8).

Spermatozoa can be considered a holocrine secretory product of the testes, and some 200 to 300 million are contained in each ejaculate. The total time required to produce a mature human spermatozoon is estimated at ~70 days.

GERM CELLS: MEIOSIS AND SPERMATOGENESIS

The seminiferous tubules contain all the spermatogenic cells. These cells are arranged within the wall in sequence, with the earliest cells at the periphery and the latest ones at the lumen. The wall of the seminiferous tubule is thus lined by a stratified layer of germinal cells (Plate 63A,B; Fig. 23.4). The diploid *spermatogonia* are basally located in the seminiferous epithelium and are in contact with the basement membrane. Several populations of spermatogonia are usually denoted. A type A spermatogonium is highly proliferative and undergoes mitosis to provide for an extensive pool of cells for subsequent meiosis. The type A spermatogonia have a lightly staining, euchromatic nucleus, and the cells are located in the *basal compartment* of the seminiferous epithelium. Some investigators have found a dark type A spermatogonia with darker-stained nuclei that may represent quiescent cells that become activated to proliferate only under certain unusual conditions. The *type B spermatogonia* are those that will differentiate into primary spermatocytes. They become located in an *adluminal compartment* of the seminiferous tubule prior to prophase of meiosis I.

A number of different nuclear stages during prophase of meiosis I can be denoted. The initial stage

Figure 23.6A. Diagram of the action of LH on the interstitial cells of Leydig, causing them to produce testosterone. A rising testosterone level depresses LH release. FSH stimulates Sertoli cells to synthesize ABP. 6B. Diagram of the relationship between the Sertoli cell and the spermatogonia, spermatocytes, and spermatids. Circumferential tight junctions form basal and adluminal compartments for the seminiferous epithelium.

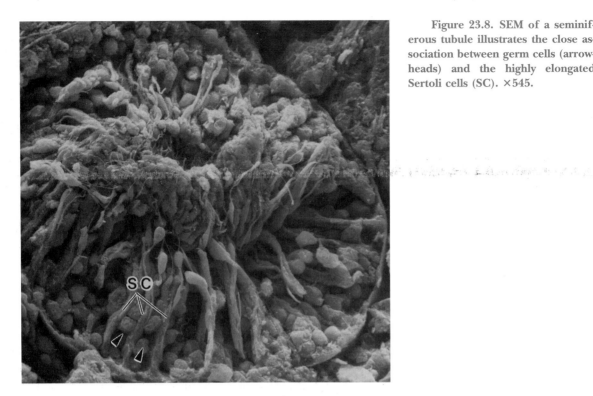

is called *leptotene*, and the *double (d)-chromosomes* are extremely thin. The d-chromosomes then undergo pairing and are known as *bivalents*. It is near the end of leptotene that a parallel, ribbon-like structure called a
synaptonemal complex becomes associated with and holds
each of the paired chromosomes. Each end of the synaptonemal complex is attached to the inner nuclear membrane. The d-chromosomes become still thicker and
shorter (i.e., more condensed) during *pachytene*. Then,
during *diplotene*, the two d-chromosomes of each bivalent separate slightly so that *chiasmata* can be observed.
The final stage of prophase I is called *diakinesis*, and
there is further thickening of the chromosomes.

The primary spermatocytes then enter *metaphase I*,
and the chromosomes become positioned on an equatorial plate. In the anaphase that follows, the d-chromosomes of the bivalent separate and move to opposite
poles. Since each single chromosome (s-chromosome)
of each d-chromosome remains attached at the centromere region throughout prophase of meiosis I, each
of the resulting secondary spermatocytes receives the
haploid number of d-chromosomes.

Secondary spermatocytes are smaller than primary
spermatocytes. Since the secondary spermatocytes have
no S phase, they rapidly complete the second maturation (meiosis II) and are usually not apparent as interphase cells in the seminiferous epithelium. The two cells
resulting from the division of one secondary spermatocyte are called *spermatids*.

Spermatids are located adjacent to the lumen of
the seminiferous tubule. These cells have small, spherical nuclei initially, but they then undergo *spermiogene-*

sis. During this process a number of events occur, including *condensation* of *chromatin*, *elongation* of the *nucleus*, and development of a *streamlined motile cell.*

Throughout the process of cell differentiation during spermatogenesis, all the progeny of B-type spermatogonia remain attached to each other because of incomplete cytokinesis (Figs. 23.6A,B). Thus, the clonal
descendants of each spermatogonium are interconnected by narrow *intercellular bridges,* and these connections cause synchrony in subsequent divisions. The cells
completely separate in the spermatid stage.

It requires more than 2 months (~70 days) to
progress from the spermatogonium stage to the spermatozoon stage of differentiation. In humans, each mil-
liliter of semen contains ~100 million sperm, but the
number can be variable. On average, ~3 ml of semen
is contained in each ejaculate.

SUMMARY OF CHROMOSOME CHANGES

It seems worthwhile to summarize the changes in chromosomes that occur during meiosis I and meiosis II.
Prior to the first meiotic division of spermatogonia, as
in all mitotic divisions, the chromosomes have replicated in the previous S phase. Thus, at the onset of meiosis, they are d-chromosomes. During meiosis I, the chromosomes remain double; *homologs separate,* but *sister
chromatids do not.* The secondary spermatocytes each receive a haploid number of chromosomes that are double. When the secondary spermatocytes undergo meiosis II the sister chromatids separate, leading to

spermatids that have the haploid number of chromosmes, which are now single.

SPERMIOGENESIS

The term *spermiogenesis* denotes the morphologic transformation of a spherical haploid spermatid into an elongate, streamlined spermatozoon. During spermiogenesis, the size of the cell decreases and there is a change in the shape of the cell and the nucleus. The cell elongates and the chromatin undergoes marked condensation. The Golgi apparatus synthesizes and packages an *acrosome*, which migrates toward the anterior tip of the sperm and becomes flattened (Fig. 23.9). The *acrosome* is important for fertilization of the egg and contains such substances as *aryl sulfatase, acid phosphatase, neuraminidase, hyaluronidase,* and *proteolytic enzymes* (Fig. 23.9). One of the paired centrioles located next to the posterior pole of the nucleus sprouts a flagellum (Fig. 23.10). The mitochondria cluster and become organized in a characteristic manner around the flagellum. The excess cytoplasm is removed during the streamlining process of the cell and released as a *residual body* that is ingested and digested by the Sertoli cells (Fig. 23.6B). Microtubules comprising what is called the *manchette* (Fig. 23.11) become closely associated with the spermatid nucleus during its elongation. Figure 23.12 illustrates a section of a mature hamster sperm to illustrate the acrosome and condensed nuclear chromatin.

Fig. 23.13 illustrates a mature human spermatozoon by SEM.

SERTOLI CELLS

Sertoli cells are supporting (sustentacular) cells in the seminiferous tubule that have a number of important functions. They arise from the epithelial cords in the developing gonad. They are columnar in shape; basally they are in contact with the basement membrane and extend to the lumen of the seminiferous tubule (Figs. 23.6, 23.8, 23.15). The Sertoli cells are nonproliferating cells. All Sertoli cells in a seminiferous tubule contact adjacent Sertoli cells, although only in localized focal areas. Although not apparent in LM sections, the Sertoli cells actually touch adjacent Sertoli cells and prominent circumferential tight junctions are located here (Fig. 23.6A,B). The remaining area between each of the Sertoli cells is packed with male germ cells in different stages of spermatogenesis. The sides of the Sertoli cells may be rounded or indented and partially invest the developing male germ cells. The Sertoli cells are thus intimately associated with the germ cells during their differentiation, but this is not apparent in LM preparations because the membranes of Sertoli cells are indistinct.

The Sertoli cell has a large, pale-staining nucleus that is located basally in the cell and that has indentations. The nucleus contains a large, prominent nucleolus. The cytoplasm contains prominent Golgi com-

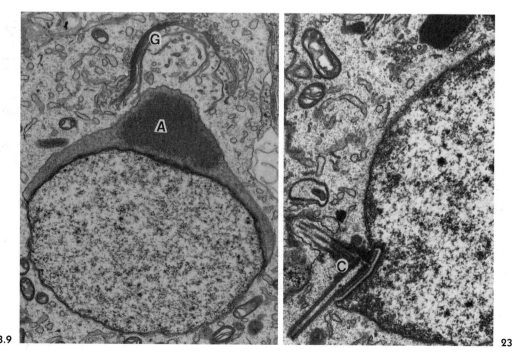

Figures 23.9, 23.10. TEM of spermatids during spermiogenesis. Golgi complexes (G), forming acrosomes (A) and proximal centrioles (C), are denoted. Figure 23.9 (left), ×12,600; Figure 23.10 (right), ×9600.

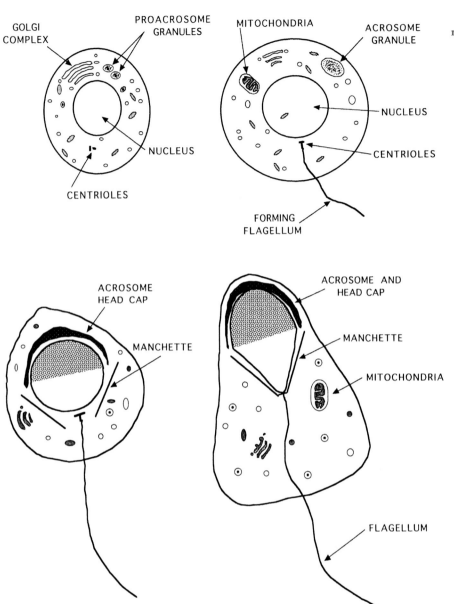

Figure 23.11. Diagrams of the major events in spermiogenesis.

plexes, mitochondria, sER, rER, lipid droplets, lysosomes, residual bodies, and a lipochrome pigment (Fig. 23.15). Microfilaments and microtubules are also present. The cytoplasm of Sertoli cells may contain crystalline inclusions (the Charcot-Böttcher crystals or crystalloids), whose functional significance is unknown.

The Sertoli cells produce a secretion called *testicular fluid*, which is released into the lumen of the seminiferous tubules. This fluid appears to be important for sperm survival; it is especially rich in *potassium, glutamate,* and *inositol*. The Sertoli cells are responsive to FSH since they possess cell surface receptors for this hormone. In response to FSH, Sertoli cells synthesize and secrete an *ABP* that binds *testosterone* so that a microenvironment consisting of a high concentration of testos-

terone is maintained in the seminiferous tubules. In order for spermatogenesis to occur, a high concentration of testosterone must be maintained in the seminiferous tubules. Sertoli cells (1) play an important role in providing the proper microenvironment for sperm differentiation, (2) are important in the movement of the interconnected germ cells, (3) play a role in the release (spermiation) of the spermatozoa into the seminiferous tubule lumen (Fig. 23.15), and (4) phagocytize degenerating sperm or residual bodies that are sloughed from spermatids and digest them intracellularly. Still another important function (5) is the role of Sertoli cells in the formation of a *blood-testis barrier*. Sertoli cells (6) have a *nutritive function* and provide a route for the passage of nutrients from the capillaries outside the basement

Figure 23.11. continued

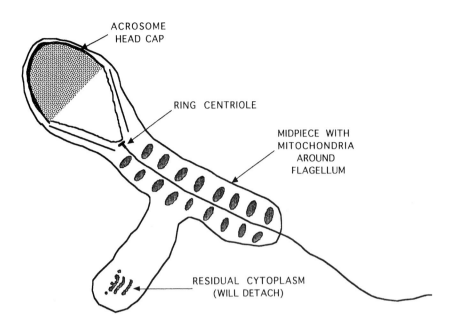

ACROSOME
HEAD CAP

RING CENTRIOLE

MIDPIECE WITH
MITOCHONDRIA
AROUND
FLAGELLUM

RESIDUAL CYTOPLASM
(WILL DETACH)

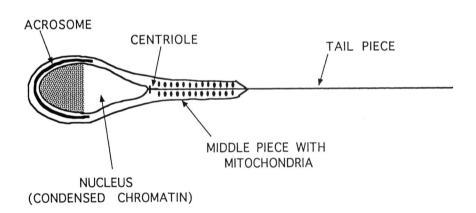

ACROSOME

CENTRIOLE

TAIL PIECE

MIDDLE PIECE WITH
MITOCHONDRIA

NUCLEUS
(CONDENSED CHROMATIN)

membrane of the seminiferous epithelium to the developing germ cells in the basal compartment. The seminiferous epithelium, like other epithelia, is avascular.

The spermatids are located in deep, narrow indentations at the apical end of the Sertoli cell (Figs. 23.15, 23.16). At the end of spermiogenesis, the spermatozoa are released from their intimate association with the Sertoli cells (spermiation). It has been suggested that sperm release from Sertoli cells occurs as a result of fusion of elements of the *sER* at the apical end of Sertoli cells so that the apical end undergoes a type of lysis or dissociation, releasing the sperm. In amphibians, for example, injection of LH causes swelling of the sER and lysis of the apical end of the Sertoli cell.

BLOOD-TESTIS BARRIER

The blood-testis barrier results from the presence of extensive *circumferential zonulae occludentes* (tight junctions) between adjacent Sertoli cells near their base. As a result of these many sealing strands, the seminiferous tubule is divided into a *basal compartment*, which contains proliferating type A spermatogonia, and an *adluminal compartment*, which contains type B spermatogonia that are committed to become spermatocytes (Fig. 23.6B). The presence of a blood-testis barrier means that it is possible for the Sertoli cells to direct the flow of fluid to the lumen of the seminferous tubule so that it does not pass back into the interstitium. Therefore, a special microenvironment can be maintained for the

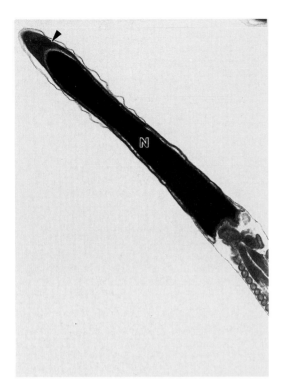

Figure 23.12. TEM. Longitudinal section of a mature hamster sperm showing an acrosome (arrowhead) and condensed chromatin in the nucleus (N). ×14,700.

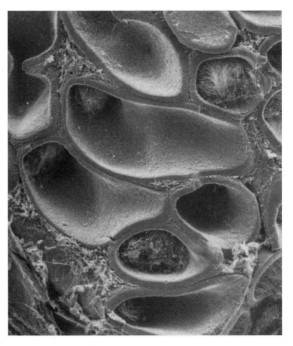

Figure 23.14. SEM in transverse section of highly coiled epididymis. Sperm tails are located in the lumen. (From R. Kessel and R. Kardon, *Tissues and Organs: A Text-Atlas of Scanning Electron Microscopy*, W.H. Freeman, New York, 1979, with permission)

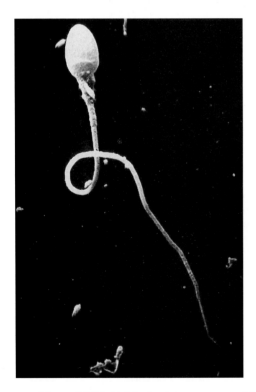

Figure 23.13. SEM of a human sperm. The acrosome and nucleus are located at the top. Midpiece, principal piece, and tail extend posteriorly from the nucleus. ×4620. (From R. Kessel and R. Kardon, *Tissues and Organs: A Text-Atlas of Scanning Electron Microscopy*, W.H. Freeman, New York, 1979, with permission)

spermatids in the adluminal compartment of the seminiferous tubule. This *testicular fluid* contains a high concentration of *ABP* and has a high concentration of K^+ ions but a low concentration of Na^+ ions. Since the haploid primary spermatocytes that have completed meiosis are genetically different from the parent or host, a barrier could prevent foreign proteins associated with the spermatocyte or spermatids from reaching the host's bloodstream and perhaps inducing antibody formation. Genetic recombination can occur during diplotene of prophase I; therefore, antigens could be expressed on the surface of the primary spermatocytes that might potentially cause a self-directed immune response. Since the spermatocytes are segregated to an adluminal compartment, these foreign antigens are restricted from the host's immune cells. In addition, passage of humoral antibodies is restricted from the adluminal compartment by the sealing strands of the barrier so that they would not come into contact with the developing spermatocytes and spermatids.

INTERSTITIAL CELLS OF LEYDIG

Clusters of endocrine cells called the *interstitial cells of Leydig* are located in the connective tissue (septuli testis) between the seminiferous tubules (Fig. 23.6A). These cells contain mitochondria, sER, and lipid droplets characteristic of endocrine-producing cells.

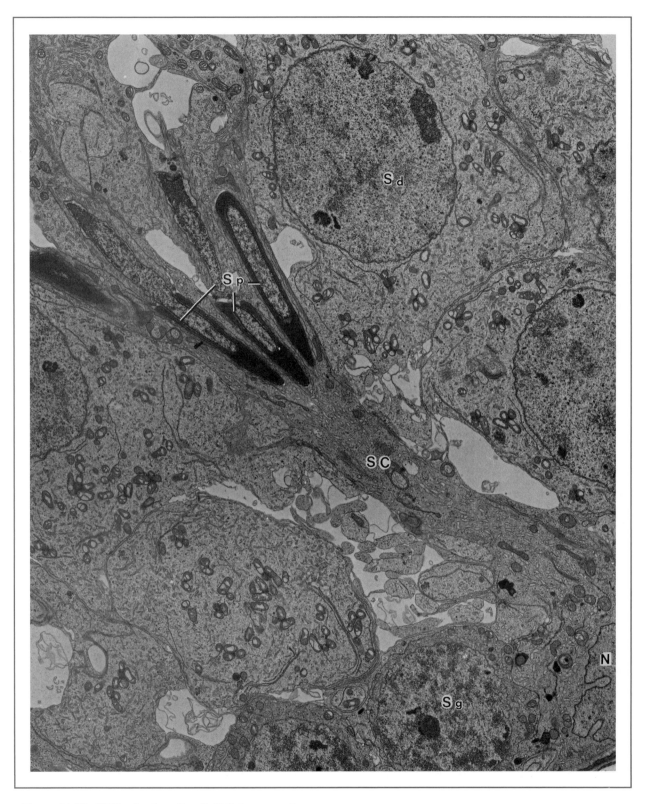

Figure 23.15. TEM of a Sertoli cell (SC) in rat testis. The nucleus (N) is located near the cell base (lower right). Several spermatids (Sp) are invested in a hand-and-glove arrangement at the apical end of the cell. Early spermatids (Sd) and a spermatogonium (Sg) are identified. ×6600. (From R. Roberts, R. Kessel, and H. Tung, *Freeze Fracture Images of Cells and Tissues*, Oxford University Press, New York, 1991, with permission)

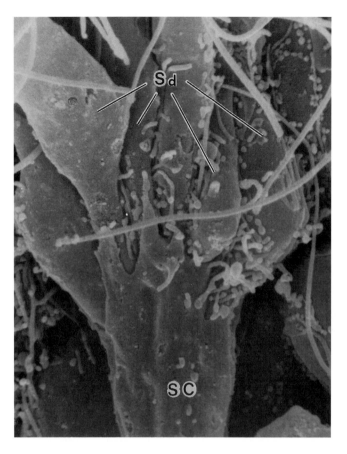

Figure 23.16. SEM of the apical end of a Sertoli cell (SC). Several spermatids (Sd) are closely invested by the apical end of the Sertoli cell. ×1290. (From R. Kessel and R. Kardon, *Tissues and Organs: A Text-Atlas of Scanning Electron Microscopy*, W.H. Freeman, New York, 1979, with permission)

The cells synthesize *testosterone* (Fig. 23.17). These cells develop from mesenchyme. In humans, relatively large crystalloids called the *crystalloids of Reinke* may be located in the cytoplasm of some cells, but their significance is unclear. In response to LH, the interstitial cells of Leydig produce androgens, the principal one being *testosterone*. Testosterone has several important effects, including (1) *stimulation of spermatogenesis*, (2) *stimulation* of *secretion* of *accessory glands*, and (3) *development* of *secondary male sex characteristics*. Both *LH* and *FSH* are necessary for normal spermatogenesis.

TUBULI RECTI AND RETE TESTIS

The *tubuli recti* are connected to the ends of the seminiferous tubules. These small, short tubules are lined with simple cuboidal or columnar epithelial cells that are similar to Sertoli cells. The tubuli recti are continuous with the *rete testis* (Fig. 23.2). The rete testis is lined by simple cuboidal or simple columnar epithelium similar to that in the tubuli recti. The rete testis tubules are located in connective tissue called the *mediastinum testis*.

DUCTULI EFFERENTES

Some 15–20 tubules lead from the rete testis into the head of the nearby epididymis (caput epididymidis) (Fig. 23.2). These tubules are called the *ductuli efferentes* and are lined by a simple epithelium containing cells with different heights. Some cells are tall and have cilia, while others are shorter (Plate 63C). This variation in cell height gives the epithelium a festooned or garland-like appearance. The ciliated cells propel the nonmotile sperm from the seminiferous tubules into the epididymis. The ductuli efferentes represent the only region where cilia are present in the male reproductive tract. The nonciliated cells play a role in absorbing some of the testicular fluid. The epithelium of the tubular ductuli efferentes is surrounded by a basement membrane, circular smooth muscle and elastic fibers, and an outer vascularized layer of loose connective tissue.

DUCTUS EPIDIDYMIDIS

The ductus epididymidis is divided into *head* (caput), *body* (corpus), and *tail* (cauda) regions. The ductuli ef-

Figure 23.17. Diagram of the pathway in testosterone synthesis.

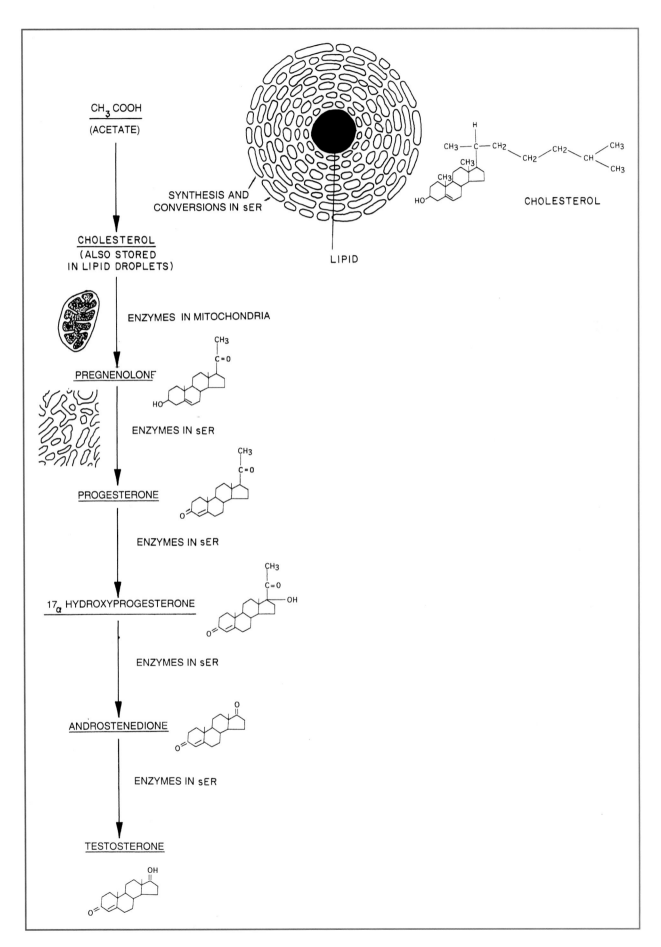

CH₃ COOH
(ACETATE)

SYNTHESIS AND
CONVERSIONS IN sER

LIPID

CHOLESTEROL

CHOLESTEROL
(ALSO STORED
IN LIPID DROPLETS)

ENZYMES IN MITOCHONDRIA

PREGNENOLONE

ENZYMES IN sER

PROGESTERONE

ENZYMES IN sER

17α HYDROXYPROGESTERONE

ENZYMES IN sER

ANDROSTENEDIONE

ENZYMES IN sER

TESTOSTERONE

509

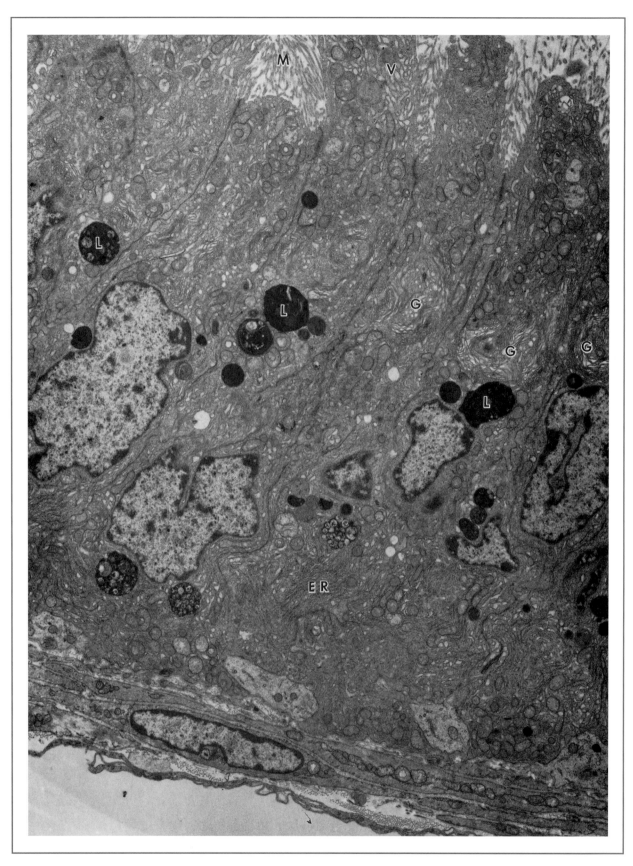

Figure 23.18. TEM of a columnar epithelial cell from the ductus epididymidis. Microvilli (M), Golgi complex (G), lysosomes (L), vesicles (V) and rER are identified. ×5260.

ferentes converge in the head of the ductus epididymidis, and the resulting single tubule becomes highly convoluted and coiled (Plate 64A; Fig. 23.14). The epithelium is pseudostratified columnar, and the cells contain long apical microvilli that are sometimes called *stereocilia* (Fig. 23.18). However, the epididymis and all distal conducting passageways lack true cilia. Prominent sealing strands of circumferential tight junctions are located at the apical ends of adjacent epithelial cells and prevent material from moving from the lumen between the cells. The epithelial cells are both secretory and absorptive (Fig. 23.18). Numerous coated vesicles are associated with the apical cell surface and appear to play a role in absorbing testicular fluid. The epithelium is surrounded by *connective tissue* and *circular smooth muscle*. Although an ABP is produced in the testis by Sertoli cells, it circulates in the testicular fluid into the epididymis.

The spermatozoa that emerge from the testis are stored in the ductus epididymidis. The spermatozoa that enter the epididymis are not motile and are not yet capable of fertilization. These spermatozoa undergo a *capacitation* process in the epididymis before they are capable of fertilization. It is thought that the secretory epithelial cells in the epididymis produce a protein that cause the spermatozoa to become motile and undergo forward motion. The secretions of other accessory glands are also important to the forward motility of the spermatozoa.

DUCTUS DEFERENS (VAS DEFERENS)

The *ductus deferens* (or vas deferens) is a long, thick-walled, muscular tube (Fig. 23.19). The folded mucosa consists of pseudostratified columnar epithelium and a connective tissue lamina propria layer. The epithelial cells typically contain apical, long microvilli called *stereocilia*. The lumen is quite small compared to the wall thickness. A submucosa layer is not well defined, but the muscularis layer is quite thick and consists of three layers of smooth muscle. An extensive network of autonomic nerve fibers innervates this thick, smooth muscle layer, and during ejaculation, peristaltic contractions of the smooth muscle layers conduct the spermatozoa from the epididymis to the urethra.

SEMINAL VESICLE

The paired seminal vesicles are ~5–7 cm in length and empty into the distal end of each ductus deferens (Fig. 23.1). Because the seminal vesicle is such a highly coiled tube, it appears glandular in section (Plate 64D). The tube consists of three layers: an outer connective tissue layer, a middle layer containing circular and longitudinal smooth muscle, and a mucosal layer that is highly folded. The primary folds can branch into secondary and tertiary folds. The epithelium is usually simple columnar but may be pseudostratified columnar, with basal cells scattered throughout the epithelium.

The seminal vesicle secretion constitutes more than half of the volume of semen in an ejaculate. The thick, yellowish secretion provides nourishment for the spermatozoa. The secretion contains significant quantities of fructose, globulins, ascorbic acid, and prostaglandins. The development and normal secretory activity of the seminal vesicles are dependent upon appropriate levels of testosterone in the blood.

Figure 23.19. SEM in Transverse section of the ductus deferens. The small lumen (L) and thick, muscular (M) wall are evident. ×50. (From R. Kessel and R. Kardon, *Tissues and Organs: A Text-Atlas of Scanning Electron Microscopy*, W.H. Freeman, New York, 1979, with permission)

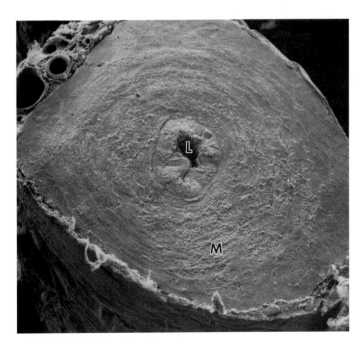

PROSTATE GLAND

The prostate gland surrounds the urethra as it emerges from the bladder (Fig. 23.1). The prostate consists of a number of individual glands (*mucosal, submucosal, main*) that open into the *prostatic urethra* by several excretory ducts (Fig. 23.20). The glands are surrounded by a stroma of connective tissue and smooth muscle (Plate 64B,C). The glands are characterized as *compound tubuloalveolar*. The epithelium consists of tall, simple columnar cells with occasional rounded or basal cells. Under certain physiologic conditions, the epithelium may be pseudostratified or simple cuboidal. The secretory epithelium is extensively folded, and substantial amounts of stored secretion are often present in the lumen of the gland. Calcified concretions may be located within the prostatic lumen in older men (Plate 64B,C). These calcified secretory masses or concretions are called *corpora amylacea*.

Testosterone is important for the development and secretory activity of the prostate. One of the constituents of the prostatic secretion is *acid phosphatase*. The prostatic secretion also contains *fructose, diastase, β-glucuronidase*, several *proteolytic enzymes*, and a potent *fibrinolysin*. Although the function of the acid phosphatase enzyme in the prostate is unclear, an elevated level of this enzyme in the blood has been used in the diagnosis of malignant tumors of the prostate. The growth of some prostatic carcinomas can be slowed by bilateral castration to deprive the carcinoma of androgen. In addition, estrogen has been used to depress the growth of prostatic carcinoma since sufficient estrogen inhibits the release of LH and therefore reduces the testosterone level.

BULBOURETHRAL GLANDS OF COWPER

The glands of Cowper or the *bulbourethral glands* are paired structures, each approximately the size of a pea, and their ducts drain into the proximal portion of the penile urethra (Fig. 23.1). Cowper's glands are *compound tubuloalveolar* and have a connective tissue capsule. Connective tissue septa extend into the gland, and these septa contain elastic fibers, skeletal muscle, and smooth muscle. The epithelium of the gland varies from simple cuboidal to simple columnar, depending upon the secretory cycle of the cells. The epithelial cells contain mucigen granules, and the secretory product contains *mucus* as well as *sialoproteins* and *amino sugars*. The secretion is a clear, viscid product that is released through ducts into the penile urethra during erotic stimulation. The secretion functions as a lubricant for the penile urethra.

PENIS

The penis consists of three longitudinally oriented, cylindrical bodies of erectile tissue covered by epidermis and dermis. The paired dorsal cylindrical bodies of erectile tissue are called the *corpora cavernosa penis*, and they are surrounded by layers of dense collagen fibers that comprise a *tunica albuginea*. The single ventral cylinder of erectile tissue is called the *corpus cavernosum urethrae* or *corpus spongiosum* (Plate 64C,D). The *penile urethra* extends the length of the corpus spongiosum. The corpus spongiosum becomes expanded distally as the *glans penis*. The epidermis and dermis are loosely attached to the penis and at its distal end are modified into a *prepuce*. Modified sebaceous glands (glands of Tyson) are located on the glans penis and on the inner surface of the prepuce. They are unusual since there are no hair follicles associated with them. The epithelium of the *male* urethra is usually stratified columnar, and mucus-secreting *glands of Littré* are associated with the epithelium.

The cavernous bodies of erectile tissue consist of a sponge-like system of irregular, endothelium-lined vas-

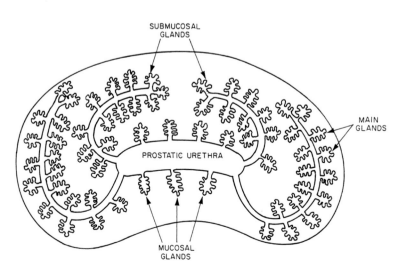

SUBMUCOSAL
GLANDS

MAIN
GLANDS

PROSTATIC URETHRA

MUCOSAL
GLANDS

Figure 23.20. Diagram of the mucosal, submucosal, and main glands comprising the prostate and prostatic urethra.

Regional Functions in the Male Reproductive Tract

Testis	Produce spermatozoa (seminiferous epithelium); *spermatogenesis, meiosis, spermiogenesis*
	Secrete *testosterone* (interstitial cells of Leydig); *inhibin* (Sertoli cells)
	Produce *testicular fluid* with high concentration of *ABP* from Sertoli cells; fluid contains *high K^+, low Na^+* concentrations, *steroid*, and *proteins*
Ductuli efferentes	Both ciliated and nonciliated epithelial cells; ciliated cells assist in moving sperm to epididymis
	Resorption of testicular fluid
Epididymis	Storage and concentration of sperm
	Secretion of protein involved in sperm motility and forward locomotion
	Maturation of sperm (motility and fertility)
Ductus deferens	Storage and concentration of sperm
	Smooth muscle layers provide major motive force for expelling sperm
Seminal vesicles	Secretion is major contributor to semen
	Secretion contains precursors (fibrinogen) for *clotting* of semen
	Secrete fructose to *nourish* ejaculated spermatozoa; secretion also contains *ascorbic acid, globulins*
	Secrete *prostaglandins* that stimulate sperm motility in female reproductive tract
Prostate gland	Secretion contains *alkaline phosphatase, fructose, diastase*
	Alkaline secretion neutralizes acidic vaginal environment
	Involved in clotting of semen to keep sperm in vagina
	Produces enzymes that convert fibrinogen to fibrin
	Fibrin-degrading enzymes (fibrinolysin) in secretion
Bulbourethral gland	Secretes *mucus*, which serves as lubricant for penile urethra and as a protective/nutritive function for sperm
	Sialoproteins and *amino sugars* present in secretion
Glands of Littré	Localized differentiations in epithelium of penile urethra; secrete *mucus*

cular spaces. The trabeculae between the vascular spaces consist of dense fibrous tissue with collagen and elastic fibers, as well as some smooth muscle. The tunica albuginea surrounding the corpora cavernosa penis is much thicker than that surrounding the corpus cavernosum urethrae.

In the flaccid state, blood flows toward the corpora cavernosa in the deep artery of the penis, which has intimal cushions that tend to regulate blood flow. Virtually all of the blood passes directly into an arteriovenous anastomosis that is usually dilated in the flaccid state and connects with efferent veins. Under such conditions, minimal amounts of blood pass into the spaces of the corpora cavernosa. Inside the corpora cavernosa, the deep artery divides into two branches: the *helicine artery*, which empties almost directly into the blood spaces of the erectile tissue, and the *nutritive artery* of the trabeculae, which, after breaking down into a capillary network, re-forms into a small vein and empties into the cavernous space. Cavernous spaces are drained by veins that have *intimal cushions*, and they pierce the tunica albuginea and constitute the efferent venous return. In erection,

blood flow in the deep artery of the penis increases. The opening of the arteriovenous anastomosis is reduced by active vasoconstriction, resulting in a slightly dilated artery passing through the tunica albuginea into the cavernous body. The helicine arteries dilate and the cavernous spaces fill with blood, while the nutritive vessel and its venous junction with the cavernous space become compressed. Blood flow exiting the cavernous body is not reduced despite the internal structure of the emergent veins.

Regional functions in the male reproductive tract are summarized in the accompanying table.

SELECTED BIBLIOGRAPHY

Aumuller, G., and Seitz, J. (1990). Protein secretion and secretory processes in male accessory sex glands. *Int. Rev. Cytol.* **121**, 127–231.

Bearer, E.L., and Friend, D.S. (1990). Morphology of mammalian sperm membranes during differentiation, maturation, and capacitation. *J. Electron Microscopy Tech.* **16**, 281–297.

Braun, R.E., Behringer, R.R., Peschon, J.J., Brinster, R.L., and Palmiter, R.D. (1989). Genetically haploid spermatids are phenotypically diploid. *Nature* **337**, 373–376.

Cooke, B.A., and Sharpe, R.M. (1988). *The Molecular and Cellular Endocrinology of the Testis.* Raven Press, New York.

DeJong, F.H. (1988). Inhibin. *Physiol. Rev.* **68**, 555–607.

Dufau, M.L. (1988). Endocrine regulation and communicating functions of the Leydig cell. *Annu. Rev. Physiol.* **50**, 483–508.

Gehring, U. (1987). Steroid hormone receptors: biochemistry, genetics, and molecular biology. *Trends Biochem. Sci.* **12**, 399–402.

Hafex, E.S.E., and Spring-Mills, E., eds. (1979). *Accessory Glands of the Male Reproductive Tract.* Ann Arbor Science, Ann Arbor, MI.

Holstein, A.F., and Roosen-Runge, E.C. (1981). *Atlas of Human Spermatogenesis.* Grosse Verlag, Berlin.

Jegou, B. (1992). The Sertoli cell. *Bailliere's Clin. Endocrinol. Metab.* **6**, 273–311.

Johnson, M.H., and Everitt, B.J. (1980). *Essential Reproduction.* Blackwell Scientific, Oxford.

Jones, R. (1989). Membrane remodelling during sperm maturation in the epididymis. *Oxford Rev. Reprod. Biol.* **11**, 285–337.

Linder, C.C., Heckert, L.L., Roberts, K.P., Kim, K.H., and Griswold, M.D. (1991). Expression of receptors during the cycle of the seminiferous epithelium. *Ann. N.Y. Acad. Sci.* **637**, 313–321.

Moudgil, V.K., ed. (1988). *Steroid Receptors in Health and Disease.* Plenum, New York.

Plant, T.M. (1986). Gonadal regulation of hypothalamic releasing hormone release in primates. *Endocrinol. Rev.* **7**, 75–88.

Setchell, B.P. (1980). The functional significance of the blood-testis barrier. *J. Androl.* **1**, 3.

Tindall, D.J., et al. (1985). Structure and biochemistry of the Sertoli cell. *Int. Rev. Cytol.* **94**, 127.

Trainer, T.D. (1987). Histology of the normal testis, *Am. J. Surg. Pathol.* **11**, 797.

Turner, T.T. (1991). Spermatozoa are exposed to a complex microenvironment as they traverse the epididymis. *Ann. N.Y. Acad. Sci.* **637**, 364–383.

Glossary

Acetylcholine (ACh). A neurotransmitter released at the myoneural junction that binds to nicotinic acetylcholine receptors to cause contraction; binds to muscarinic acetylcholine receptors in cardiac muscle to slow the heartbeat.

Acidophil. A cell that stains with an acid dye, such as acidophils in the anterior lobe of the pituitary gland.

Acidophilic. Affinity of a cell or cell component for staining with an acid dye such as eosin or light green.

Acinus (pl. acini). A rounded, grape-shaped secretory unit composed of acinar cells; found in a variety of secretory glands such as the pancreas and salivary glands; the term *alveolus* (pl. *alveoli*) sometimes is used as a synonym.

Acrosome. A flattened cap closely applied to the anterior end of a spermatozoon; contains hydrolytic enzymes and facilitates penetration of the egg zona pellucida and egg plasma membrane.

Actin. A globular protein, many subunits of which are organized into thin filaments of muscle and microfilaments in motile, nonmuscle cells.

α-Actinin. An actin cross-linking protein that is present in the Z band or Z disk in skeletal muscle.

Action Potential. An electrical signal involving a wave of depolarization that spreads along the axolemma of nerve cells and the sarcolemma of muscle fibers; involves movements of sodium and potassium ions across these membranes by operation of the sodium-potassium ATP pump, as well as sodium and potassium channels.

Active transport. The energy-requiring pumping of substances such as certain ions, sugars, and amino acids across biologic membranes against a concentration gradient.

Adenohypophysis (anterior lobe). The portion of the pituitary gland that is derived from oral ectoderm and consists of the pars distalis, pars tuberalis, and pars intermedia.

Adenylyl cyclase. An enzyme in the plasma membrane that catalyzes conversion of ATP to cAMP.

Adipocyte. A connective tissue cell type derived from mesenchyme that can store or mobilize fat in response to certain hormones.

Adrenal cortex. The outer portion of the adrenal gland, consisting of three histologically distinct regions: zona glomerulosa, zona fasciculata, and zona reticularis; cells are derived from mesoderm and secrete different kinds of corticosteroids.

Adrenal medulla. The inner portion of the adrenal gland that secretes epinephrine and norepinephrine; derived embryologically from neural crest cells.

Adrenergic receptor. A receptor that binds epinephrine.

Adrenocorticotropic hormone (ACTH). A hormone released from the anterior lobe of the pituitary gland in response to a releasing factor produced by neurons in the hypothalamus; the hormone stimulates cells in the adrenal cortex, principally those in the zona fasciculata and zona glomerulosa, to secrete their products.

Adventitia. An outer covering of certain organs or parts of organs (e.g., most of the esophagus) that consists of loose connective tissue; also the outer layer of connective tissue surrounding arteries and veins.

Afferent. A structure, such as a blood vessel or nerve, that carries materials or an action potential in a central direction, from the periphery inward.

Agranulocyte. A white blood cell that lacks specific staining cytoplasmic granules, such as lymphocytes and monocytes, even though a small population of these cells may contain nonspecific cytoplasmic, azurophilic granules.

Aldosterone. A steroid hormone produced by cells in the zona glomerulosa of the adrenal cortex that stimulates cells in the distal portion of the nephron to conserve sodium by pumping ions back into the bloodstream.

Alveolus (pl. alveoli). Literally "a little hollow," a term used to denote a thin-walled, air-filled sac within the lung; gas exchange occurs between air in the alveolus and nearby capillaries. May also refer to grape-like secretory units comprising compound alveolar glands.

Amacrine cell. An interneuron in the retina that interconnects ganglion cells, thereby promoting or spreading intercellular communication.

Ameloblast (ganoblast). An epithelial cell in a developing tooth that secretes enamel in a polarized direction and results in enamel prisms in the tooth; cells lost at eruption of tooth.

Amino acid. Building blocks for proteins; although there are many different possible types, 20 amino acids are common in proteins; long linear polymers of amino acids are joined head to tail by a peptide bond between the carboxylic acid group of one amino acid and the amino acid group of the next amino acid in the synthesis of proteins.

Ampulla. A localized expansion or dilation of a canal or duct (e.g., the ampulla of a semicircular canal and a semicircular duct in the inner ear).

Ampulla of oviduct. The longest part of the oviducts that connect the infundibulum and isthmus.

Amylase. An enzyme in saliva and exocrine pancreas secretion that catalyzes the hydrolysis of starch into smaller molecules.

Androgen. A male sex steroid hormone such as testosterone.

Androstenedione. A precursor of estrogen; produced, for example, in cells of the theca interna of the developing ovarian follicle.

Angiogenesis. The growth of new blood vessels.

Angström unit. A unit of measure equal to 1/10th of a nanometer, 1/10,000th of a micrometer, or 1/10,000,000th of a millimeter.

Anion. A negatively charged molecule or atom.

Ankyrin. A peripheral protein in the erythrocyte plasma membrane that links spectrin to band III protein, which is an integral membrane protein.

Annexins. A group of calcium-binding proteins involved in the binding of cell membranes.

Antibody. A wide array of Y-shaped molecules with diverse amino acid sequences and binding sites for antigens; antibodies are collectively called *immunoglobulins* and comprise the most abundant blood protein; each distinct antibody has specific amino acid sequences that bind to specific antigens that induce antibody production.

Antigen. A protein, usually unlike any of those present in the body, that is recognized as foreign by immune cells in that body; antigens may induce the formation of specific antibodies that destroy or inactivate the antigen.

Antrum. A cavity in the developing ovarian follicle that increases in size during folliculogenesis; contains a variety of bioactive molecules including glycoproteins, estrogen, oocyte maturation inhibitor, and others.

Apocrine sweat gland. A type of sweat gland consisting of a coiled tubular gland located in the armpits and anogenital areas, that produces an odoriferous secretion; ducts open into hair follicles, not involved in temperature regulation.

Apoptosis. A type of programmed cell death.

Aqueous humor. A fluid present in the posterior and anterior chambers of the eye; secreted by inner, nonpigmented epithelium of the ciliary processes; circulates from the posterior chamber through the pupil into the anterior chamber and exits the eye by way of the trabecular meshwork and canal of Schlemm into the anterior ciliary veins.

Areolar glands of Montgomery. Modified sweat glands that open onto the surface of the mammary gland.

Arrector pili. Smooth muscle that extends from the undersurface of epidermis to the lower part of a hair shaft in the dermis; when muscle contracts, the hair follicle tends to be elevated; cold may cause reflexive contraction of large numbers of these muscles and may result in "goose bumps."

Arteriole. The smallest division of arteries in the vascular system; vessels are usually less then 10 μm in diameter and have one to three layers of smooth muscle in their walls; incomplete relaxation may result in hypertension.

Astral spindle microtubules. Microtubules that radiate from centrioles of the centrosome at the spindle poles toward the plasma membrane during mitosis.

ATP. Adenosine triphosphate, a molecule that serves as a source of energy for cellular activities that require energy. Approximately 7300 calories per mole of energy reside in the phosphate bond, which are released during the hydrolysis of ATP to ADP.

Atresia. The death of ovarian follicles, which may occur throughout the reproductive life of a female; can occur at any stage of follicle development; in antral follicles, granulosa cells may become pyknotic and float in the follicular liquor of the antrum; eventually replaced by ovarian stroma; cause unclear but seems to occur in follicles with maximum luteinizing (LH) receptors at a time when blood LH levels are low.

Atrium (auricle). A chamber of the heart; the right atrium receives venous blood from the body; the blood then passes into the right heart ventricle, to be pumped to the lungs, where the blood is oxygenated; oxygenated blood in the pulmonary veins returns to the left atrium or auricle and then to the left ventricle, to be pumped throughtout the body.

Auerbach's plexus. The autonomic nervous innervation of the muscularis layer of the digestive tract; consists of preganglionic terminals, postganglionic nerve cell bodies, and postganglioinc fibers of the parasympathetic division and postganglioinic fibers of the sympathetic division of the autonomic nervous system.

Autocrine. A situation in which a cell secretes a substance that acts on itself to effect a response.

Autonomic nervous system (ANS). Includes the efferent innervation of smooth muscle, glands, and the heart; consists of two divisions, the parasympathetic or cranial-sacral outflow division and the sympathetic or thoracolumbar division; the two divisions are antagonistic in their actions.

Axon. The process extending from the cell body or perikaryon of a neuron that generally carries impulses away from the nerve cell body.

Axoneme. The tubular constituents of a cilium or flagellum, which include nine peripheral doublet microtubules and a central pair of microtubules.

Axoplasmic transport. The movement of materials through an axon; movement may be anterograde (toward the axon ending) or retrograde (toward the cell body); the rate of movement may be variable, including a slow stream and a fast stream, or intermediate.

Azurophilic granules. A cytoplasmic granule present in promyelocytes, some myelocytes, and a small percentage of circulating neutrophils, lymphocytes, and monocytes; granules stain with methylene azure, hence their name; granules contain lysosomal enzymes and peroxidase.

B-Lymphocyte. A nongranular leukocyte of blood derived from the bone marrow. When appropriately stimulated by or introduced to a specific molecule (antigen) that it can recognize (involving helper T lymphocytes and macrophages in many cases), these cells proliferate (B lymphoblasts) and produce memory B lymphocytes and numerous antibody-producing plasma cells.

Barr body. One of the X chromosomes in the female that does not uncoil at the end of mitosis.

Basal body. A tubular organelle consisting of nine peripheral triplet tubules in the form of a cyclinder or barrel that is connected at one end to the proximal end of a cilium or flagellum.

Basal lamina. A differentiation of the cell coat at the base of epithelial cells (visible by TEM) that consists of a lamina lucida adjacent to the plasma membrane and an outer thin lamina densa; the basal lamina contains molecules (e.g., laminin, fibronectin, entactin-nodogen, and type IV collagen) that are synthesized by the epithelial cell (Schwann cells, endothelium, and muscle fibers also produce a basal lamina); the epithelium-produced basal lamina, in conjunction with type III collagen produced by adjacent connective tissue fibroblasts, comprises a layer (agyrophilic, PAS positive) called the *basement membrane* that is visible in LM preparations.

Basal striations. Fine vertical striations that may be evident in the basal region of certain columnar epithelial or gland cells with high magnification (oil immersion) using the LM; image due to many basal infoldings of the plasma membrane and associated mitochondria that are present among these infoldings; the plasma membrane and its molecules (including sodium pumps) are increased or amplified for transport in this region, and mitochondria provide the necessary energy for the active transport.

Basalis. A thin portion of the endometrium adjacent to the myometrium; this layer is not shed or lost during menstruation because it has a blood supply different from that of the thicker functionalis layer, which is shed during menstruation; the basalis regenerates the shed functionalis during the proliferative or estrogenic phase of uterine endometrial activity following menstruation.

Basement membrane. A thin layer applied to the basal surface of epithelial cells that consists of a basal lamina produced by the epithelial cells and a lamina fibroreticularis composed of reticular fibers produced by connective tissue fibroblasts. This layer anchors epithelium to connective tissue; it also surrounds Schwann cells and muscle fibers.

Basilar membrane. A resonant structure in the membranous cochlea on which the organ of Corti resides; it consist of scleroprotein fibers with bipolar epithelial cells associated with the undersurface adjacent to the scala tympani.

Basket cell. A myoepithelial cell associated with secretory alveoli and small ducts (as in salivary glands, mammary glands, sweat glands and ducts); cells are primitively contractile and may serve to move secretory contents.

Basophil. A cell or substance within a cell that stains with basic dyes such as hematoxylin.

Bile. A fluid secreted by hepatocytes into bile canaliculi that join to form bile ducts, which convey bile to the gallbladder for concentration; concentrated bile is then released into the common bile duct, which enters the duodenum, where bile is involved in emulsification of fats.

Bile canaliculus. A small intercellular channel between adjacent hepatocytes into which bile is secreted and through which bile is transported to bile ducts in portal areas of the liver lobules.

Blastocyst. A very small mammalian embryo approximately 3–4 days after fertilization; stage at which implantation usually occurs.

Bowman's capsule. A two-layered structure in the renal corpuscle consisting of simple squamous epithelium intimately associated with the glomerulus; the two layers are an outer parietal layer and an inner visceral layer; the space between the two layers is called the *urinary space.*

Brunner's glands. Mucous secreting glands in the submucosa of the duodenum; open into the base of crypts of Lieberkuhn; bicarbonate in secretion helps to neutralize gastric acid entering the duodenum; secretion also contains urogastrone, which is a peptide that inhibits secretion of hydrochloric acid and stimulates epithelial cell proliferation.

Calcitonin. A hormone secreted by parafollicular or C cells scattered throughout the thyroid gland; inhibits osteoclast activity, thereby lowering the blood calcium level.

Callus. A firm, bone-like substance that covers the ends of a fractured bone during its healing.

Calmodulin. A calcium-binding protein that mediates many effects of calcium ions.

Capacitation. A physiologic maturation process in which spermatozoa acquire fertilizing capacity and the ability for forward locomotion; occurs principally in epididymis.

Cardiac muscle fiber. A cellular, contractile unit of cardiac muscle containing myofibrils and centrally located nucleus; fibers may branch; some cells may be binucleate.

Catecholamine. A class of neurosecretory material that includes dopamine, norepinephrine, and epinephrine; may constitute a type of neurotransmitter.

Caveolae. Small depressions or invaginations in the plasma membrane; may pinch off the plasma membrane, as occurs in a type of endocytosis called *micropinocytosis*, or may be rather permanent, such as the permanent pits of smooth muscle cell plasma membrane.

CD4. A plasma membrane glycoprotein that, in conjunction with a receptor on a T cell, binds helper T cells and antigen-MHC II complexes.

CD8. A plasma membrane glycoprotein that acts in conjunction with T-cell antigen receptors to bind killer T cells and antigen-MHC I complexes.

Cell membrane. Bimolecular layer of lipids with which integral and peripheral membrane proteins are associated; mediates the interaction of the cell with its environment; appears as a trilaminar structure with TEM and has a total width ranging from 7.5 to 9 nm; also called the *plasma membrane* or *plasmalemma*.

Cementum. A substance that surrounds the dentin or that portion of the tooth residing in its socket; consists of cell-free and cellular cementum with cementocytes much like osteocytes; collagen fibers (fibers of Sharpey) embedded in cementum anchor the tooth in the socket.

Central vein (venule). A venule located in the center of hepatic lobules in the liver; plates of hepatocytes and intervening sinusoids radiate from the central venule to portal areas at the apices of the lobule; blood flows through sinusoids to the central venule.

Centriole. A cylindrical- or barrel-shaped organelle consisting of nine triplet tubules; two closely positioned centrioles (a diplosome) at right angles to each other are located in the juxtanuclear cytocentrum; may have microtubule-associated proteins and a diffuse, amorphous material located in close proximity; paired centrioles divide prior to mitosis, and pairs migrate to opposite poles of the future spindle.

Centroacinar cell. A cell located in the center of secretory units (acini) in the exocrine pancreas; does not stain and represents initial duct cells (intercalated duct) connected to the secretory units.

Centromere. Region of a chromosome that attaches DNA to the mitotic spindle.

Chemically gated channels. Integral membrane channel proteins that open when a molecule such as a neurotransmitter binds to a specific receptor or channel protein, as in the postsynaptic membrane of a synapse.

Chief cell. The principal cell type in a gland (organ); examples include chief cells in parathyroid and chief (zymogenic) cells in the stomach.

Cholecystokinin. A peptide hormone produced by enteroendocrine cells in the intestinal glands of the duodenum and jejunum; causes gallbladder contraction after ingestion of fats; stimulates secretion of pancreatic digestive enzymes and enterokinase.

Cholesterol. A steroid that is widely distributed in animal cells and used in plasma membranes and in the synthesis of such steroids as sex steroids and adrenal corticosteroids.

Chondroblast. A young cartilage-forming cell derived from mesenchyme cells that is active in the synthesis of the constituents of cartilage matrix.

Chondrocyte. A more mature cartilage cell that is usually less active in the formation of cartilage matrix than the chondroblast but important in the maintenance of the matrix.

Choriocapillaris. Small blood vessels (capillaries) in the inner portion of the choroid layer of the eye adjacent to Bruch's membrane and the pigmented epithelium of the retina; the basal lamina of the endothelial cells of the choriocapillaris comprises only one layer of Bruch's membrane.

Chorionic gonadotropin (human, hCG). A glycoprotein produced shortly after implantation of the embryo by syncytiotrophoblast cells; has LH activity, so corpus luteum continues to produce progesterone until the fetal placenta begins progesterone production.

Choroid. A middle tunic of the eye between the retina and sclera; consists of connective tissue with pigment and is highly vascularized; anteriorly, the choroid is continuous with the ciliary body and iris; collectively these structures comprise the uvea of the eye.

Chromaffin cells. Neurosecretory cells that stain with chromaffin salts and are located in the adrenal medulla; are formed from neural crest cells in embryonic development; produce epinephrine or norepinephrine.

Chromophobe. A cell type in the anterior lobe of the pituitary gland that does not stain with most stains, such as H&E; functional significance is uncertain, but may represent reserve cells or a chromophil cell that has lost its cytoplasmic granules.

Chromosomal spindle microtubules. Microtubules that extend from centrioles of spindle poles to attach to chromosomal kinetochores.

Chromosome. A structural unit containing DNA located in the nucleus of eukaryotic cells and the basis for heredity; there are 46 chromosomes in humans; histones in a precise form and other proteins are associated with the paired helical strands of DNA.

Chyme. The acidic content that exits from the stomach into the duodenum.

Cilium. A long, slender structure, usually motile, that extends from the basal body; it consists of nine peripheral doublet microtubules and two central ones; during movement of cilium, ciliary doublets slide past each other; their movement is powered by ATP/ATPase associated with the paired dynein arms extending between ciliary doublets; cilia move in metachronal waves; some cilia may be nonmotile, especially a single cilium on some cells and cilia comprising modified dendrites of sensory cells (e.g., bipolar neurons in the olfactory epithelium).

Circumvallate papilla. Large, circular structures located at the sulcus terminalis at the base of the tongue that contain many taste buds; serous glands of von Ebner flush the vallum around the papilla.

Cisternae. Membrane-bound, flattened sacs comprising the rER, sER, and Golgi apparatus.

Clara cell. A nonciliated, dome-shaped cell found in the epithelium of the terminal bronchiole; its secretory product may be a component of surfactant.

Collagen. Widely distributed fibrous protein; rich in glycine, hydroxylysine, and hydroxyproline; secreted by fibroblasts; comprises the main fibrous element of loose connective tissue, tendons, and ligaments.

Collagenous fibers. Acidophilic, connective tissue fibers 1–20 μm wide, visible with LM; consist of fibrils ranging from 0.3 to 0.5 μm wide.

Collecting duct. A large duct in the uriniferous tubule into which the nephrons drain.

Colloid. A viscous glycoprotein material produced by thyroid follicle cells and stored in the lumens of the follicles. When follicle cells are stimulated by thyroid-stimulating hormone, cells endocytose the colloid and break the colloid down into triiodothyronine T_3 and T_4 (thyroxine), which are released into capillaries at cell base.

Columnar epithelium. A simple epithelium containing cells whose height exceeds both their length and their width; line the stomach and small intestine, where some cells may be differentiated into goblet cells (unicellular mucous glands) for amplification of mucous secretion.

Compact bone. Bone that appears solid when grossly examined but consists of microscopic channels (haver-sian and Volkmann canals) containing blood vessels; usually organized into haversian systems as well as outer circumferential lamellae, inner circumferential lamellae, and interstitial lamellae; located in shafts of long bones and in plates of skull bones.

Complement. A series of enzymatic proteins in normal blood serum that interact with antigen-antibody complexes to produce lysis when the antigen is an intact cell; when complement is activated, neutrophils are attracted and become phagocytic.

Cone. One type of retinal photoreceptor that is involved in color vision, bright light vision, and visual acuity; concentrated in the fovea centralis and macula lutea.

Confocal microscope. A microscope with which one can focus on a selected plane in a thick specimen and eliminate any illumination that comes from out-of-focus areas above or below the selected plane; thus one can visualize images, including fluorescent molecules, in a single focus plane, which gives much sharper images.

Confocal scanning microscope. A fluorescence light microscope that permits focusing of an illuminating beam in a single plane within a specimen, thus eliminating adverse effects of specimen thickness.

Cords of Billroth. One component of the red pulp of the spleen; the other is the splenic sinusoids. The red pulp cords contain many erythrocytes and other cells of the circulating blood; macrophages abound and remove worn-out red blood cells; is a place for blood storage; cells can easily pass between cells of the sinusoidal walls.

Corona radiata. Referring to the granulosa follicle cells that immediately surround the zona pellucida of the primary oocyte.

Corpora cavernosa penis. Paired dorsal cylindrical bodies of erectile tissue (endothelium-lined vascular spaces) in the penis.

Corpus luteum. A large cell mass formed from the components of the Graafian follicle after ovulation of the oocyte and cumulus mass; it is a large, yellowish, highly vascularized cellular mass that produces progesterone to maintain the progestational uterine endometrial phase; some estrogen is also produced.

Corpus spongiosum. A single ventral cylinder of erectile tissue that contains the penile urethra.

Cortical sinus. System of spaces in the cortex of a lymph node that contains reticular cells, macrophages, and lymph; is continuous with the subcapsular sinus and medullary sinus of the lymph node.

Cortisol (hydrocortisone). An adrenocorticosteroid hormone produced by cells in the zona fasciculata of the adrenal cortex; regulates carbohydrate and protein metabolism; promotes gluconeogenesis; used as an anti-inflammatory.

Crista ampullaris. Three neurosensory areas located in the wall of the membranous ampullae of the semicircular canals; concerned with angular acceleration and deceleration.

Cristae. Foldings of the inner mitochondrial membrane into the matrix; may be tubular, vesicular, or shelf-like in form; increase the surface of inner membrane subunits that generate ATP.

Crown. That portion of the tooth above the gum.

Cryps of Lieberkuhn (intestinal glands). Simple tubular glands in the mucosa or mucous membrane of the small and large intestines; lined by simple columnar epithelium containing many goblet cells, Paneth cells, enteroendocrine cells, and basal proliferative cells.

Cuboidal epithelium. An epithelium in which the closely packed cells are equal in length, width, and height; comprise the lens epithelium, pigmented epithelium of retina, choroid plexus epithelium, and thyroid gland follicles, for example.

Cumulus oophorus. Granulosa cells that surround and suspend the oocyte into the antrum of a tertiary or Graafian follicle.

Cyclic amp. A nucleotide that acts as a second messenger in certain signaling pathways; may act by activating protein kinase A.

Cyclins. A group of proteins that activate protein kinases involved in progression through the cell cycle.

Cytokinesis. That portion of cell division in which cytoplasmic division results in the separation of one cell into two; may involve a contractile ring of actin-containing microfilaments; usually follows nuclear division (karyokinesis).

Cytoplasm. That portion of a eukaryotic cell that consists of organelles, formed elements, and cytosol.

Cytoskeleton. Tubular (microtubules) and fibrillar (intermediate filaments, actin-containing microfilaments) elements that support internal cell structures and maintain (and sometimes alter) cell shape.

Dendrite. In a multipolar neuron, a number of thin cytoplasmic extensions that conduct impulses toward the cell body of the neuron.

Dense irregular connective tissue. A type of connective tissue usually consisting of collagen fibers that have a variety of orientations in a connective tissue sheet; fibers more irregular in orientation than those of dense regular connective tissue.

Dense regular connective tissue. A type of connective tissue usually consisting of collagen (white fibers) but can include elastic fibers (yellow elastic) that are closely packed, with similar parallel orientation, as occurs in tendons and ligaments.

Dentin. A hard, mineralized substance that comprises the majority of the tooth; formed by odontoblasts and contains dentinal tubules; covered by enamel and cementum.

Dermis (corium). A dense, irregular connective tissue layer that underlies the epidermis; a component of the integument; derived from mesoderm.

Desmosome (spot desmosome, macula adherens). A type of intercellular junction that plays an important role in holding cells together, as in cells in the stratum spinosum of epidermis; consists of keratin intermediate filaments that loop into electron-dense plaques adjacent to the plasma membrane; also includes transmembrane linkers and several cell adhesion molecules.

Diastole. Phase of heartbeat during which the left ventricle relaxes; time when blood is pumped to the body but not the lungs.

Distal convoluted tubule. Portion of uriniferous tubule that connects the loop of Henle with the collecting duct; provides active transport of Na^+ from filtrate to interstitium; NH_3 ions excreted here.

Diploid. The $2n$ number of chromosomes; in human somatic cells, this number is 46.

DNA. Deoxyribonucleic acid arranged in a double helix with base pairing of nucleotides (uridine, cytidine, guanosine, adenine); the genetic material comprising the chromosomes.

Ductus deferens (Vas deferens). A thick-walled, muscular tube that propels spermatozoa from the ducts of the epididymis to the urethra.

Dust cell. Name sometimes used for a pulmonary alveolar macrophage.

Dynein arm. An ATPase that takes the form of small projections from the microtubule doublets of the ciliary axonemes; provides motive force for ciliary movement.

Dystrophin. A protein associated with the inner surface of the sarcolemma that can result in muscular dystrophy when altered.

Early endosome. A membrane-bound structure resulting from endocytosis of material; located close to the plasma membrane; has H^+-ATPase for acidifying contents; some constituents may be recycled back to the plasma membrane via transport vesicles.

Eccrine sweat gland. A coiled tubular gland derived from epidermis of the integument; consists of a secretory portion and a duct portion; the duct opens onto the surface of the integument; functionally associated with temperature regulation.

Efferent. A nerve process, blood vessel, or duct that conveys a nerve impulse or product toward the periphery.

Elastic cartilage. A type of cartilage in which matrix contains elastic fibers that give flexibility to the cartilage; found in the pinna of the ear, for example.

Elastic fiber. A type of connective tissue fiber containing the protein elastin; is able to recoil after being stretched; elastic fibers are present in the aorta, elastic cartilage, and certain ligaments.

Elastin. A protein in the elastic fibers containing the amino acids desmocine and isodesmocine.

Electrophoresis. A technique in which charged molecules are separated by an electric field applied to gels made of polyacrylamide or agarose.

Endocardium. The lining of the auricles and ventricles of the heart; the innermost layer of the heart, consisting of endothelium as well as a thin layer of loose connective tissue.

Endochondral (intracartilaginous) ossification. A type of bone formation in which hyaline cartilage models of future bones are slowly eroded and replaced by bone, but continued growth is made possible by a proliferating plate of cartilage until growth is complete.

Endometrial (uterine) glands. Tubular glands in the endometrium of the uterus; also called *uterine glands.*

Endometrium. The inner layer of the uterus, divided into a thicker, functionalis layer and a basalis layer adjacent to the myometrium; the functionalis layer is shed at menstruation, to be regenerated by the basalis layer; layer of the uterus in which the blastocyst implants.

Endomysium. A thin connective tissue sheath that surrounds each muscle fiber in a muscle; conveys blood vessels and nerves.

Endoneurium. A thin connective tissue sheath that surrounds individual axons in a nerve.

Endoplasmic reticulum (ER). A membranous cytoplasmic organelle that may be coated with polyribosomes, called the *granular* or *rough-surfaced ER,* or that may lack attached ribosomes, called the *agranular* or *smooth-surfaced ER.*

Endorphins. Peptide hormones that inhibit pain in the nervous system by binding to opiate receptors on the neurons.

Enkephalins. Peptide neurotransmitters that inhibit pain-signaling neurons by binding to opiate receptors.

Enteroendocrine cells. Cells in the gastric and intestinal glands that produce a variety of substances such as secretin, gastrin, cholecystokinin, and serotonin, for example.

Enzyme. A protein that is capable of producing or accelerating by catalytic action a change in a substrate for which it is specific.

Eosinophil. A type of granular leukocyte that may be capable of phagocytizing antigen-antibody complexes; contains specific eosinophilic (acidophilic) granules that contain lysosomal enzymes, histaminase, aryl sulfatase; the eosinophil number is elevated in parasitic infections.

Ependyma cells. Ciliated cells that line the ventricles of the brain and the central canal of the spinal cord.

Epicardium. The outermost layer of the heart; consists of fibroelastic connective tissue that is covered externally by a single layer of mesothelium; the layer is continuous with the tunica adventitia of attached vessels.

Epidermis. The stratified squamous (keratinized) layer of the integument that is derived from ectoderm and covers the dermis of the integument; can give rise to hair follicles, sebaceous glands, sweat glands, and nails.

Epididymis (ductus epididymidis). A long, coiled tube that is divided into a head (caput) region, a body (corpus) region, and a tail (cauda) region that conveys sperm from the efferent ductules to the vas deferens; secretion is important for acquisition of forward motiltiy by spermatozoa (capacitation).

Epinephrine. Also called *adrenaline;* a catecholamine released by the adrenal medulla; a transmitter in the sympathetic nervous system; causes increased heart rate, increased respiration, and breakdown of glycogen to glucose in liver.

Epineurium. A connective tissue sheath that surrounds an entire nerve such as the brachial or sciatic nerve.

Epiphyseal plate. A persistent plate of hyaline cartilage in a developing bone that is responsible for continued growth in the bone through interstitial growth; disappears when growth is completed.

Epitope. That part of an antigen that is capable of eliciting its specific immune response.

Erythrocyte. A red blood cell or corpuscle that is filled with iron-containing hemoglobin that reversibly binds oxygen and carbon dioxide; binconcave disc; enucleate in mammals.

Erythropoietin. A hormone produced in the kidney that stimulates differention of erythrocytes.

Estradiol. A form of estrogen that is most potent.

Estrogen. A female steroid sex hormone.

Euchromatin. Lightly staining chromatin in the interphase nucleus; it represents those chromosomes or portions of chromosomes that become uncoiled after mitosis; usually the form of chromatin in more active cells.

Exocytosis. The process in which secretory granules or other cell products are discharged from a cell; an energy-requiring process.

Extracellular matrix. Includes the fibrous and amorphous intercellular substances synthesized and exported by cells.

F_0. Membrane proteins of mitochondria that anchor F_1 particles to the inner mitochondrial membrane; also serve as a proton channel for ATP synthase.

F_1 particle. Protein subunits of the inner mitochondrial membrane that contain ATP-synthase for phosphorylating ADP to ATP.

Facilitated diffusion. Solute transport across cell membranes in which the solute transported moves down an electrochemical gradient; involves membrane transport proteins; does not require energy.

Fallopian tube. A synonym for the oviduct; is open at one end close to the ovary, to which the ovulated egg and cumulus mass become attached in preparation for a journey through this tube, which connects with and opens into the body of the uterus.

Fascicle. A general term denoting a bundle, as in the case of a muscle bundle (fascicle) or nerve bundle (fascicle); fascicles are surrounded by a connective tissue layer called the *perimysium* (muscle) or *perineurium* (nerve).

Fast axonal transport. Refers to rapid movement of vesicles in an anterograde direction guided by microtubules.

Fenestrated capillary. A capillary that contains openings or fenestrations that facilitate rapid transport of materials across the capillary wall; located in, for example, the adrenal cortex, glomerular capillary, sinusoidal endothelium of the liver, and other locations.

Fiber. A long, slender structure or cell such as a muscle fiber or nerve fiber or a process of it; may refer to products made and exported by cells, such as collagen, elastic, and reticular fibers.

Fibril. A thinner structure that may make up a larger fiber; for example, collagen fibers are composed of smaller fibrils.

Fibroblast. A connective tissue cell derived from mesoderm that is able to synthesize collagen fibers, elastic fibers, and reticular fibers, as well as the amorphous components (glycosaminoglycans and proteoglycans) of connective tissue intercellular substance.

Fibrocartilage. A type of hyaline cartilage in which numerous collagen fibers are present in the cartilage matrix; this type of cartilage (as in intervertebral disks) may result when collagen fibers of tendons and ligaments insert into the cartilage of intervertebral disks; fibers tend to cause alignment of chondrocytes in rows; no true perichondrium.

Fibronectin. A glycoprotein in the extracellular matrix; fibronectin occurs in the basal lamina of epithelial cells and binds to fibronectin receptors in the plasma membrane; important in cell migration.

Fila olfactoria. Long, slender dendrites of bipolar olfactory neurons that are modified cilia; axons of neurons form the olfactory nerve.

Filiform papillae. Slender, pointed projections of the mucous membrane on the dorsum of the tongue.

Flagellum. A long, motile structure similar to a cilium and attached to a basal body at one end; movement is by a whip-like motion; provides motility for spermatozoa, for example.

Fluorescence microscope. A type of microscope that permits visualization of fluorescent substances in cells, including fluorescent-labeled antibodies and fluorescent stains.

Follicle cells. Cells surrounding the primary oocyte that multiply during folliculogenesis; also called *granulosa cells*; divided into membrana granulosa cells and cumulus oophorous (discus proligerus) cells in the late antral follicle; membrana granulosa cells surround the antrum, while cumulus oophorous cells surround and suspend the oocyte into the antrum.

Follicle-stimulating hormone (FSH). A hormone synthesized and released from a population of basophils (gonadotrops) in response to gonadotropin-releasing hormone (GnRH), which is made in neurons in the hypothalamus and which travels in a pituitary portal system to the anterior pituitary to exert it effect on gonadotrops; hormone causes folliculogenesis in the ovary.

Follicular fluid. The fluid, also called *liquor folliculi*, that accumulates in the antrum during folliculogenesis.

Fovea centralis. A thin region or depression of the retina that contains a concentration of cones involved in color vision and visual acuity.

Functionalis. The layer of the uterine endometrium that is shed at menstruation; consists of uterine stroma, uterine glands, and blood vessels; the narrower basalis layer of the endometrium regenerates a new functionalis layer that is complete prior to ovulation.

Fungiform papillae. Rounded projections of the epithelium and lamina propria on the dorsum of the tongue; may have a few taste buds in epithelium.

G proteins. A group of membrane-associated, GTP-binding proteins that play a role in signal transduction.

Ganglion. A region of concentration of nerve cell bodies outside the central nervous system; examples include dorsal root ganglia, autonomic ganglia, and cranial (parasympathetic) ganglia.

Gap junction (nexus, communicating junction). A specialized region between adjacent cells in which the intercellular space is only about 3 nm and containing connexons, consisting of pore-like hexagonal subunits aligned from one cell to another and permitting small ions and molecules (less than 1200 D) to move from one cell to a neighboring cell.

Gastric gland. A simple tubular or branched tubular gland of the gastric mucosa; contains chief cells that secrete enzymes, parietal cells that secrete hydrochloric acid, mucus-secreting cells, and enteroendocrine cells.

Gastric juice. The fluid produced by the gastric mucosa that is released into the stomach cavity; includes digestive enzymes, hydrochloric acid, and mucus.

Gastric pits. Invaginations of the gastric mucosa continuous with the gastric gland; also called *foveolae*; lined by simple columnar epithelial cells that secrete mucus.

Gastrin. A hormone secreted by enteroendocrine cells in the pyloric stomach mucosa; stimulates secretion of gastric acid and pepsin; weakly stimulates pancreatic enzymes and gallbladder contraction.

Gene. A nucleotide sequence in a DNA molecule that produces an RNA molecule to encode a polypeptide chain.

Germinal center. The central region of a lymphatic nodule in the lymph node, tonsils, or spleen in which B lymphocytes enlarge into B lymphoblasts and divide to produce many progeny; some may become B memory cells, while others may differentiate into plasma cells; macrophages and reticular cells may also be present in the germinal center of a lymphatic nodule.

Germinal epithelium. The covering epithelium of the ovary, once believed to be the source of germ cells for the ovary; forms a layer of squamous follicle epithelial cells for the germ cells that migrate into the ovarian cortex from other sources.

Glands of Tyson. Modified sebaceous glands located on the glans penis and inner surface of the prepuce.

Glomerular filtrate. The ultrafiltrate of blood that passes through the fenestrated endothelium, glomerular basement membrane, and filtration slit diaphragms into the urinary space and proximal convoluted tubule.

Glomerulus. A tuft of capillaries interposed between the afferent and efferent arterioles in the kidney; capillaries are invested by cells called *podocytes*, which comprise the visceral layer of Bowman's capsule of the renal corpuscle.

Glucagon. A hormone produced by alpha cells in the pancreatic islets of Langerhans that causes glycogen in the liver to be transformed into glucose, which enters the bloodstream; acts antagonistically to insulin; elevates blood glucose level.

Gluconeogenesis. Synthesis of carbohydrates from lipids.

Glycogen. The major storage form of sugar.

Glycoprotein. A substance composed of protein and carbohydrate joined together.

Goblet cell. A modified epithelial cell that synthesizes and exports the glycoprotein mucus; an example of a unicellar gland cell; the apical end of the cell is rounded and often filled with mucigen granules; the cell narrows toward the base.

Golgi apparatus (Golgi complex). An organelle that consists of stacked, flattened saccules enclosing a small cisterna or space, as well as many small, membrane-bound Golgi vesicles; involved in certain glycosylation reactions (glycosyl transferase enzymes), in carbohydrate synthesis, and in joining of the carbohydrate to protein made in the rER and sent to the Golgi; also involved in packaging of lysosomal enzymes and in both regulated and constitutive secretion.

Graafian follicle. A mature ovarian follicle that has completed folliculogenesis and is ready for ovulation;

when the oocyte is ovulated with its cumulus mass, the remaining theca and granulosa cells of the follicle become a yellow body (corpus luteum), an endocrine gland that produces progesterone and some estrogen.

Granulocyte. A leukocyte in the blood that contains specific staining cytoplasmic granules identifiable with LM; includes neutrophilic, eosinophilic, and basophilic granular leukocytes.

Granulosa cell. Follicle cells that surround the oocyte during folliculogenesis; divided into membrana granulosa cells around the antrum and cumulus oophorus (discus proligerus) cells that invest and suspend the oocyte in the antrum.

Growth hormone. Also called *somatotropin* or *somatotropic hormone*; a protein hormone secreted by a population of acidophils in the anterior pituitary in response to releasing hormone made by neurons in the hypothalamus; promotes general body growth.

Haploid. A condition in which one-half (23) of the normal chromosome number is present; occurs in mature spermatozoa and ova after oogenesis and spermatogenesis; when the egg is fertilized by the spermatozoon, the diploid chromosome number is reestablished.

Hassal's corpuscle. Structure usually found in the medulla of the thymus; consists of keratin and keratohyalin surrounded by epithelial-reticular cells derived from endoderm; although characteristic of the thymus, its functional significance is unclear.

Haversian system. Also called an *osteon*; located in compact bone; consists of a central haversian canal with a blood vessel and endosteum surrounded by concentric layers of bone matrix with osteocytes in lacunae; osteocyte processes in small canals called *canaliculi* in adjacent orbits may touch; bone matrix in the haversian system contains collagen fibers with different orientation to increase the strength of bone.

Helper T cell. A type of T lymphocyte that is activated by binding to antigen-MHC II complexes; after activation, helper T cells may activate B cells and killer T cells.

Hemoglobin. The iron-containing protein that fills the fully differentiated erythrocyte.

Hemosiderin. An insoluble protein produced during the intracellular digestion of erythrocytes by macrophages.

Heparin. An anticoagulant that is present in many mast cell granules.

Hepatic artery. A branch of the abdominal aorta that conveys oxygenated blood to the liver; branches of this artery convey blood to the sinusoids in liver lobules.

Hepatocyte. The principal cell comprising the parenchyma of the liver; organized into plates surrounding a central venule; performs a multitude of important functions.

Heterochromatin. The darkly staining chromatin in the interphase nucleus; represents those chromosomes or portions of chromosomes that do not uncoil appreciably after mitosis.

Histamine. A constituent of mast cell granules; can cause vasodilatation, bronchial constriction, and increased capillary permeability.

Histones. Nuclear proteins that have an important role in the orderly packing of the DNA double helix; have a role in gene activity.

Holocrine secretion. A type of secretion in which the entire cells, with their secretory product, are released, as is the case for sebaceous glands.

Horizontal cell. A cell in the retina that interconnects adjacent photoreceptors.

Howship's lacuna. A localized depression in the surface of bone containing a multinucleate osteoclast that resorbs bone locally; the term *resorption bay* is a synonym.

Hyaline cartilage. The most abundant form of cartilage, consisting of chondroblasts, chondrocytes, and cartilage matrix surrounded by a fibrocellular sheath called the *perichondrium*; this type of cartilage occurs in the trachea, costal cartilages, bronchi, articular surfaces of joints, and other places; in addition, most of the bones of the body begin as small hyaline cartilage models before ossification occurs.

Hydrolysis. A process in which complex substances are cleaved or digested into smaller molecules; hydrolytic enzymes in lysosomes hydrolyze or digest substances ingested into cells.

Hyperopia. Farsightedness or refractive deviation resulting when the axial length of the eye is decreased by a single millimeter.

Hyperpolarized. A condition in which negative ions, such as chloride ions, may enter the axolemma at the synapse, increasing the electronegativity of the interior and thus making the neuron more difficult to fire.

Hypophysis cerebri. A synonym for the pituitary gland.

Hypothalamic-hypophyseal portal circulatory system. A network of capillaries that begin and end as veins; by means of this system, hormones released by neurons of the hypothalamus travel to the anterior pituitary and cause specific cells to release their hormone.

Immunoglobulin. Proteins that may be located in all body fluids that function as specific antibodies and are responsible for the humoral aspects of immunity.

Implantation. The attachment and erosion of the blastocyst (early embryonic stage of development) into the highly secretory progestational endometrium approximately 6–7 days after ovulation and fertilization.

Inner nuclear layer. A layer of the retina (layer 6) that contains the nuclei and cell bodies of the bipolar neurons; also contains nuclei of amacrine and horizontal cells in the retina.

Inner plexiform layer. A layer of nerve cell processes (layer 7) of the retina that consists of axons of bipolar neurons and dendrites of ganglion cells.

Inner segment. That portion of the rod or cone cell that contains the mitochondria and rER; it is connected to the outer segment by a narrow stalk that contains a modified cilium.

Inositol triphosphate (IP$_3$). A second messenger that under appropriate conditions can cause the release of calcium ions from ER vesicles into the cytosol.

Insulin. A hormone produced by beta cells in the islets of Langerhans that reduces the blood sugar level by facilitating passage of glucose into cells.

Interalveolar pores of Kohn. Pores or interruptions in the interalveolar septa of the lung that permit or facilitate passage of air between adjacent alveolar ducts.

Interalveolar septum. The thin wall that separates alveoli of adjacent alveolar ducts; includes epithelium of air sacs, basement membranes, and endothelium of capillaries; narrow diffusion distance between air in alveoli and capillaries in alveolar septa.

Intercalated disk. The boundary between adjacent cardiac muscle cells; stains with Heidenhain's iron hematoxylin in LM preparations; with TEM, this differentiated region includes a fascia adherens (where many actin microfilaments of muscle cell insert into plasma membrane), gap junctions, and spot desmosomes.

Intercalated duct. The smallest of the intralobular ducts in a compound gland at the attachment to the secretory cells of an acinus; usually constructed of low cuboidal epithelium.

Interferons. Lymphokines that can activate killer T lymphocytes; inhibit viral replication.

Intermediate junction. Also known as a *zonula adherens*; a junctional complex that completely invests adjacent epithelial cells at the apical end; thought to play a role in cell adhesion.

Internal elastic lamina. A rather thick but fenestrated elastic membrane forming the inner extent of the tunica intima of blood vessels adjacent to the tunica media.

Interstitial cells (of Leydig). Large cells occurring in clusters in the connective tissue (septuli testis) of the testis; cells synthesize testosterone; contain large quantities of sER, mitochondria, and lipid droplets; cells synthesize testosterone in response to LH.

Interstital fluid. Tissue fluid located in interstitial spaces surrounding cells, fibers, and amorphous intercellular substances.

Interstitial gland cells. Appear to be derived from the theca interna cells of developing follicles that have undergone atresia; cells make androgen for use by granulosa cells in producing estrogen.

Intramembranous ossification. A type of ossification (bone formation), as occurs in the flat bones of the vault of the skull; does not involve hyaline cartilage models; mesenchyme cells in richly vascularized area transform into osteoblasts and begin to secrete bone matrix and collagen fibers as spicules that become calcified.

Islets of Langerhans. Nearly 1 million clusters of endocrine cells concentrated in the tail of the pancreas; contain several cell types; the most numerous are the glucagon-producing alpha cells and the insulin-producing beta cells.

Isoform. A closely related set of polypeptide chains.

Juxtaglomerular cells. Modified smooth muscle cells in the wall of the afferent arteriole of the kidney; contain acidophilic-staining granules that contain renin and erythropoietin.

Karyotype. A preparation that illustrates the paired chromatids of all chromosomes in somatic cell of an organism.

Keratin. A tough albuminoid protein that forms a waterproof layer of the body; two types of keratin exist; soft keratin in skin desquamates, but hard keratin in nails and hair does not desquamate and therefore must be trimmed.

Keratinocyte. The most numerous type of cell in the epidermis of the integument; transforms into a nonliving cell called a *corneocyte* filled with keratin.

Keratohyalin granules. Basophilic-staining granules of soft keratin in cells of the stratum granulosum layer of the epidermis; keratohyalin granules interact with tonofilaments in the cells to form keratin.

Killer T cells. A type of T lymphocyte that plays an important role in cell-mediated immunity; killer T cells can recognize other cells with foreign antigens on their surface (like virus-infected cells) and kill these cells by causing cell lysis.

Kinesin. A motor molecule (ATPase) that moves organelles or particles toward the (+) end of microtubules; energy derived from ATP hydrolysis.

Kupffer cell. A stellate phagocytic cell that is present in the sinusoids of the liver.

Lacteal. A large lymphatic capillary that arises in the core of villi in the small intestine.

Lacuna (pl. lacunae). A small space or cavity such as bone lacunae in which osteocyte cell bodies reside.

Lamina cribrosa. A region of the eye where optic nerve fibers exit through fenestrated layers of collagen fibers in the sclera.

Lamina propria. A layer of connective tissue comprising the inner mucous membrane or mucosa layer of the tubular digestive tract; contains fibroblasts, plasma cells, mast cells, macrophages, collagen fibers, blood vessels, nerves, and lymphatics; located between the epithelial layer and muscularis mucosa of the mucosa.

Late endosome. A membrane structure similar to an early endosome but located close to the Golgi complex; also has ATP-driven H^+ pumps in the membrane; more acidic than the early endosome; may become mixed with acid hydrolases and transform into lysosome.

Lens. A biconvex, transparent structure consisting of highly elongate lens fibers (cells) that is held in place in the eye by a system of zonule filaments and brings images into focus on the retina.

Ligament. A band of connective tissue fibers (collagen, elastin) and fibrocytes that connects bones or cartilages and connects adjacent bones in a joint and vertebrae in the vertebral column; supports and strengthens joints.

Ligaments of Cooper. Elastic fibers that attach the breast to the integument.

Ligaments of Zinn (zonule fibers). Suspensory ligaments that connect at one end with the lens capsule at its equator and at the other end with the pars plica and pars plana of the ciliary body.

Limbus. The region of the junction of the cornea and sclera in the eye.

Limbus spiralis. The medial margin of the membranous cochlear duct; extends two lateral projections, an upward projection called the *vestibular lip* and a lower projection called the *tympanic lip.*

Lipase. An enzyme that hydrolyzes fats.

Lipids. Amphipathic molecules of three main types: phospholipids, cholesterol, and glycolipids; membrane lipids have hydrophilic and hydrophobic constituents.

Lipofuscin pigment granules. Membrane-bound pigment granules that represent remains of lyosomes called *residual bodies* filled with indigestible material; also called *aging pigment;* found in a variety of cells including neurons.

Liquor folliculi (follicular fluid). The fluid that initially appears in Call-Exner vacuoles of the secondary ovarian follicle and that accumulates in a large antrum in the growing and mature follicle; lost at ovulation.

Littoral cell. A sinus-lining cell in the lymph node and bone marrow.

Lobule. Structure comprising lobes of glands; consists of secretory units and intralobular ducts; surrounded by connective tissue of interlobular septa; examples occur in salivary glands, pancreas, and liver.

Loop of Henle. A hairpin loop of the uriniferous tubule that connects the proximal and distal convoluted tubules; consists of thick and thin descending and ascending portions.

Luteinizing hormone (LH). A hormone secreted by basophils in the anterior pituitary in response to LHRH;

causes ovulation and stimulates development of a corpus luteum after ovulation from the remains of the ovarian follicle.

Lymphoblast. A large mitotic cell that may be either a B lymphoblast or a T lymphoblast; results when a T or B lymphocyte that has been stimulated by the appropriate antigen and MHC molecules enlarges, divides, and differentiates appropriately.

Lymphocyte. An agranular leukocyte that lacks specific cytoplasmic granules; a small percentage may contain a few azurophilic granules; includes bone marrow-derived lymphocytes (B lymphocytes), thymus-derived lymphocytes (T cells), or NK cells.

Lymphokines. Substances released by activated lymphocytes that stimulate monocytes and macrophages.

Lysosome. A membrane-bound organelle that contains acid hydrolases; can fuse with and destroy ingested material (heterophagy) or senescent intracellular organelles (autophagy).

Lysozyme. An enzyme that can kill bacteria by destroying their cell walls; produced by Paneth cells, macrophages, and other cells.

M phase promoting factor (MPF). A very large protein with two subunits, one of which is a protein kinase; triggering of MPF requires synthesis of a protein called cyclin.

Macrophage. A large, usually migratory cell that is phagocytic, may ingest particulate material, and may also ingest, digest, and present antigen together with MHC molecules for the activation of certain T cells, such as T helper cells.

Macula sacculi. A localized neurosensory region in the sacculus that helps to promote static equilibrium, acts as a sensor of gravity and linear acceleration.

Macula utriculi. A localized neurosensory region in the utriculus that functions in static equilibrium, a sensor of gravity, and linear acceleration.

Mast cell. A large connective tissue cell type usually filled with cytoplasmic granules; granules may contain heparin, histamine (involved in anaphylactic shock), the slow-reacting substance of anaphylaxis (SRS-A), and an eosinophilic chemotactic factor (ECF-A); the cell surface has receptors with an affinity for IgE.

Medulla. The central region of an organ such as the medulla of the kidney, the adrenal medulla, or the medulla of the ovary.

Medullary rays (of Ferrein). Close aggregations of collecting ducts and ascending and descending limbs of the loop of Henle that extend into the cortex from the medulla of the kidney.

Megakaryocyte. A large cell containing a large nucleus that is lobated; located in bone marrow and forms blood platelets.

Meiosis. A process involving two cell divisions, one of which has a complex prophase that results in a reduction division during which the number of chromosomes is reduced by one-half in the formation of eggs and sperm; the diploid chromosome number is restored when the egg and sperm fuse (fertilization).

Meissner's corpuscle. A type of mechanoreceptor located in the dermis and some mucous membranes that is a tactile or touch receptor.

Meissner's plexus. Autonomic innervation of the smooth muscle in the muscularis mucosa layer of the digestive tract; consists of postganglionic fibers of postganglionic neurons of the sympathetic division and the preganglionic fibers and postganglionic cells and fibers of the parasympathetic division of the ANS.

Melanin. A pigment produced by melanocytes that provides color to the skin, hair, and eyes.

Melanocyte. A cell that can synthesize melanin using amino acid tyrosine; in epidermis cells are derived from the neural crest.

Menarche. The beginning of puberty, marked by the initiation of menstruation.

Merkel cell. A type of cell in the epidermis of the integument that is thought to function as a mechanoreceptor.

Meromyosin. Results when the myosin molecule is subjected to tryptic digestion; results in two parts of the molecule: a light meromysin fragment and a heavy meromysin fragment.

Mesenchyme. The middle layer of the embryo derived from mesoderm and forming a packing between the endoderm and ectoderm; gives rise to elements of the connective tissue.

Mesothelial cell. A simple squamous epithelial cell; in connection with a thin layer of loose connective tissue, the layer is called a *serosa* and forms a thin external layer for most of the digestive tract and certain other organs.

Metaphase. A stage of mitosis in which chromosomes become aligned on the equatorial plate prior to separation and migration to opposite poles at anaphase.

Microfilaments. A filament approximately 7 nm in diameter composed of the protein actin; important constituent of the cytoskeleton involved in cell motiltiy.

Micrometer (μm). A unit of measure formerly called the *micron*; equals 1/1000th of a millimeter; now replaced by the term *nanometer*, which is 0.1 micrometer (i.e., 100 Å = 10 nm).

Microtubule. A tubular organelle ~25 nm in diameter constructed of protein tubulin; the wall of the microtubule contains 13 protofilaments consisting of an α,β tubulin heterodimer; forms spindle microtubules and cytoplasmic microtubules that are important components of the cytoskeleton; involved in development and maintenance of cellular asymmetry and may direct intracellular movements.

Microtubule-organizing center. Structures such as the centrosome that initiate microtubule assembly.

Microvilli. Finger-like projections from the apical surface of many epithelial cells; contain a complex internal structure of actin microfilaments and other proteins; greatly amplify the plasma membrane locally for enhanced numbers of important molecules involved in transport and other processes.

Mineralocorticoids. A class of adrenal corticosteroid hormone produced by cells in the zona glomerulosa; the major mineralocorticoid is aldosterone, which is secreted in response to renin release by juxtaglomerular cells in the kidney; aldosterone promotes sodium resorption in the kidney and increases blood pressure.

Mitochondria. An organelle consisting of two membranes, the inner one of which is usually folded into shelves or cristae; contains Kreb's cycle enzymes; electron transport and oxidative phosphorylation are coupled to the phosphorylation of ADP to form ATP; thus the mitochondria are the "powerhouses" of the cell.

Monocyte. A circulating agranular leukocyte comprising 3–8% of the leukocytes; usually enters the tissues and transforms into a macrophage.

Morula. An embryonic stage consisting of many cells just prior to the blastula stage.

Motor end plate (myoneural junction). An effector structure consisting of a sensory nerve that ends in relation to a specialized region of the sarcolemma of a muscle fiber; a "synaptic region" between nerve and a muscle.

Motor neuron. An efferent (effector) nerve cell; the cell body is isolated in the gray matter of the CNS; axon extends through a peripheral nerve to innervate muscle fibers, glands, and epithelium.

Mucosa (mucous membrane). The inner layer of many tubular organs; consists of three layers: an inner epithelium, a middle lamina propria of connective tissue, and an outer layer of smooth muscle called the *muscularis mucosa*; the epithelial layer in some organs (e.g., stomach, intestine) may be modified into glands.

Mucous neck cell. A type of epithelial cell in gastric glands of the stomach that secrete mucus.

Mucus. A glycoprotein secretory product that is produced by goblet cells and mucous gland cells (*mucous* is the adjective form).

Müller cell. A highly branched, neuroglia-type cell that is widespread in the retina; has many processes that form an interlinking network among the neural cells in the retina; functional roles unclear; may have nutritive and other functions.

Multinucleate. A condition in which a cell has more than one nucleus.

Muscarinic acetylcholine receptor. A receptor for ACh that causes potassium channels to open, permitting potassium to exit the cell and hyperpolarizing the plasma membrane.

Muscle fiber. In striated skeletal muscle, a long, isodiametric structure, usually 1–2 mm in length, with many nuclei (multinucleate) located just inside the sarcolemma or plasma membrane of the muscle fiber.

Muscularis mucosa. A layer of the mucosa usually consisting of two layers of smooth muscle: an inner circular one and an outer longitudinal one; in the stomach, three layers may be present in the muscularis mucosa; layer permits independent movements of the mucosa.

Myeloid tissue. A type of hemopoietic (bone-forming) tissue represented by the red (active) bone marrow.

Myoblast. A cell that can form a muscle fiber by the fusion of many myoblasts; can synthesize actin and myosin myofilaments and other proteins.

Myocardium. The middle muscular layer of the heart; the thickest layer of the heart, located between the inner endocardium and the outer epicardium.

Myoepithelial cell. An epithelial cell that is highly branched, contains contractile filaments, and surrounds secretory alveoli and the smallest ducts (intercalated ducts) of certain glands; the cell surrounds the secretory alveolus the way a hand surrounds a baseball.

Myofibril. A unit of structural organization within the muscle fiber; appears as numerous "dots" in transverse sections of muscle fibers with the LM; with the TEM, the myofibril contains a large (variable) number of actin and myosin myofilaments.

Myofilament. Constituents of the myofibril of muscle; actin thin myofilaments are approximately 7 nm in diameter and 1 μm long; myosin thick myofilaments are about 15 nm in diameter and 1.5 μm long.

Myometrium. The thick middle muscular layer of the uterus.

Myopia. Nearsightedness that occurs if the axial length of the eye is increased by only a single millimeter.

Myosin. The principal protein comprising the thick filaments in the A band of striated muscle (skeletal and cardiac).

Myosin light chain kinase. An enzyme that phosphorylates myosin in smooth muscle cells, which is necessary for the myosin-actin interaction (contraction) in smooth muscle.

Myotube. An early stage in the formation of a muscle fiber; results from the fusion of many myoblasts end to end.

N-linked glycosylation. The addition of sugar chains to amino groups of asparagine in proteins.

Nephron. That part of the uriniferous tubule in the kidney that consists of a renal corpuscle and a complex tubular portion.

Neurofilaments. Filamentous components in the axoplasm of neurons that are approximately 10 nm diameter and represent the intermediate filaments of nerve cells.

Neuroglia. Nonnervous cells in the nervous system; exist as protoplasmic and fibrous astrocytes, oligodendroglia, and microglia; play a variety of functional roles in nervous tissue.

Neurohypophysis (pars nervosa). That portion of the pituitary gland derived from a downgrowth of the diencephalon in the embryo; contains many nerve processes of neurons located in the hypothalamus; these neurons secrete vasopressin and oxytocin which travel along the axons to blood vessels in the pars nervosa, where they are released into the circulation.

Neuron. A nerve cell, the fundamental unit of nervous tissue; the basic unit of information that is transmitted throughout the nervous system is an action potential; the cell consists of a cell body (perikaryon) and usually several branches called *dendrites* and a single axon.

Neurosecretory cell. A nerve cell that synthesizes and releases a product (possibly a hormone) from its axon; examples include neurosecretory cells in the hypothalamus and adrenal medullary chromaffin cells.

Neurotransmitter. A chemical released at the synapse that affects the ion permeability of the postsynaptic cell or membrane; examples include norepinephrine, acetylcholine, glycine, GABA, and others.

Neutrophil (polymorphonuclear leukocyte). The most numerous of the white blood cells; usually contains a lobated nucleus of three to five lobes; contains specific cytoplasmic granules called *neutrophilic granules* that contain bactericidal substances permitting destruction of ingested bacteria.

Nissl substance. Stacks of rER in the perikaryon of a neuron that stain as basophilic clumps (Nissl substance) in the LM.

Node of Ranvier. Interruptions in the myelin sheath along a myelinated nerve process (axon); in saltatory conduction of nerve impulses, ion changes occur in the region of the nodes.

Norepinephrine. A hormone produced by some cells in the adrenal medulla; this catecholamine may also be a neurotransmitter in postganglionic synaptic regions of the sympathetic nervous system.

Nuclear envelope. An organelle characteristic of the eukaryotic cell that consists of an inner membrane closely associated with a nuclear lamina, an outer membrane that may contain ribosomes and be continuous in places with the rER, and complex apertures called *nuclear pores* or *nuclear pore complexes.*

Nuclear lamina. A thin, homogeneous layer of lamins attached to the inner nuclear membrane; consists of lamins, which form a meshwork of intermediate filaments; phosphorylation of serine residues on lamins causes reversible disassembly at mitosis.

Nuclear matrix. An insoluble structural skeleton in the nucleus that is important in arranging DNA into an organized configuration.

Nuclear pore. A complex region in the nuclear envelope through which substances may exit or enter the nucleus; proteins are imported into the nucleus from the cytoplasm, and ribonucleoprotein is translocated into the cytoplasm from the nucleus (requires energy).

Nucleolar organizer (secondary constriction). A region of chromosomal DNA that encodes for ribosomal RNA; in humans, located on chromosomes 13, 14, 15, 21, and 22.

Nucleolus. An organelle in the nucleus formed by the nucleolus-organizing region(s) of specific chromosomes; ribosome subunits for cytoplasmic ribosomes are synthesized in the nucleolus.

Nucleosomes. DNA-protein particles that are the unit particles of chromatin.

Nucleus. A portion of the eukaryotic cell that contains the chromosomes (DNA and histones), nucleolus (ribosome formation), nuclear lamina (involved in chromosome attachment and breakdown of nuclear envelope at mitosis), and proteins comprising the nuclear matrix.

O-linked glycosylation. Process occurring in the Golgi apparatus in which some proteins have sugars added to OH groups of selected serine or threonine side chains; catalyzed by a series of glycosyl transferase enzymes; sugars added to a protein sequentially; usually N-acetylgalactosamine is added, followed by other sugars (ranging from only a few to a dozen or more).

Odontoblast. A cell derived from the cranial neural crest that synthesizes and secretes dentin in a polarized fashion; dentin is a calcified matrix that comprises most of the tooth; in the adult, odontoblasts line the pulp cavity.

Olfactory bulb. The expanded dendrite portion of an olfactory neuron, from which modified cilia extend into the nasal cavity.

Olfactory cilia. Cilia that extend from olfactory neurons in the olfactory epithelia; modified dendrites; cilia lack the two central microtubules and are not motile; membranes of cilia contain odor receptors.

Olfactory nerve. The first cranial nerve; formed by the axons of olfactory neurons in the olfactory epithelium in the upper portion of the nasal cavities; axons extend to the olfactory region of the brain.

Oligodendroglia (oligodendrocyte). A type of branched neuroglia cell that produces myelin for myelinated nerves in the CNS; each oligodendrocyte can myelinate a portion of several nerve processes.

Oocyte. A name for the immature female germ cell; primary oocyte designation during meiosis I, secondary oocyte designation in meiosis II.

Optic nerve. The second cranial nerve that is formed from the axons of ganglion cells in the retina.

Ora serrata. The anteriormost extent of the retina.

Organ of corti. The neurosensory area in the cochlear duct that is responsible for hearing; consists of innervated "hair" cells and supporting cells that reside on a resilient basilar membrane.

Osmosis. Movement of a solvent through a semipermeable membrane from a region of lesser solute concentration to a region of greater solute concentration.

Osteoblast. A bone-forming cell that actively synthesizes and exports the organic constituents of bone matrix, i.e., collagen and sulfated protoglycans and other proteins; when trapped by the product of its secretion, it becomes an osteocyte with long processes and bone production ceases.

Osteoclast. A large, multinucleate cell that digests bone matrix; activated by parathyroid hormone, inactivated by calcitonin; resides in depressions of bone (called *resorption bays* or *Howship's lacunae*), and the plasma membrane is folded in this region; cells contain many lysosomes for digesting bone matrix by both extracellular and intracellular means.

Osteocyte. A bone cell that is completely trapped by bone matrix and is inactive in bone matrix formation.

Osteoid. Newly secreted bone matrix next to an osteocyte that has not yet become calcified and therefore lacks hydroxyapatite crystals.

Outer nuclear layer. A layer of closely packed nuclei of photoreceptor cells (rods and cones) in the retina.

Outer plexiform layer. A layer of nerve cell processes in the retina that contains synaptic terminations of the photoreceptors with the dendrites of the bipolar neurons.

Outer segment. A portion of the rod and cone photoreceptor that consists of many flattened, membranous sacs or disks in which the visual pigment is located.

Ovary. One of the paired female reproductive organs in which germ cells mature (folliculogenesis) and from which ovulation occurs; may also contain a corpus luteum or corpus albicans.

Ovulation. The process by which the oocyte and surrounding cumulus mass rupture through the ovarian surface to be received by the fimbriated lips of the oviduct; caused by luteinizing hormone (LH).

Oxidative phosphorylation. Process in which ATP synthesis is coupled to electron transport in the respiratory chain, which is mediated by an electrochemical proton gradient during electron transfer.

Oxytocin. A hormone produced by neurons in the hypothalamus that is released from the pars nervosa; causes milk letdown and contraction of the uterine endometrium.

Pacinian corpuscle. A large, spherical mechanoreceptor located in the dermis of the integument and in other places in connective tissue; a deep pressure receptor.

Pancreatic duct. The main duct (duct of Wirsung) that conducts secretions of the exocrine pancreas to the duodenum; the minor pancreatic duct is the duct of Santorini.

Paneth cell. A cell located in the base of the crypt of Leiberkuhn; contains eosinophilic-staining granules containing lysozyme and zinc; may phagocytize certain microorganisms.

Paracrine. A condition in which a cell releases a substance that diffuses and acts on nearby cells.

Parafollicular (C) cell. Individual cells or cell clusters distributed throughout the thyroid, but not a part of the follicles; derived from the neural crest; produce calcitonin (thyrocalcitonin), which shuts down osteoclast activity, thereby lowering the blood calcium level.

Parasympathetic nervous system. A part of the ANS; called the *cranial sacral outflow* since the preganglionic neurons have their origin in the brain stem and sacral region of the spinal cord; cholinergic endings; increases contractility of smooth muscle in gut (peristalsis).

Parathyroid gland. Usually includes four small glands embedded in the connective tissue covering the posterior surface of the thyroid gland; consists of chief and oxyphil cells; chief or principal cells produce parathyroid hormone when the blood calcium level is lowered; acts indirectly to cause increased bone resorption and thus raise the blood calcium level.

Parietal cells (oxyntic cells). Large, eosinophilic cells in the gastric glands; contain the intracellular canaliculus and numerous mitochondria; secrete hydrochloric acid and gastric intrinsic factor.

Parietal layer. The outer layer of two-layered structures; examples include the parietal pleura (an inner visceral pleura is also present) and the parietal layer of Bowman's capsule in the renal corpuscle (an inner, visceral layer of Bowman's capsule also exists).

Parotid gland. Pair of compound alveolar salivary glands located anterior to the ears; produces a serous type of secretion.

Pars distalis. Comprises the largest part of the anterior pituitary or adenohypophysis; consists of cells (acidophils, basophils, chromophobes) and well-vascularized connective tissue; cells synthesize a number of hormones, including growth hormone, prolactin, luteinizing hormone (LH), follicle-stimulating hormone (FSH), thyroid-stimulating hormone (TSH), and adrenocorticotropic hormone (ACTH).

Pars intermedia. A narrow region of the pituitary gland between the pars distalis and the pars nervosa; is not well developed in humans; consists of a row of fluid-filled follicles.

Pars tuberalis. An upward extension of the pars distalis of the pituitary gland.

Pedicel. A terminal or foot process of a podocyte; pedicels of different podocytes interdigitate and surround or invest the capillary tuft of the renal glomerulus in Bowman's capsule; thin slits between adjacent pedicels are filtration slits.

Pepsin, pepsinogen. The inactive proenzyme pepsinogen is secreted by chief cells in the gastric glands of the stomach; acid in the stomach converts the inactive pepsinogen into the active proteolytic enzyme pepsin.

Perforin. A protein produced by T killer cells that causes pores in the target cell and results in its death.

Perichondrium. A fibrous layer consisting of dense collagen fibers and fibroblasts that surround hyaline and elastic cartilage (except for articular cartilage at joints); an inner layer of the perichondrium may contain immature chondrogenic cells with the potential to become chondroblasts and secrete new cartilage matrix on the surface (appositional growth).

Perikaryon. The cell body of a neuron contains a nucleus (and nucleolus), Golgi complexes, rER (Nissl substance), lysosomes, centrioles, neurotubules, and neurofilaments; dendrites and single axon connected to the neuronal perikaryon.

Periodontal ligament. A ligament consisting of collagen fibers that anchor the tooth in its socket; collagen fibers insert in bone at one end and into the cementum of the tooth root at the other end.

Periosteum. A fibrocellular membrane surrounding bone; consists of an outer fibrous layer of collagen fibers and fibrocytes and an inner layer of osteogenic cells with the potential to become osteoblasts and form new bone on the surface of preexisting bone (appositional growth).

Peripheral nervous system. Portion of the nervous system consisting of paired cranial and spinal nerves that connect the CNS to the periphery.

Peristalsis. The process by which food is moved through a muscular tube such as the intestine; occurs by the alternate contraction and relaxation of circular and longitudinal smooth muscle bands in the muscularis externa of the digestive tract.

Peroxisome. A membrane-bound organelle, as in liver and kidney cells, that may contain a central crystalline nucleoid containing urate oxidase; other enzymes that may be present include *d*-amino acid oxidase, α-hy-

droxy-acid oxidase involved in production of hydrogen peroxide, and catalase, which is involved in destruction of hydrogen peroxide; in plants called *glyoxysome* and may play a role in conversion of fat to carbohydrate.

Peyer's patches. A region of the ileum of the small intestine in which a number of lymphatic nodules are present in the submucosa layer.

Phagocytosis. A type of endocytosis in which rather large pieces of particulate material such as bacteria may be ingested into a cell.

Phalangeal cells. Supporting cells for the inner and outer hair cells located in the organ of Corti; also called *Deiter's cells.*

Phospholipase C. An enzyme that cleaves phosphatidylinositol biphosphate into inositol triphosphate and diacylglycerol.

Pigmented epithelium. A layer of simple cuboidal epithelial cells in the retina that contain melanin that reflects light; cells are intimately associated with the tips of photoreceptors and phagocytize and digest worn-out membranous disks from the tips of the photoreceptors.

Pillar cells. Inner and outer pillar cells reside on the basilar membrane of the organ of Corti and enclose the tunnel of Corti; they are supporting cells.

Pinocytosis (micropinocytosis). A form of endocytosis, which means "cell drinking on a small scale"; material in the plasma membrane pits pinch off as an isolated vesicle in the cytosol.

Pituicytes. A type of supporting neuroglia cell that is present in the pars nervosa and closely surrounds the axons from neurosecretory neurons in the hypothalamus.

Placenta. A highly vascular organ, composed of both maternal and fetal portions, that provides for interchange of nutrients and gases between the mother and fetus via the extensive vascular system.

Plasma. The fluid portion of the blood, exclusive of erythrocytes, leukocytes, and platelets.

Plasma cell. An immunoglobulin-producing cell that contains extensive rER and results from the stimulation of a B lymphocyte by an appropriate antigen; produces humoral (circulating) antibodies associated with the humoral immune response.

Platelet. A biconvex disk, 2–3 μm in diameter, produced by megakaryocytes in the bone marrow; approximately 250,000 per cubic millimeter of blood; involved in blood clotting.

Platelet-derived growth factor. A proteinaceous growth factor that stimulates proliferation of connective tissue and smooth muscle cells.

Plicae circulares (valves of Kerckring). Permanent folds of the mucosa and submucosa of the small intestine; increase the surface area for digestion and absorption.

Pneumocyte II (septal cell, great alveolar cell). An epithelial cell in the wall of the alveoli of the lung with lamellar bodies containing dipalmitoyl lecithin or pulmonary sufactant that is released to coat the alveolar surface of the epithelium; alveolar surfactant reduces surface tension (therefore reducing required inspirational force) and permits easier inflation of the lung alveoli.

Podocyte. The name given to the visceral layer of Bowman's capsule because the cells are highly branched; have primary, secondary, and tertiary processes or pedicels; pedicels interdigitate with those of adjacent cells and form the filtration slits that cover the glomerular capillary.

Polar spindle microtubules. Microtubules that extend from opposite poles and overlap in the metaphase plate region during mitosis.

Polysaccharide. A carbohydrate that can be hydrolyzed into two or more monosaccharides; the major storage polysaccharide of animal cells is glycogen.

Portal triad. Also called a *portal tract, area,* or *radicle;* denotes regions at the apices of the polygonal portal lobule, which contains branches of the hepatic artery, hepatic portal vein, bile duct, and a lymphatic vessel.

Portal vein. A vein that originates in capillaries and breaks down into capillaries; portal veins are present in the liver and pituitary gland, for example; capillaries in the digestive tract form the hepatic portal vein, which travels to the liver to break down once again into a multitude of branches communicating with hepatic sinusoids or capillaries.

Predentin. The most recently secreted, uncalcified dentin released by odontoblasts; predentin is calcified after it is secreted and becomes dentin.

Primary follicle. An early stage of ovarian follicle development in which the primary oocyte is surrounded by one layer of simple squamous follicle cells (inactive primordial follicle) or a single layer of cuboidal or columnar epithelial cells (activated primary follicle).

Primary spermatocyte. A stage in the process of spermatogenesis when spermatogonia located in the basal compartment of the seminiferous tubule initiate meiotic prophase; they move through circumferential tight junctions between Sertoli cells and become located in the adluminal compartment of the seminiferous tubule; primary spermatocytes divide in a reduction division to produce secondary spermatocytes, which immediately divide mitotically to form spermatids.

Principal cell. The most widespread cell within a gland; for example, the principal cell in the parathyroid gland, which secretes parathyroid hormone.

Progesterone. A steroid hormone secreted by granulosa lutein cells in the corpus luteum; the hormone acts on the endometrium of the uterus to cause secretion of uterine glands for possible implantation of an early embryo; depresses follicle-stimulating hormone (FSH) so that folliculogensesis is prevented.

Prolactin. A protein hormone produced by a population of acidophils in the anterior pituitary and released in response to a releasing hormone (PRH) produced by neurosecretory cells in the hypothalamus; stimulates secretion by mammary glands.

Proliferative phase. The phase of uterine endometrium in the menstrual cycle during which the entire functionalis layer is regenerated from the narrow basalis layer following menstruation; largely due to the influence of estrogen; sometimes also called *estrogenic* or *follicular phase* of the uterine endometrium.

Prostaglandins. Long chain fatty acids that have a hormone-like function; especially associated with smooth muscle contraction and blood pressure changes.

Prostate gland. A large gland in the male reproductive tract that surrounds and opens into the prostatic urethra immediately below the urinary bladder; secretion contains acid phosphatase, fructose, diastase, proteolytic enzymes, and other substances.

Prostatic concretions (corpora amylacea). Calcified secretory material in the lumen of the prostate gland; more numerous in older males; their significance is unclear.

Protein. A macromolecule constructed from a series of amino acids.

Protein kinases. A large group of enzymes that catalyze the transfer of a phosphate group from ATP to an amino acid in a protein.

Proximal convoluted tubule. The initial portion of the uriniferous tubule that begins at the urinary pole of Bowman's capsule; in this region, approximately seven-eighths of the proteins, amino acids, glucose, and salts in the lumen are reabsorbed into the capillaries surrounding the proximal convoluted tubule.

Pseudopodia. Literally, "false feet"; transient extensions of the cell cortex that surround material during phagocytosis; also formed during cell locomotion.

Ptyalin. An enzyme in saliva that converts starches into sugars; salivary amylase.

Pulmonary macrophage (alveolar phagocyte, dust cell). A migratory macrophage in the alveoli and interalveolar septa of the lung; can ingest particulate material.

Pulp cavity. The central cavity of a tooth that contains connective tissue, blood vessels, and nerves; lined by odontoblasts.

Radial spokes. Thin, filamentous structures that extend from each microtubule doublet in a ciliary axoneme to a central sheath that surrounds the central doublet microtubules of the cilium.

Red pulp. One structural component of the spleen that consists of many splenic sinusoids and intervening red pulp cords (of Billroth); cells can move easily between these two compartments of the splenic red pulp.

Relaxin. A polypeptide hormone formed by lutein cells in the corpus luteum late in pregnancy that promotes dilation of the cervix and, in some species, loosens the symphysis pubis, facilitating parturition.

Renal corpuscle. That portion of the nephron in the kidney that consists of Bowman's capsule (parietal and visceral layers) and the enclosed glomerular capillary tuft.

Renal pelvis. A funnel-shaped structure into which urine enters from the kidney and that conveys urine to the ureter.

Renin. An enzyme produced and released by juxtaglomerular cells in the kidney in response to a reduced sodium concentration in an ultrafiltrate or reduced blood pressure; renin acts on the blood protein angiotensinogen, which is converted to angiotensin I; angiotensin I is converted to angiotensin II by a converting enzyme that is produced by pumonary endothelial cells; angiotensin II acts on zona glomerulosa cells in the adrenal cortex to release aldosterone, which stimulates the distal nephron to reabsorb more sodium ions and water.

Residual bodies. A form of lysosome in which the digestive process is complete; residual bodies may be discharged from the cell, but in some cells they may persist and transform slowly into aging pigment.

Reticular fiber. A type of connective tissue fiber that is a specialized collagen fiber (type III collagen) that stains with silver (argyrophilic); may be formed by reticular cells, fibroblasts, or smooth muscle cells in certain blood vessels; especially numerous in lymph nodes, spleen, and bone marrow.

Reticulocyte. An immature erythrocyte that still contains polyribosomes that, when stained, may precipitate in the form of a fine reticulum; also called a *polychromatophilic erythrocyte.*

Ribosome. An organelle consisting of tRNA, mRNA, and rRNA and involved in protein synthesis; may be free in the cytoplasm or attached to membranes of the rER.

Rod photoreceptor. In the vertebrate retina, an elongate cell involved in black and white vision and dim light vision.

Romanovsky stain. A commonly used stain for blood smears and bone marrow smears; contains a basic dye (methylene blue), an acid dye (eosin), and alcohol for fixation; another commonly used blood smear stain is Wright's stain.

Rough endoplasmic reticulum (rER). An organelle consisting of membranous compartments that enclose spaces (cisternae); coated with polyribosomes; involved in protein synthesis for export; newly synthesized protein is usually transported to the Golgi complex for packaging and addition of other constituents.

Sarcolemma. The plasma membrane of the muscle fiber; surrounded by a basal lamina or basement membrane; many invaginations form transverse tubules.

Sarcomere. The region between adjacent Z bands in skeletal and cardiac muscle; sarcomere shortening occurs during muscle contraction.

Sarcoplasmic reticulum. A system of smooth, membranous tubules and cisternae in skeletal and cardiac muscle that surround all myofibrils in a muscle fiber; a specialized sER; stores calcium between contractions but releases calcium to the myofibrils as necessary for contraction when an impulse travels along the sarcolemma into the transverse tubules; terminal cisternae of the SR are closely associated with the transverse tubules.

Schwann cell. Cells derived from the neural crest that function in forming myelin for peripheral nerves; a number of Schwann cells must align along a nerve and form the myelin by wrapping around and around the nerve process.

Sclera. The outer layer of the eyeball, consisting of dense collagenic fibers; protects the eye and attaches the extraocular muscles.

Sebaceous gland. Glands that usually form from a hair follicle and synthesize an oily substance called *sebum*; cells die as they become filled with secretion and are discharged whole (called *holocrine secretion*).

Secondary follicle. A stage in folliculogenesis characterized by a number of follicle or granulosa cells surrounding an oocyte; a multilaminar follicle.

Secondary papillae. Vascularized connective tissue extensions of the papillary layer of the dermis into the undersurface of epidermal folds.

Secondary spermatocyte. A stage of spermatogenesis between primary spermatocyte and spermatid; this division is equational and rapid in humans.

Secretory phase. The phase of the menstrual cycle in which the uterine glands are active in the secretion of glycogen, mucus, fat, and other substances and the endometrium is ready for implantation of a blastocyst; also called the *progestational phase* of the uterine endometrium because changes are due to this hormone.

Secretory (zymogen) granules. The membrane-delimited secretory material to be exported from the apical surface of the cell by exocytosis.

Semen. The material containing seminal fluid and spermatozoa released by the male during ejaculation.

Seminal fluid. A complex nutritive fluid produced primarily by the seminal vesicles and prostate gland in which spermatozoa are suspended.

Seminal vesicle. An accessory gland of the male reproductive tract; an outpocketing of the vas deferens near the junction with the ejaculatory duct; the secretion contains fructose, prostaglandins, ascorbic acid, and other materials; the major contributor to the seminal fluid.

Seminiferous tubule. Highly folded tubules, approximately 500 per testis, in which spermatogenesis occurs; contains spermatogonia, spermatocytes, spermatids, and Sertoli cells.

Serosa. The outer layer of organs of the coelom; consists of an inner thin layer of connective tissue and an outer layer of simple squamous epithelial cells called *mesothelium*.

Serous cell. A cell that produces a proteinaceous secretory product; the parotid gland is an entirely serous gland.

Serous demilune. A cap of serous-secreting cells that "cap" mucus-secreting alveoli or acini; occurs in sublingual and submandibular salivary glands.

Sertoli (sustentacular) cell. A highly irregularly shaped cell in the seminiferous tubule; extensive circumferential tight junctions are formed between extensions of adjacent Sertoli cells and comprise the basis of the blood-testis barrier; cells permits a basal and an adluminal compartment for the testis; synthesize testicular fluid; ingest and digest residual bodies of spermatids.

Sinusoid. A large capillary-like space in the blood vascular system; cells may be fenestrated and the basal lamina may be incomplete, facilitating rapid transsinusoidal transport, as in liver.

Skeletal muscle fiber. The contractile unit of striated skeletal muscle; consists of multicellular fibers (a syncytium), contraction is voluntary, innervated by cerebrospinal nerves.

Smooth endoplasmic reticulum (sER). A system of smooth-surfaced membranes in the cytoplasm that has several functions; plays a role in glycogen utilization, steroid biosynthesis, and triglyceride synthesis; in striated muscle, acts as a storage area for calcium ions.

Smooth muscle. A type of involuntary muscle consisting of spindle-shaped cells that may be closely packed into sheets; sheets of smooth muscle are arranged into circular and longitudinal layers in the digestive tract; innervated by the ANS.

Sodium-potassium pump (Na^+-K^+-ATPase). An ATP-driven membrane transport protein that couples the active transport of sodium out of cells to the active transport of potassium ions into cells.

Somatotropes. A population of acidophils in the anterior pituitary that secretes growth hormone (GH) in response to a growth hormone-releasing factor produced by neurosecretory cells in the hypothalamus and travels to the anterior lobe in a portal circulatory system.

Spermatid. A haploid germ cell derived from secondary spermatocyte in the seminiferous tubules during spermatogenesis; the spherical spermatid undergoes

changes in shape, condensation of chromatin in the nucleus, formation of an acrosome, and formation of a flagellum for locomotion; spermatids in seminiferous tubules are incapable of forward locomotion.

Spermatocyte. A type of cell, including the primary and secondary spermatocytes, that results from a spermatogonium; the primary spermatocyte undergoes a complicated series of changes during meiotic prophase; when these changes are completed, the primary spermatocyte divides into two secondary spermatocytes, each of which then rapidly divides into two spermatids.

Spermatogenesis. The process by which spermatogonia transform into spermatozoa.

Spermatogonia. Proliferative stem cells in the seminiferous epithelium of the seminiferous tubules that give rise to primary spermatocytes.

Spermatozoon. A mature sperm that has an acrosome, condensed chromatin, and a mitochondrial sheath surrounding a flagellum; functions to fertilize an ovum.

Spermiogenesis. The morphologic transformation of a spherical spermatid into an enlongate, flagellated spermatozoon.

Spicules. Small slivers of bone matrix formed in the early stages of cancellous or spongy bone formation.

Spiral ganglion. A region of concentration of bipolar neurons between the thin bony plates of the osseous spiral lamina in the ear; dendrites innervate hair cells in the organ of Corti, and axons enter the brain stem.

Splenic cords (red pulp cords of Billroth). That part of the red pulp of the spleen that contains reticular cells and fibers, macrophages, and all possible types of blood cells; a region of blood storage and destruction of worn-out erythrocytes.

Spongy (cancellous, trabeculated) bone. A type of bone that consists of a grating of bone matrix and bone cells (osteoblasts, osteocytes); does not contain haversian systems.

Squames. Flattened, dead cells full of keratin, sometimes called *corneocytes*, that continually desquamate (shed) from the surface of the epidermis of the integument and other regions.

Squamous epithelium. A type of epithelium; may exist in the form of simple epithelium, which is a single layer of flattened cells, or a stratified epithelium, in which a number of cell layers are present but the surface cells are flattened.

Stereocilia. Long, finger-like extensions of certain columnar epithelial cells; actually are microvilli; initially, with LM, were thought to be long, nonmotile cilia.

Stratum basale. The most basally located cells in the epidermis of the integument; these cells are mitotic and generate new cells that move superficially in the process of producing a waterproofing layer of keratin for the integument.

Stratum corneum. Highly flattened, dead cells filled with keratin and known as a *corneocytes*.

Stratum granulosum. A layer of cells in the epidermis of the integument that contains basophilic-staining soft keratin granules called *keratohyalin*, which are involved in the formation of keratin.

Stratum lucidum. A thin layer in thick skin located between the stratum granulosum and the stratum corneum; consists of dead or pyknotic cells transforming from keratinocytes to corneocytes.

Stratum spinosum. A rather thick layer of polygonal cells superficial to the stratum basale in the integument; cells are anchored by large numbers of spot desmosomes or maculae adherentes.

Striated border (brush border, microvillus border). A specialized region of the apical plasma membrane of certain epithelial cells that consists of many finger-like evaginations of the plasma membrane that contain a complex cytoskeleton involving long actin microfilaments; amplifies the apical plasma membrane for special membrane molecules.

Subcapsular sinus. The lymph sinus beneath the capsule of a lymph node; receives lymph from afferent lymphatic vessels.

Sublingual gland. Paired salivary glands located below the tongue; a mixed gland containing mucous and serous secreting cells but mainly mucous alveoli.

Submandibular gland. Paired salivary glands located below the mandible; a mixed gland but mainly serous-secreting alveoli.

Submucosa. A layer of loose connective tissue between the mucosa and muscularis externa layers of many organs, including the digestive tract.

Substantia propria (corneal stroma). A layer of the cornea that consists of a highly ordered arrangement of collagen fibers and fibrocytes.

Suppressor T cell. A type of T lymphocyte that can inhibit the ability of other lymphocytes to respond to antigen stimulation.

Surfactant. A layer coating the alveolar surface of the lung; contains dipalmitoyl lecithin, which reduces surface tension and permits easier inflation of the alveoli; produced mainly by pneumocyte II cells of the alveolar epithelium.

Sustentacular cell. A cell that supports other cells.

Sympathetic nervous system. One division of the ANS that consists of two efferent neurons (preganglionic and postganglionic neurons); preganglionic neurons arise in the lateral horn of gray matter in the thoracic and lumbar portions of the spinal cord; the second efferent neuron (the postganglionic neuron) is located in the prevertebral or paravertebral ganglion; postganglionic

fibers innervate epithelium, glands, smooth muscle, the heart muscle; adrenergic fibers often reduce secretion, decrease contractility of smooth muscle, and cause vasoconstriction.

Synapse. A region of close apposition of nerves where the nerve impulse passes; involves presynaptic and postsynaptic neurons; a region where synaptic vesicles are released from the presynaptic neuron under appropriate conditions and neurotransmitter in the vesicles is released into the synaptic cleft, which causes depolarization or hyperpolarization of the postsynaptic neuron.

Synapsin I. Integral membrane protein of synaptic vesicles that connects them to each other, to microtubules, or to actin filaments in the synapse region; during depolarization, synapsin is phosphorylated by a calcium-calmodulin-dependent kinase, which causes synapsin to dissociate from the vesicles; vesicles can then move to presynaptic membrane and undergo exocytosis.

Synaptic cleft. A narrow space between two neurons in a synaptic series.

Synaptic vesicle. A small membrane-bound vesicle in the presynaptic nerve terminal that contains neurotransmitter.

Syncytium. A multinucleate cell that may result from nuclear division without cytoplasmic division or may result from the fusion of separate cells into a single cell.

Synovial fluid. The fluid in a joint that is formed by the epithelium of a synovial membrane; lubricates and facilitates movement at the joint.

Systole. The pressure (pulse) that is created when the left ventricle of the heart contracts.

T lymphocyte. A lymphocyte that matures in the thymus and is involved in cell-mediated immunity.

T system. A system in skeletal muscle that includes transverse tubules and terminal cisternae of the SR.

Taste bud. Modified neuroepithelial cells and supporting cells located on circumvallate papillae (and some fungiform papillae); involved in taste discrimination.

Taste pore. A small opening into a taste bud; microvilli of the neuroepithelial cell extend into the pore.

Tectorial membrane. A gelatinous sheet in the organ of Corti that is formed by interdental cells. The undersurface of the membrane is in contact with the hair tufts of the outer hair cells in the organ of Corti.

Telomeres. Nucleotide sequences in chromosomal DNA that permit DNA to be replicated; special DNA sequences at each end of eukaryotic chromosomes that block neighboring G nucleotides.

Tendon. A dense, regularly arranged white, fibrous connective tissue (usually collagen but may be elastic fibers) that connects muscle to bone.

Terminal cisternae. Dilated regions of the SR of striated muscle that occur adjacent to the transverse tubules; membranes are rich in calcium pumps and calcium channels for calcium, which is stored in the terminal cisternae and released from them during contraction.

Tertiary follicle. A stage in folliculogenesis in which a fluid-filled antrum is prominent, becomes a Graafian follicle.

Testis. Compound tubular gland containing seminiferous tubules in which spermatogenesis occurs; located in the scrotum outside of the body cavity.

Theca externa. The outer layer of the theca folliculi, which invests the granulosa cells; consists principally of connective tissue cells and fibers.

Theca folliculi. A connective tissue sheath that invests the granulosa cells and contained oocye; differentiates into the theca interna and theca externa.

Theca interna. Inner layer of the theca folliculi, containing theca interna cells that are highly vascularized and contain sER, lipid, and mitochondria for steroid synthesis; synthetic products include estrogen.

Theca lutein cells. Cells in the vascularized corpus luteum that are formed after ovulation from remnants of the Graafian follicle.

Thymus. An endodermal derivative of the pharyngeal pouches in the embryo; consists of numerous T lymphocytes, macrophages, and epithelial reticular cells; place where many T cells are produced and sent to colonize other lymphoid organs.

Thyroglobulin. Glycoprotein secretion comprising the colloid of thyroid follicles; storage form of hormone.

Thyrotrope. A population of basophils in the anterior pituitary that produces thyroid-stimulating hormone (TSH) in response to a thyrotropin-releasing factor produced by neurosecretory cells in the hypothalamus.

Thyrotropin-releasing factor. A hormone secreted by neurons in the hypothalamus; travels in the portal circulatory system to the anterior pituitary, where it causes thyrotrops to release TSH.

Thyroxine (T_4). The principal form of the thyroid hormone tetraiodothryronine, which has a profound effect on the metabolic rate of cells in the body. Triiodothyronine (T_3) is a more potent form of the hormone, produced during iodine insufficiency.

Tight junction (zonula occludens). A junctional complex located at the apical end of adjacent epithelial cells in a sheet; completely invests the cells (belt-like) and is marked by the fusion of the outer leaflets of the plasma membrane of adjacent cells, thus obliterating the intercellular space in this region; this restricts movement of materials through the intercellular space and movement of integral membrane proteins in the apical plasma membrane.

Topoisomerase. An enzyme concentrated in kinetochores that facilitates the untangling of DNA so that chromosomes can move toward the poles during mitosis.

Trabeculae. Supporting material of organs; connective tissue in capsules surrounding organs may extend in places into the interior of the organ, forming connective tissue trabeculae; also denotes thin, branching plates of cancellous bone.

Transcription. A process in which the genetic information of DNA is transferred to complementary sequences of bases in an RNA chain.

Transcytosis. The process of incorporating material into the apical end of a cell in vesicles and the movement of these vesicles to the basolateral plasma membrane, where exocytosis or release into the intercellular space occurs.

Transfer (transition) vesicles. Small, membrane-bound vesicles that bud from the partial sER and partial rER adjacent to the forming face of the Golgi complex; protein is shuttled from the ER to the Golgi complex by these vesicles.

Transitional epitheluim. A layered or compound epithelium in which the surface cells may be rounded or dome-shaped (when the structure is collapsed) or flattened when the structure is dilated from within; type of epithelium in renal calices, renal pelvis, ureters, and urinary bladder.

Tropic hormone. A hormone secreted by one gland cell that may cause another cell or organ to produce a different hormone.

Tropomyosin. A two-stranded alpha helical rod (70-kD protein) oriented along the axis of the thin myofilament; a regulatory protein associated with actin filament that blocks actin-myosin interaction without the presence of calcium ions.

Troponin. A calcium-binding regulatory protein in muscle; a complex of three polypeptides—TnC (calcium binding), TnI (actin binding), and TnT (tropomyosin binding)—that is located in the thin filament at intervals of 385 Å; a troponin complex is bound to a molecule of tropomyosin, which regulates the activity of about seven actin monomers; after TnC binds calcium, tropomyosin moves slightly to uncover the reactive sites on the actin for interaction with myosin heads during contraction.

Trypsin. A pancreatic enzyme involved in digestion of proteins; is secreted in an inactive form called *trypsinogen*, which is activated by enterokinase; trypsin cleaves partially digested proteins into peptides.

Tunica adventitia. An outer layer or tunic of arteries and veins; consists of connective tissue (in arteries), but the vena cava may have smooth muscle in the tunica adventitia.

Tunica albuginea. A dense connective tissue layer that invests certain organs, such as the paired testes.

Tunica intima. The inner layer of an artery or vein that consists of endothelium, a possible thin subendothelial connective tissue layer, and a thick internal elastic lamina.

Tunica media. The middle layer of arteries and veins; usually contains variable amounts of smooth muscle in elastic arteries and arterioles, contains many elastic fibers in elastic arteries (e.g., the aorta).

Ureter. A muscular tube that conducts urine from each kidney to the urinary bladder.

Urethra. Channel conducting urine from the urinary bladder to the outside; is short in females and longer in males, in whom there are prostatic and penile portions.

Urinary space. A space between the visceral and parietal layers of Bowman's capsule in the kidney; it is continuous with the lumen of the proximal convoluted tubule and receives the glomerular filtrate.

Uterus. The organ in the female that undergoes cyclic changes during the menstrual cycle; the organ in which implantation of an embryo occurs; consists of an inner endometrial layer, a middle muscular myometrium, and thin outer perimetrium or epimetrium.

Vasa recta. A system of small, hairpin-like blood vessels that extends into the medulla of the kidney and is closely associated with the loops of Henle and collecting ducts.

Vasopressin (antidiuretic hormone). A hormone that is synthesized in the hypothalamus and travels down axons into the pars nervosa, where it is released into blood vessels; promotes water resorption from collecting ducts and may also elevate blood pressure by causing smooth muscle contraction in arterioles.

Venous sinus. A large capillary found in areas such as the liver, spleen, and bone marrow; capillaries may be fenestrated and lack complete basal lamina, making it easier for materials to move across the capillary wall.

Villus (pl. villi). Evaginations of the mucosa of the small intestine that increase the absorptive surface area; villi are lined by epithelium (simple columnar absorptive cells and goblet cells) and have a core of lamina propria.

Visceral layer. The inner layer of Bowman's capsule, consisting of podocytes that closely invest the glomerular capillary; may also denote the inner layer of the pleura, which invests the lungs.

Vitreous humor. A watery material containing hydrophilic polysaccharides and fine collagenic fibrils in the vitreous body of the eye.

Voltage-gated channels. Integral membrane protein channels for ions that open and close in response to voltage differences across the membrane.

White pulp. That portion of the spleen that includes periarterial lymphatic sheaths and splenic (Malpighian) nodules; heavily cellular regions of the spleen and includes many B lymphoblasts, B lymphocytes, and T lymphocytes, as well as macrophages and reticular cells.

Zona fasciculata. A middle layer of the adrenal cortex that secretes glucocorticoids such as cortisol; glucocorticoids play a role in regulating protein and carbohydrate metabolism, suppress the inflammatory response, and provide resistance to stress.

Zona glomerulosa. The outer layer of the adrenal cortex; cells secrete aldosterone (a mineralocorticoid) when stimulated to do so by renin release from the kidney; aldosterone promotes sodium resorption from the distal tubule and the collecting duct.

Zona pellucida. A thick extracellular layer that is secreted between the oocyte and the investing layer of follicle cells; contains microvilli of the oocyte plasma membrane and granulosa cell membranes; the zona pellucida accompanies the oocyte after ovulation, and sperm penetrate this layer during fertilization; the layer disappears just prior to implantation.

Zona reticularis. The innermost layer of the adrenal cortex; cells secrete sex steroid hormones.

Zygote. The fertilized egg after sperm has been incorporated into the egg; followed by cleavage stages.

Zymogen granule. A secretory granule of a cell; discharged from the cell by exocytosis in response to appropriate stimulation.